OXFORD MEDICAL PUBLICATIONS

Essentials of human nutrition

Essentials of human nutrition

Edited by
JIM MANN

*Professor of Human Nutrition, University of Otago,
New Zealand*

and

A. STEWART TRUSWELL

*Professor of Human Nutrition, University of Sydney,
Australia*

Oxford   New York   Tokyo
OXFORD UNIVERSITY PRESS
1998

Oxford University Press, Great Clarendon Street, Oxford OX2 6DP

Oxford New York

Athens Auckland Bangkok Bogota Bombay
Buenos Aires Calcutta Cape Town Dar es Salaam
Delhi Florence Hong Kong Istanbul Karachi
Kuala Lumpur Madras Madrid Melbourne
Mexico City Nairobi Paris Singapore
Taipei Tokyo Toronto Warsaw

and associated companies in
Berlin Ibadan

Oxford is a trade mark of Oxford University Press

Published in the United States
by Oxford University Press, Inc., New York

© Oxford University Press, 1998

A catalogue record for this book is available from the British Library

Library of Congress Cataloging in Publication Data

Essentials of human nutrition/edited by J.I. Mann and A. Stewart Truswell
1. Nutrition.   I. Mann, Jim.   II. Truswell, A. Stewart.
QP141.E82 1998   612.3'9–dc21   97-28309

ISBN 0 19 262757 0 (Hbk)
ISBN 0 19 262756 2 (Pbk)

Typeset by Newgen Imaging Systems (P) Ltd, Chennai, India

Printed in Great Britain
by Bookcraft (Bath) Ltd,
Midsomer Norton, Avon

PREFACE

Several excellent textbooks of human nutrition are available. We have attempted to produce a new book which differs from most of them by asking our contributors to describe what they regard as those aspects of their topics which are essential to the understanding and practice of human nutrition. Most of the authors are international authorities on the subjects on which they have written and all are very experienced teachers. We were initially reluctant to accept the offer of the publishers to produce yet another textbook of human nutrition. We were persuaded to do so because we felt there was a need for a book which described the essential information required by students embarking on a University course in human nutrition, and by those in training in the health and food science professions where the importance of nutrition is being increasingly recognized. Many of our clinical colleagues in medicine, dentistry, nursing and physiotherapy, and school teachers, provided strong encouragement for this project since they too required a simple reference volume, having themselves received little formal training in nutrition. An increasingly informed public expects its health providers to have knowledge of one of the most important determinants of individual and public health. Health professionals and food scientists need to be able to disentangle scientifically established nutrition principles from the morass of misinformation available in the public domain. The book may also be of value to those in the fitness industry and last but not least individual members of the public who have sufficient knowledge of biology and chemistry and who wish to be informed of the essentials of human nutrition. The book is not intended to be a detailed reference volume and each chapter contains further reading for those wishing to extend the information provided in the text.

We have tried to emphasize that nutritional science encompasses a spectrum of disciplines and involves the use of many methodologies. In the past, the major advances in nutrition were made at the level of organs and organisms, many from studies of experimental animals. Most present advances have been at the population level and, even more recently, at the molecular level. The discovery that dietary alteration can modify gene expression suggests that what we eat has even more profound implications than had previously been believed. These disciplines now need to be integrated at the human level to promote the practical application of nutritional science in metabolic, clinical, and public health nutrition.

It has not been easy to integrate the findings from these diverse methodologies and disciplines in a relatively brief volume purporting to describe the essentials of human nutrition. We are grateful to our authors for their attempts to do so despite the many constraints which were placed upon them by the editors. We believe they have succeeded in providing the students and practitioners in human nutrition and the health sciences with what might be regarded as consensus opinions regarding most of the key issues. There will always be differences of opinion, particularly with regard to the practical implementation of nutrition knowledge and some of the views they have expressed may be modified in the future. However, there is little doubt concerning the profound health benefits which would accrue worldwide if even half the recommendations offered here were to be implemented.

New Zealand   Jim Mann
Australia   Stewart Truswell
October 1997

Contents

LIST OF CONTRIBUTORS

Margaret ALLMAN-FARINELLI PhD, Dip Nutr Diet, Senior Lecturer, Human Nutrition Unit, University of Sydney, NSW 2006, Australia

Soumela AMANATIDIS BSc, Dip Nutr Diet, Community Nutritionist, Central Sydney Area Health Service, Queen Mary Building, Grose Street, Camperdown 2050 NSW, Australia

Madeleine J. BALL MD, MRCP, FRCPath, Professor of Human Nutrition, Deakin University, 336 Glenferrie Road, Malvern Vic 3144, Australia

Sarah E. BETHELL BSc, Dip Sci, PG Dip Diet, Department of Human Nutrition, University of Otago, Dunedin, New Zealand

Sheila BINGHAM BSc, MA, PhD, Head, Diet and Cancer, Dunn Clinical Nutrition Centre, Cambridge, United Kingdom

Janette C. BRAND-MILLER PhD, Associate Professor, Human Nutrition Unit G08, University of Sydney 2006 NSW, Australia

David BRIGGS PhD, Associate Professor, Department of Human Nutrition, Deakin University, Geelong Vic 3217, Australia

Ian CATERSON MB,BS, PhD, FRACP, Boden Professor of Human Nutrition, Department of Biochemistry G08, University of Sydney 2006, NSW, Australia

Christopher G. FAIRBURN DM, MPhil, FRCPsych, Wellcome Principal Research Fellow and Professor, Department of Psychiatry, University of Oxford, Oxford, United Kingdom

Rosalind S. GIBSON BSc, MS, PhD, Professor in Human Nutrition, Department of Human Nutrition, University of Otago, Dunedin, New Zealand

Ailsa GOULDING BSc, PhD, FACN, Senior Research Fellow, Department of Medicine, Otago Medical School, Dunedin, New Zealand

Trish GRIFFITHS BSc, Dip Nutr Diet, MPH, Nutrition Services Manager, Bread Research Institute, North Ryde, 2113 NSW, Australia

Barbara GUTHRIE MHSc, PhD, Senior Lecturer in Human Nutrition, Department of Human Nutrition, University of Otago, Dunedin, New Zealand

Basil HETZEL AO, MD, FRACP, Chairman ICCID, c/-Health Department Foundation, 72 King William Road, North Adelaide 5006, SA, Australia

Caroline HORWATH BSc(Hons), PhD, Senior Lecturer in Human Nutrition, Department of Human Nutrition, University of Otago, Dunedin, New Zealand

Alan A. JACKSON MA, MD, FRCP, FRCPCH, Professor of Human Nutrition, Institute of Human Nutrition, University of Southampton, United Kingdom

W. Philip T. JAMES CBE, MA, MD, DSc, FRCP, FRCP (Edin), FRSE, Director, Rowett Research Institute, Bucksburn, Aberdeen, United Kingdom

Elizabeth M. JOHNSTON BSc, MS, PhD, FCDA, PDt, Director, School of Nutrition and Food Science, Acadia University, Wolfville, Nova Scotia, Canada

Helen M. LEACH MA, PhD, Associate Professor in Anthropology, Department of Anthropology, University of Otago, Dunedin, New Zealand

Philippa M. LYONS WALL PhD, Dip Nutr Diet, Lecturer, Human Nutrition Unit G08, University of Sydney 2006 NSW, Australia

A. Patrick MacPHAIL MB, BCh, PhD, FCP, Professor of Medicine, Medical School, University of the Witwatersrand, Johannesburg, South Africa

Louise MACAN M Nutr Diet, Nutritionist, Meadow Lea Foods Ltd, Mascot 2020 NSW, Australia

Jim I. MANN MA, DM, PhD, FRACP, FRSNZ, Professor in Human Nutrition and Medicine, Department of Human Nutrition, University of Otago; Head of Endocrinology, Dunedin Hospital, Dunedin, New Zealand

Robyn MILNE BSc(Hons), PhD, Lecturer in Human Nutrition, Department of Human Nutrition, University of Otago, Dunedin, New Zealand

Losa MOATA'ANE BN, NZRN, Research Nurse, Department of Human Nutrition, University of Otago, Dunedin, New Zealand

So'ana MUIMUI-HEATA BHSc, BSc, PG Dip Diet, Dietitian, Department of Health, Tonga

Sue MUNRO BSc, Dip Nutr Diet, Associate Lecturer, Human Nutrition Unit G08, University of Sydney 2006 NSW, Australia

Winsome R. PARNELL BHSc, MSc, NZ Reg Dietitian, Senior Lecturer in Human Nutrition, Department of Human Nutrition, University of Otago, Dunedin, New Zealand

Aileen ROBERTSON PhD, Acting Regional Adviser for Nutrition, Programme for Nutrition Policy, Infant Feeding and Food Security (NIF), Lifestyles and Health Unit, World Health Organisation, Copenhagen, Denmark

James ROBINSON MD, ScD, FRACP, FRSNZ, Emeritus Professor in Physiology, Department of Physiology, Otago Medical School, Dunedin, New Zealand

Marion ROBINSON CBE, MHSc, PhD, FNZIC, FRSNZ, Emeritus Professor in Human Nutrition, Department of Human Nutrition, University of Otago, Dunedin, New Zealand

Samir SAMMAN PhD, Senior Lecturer, Human Nutrition Unit G08, University of Sydney 2006 NSW, Australia

Sue SCARLET Dip HSc, Dip Sc, NZ Reg Dietitian, Dietitian/Nutritionist, Wellington, New Zealand

Vicky SCOTT BSc, BHSc, PhD, Department of Human Nutrition, University of Otago, Dunedin, New Zealand

Donna SECKER RD, MSc, Clinical Dietitian, Hospital for Sick Children, University of Toronto, Toronto, Ontario, Canada

C. Murray SKEAFF BSc, PhD, Senior Lecturer in Human Nutrition, Department of Human Nutrition, University of Otago, Dunedin, New Zealand

Christine D. THOMSON MHSc, PhD, Senior Lecturer in Human Nutrition, Department of Human Nutrition, University of Otago, Dunedin, New Zealand

Viliami TOAFA BSc, DPH, Researcher, Department of Human Nutrition, University of Otago, Dunedin, New Zealand

A. Stewart TRUSWELL MD, FRCP, FRACP, FFPHM, Professor of Human Nutrition, University of Sydney 2006 NSW, Australia

Cynthia R. TUTTLE BSc, PhD, MPH, Lecturer in Human Nutrition, Department of Human Nutrition, University of Otago, Dunedin, New Zealand

JOOP VAN RAAIJ PhD, Lecturer, Department of Human Nutrition, Wageningen Agricultural University, 6700 EV Wageningen, The Netherlands

Mark L. WAHLQVIST MD, MD, FRACP, Professor of Medicine, Monash University Medical School, Clayton Vic 3168, Australia

Clive E. WEST PhD, DSc, Associate Professor, Division of Human Nutrition and Epidemiology, Wageningen Agricultural University, 6700 EV Wageningen, The Netherlands (also Visiting Professor, Department of International Health, Rollins School of Public Health of Emory University, Atlanta, GA 30322, USA.

Peter WILLIAMS PhD, Dip Nutr Diet, Science and Regulatory Affairs Manager, Kellogg (Australia) Pty Ltd, Pagewood 2019 NSW, Australia

William WOODWARD PhD, Associate Professor, Department of Human Biology and Nutritional Sciences, University of Guelph, Guelph, Ontario, Canada

Stanley H. ZLOTKIN MD, PhD, Professor, Departments of Paediatrics and of Nutritional Sciences, University of Toronto and Research Institute and Division of Gastroenterology, Hospital for Sick Children, Toronto, Ontario, Canada

ACKNOWLEDGEMENTS

Many people have made substantial contributions towards the production of this book, but some warrant special mention. Professors Marion and James Robinson and Rosalind Gibson have been involved with this project from its inception and have participated in all aspects of its production, most especially in the lengthy editorial process involved in attempting to achieve a degree of consistency throughout the text. They have also helped with final proof reading. Indeed, the book is unlikely to have seen the light of day without their unfailing support. Dr Clare Casey also provided valuable editorial help. In the Sydney office Marianne Alexander and Isa Hopwood provided expert secretarial support. Professor Ian Gibson also provided considerable help with regard to the format of the text and illustrations. Many of the figures were drawn by Peter Scott. We are, last but not least, grateful to our families who have been tolerant and supportive of ourselves and this project, which was far more time consuming than we imagined it would be when we first embarked upon it.

Miss Elizabeth Gray acted as editorial assistant. She typed many of the chapters and amended most of the others after the editorial process. She also had the unenviable task of converting the entire text and tables into a standardized format. We are immensely grateful to her for this key role in the production of this book.

PERMISSIONS

Table 2.1: Adapted, with permission, from Asp N-G. Nutritional classification and analysis of food carbohydrates. *Am J Clin Nutr* 1994; 59 (suppl.): 679S–81S.

Table 2.2: Reproduced with permission: Englyst HN et al. Classification and measurement of nutritionally important starch fractions. *Europ J Clin Nutr* 1994; 46: S33–50.

Table 2.3: Reprinted with permission of Macmillan Press Ltd, from Woodward M and Walker ARP. Sugar consumption and dental caries: evidence from 90 countries. *Br Dent J* 1994; 176: 297–302.

Table 2.4: Foster-Powell K, Brand Miller J. International tables of glycemic index. *Am J Clin Nutr* 1995; 62: 871S–893S. © Am J Clin Nutr American Society for Clinical Nutrition.

Tables 3.2, 3.3, 8.2, 13.2, 13.5, 22.6, 22.8: Reproduced with permission of NZ Institute for Crop & Food Research Limited. A Crown research institute.

Figure 5.3: Reprinted with permission of Macmillan Press Ltd, from Murgatroyd PR et al. Techniques for the measurement of human energy and expenditure: a practical guide. *Int J Obesity* 1993; 17: 549–68.

Table 5.7: Reprinted with permission of World Health Organization, from: FAO/WHO/UNU. Energy and protein requirements, Technical report series No. 724, 1985.

Table 6.2: Reprinted with permission. Boffeta P and Garfinkel L. Alcohol drinking and mortality among men enrolled in an American Cancer Society Prospective Study. *Epidemiology* 1990; 1: 342–48.

Table 7.1: Adapted, with permission of Blackwell Science Ltd from Bray JJ et al. *Lecture notes on human physiology*, 3rd edition; 1994.

Box 7.1: Reproduced with permission of GP Publications, Wellington, New Zealand.

Table 9.2: Reprinted with permission of Food and Agriculture Organization of the United Nations, from Food and Nutrition Series No. 23, 1988—Requirements of vitamin A, iron, folate, and vitamin B12.

Figure 10.1: Reproduced with permission of Cambridge University Press from: Hercus CE et al. Endemic goitre in New Zealand and its relation to soil iodine. *J Hygiene*, 24: 321–402.

Figure 10.3: Thomson CD and Robinson MF. Blood selenium levels report in healthy adults reported in various countries. *Am J Clin Nutr* 1980; 33: 303–23. © Am J Clin Nutr American Society for Clinical Nutrition.

Figure 10.4: Reprinted with permission of the *British Journal of Nutrition*.

Table 10.4: Reprinted with permission of Australian Professional Publications, from Dreosti I. Recommended nutrient intakes, Australian Papers, 1990.

Table 15.2: Reprinted with permission from Burdock GA. *Fenarol's handbook of flavour ingredients*, vol 2, 3rd ed, 1995. Copyright CRC Press, Boca Raton, Florida © 1995.

Table 15.5: Reprinted with permission from Duke JA. *Handbook of phytochemical constitutenmts of GRAS herbs and other economic plants*, 1992. Copyright CRC Press, Boca Raton, Florida © 1992.

Table 18.2: Lewis B. Disorders of lipid transport. In: Weatherall DJ, Ledingham JGG, Warrell DA (eds). *Oxford textbook of medicine*. 2nd ed. By permission of Oxford University Press.

Figure 18.4: Reprinted with permission of the publisher from Seven Countries: a multivariate analysis of death and coronary heart disease by Ancel Keys, Cambridge, Mass.: Harvard University Press, Copyright © 1980 by the Presidents and Fellows of Harvard College.

Figure 18.5: Martin MJ et al. Serum cholesterol, blood pressure and mortality: implications from a cohort of 361662 men. 2: 933–36. © The Lancet, 1986.

Figure 18.7: Ulbricht TLV, Southgate DAT. Coronary heart disease: seven dietary factors. 338: 985–92. © The Lancet 1991.

Figure 18.8: Reprinted with permission of World Health Organization, from Technical Report Series 678, Prevention of coronary heart disease, 1982.

Figure 18.9: Reprinted with permission of Nature Medicine, New York, USA.

Figure 18.10: Beilin LJ, et al. Vegetarian diet and blood pressure levels: incidental or causal association? *Am J Clin Nutr* 1988; 48: 806–10. © Am J Clin Nutr American Society for Clinical Nutrition.

Table 18.2: Weatherall D et al. Disorders of lipid transport. In: Oxford Textbook of Medicine, 2nd edition. 1987. By permission of Oxford University Press, Oxford.

Table 18.4: Adapted, with permission from *Australian and New Zealand Journal of Medicine*.

Table 18.5: Department of Health. Dietary reference values for food energy and nutrients for the United Kingdom. 1991, No. 41. Crown copyright is reproduced with the permission of the Controller of Her Majesty's Stationery Office.

Figure 19.1: Reproduced with permission of International Agency for Research on Cancer, World Health Organization.

Figure 19.2: Reproduced with permission of International Agency for Research on Cancer, World Health Organization.

Figure 19.5: Reproduced with permission of Cell Press, Cambridge MA, USA.

Figure 19.6: Reproduced with permission of the British Journal of Nutrition.

Figure 20.1: Reproduced with permission of World Health Organization.

Figure 20.2: Reprinted with permission, from: Knowler WC et al. Diabetes incidence in Pima Indians: contributions of obesity and parental diabetes. *Am J Epidemiol* 1981; 113: 144–56.

Figure 20.3: Reprinted with permission, from: LaPorte RE et al. Geographic differences in the risk of insulin-dependent diabetes mellitus: the importance of registries. *Diabetes Care* 1985; 8: 101–7.

Figure 20.4: Toeller M et al. Nutritional intake of 2868 IDDM patients from 30 centres in Europe. *Diabetologia* 1996; 39: 929–39. © Springer-Verlag GmbH & Co. KG.

Table 22.1: Reprinted by courtesy of Marcel Dekker Inc., from Lorenz KJ and Kulp K (eds.) Handbook of cereal science and technology, 1991.

Table 22.1: Reprinted with permission from: Mugford DC and Batey IL. Composition of Australian flour mill products from bakers' wheat grist. Food Australia; 1995. Bread Research Institute of Australia; and Mugford D. Nutritional composition of Australian wheat and bakers' flour. Bakers and Millers Journal, 1983; February.

Tables 22.2, 22.5, 22.9, 22.14: English R and Lewis J. The composition of foods Australia, Canberra: AGPS. Commonwealth of Australia copyright reproduced with permission.

Tables 22.3, 22.4, 22.7, 22.14: Data from The Composition of Foods 5th edition and supplements are reproduced with the permission of The Royal Society of Chemistry and the Controller of Her Majesty's Stationery Office.

Table 23.3: Reprinted from the *Journal of Food Protection* 1993; 56: 1077, with permission of the International Association of Milk, Food and Environmental Sanitarians., 6200 Aurora Avenue, Suite 200W, Des Moines, IA 50322-2863; 515-276-3344; US or Canada: 800-369-6337; Fax: 515-276-8655.

Table 24.4: English R and Lewis J. Nutritional values of Australian foods, Canberra, AGPS (AOAC Prosky and Asp 2, method of estimating dietary fibre content of dried kidney beans). Commonwealth of Australia copyrights reproduced with permission.

Table 24.7: Reproduced with permission of Academic Press Inc., Orlando, Florida, USA.

Figure 25.3: Adapted from Nutrition recommendations, Health Canada, 1997. With permission.

Table 25.5: Modified with permission from: Block G et al. A data-based approach to diet questionnaire design and testing. *Am J Epid* 1986; 124: 434–69.

Table 25.6: Beaton. Uses and limits of the use of the Recommended Dietary Allowances for evaluating dietary intake data. *Am J Clin Nutr* 1985; 41: 155–64. © Am J Clin Nutr American Society for Clinical Nutrition.

Table 26.1: Reprinted with permission of Macmillan Press Ltd, from: Ferro-Luzzi A. A simplified approach of assessing adult chronic energy deficiency. *Euro J Clin Nutr* 1992; 46: 173–86.

Table 26.3: Reprinted with permission of Mosby-Year Book Inc., St Louis, MO, USA.

Table 26.4: Adapted with permission of the American Public Health Association, and adapted from: Cristakis G. Nutritional assessment in health programs: physical signs and symptoms related to malnutrition. *Am J Pub Health* 1973; 63: 1–82.

Tables 29.1, 29.2, 29.3: Crown copyright is reproduced with the permission of the Controller of Her Majesty's Stationery Office.

Figure 29.2: Reprinted with permission of Mosby-Year Book Inc., St Louis, MO, USA.

Table 29.4: Reprinted with permission of Macmillan Press Ltd, from: Scrimshaw NS et al. Energy and protein requirements. Mean energy intakes for 17–18 years and energy expenditure of adults. *Eur J Clin Nutr* 1996; 50 (suppl.).

Table 31.1: Reprinted with permission of Ambio.

Figure 31.2: Reprinted with permission of Plenum Publishing Corp, New York, NY, USA.

Figure 31.3: Reprinted with permission of The Gerontological Society of America, from McGandy RB et al. Nutrient intakes and energy expenditure in men of different ages. *J Geront* 1966; 21: 581–7.

Figure 31.4: Holick M. Vitamin D—new horizons for the 21st century. *Am J Clin Nutr* 1994; 60: 619–30. © Am J Clin Nutr American Society for Clinical Nutrition.

Table 35.3: Greene GW et al. Stages of change for reducing dietary fat to 30% of energy or less. Copyright The American Dietetic Association. Reprinted with permission from *Journal of the American Dietetic Association* 1994; 94: 1105–10.

Figures 39.1, 39.2, 39.3: Reproduced with permission of the National Heart Foundation of New Zealand.

DEDICATION

The Editors would like to dedicate this book to Marion Robinson, whose outstanding contribution to teaching and research in human nutrition is acknowledged.

1
INTRODUCTION

Stewart Truswell and Jim Mann

1.1 DEFINITION

This book is about what we consider to be the essentials of human nutrition.

The science of human nutrition deals with all the effects on people of any component found in food. This starts with the physiological and biochemical processes involved in nourishment—how substances in food yield work or are converted into body tissues, and the diseases that result from insufficiency or excess of essential nutrients (malnutrition). The role of food components in the development of chronic degenerative disease like coronary heart disease, cancers, dental caries, etc., are major targets of research activity nowadays. The scope of nutrition extends to any effect of food on human function: fetal health and development, resistance to infection, mental function and athletic performance. There is growing interaction between nutritional science and molecular biology which may help to explain the action of food components at the cellular level and the diversity of human biochemical responses.

Nutrition is also about why people choose to eat the foods they do, even if they have been advised that doing so may be unhealthy. The study of food habits thus overlaps with the social sciences of psychology, anthropology, sociology and economics. Dietetics and community nutrition are the application of nutritional knowledge to promote health and wellbeing. Dietitians advise people how to modify what they eat in order to maintain or restore optimal health, and to help in the treatment of disease. People expect to enjoy eating the foods that promote these things; and the production, preparation and distribution of foods provides many people with employment.

A healthy diet means different things to different people. Those concerned with children's nutrition—parents, teachers and paediatricians-aim to promote healthy growth and development. For adults in affluent communities nutrition research has become focused on attaining optimal health and 'preventing'—which mostly means delaying—chronic degenerative diseases of complex causation, especially obesity (Chapter 16), cardiovascular diseases (Chapter 18), cancer (Chapter 19) and diabetes (Chapter 20).

Apart from behavioural and sociological aspects of eating there are two broad groups of questions in human nutrition, with appropriate methods for answering them:

First, what are the essential nutrients, the substances that are needed in the diet for normal function of the human body? How do they work in the body and in which foods can we obtain each of them? Many of the answers to these questions have been established.

Second, can we delay or even prevent the chronic degenerative diseases by modifying what we usually eat? These diseases, like coronary heart disease, have multiple causes, so nutrition can only be expected to make a contribution—causative or protective. The answers to these questions are at best provisional; much still has to be disentangled and confirmed.

1.2 ESSENTIAL NUTRIENTS

Essential nutrients have been defined as chemical substances found in food that cannot be synthesized at all or in sufficient amounts in the body, and are necessary for life, growth, and tissue repair. Water is the most important nutrient for survival. By the end of the nineteenth century the essential amino acids in proteins had been mainly identified, as well as the major inorganic nutrients such as calcium, potassium, iodine, and iron.

The period 1890 to 1940 saw the discovery of 13 vitamins, organic compounds essential in small amounts. Each discovery was quite different; several are fascinating stories. The research methods have been observations in poorly nourished humans, animal models, chemical fractionation of foods, biochemical research with tissues in the laboratory, and human trials.

Animal experiments played a major role in discovering which fraction of a curative diet was the missing essential food factor and then how this fraction functions biochemically inside the body. The laboratory white rat is not suitable for experimental deficiency of all nutrients; the right animal model has to be found. Lind had demonstrated as early as 1747, in a controlled trial on board HMS Salisbury, that *scurvy* could be cured by a few oranges and lemons but progress towards identifying vitamin C had to wait until the guinea-pig was found, in 1907, to be susceptible to an illness like scurvy. Rats and other laboratory animals do not become ill on a diet lacking fruit and vegetables; they make their own vitamin C in the liver from glucose.

For thiamin (vitamin B_1) deficiency, birds provide good animal models. The first step in discovery of this vitamin was the chance observation in 1890 by Eijkman in Java, while looking for what was expected to be a bacterial cause of *beri-beri*, that chickens became ill with polyneuritis on a diet of cooked polished rice but were well if they were fed cheap unhusked rice. Human trials in Java, Malaysia and the Philippines showed that beri-beri could be prevented or cured with rice bran (or 'polish'). A bird that is unusually sensitive to thiamin deficiency, a type of rice bird, was used by Dutch workers in Java to test the different fractions in rice polish. The antiberi-beri vitamin was first isolated in crystalline form in 1926. It took another 10 years of work before two teams of chemists in the United States and Germany were able to synthesize vitamin B_1, which was given the chemical name thiamin.

To find the cause of *pellagra*, which was endemic among the rural poor in the southeastern states of the United States at the beginning of this century, Goldberger gave restricted maize diets to healthy volunteers and some developed early signs of the disease. But the missing substance, niacin, could not be identified until there was an animal model, 'black tongue' in dogs.

In the 1920s, linoleic and linolenic acids were identified as essential fatty acids. Then followed the development of analytical techniques for determining micro amounts of trace elements in foods and tissues. Thus emerged the other group of essential micro nutrients, the trace elements such as copper, zinc, manganese, selenium, molybdenum, chromium, and cobalt.

There is an additional group of food components such as dietary fibre, carotenoids and ultra trace elements, such as boron, which are not considered to be essential but which are important for maintenance of health and possibly also for reducing the risk of chronic disease.

1.3   RELATION OF DIET TO CHRONIC DISEASES

The realization is more recent that environmental factors, including dietary factors, are of importance in many of the chronic degenerative diseases that are major causes of ill health and death in affluent societies. The nutritional component of these is more difficult to study than is usually the case with classical nutrition deficiency diseases because these conditions have multiple causes and take years to develop. The dietary factor may be a 'risk factor' rather than a direct cause but for some of these diseases there is sufficient evidence to show that dietary change can appreciably reduce the risk of developing the condition. The scientific methods for investigating these conditions, their causes, treatment and prevention, differ appreciably from those used for studying adequacy of nutrient intakes.

Very often the first clue to the association between a food or nutrient and a disease comes from observing striking differences in disease incidence between countries (or groups within a country) which correlate with differences in intake of dietary components. Sometimes dietary changes over time in a single country have been found to coincide with changes in disease rates. Such observations give rise to hypotheses (i.e. theories) about possible diet–disease links rather than proof of causation because many potential causative factors may change in parallel with dietary change and it is impossible to disentangle separate effects.

Animal experiments, being usually short term, are not as useful for investigating diet and chronic diseases and can be misleading. More information has come, and is continuing to come, from well-designed (human) *epidemiological* studies which record the relationship between dietary intake, or variables known to be related to diet, and incidence of the chronic disease under question. Studies can either investigate subjects after diagnosis of the disease (retrospective studies) or before diagnosis (prospective studies).

Retrospective or case-control studies are quicker and less expensive to carry out but are less reliable than prospective studies. A series of people who have been diagnosed with for example cancer of the large bowel, are asked what they usually eat, or what they ate before they became ill. These are the 'cases'. They are compared with at least an equal number of 'controls', people without bowel cancer but of the same age, gender and, if possible, social condition. Weaknesses of the method include the possibility that the disease may affect food habits, that cases cannot recall their diet accurately before the cancer really started, that controls may have some condition that affects dietary habits, or that food intakes are recorded from cases and controls in a different way ('bias').

Prospective or cohort studies avoid the biases involved in asking people to recall past eating habits. Information about food intake and other characteristics are collected well before onset of the disease. Large numbers of people must therefore be interviewed and examined; they must be of an age at which bowel cancer (say) starts to be fairly common (i.e. middle aged), and in a population which has a fairly high rate of this disease. The healthy cohort thus examined and recorded is then followed up for five or more years. Eventually, a proportion will be diagnosed with bowel cancer and the original dietary details of those who develop cancer can be compared with the diets of the majority who have not developed the disease. Usually a number of dietary and other environmental factors are found to be more, or less, frequent in those who develop the disease. These then are apparent risk factors, or protective factors. But they are not necessarily the operative factor. Fruit consumption may appear to be protective but perhaps in this cohort, smokers eat less fruit and smoking may be more directly related. This confounding has to be analysed by, in effect, analysing the data to see the relationship of fruit to the disease at different levels of smoking.

Prospective studies usually provide stronger evidence of a diet-disease association than case-control studies, and where several prospective studies produce similar findings from different parts of the world this is impressive evidence of association (positive or negative) but still not final proof of causation. If an association is deemed not due to bias or confounding, is qualitatively strong, biologically credible, follows a plausible time sequence, and especially if there is evidence of a dose–response relationship, it is likely that the association is causal.

Definitive proof that a dietary characteristic is a direct causative or protective factor requires one or more *randomized controlled prevention trial*. These involve either the addition of a nutrient or other food component as a supplement to those in the experimental group and a placebo (dummy) capsule or tablet taken by the control group, or the prescription of a dietary regime to the experimental group while the controls continue to follow their usual diet. Disease (and death) outcomes in the two groups are compared. Such trials have the advantage of being able to prove causality as well as potential cost/benefit of the dietary change. However, they are costly to carry out because it is usually necessary to study large numbers of people over a prolonged period of time.

Quite often a single trial does not in itself produce a definitive answer, but by combining the results of all completed trials in a *meta-analysis* more meaningful answers are obtained. For example, none of the individual trials of diet for the primary and secondary prevention of coronary heart disease contained enough subjects to give a statistically significant answer with regard to differences in total death rate between experimental diet and control groups. In most trials there were fewer cases of coronary heart disease on the experimental diet, but deaths from all causes were not always fewer. However, by combining all the 15 trials in a meta-analysis there are sufficient numbers to see that deaths from all causes were significantly reduced (see Chapter 18).

In addition to epidemiological studies and trials, much research involving the role of diet in chronic degenerative disease has centred around the effects of diet on modifying risk factors rather than the disease itself. For many chronic diseases there are biochemical markers of risk. High plasma cholesterol, for example, is an important risk factor for coronary heart disease. Innumerable studies have examined the role of different nutrients and foods on plasma cholesterol or other risk factors. Such studies are cheaper and easier to undertake than epidemiological studies and randomized controlled trials since far fewer people are studied over a relatively short period of time. They have helped to find which foods lower cholesterol and so should help protect against coronary heart disease. It is this information which has formed the basis of the public health messages which have undoubtedly contributed to the decline in the incidence of coronary disease in most affluent societies over the last 20 years.

The statements about essential nutrients in this and other textbooks are fairly firmly established, though opinions may differ as to the importance of low intakes and subclinical 'deficiencies'. For the chronic diseases, however, it is very important to appreciate whether the link between something in the diet is:

(1) purely a suggestion or hypothesis (with no good epidemiological data)—this is interesting speculation; or
(2) based on one or two epidemiological studies—the relationship is possible; or
(3) based on several prospective studies and other mostly supportive data—the relationship is very probable; or
(4) based on much epidemiological data plus significant randomized controlled trial(s)—the relationship is causative (or protective) until proved otherwise.

We should be sure of our ground before we advise someone to change a diet to which they are accustomed.

1.4   TOOLS OF THE TRADE

As with any other science or profession, nutrition has its specialized techniques and technical terms. Those which are frequently used in research and professional work are introduced here. They are described in more detail further on in the book.

1.4.1   Measuring food and drink intake

Which foods does a person or a group of people usually eat and how many grams of each per day? Unless the subject is confined in a special hospital ward under constant observation the answer can never be 100% accurate. Information on food intake is subjective and depends on memory; people do not always notice, or know, the exact description of the foods they are given to eat (especially mixed dishes). When asked to record what they eat they may alter their diet. People do not eat the same every day so it is difficult to reach a profile of their usual diet.

The different techniques used are described in Chapter 25. One set of methods estimates the amounts of food produced and sold in a whole country and divides these by the estimated population. This is food disappearance or food moving into consumption. Obviously some of this is wasted and some eaten by tourists and pets. The main value of these data is to follow national trends and see if people appear to be eating too little or too much of some foods.

The other set of methods captures the particular foods and amounts of them that individuals say they actually ate. These methods either rely on subjects' memory or ask them to write down everything they eat or drink for (usually) several days.

1.4.2   Food composition tables (see Chapter 24)

Ideally, food tables would contain all the usual foods eaten in a country and show average numbers for the calories (food energy) and major essential nutrients measured by

5

chemical analysis in each food. A few other important food components (e.g. cholesterol, fibre) are included as well. In many smaller, less affluent countries there is no complete set of food composition data, so 'borrowed' data is used from one of the big Western countries (e.g. United Kingdom, United States, Germany). Food tables are used to calculate people's nutrient intakes from their food intake estimates. Most food tables are also available as computer software, which greatly speeds up a lot of calculations (e.g. 20 subjects × 4 days × 80 foods or drinks × 35 nutrients—224 000 computations).

1.4.3 Dietary reference values and guidelines (see Chapter 33)

The computer printout then shows (to select a small portion) that a subject was eating (say) 50 g of protein and 45 g of saturated fat. This does not mean anything without normative dietary reference values. Two sets are used; they differ somewhat from country to country. For protein, an essential nutrient, the reference is in a table of recommended nutrient intakes (recommended dietary allowances in the United States). For saturated fat (not an essential nutrient and related to risk of coronary heart disease) the reference is in recommendations called *dietary guidelines*.

1.4.4 Biomarkers: biochemical tests

For most nutrients, biochemical tests using blood or urine, are available to help estimate the amount of the nutrient functioning inside the body (see Chapter 26). If an individual (or group) is found to eat less than the recommended intake of nutrient 'A', they may not have any features of 'A' deficiency. The food intake may have been under-reported or only temporarily less than usual, and there are large body stores for some nutrients. On the other hand individuals can suffer deficiency of 'A' despite an acceptable intake if they have an unusually high requirement, perhaps because of increased losses from disease. *Biomarkers* provide a more economical method for estimating intake of some food components (e.g. salt) than food intake measurement, and can also be used to check the reliability of subjects' histories or records of food intake.

1.4.5 Human studies and trials

Most of the detailed knowledge in human nutrition comes from a range of different types of human experiments. They may last from hours to years and include from two or three subjects to thousands. The following are examples:

- Absorption studies. Some nutrients are poorly absorbed; absorption of nutrients is better from some foods than others. Many studies have been done to measure bioavailability, the percentage of the nutrient intake that is available to be used inside the body. After a test meal the increase of some nutrients can be measured in blood samples. Isotopes may be needed to label the nutrient.

- In metabolic studies, the diet is usually changed in one way only, and the result is measured in a change in blood or excreta (urine and/or faeces). One type is the balance experiment. This may measure, for example, the intake of calcium and its excretion in urine and faeces. Because of the minor variability of urine production and major variability of defaecation these measurements have to be made for a metabolic period of several days each time any dietary change is made.

- Another example is the effect of a controlled (usually single) change of diet on blood plasma cholesterol, a risk factor for coronary heart disease (see Chapter 18). Such an effect is known to take 10–14 days if it is going to appear and the experiment should include control periods before and after the dietary change being examined.

Interpreting the results of such studies is a complex matter. There is individual variation in the way people absorb and metabolize nutrients. There is also the possibility that changes observed over a short time period may not persist indefinitely as humans may adapt to dietary change. Furthermore, when one component is added or removed from the diet there are usually consequential changes to the rest of the diet as some other food is put in its place. An apparent effect of removing one food may at least in part be due to the effect of its replacement or to the energy deficit which will result if it is not replaced. Nutritionists must consider the diet as a whole and be aware of the complex dynamics of dietary change.

Part I: Energy and macronutrients

2

CARBOHYDRATES

Janette Brand-Miller

Carbohydrates hold a special place in human nutrition. They provide the largest single source of energy in the diet and satisfy our instinctual desire for sweetness. Glucose is the essential fuel for the brain and growing fetus and is the main source of energy for the muscles during strenuous exercise. Carbohydrates show a reciprocal relationship with fat in the diet so that a high carbohydrate diet is also a low fat diet. Diets high in carbohydrate are usually associated with lower prevalences of obesity, heart disease, non-insulin-dependent diabetes and some types of cancer.

2.1 DIETARY CARBOHYDRATE

Carbohydrates are substances having the empirical formula $C_x(H_2O)_y$ (e.g. $C_6(H_2O)_6 =$ glucose) (Fig. 2.1). The basic building block of carbohydrates is a monosaccharide, often glucose itself. Disaccharides are double sugars which contain two monosaccharide units linked together (e.g. sucrose, $C_{12}H_{22}O_{11}$, is composed of glucose and fructose). Oligosaccharides contain between 3 and 11 monosaccharide residues. Polysaccharides are those with longer chains of monosaccharides. Sugar alcohols are often referred to as carbohydrates too, although their empirical formula is slightly different. Carbohydrates that can be digested and absorbed in the human small intestine are referred to as available carbohydrate. Some plant polysaccharides in foods are resistant to hydrolysis by human digestive enzymes and are referred to as 'dietary fibre'. The most important food carbohydrates are listed in Table 2.1.

2.1.1 Sugars (mono-, di- and oligosaccharides)

Free glucose and fructose (Fig. 2.1) are found in relatively small amounts in natural foods; the main sources being fruit, vegetables and honey. Corn syrup (glucose syrup produced by the hydrolysis of corn starch) and high fructose corn syrups (containing mixtures of glucose and fructose) are used by the food industry.

Sucrose, the commonest disaccharide (Fig. 2.1), is extracted from sugar beet or sugar cane and is present in variable amounts in fruit and vegetables. It is hydrolyzed into glucose and fructose. Lactose, found in milk and milk products, is hydrolyzed to glucose and galactose. Maltose, a disaccharide comprising two molecules of glucose, occurs in sprouted wheat and barley, malt being used for brewing and in malted foods.

Raffinose, stachyose and verbascose are oligosaccharides made up of galactose, glucose and fructose and are found in plant seeds, especially legumes. Fructo-oligosaccharides

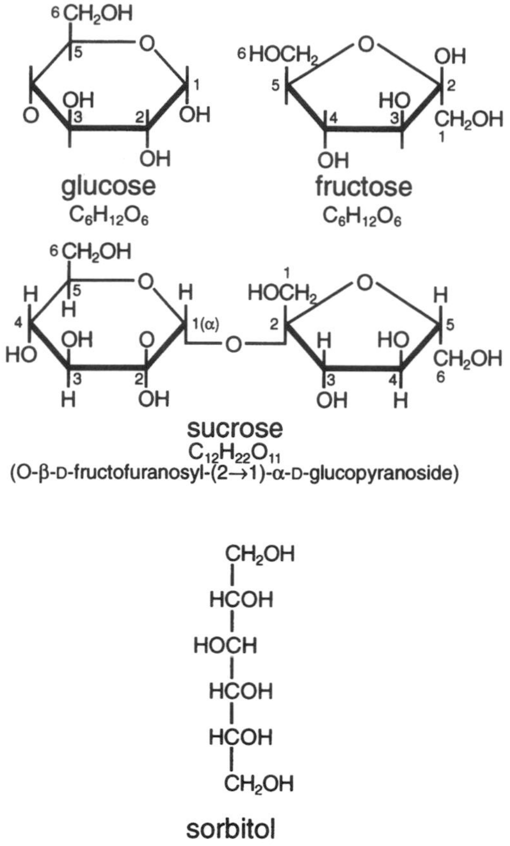

Fig. 2.1 The structure of glucose, fructose, sucrose and sorbitol.

consist of fructose residues attached to glucose. They are found naturally in cereals and vegetables, and are also produced industrially.

Sugars have also been classified in ways which do not relate to their chemical structure. For example, 'intrinsic' sugars are those which are incorporated within the intact plant cell wall, as in unprocessed fruits and vegetables. Refined sucrose, fruit juices, honey and milk are sources of 'extrinsic' sugars. Intrinsic sugars, together with milk sugars, are often referred to as 'naturally occurring' sugars and are regarded as 'healthy' sugars because their absorption tends to be slowed or because they are accompanied by significant amounts of essential nutrients. Other sugars described as 'non-milk extrinsic', 'refined' or 'added' sugars are regarded as less desirable. Although these classifications may have some merit it should be noted that there is no clear distinction between the rates of digestion and absorption of 'intrinsic' and 'extrinsic' sugars. During mastication and gastric processing, intrinsic sugars are rendered extrinsic and the body cannot distinguish the source of sugars following absorption. Added sugars in the diet perform several useful roles. They help to make bland carbohydrate foods more palatable and may thereby help to keep the fat content in the diet down. They play a role in food preservation, viscosity development,

Table 2.1 Classification of carbohydrates in the diet (modified from Asp 1994)

Available*	Unavailable*
Monosaccharides	*Oligosaccharides*
• glucose	• raffinose, stachyose, verbascose
• fructose	• human milk oligosaccharides
	• fructo-oligosaccharides
Disaccharides	
• sucrose	
• lactose	
• maltose	
• trehalose	
Polysaccharides	*Non-starch polysaccharides*
Starch[a]	*(main component of dietary fibre)*
• amylopectin	• cellulose (insoluble)
• amylose	• hemicellulose (soluble and
• modified food starches	insoluble forms)
	• β-Glucans (mainly soluble)
	• fructans (e.g. insulin)
	(these are not assayed by
	current methods)
	• gums (soluble)
	• mucilages (soluble)
	• algal polysaccharides (soluble)

Available refers to availability for digestion and absorption in the small intestine. *Unavailable* carbohydrates pass through the small intestine mostly unchanged and are fermented to varying degrees by bacteria in the large intestine.
[a] Some starch is unavailable and referred to as 'resistant starch'.

freezing point depression, osmotic balance and flavour masking. The texture and structure of products like cakes and biscuits depends upon the presence of large amounts of added sugars.

2.1.2 Sugar alcohols

Sorbitol, the alcohol of glucose (Fig. 2.1), occurs naturally in some fruit, and is made commercially from glucose using the enzyme, aldose reductase, which converts the aldehyde group of the glucose molecule to the alcohol. It is used without much justification as a replacement for sucrose in the diet of people with diabetes. Inositol hexaphosphate (phytic acid) is present in cereal bran and may reduce absorption of iron and calcium.

2.1.3 Polysaccharides

Foods containing large amounts of starch include cereals (e.g. wheat, rice, maize), root vegetables (e.g. potato) and legumes (e.g. kidney beans, baked beans). There is little starch in most fruits and other vegetables, apart from roots and tubers. Starch molecules in plants occur as granules in the form of amylose and amylopectin. Amylose is a straight chain polymer of glucose linked by α1,4-glucosidic bonds, whereas amylopectin is a branched chain polymer of glucose having as well branches of α1, 6-glucosidic bonds approximately every 25 units (Fig. 2.2). The proportion of amylose to amylopectin is 1 : 3 in most starches but 'waxy' varieties of maize and rice contain amylopectin only. The molecular weight of starch molecules varies from 10^5 to 10^8, amylopectin being larger. Glycogen, the storage form of carbohydrate in animals (including humans), has a molecule similar to amylopectin, but more highly branched.

The amylose and amylopectin in the starch granules are arranged in a crystalline structure which makes them insoluble in water and difficult to digest. The crystallinity is lost when starch is heated in the presence of water (gelatinization), enabling the amylose and amylopectin chains to be digested. Recrystallization or 'retrogradation' can take place to a variable extent after cooling.

Starches are digested by α-amylases in saliva and pancreatic juice to smaller molecules: maltose, malto-triose and α-dextrins (Fig. 2.3). Brush-border α-glucosides complete the process of digestion to glucose. Starch may also be classified according to the rate of digestion to glucose in controlled experimental conditions (Table 2.2) which probably provides a good indication of their rate of digestion in the small intestine. The rate of starch digestion is the major determinant of the plasma glucose response to the meal.

The rate of starch digestion depends upon several factors: the size of the particle (small particles in cereal flours result in full gelatinization of the starch during cooking), the

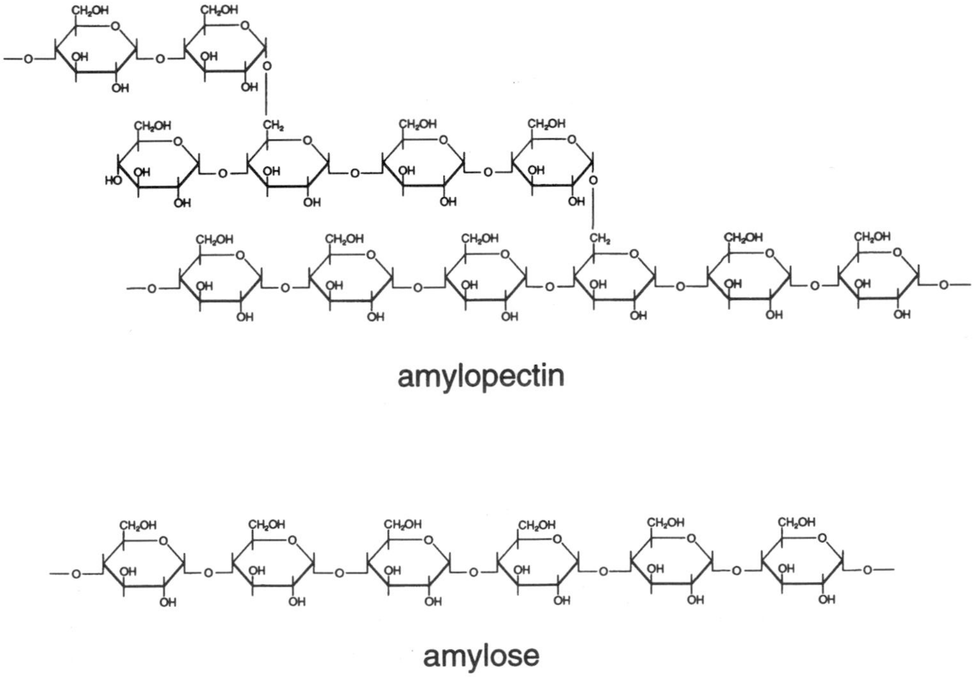

amylopectin

amylose

Fig. 2.2   The structure of amylose and amylopectin.

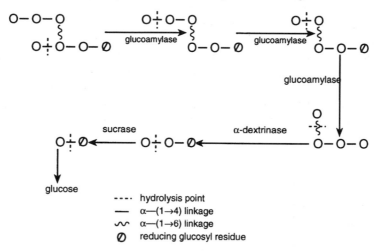

Fig. 2.3 The process of starch digestion.

ratio of amylose to amylopectin (high amylose starches digest more slowly) and the amount of dietary fibre, which can delay absorption. As much as 10–20% of dietary starch in individual foods and mixed meals escapes absorption in the small bowel and enters the large bowel. This resistant starch has important nutritional properties which are discussed later.

2.1.4   Dietary fibre (non-starch polysaccharide)

Dietary fibre was previously defined as 'plant polysaccharides and lignin which are resistant to hydrolysis by the digestive enzymes of man'. This definition includes resistant starch as part of dietary fibre. Nutrition researchers in the United Kingdom now avoid the term 'dietary fibre' and use instead 'non-starch polysaccharide' which excludes both resistant starch and lignin. Whether or not resistant starch is classed as dietary fibre, the term 'dietary fibre' includes many different types of compounds in varying concentrations,

Table 2.2 Different types of starch defined according to speed of digestion

Speed of digestion	Type of starch	Food source examples
All glucose released in under 20 min	Rapidly digestible starch (RDS)	Cooked starchy cereals, potatoes, still warm
Glucose released in 20–120 min	Slowly digestible starch (SDS)	Raw cereals Pasta Legumes
Starch not hydrolysed after 120 min	Resistant starch (RS)	Cooked potato after cooling (small fraction, not all) Under-ripe banana Partly milled grains Seeds

Source: Englyst *et al.* Europ J Clin Nutr 1992; **46** (suppl. 2): S33–S50.

depending on the food. From a nutritional point of view the most important way of grouping the components of dietary fibre is on the basis of their solubility in water.

Insoluble fibre is mainly cellulose, with some hemicelluloses. The latter contain a variety of monosaccharide residues such as glucose, galactose and xylose together with lignin (a polyphenolic compound which is not a carbohydrate). These substances are particulate by nature and individual particles can be seen with the naked eye. Soluble fibre includes pectins, some hemicelluloses, β-glucans, mucilages and gums which often, but not always, form a viscous solution in water. The particle size, viscosity and fermentability of the different types of dietary fibre are determined by the structure of the compound and the processing of the food and these in turn determine the physiological effects of fibre in the body.

2.1.5 Synthetic carbohydrates

Polydextrose is an indigestible carbohydrate used in food as a substitute for fat. It has a cream-like texture that mimics that of fat. It is produced industrially by high temperature polymerization of glucose and contains a small amount of sorbitol and citric acid. Humans are unable to break down the linkage formed so its use reduces the energy content of the food.

Neosugar (raffinose) is a fructo-oligosaccharide, non-nondigestible sweetener. It is manufactured readily from sucrose using a fungal fructosyltransferase. The resulting product is about half as sweet as sucrose and behaves like sucrose in food processing operations but is not digested by the enzymes of the small intestine. It is composed of sucrose molecules that have been lengthened by addition to the fructose unit of one, two or three molecules of fructose in a β-(2-1) glycosidic linkage.

Maltodextrins are small oligosaccharide breakdown products (5–11 glucosyl residues) from the industrial hydrolysis of starch. They are used in food as sweeteners and texture-modifying agents and as fat substitutes. They are digested and absorbed normally, but contain only 16 kJ/g versus 37 kJ/g for fat.

2.2   CONSUMPTION PATTERNS

Starch, sucrose and mixtures of glucose and fructose are the most common forms of carbohydrate in human diets. Currently, total carbohydrate intake in most relatively affluent countries averages about 40–44% energy or roughly 280 g/day for an adult male and 240 g/day for an adult female. Approximately half of this is starch (20–22% total energy). The remaining half comes from sugars—sucrose (40–80 g/day), lactose (20 g/day), glucose (10–20 g/day), fructose (10–20 g/day)—and non-starch polysaccharide (dietary fibre, 15–20 g/day). On the other hand, a traditional-living African or Asian might eat up to 400 g carbohydrate (i.e. 70–80% energy), the major part of which is starch. As incomes rise in developing countries, the proportion of energy obtained from carbohydrate falls while fat increases.

In western countries, the percentage of energy contributed by all sugars combined averages 20–22%. Of this, about half comes from naturally occurring sources such as fruits, fruit juices, milk and vegetables. The other half comes from added sugars, particularly refined sucrose, but also honey, molasses and other concentrated sugar products. Adults eat 35–70 g/day of added sugars. Young children eat 40–50 g/day. In the United States and Canada, a significant proportion of added sugars comes in the form of corn syrup solids (hydrolyzed corn starch) and high fructose corn syrups, so that per capita consumption of refined sucrose (but not added sugars) is lower than in other developed nations. Many African and Asian nations, including Japan, have low intakes of added sugars (Table 2.3).

It is difficult to quantify intakes of dietary fibre since many food tables and food labels give only figures for 'crude fibre' which is based on an early method that grossly underestimates total dietary fibre and non-starch polysaccharides. The newer 'chemical' methods are time-consuming but provide considerable information about the different chemical components of dietary fibre. These should be used increasingly in the future. At present enzymatic/'gravimetric' methods such as that of the Association of Official Analytical Chemists (AOAC) are widely used for routine analysis because they are quicker. The assay also measures some, but not all, resistant starch. Nutrition labelling in many countries is based on this method. Using information based on this enzymatic/gravimetric technique the intake of total dietary fibre in the Western diet is estimated to be around 25 g/day for adult males and 19 g/day for women. The ratio of soluble to insoluble fibre is about one : three. Among vegetarians in Western countries and in many developing countries the intake of dietary fibre may be twice as high. The intake of non-starch polysaccharide is lower: in the United Kingdom this is estimated to be about 12 g/day.

2.3   DIGESTION AND ABSORPTION OF CARBOHYDRATES

2.3.1   Sugars and digestible starch

Carbohydrates which will be absorbed in the small intestine must be hydrolyzed to their constituent monosaccharides before they can cross the intestinal wall. The enzyme which hydrolyses starch is α-amylase which is present in saliva and pancreatic juice. Salivary amylase is inhibited by the low pH in the stomach and makes a relatively small

Table 2.3 Per capita consumption (kg/head per year) of refined sucrose and estimates of numbers of decayed, missing and filled teeth at 12 years of age

Location	Year	Sugar consumption (kg/head per year)	DMFT
Developed countries			
Australia	1986	50	2.0
Canada	1988	42	4.3
Denmark	1988	48	1.6
France	1990	37	3.0
Iceland	1986	52	6.6
Italy	1985	31	3.0
Japan	1987	23	4.9
Netherlands	1988	54	2.5
Developing countries			
Barbados	1983	63	4.4
China	1984	5	0.7
Indonesia	1982	13	2.3
Philippines	1982	24	2.2
Nigeria	1983	10	2.0

Note: per capita consumption overestimates true sugar consumption by as much as 100%.
DMFT, decayed, missing and filled teeth (per individual).
Source: Woodward M, Walker ARP. Sugar consumption and dental caries: evidence from 90 countries. *Brit Dent J* 1994; **176**: 297–302.

contribution to starch digestion. α-Amylase splits starch into maltose, maltotriose and branched tri-, tetra- and penta-saccharides, producing only small amounts of glucose (Fig. 2.3). Pancreatic α-amylase acts in the lumen of the jejunum and the process is completed in the brush border of the small intestine as a result of the actions of glucoamylase, sucrose and α-dextrinase. Disaccharides are hydrolyzed by disaccharidase enzymes in the brush border: maltase, sucrase and lactase convert maltose, sucrose and lactose to their constituent monosaccharides.

The efficacy of these enzymes is so high that the rate of digestion does not limit the rate of absorption, with the exception of lactase. If too great a quantity of monosaccharide is released into the gut lumen, water is drawn into the gut by osmotic action, with subsequent diarrhoea. Glucose and galactose are absorbed rapidly with the help of specific carriers which are ATP (adenosine triphosphate)-dependent. Fructose is absorbed more slowly by facilitated diffusion and large amounts at any one time may overload the absorptive capacity of the gut, resulting in diarrhoea. For example, young children who drink a lot of apple juice whose sugar is mostly fructose (instead of milk or water) may suffer from 'toddler diarrhoea'. Fructose is absorbed better when ingested with glucose, either separately or when combined with sucrose. In most adults consuming more than 50 g of fructose may give rise to osmotic diarrhoea, whereas 250 g sucrose does not produce symptoms.

2.3.2 Resistant starch and dietary fibre

Non-starch polysaccharides and resistant starch, from foods such as wheat flour, potatoes, beans, oats and bananas, which have escaped digestion and absorption in the small intestine are fermented by microorganisms in the large bowel to short-chain fatty acids (SCFAs) and gases (Fig. 2.4). Soluble fibres (pectins, gums) are largely fermented while insoluble fibres are more difficult to degrade. Only 5% of cellulose is fermented. Finely divided bran is degraded more than coarse bran. Note that starch that has escaped absorption in the small intestine is a major substrate for fermentation in the colon.

A mixture of SCFAs is produced—mainly acetate, propionate, butyrate in the molar ratio of 57 : 22 : 21. The ratio varies slightly with the substrate. Lactic acid may be produced too if the appropriate microorganisms are present. The ratio between the individual SCFA changes with the substrate being fermented and the type of microorganisms present. The gases CO_2, H_2 and CH_4 are produced as well as water. If 20 g fermentable carbohydrate reaches the colon daily, about 200 mmol SCFA could be produced. Assuming 70% of these are absorbed, an additional 300 kJ (73 calories)/day are available. However, the amount of SCFAs actually produced varies from 220–720 mmol/day, suggesting that 20–60 g of unavailable carbohydrate reaches the colon each day. Undigested starch and unabsorbable sugars must therefore make a significant contribution to colonic fermentation.

SCFAs are taken up by the colonic epithelial cells where butyrate is selectively used for these cells' nutrition, leaving mainly acetate and propionate to pass to the portal vein

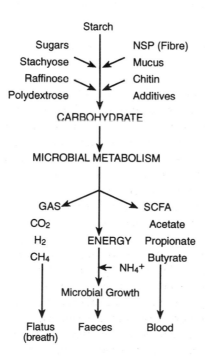

Fig. 2.4 Fermentation of carbohydrates in the large bowel. NSP, non-starch polysaccharide; GAS, gases (CO_2, H_2, CH_4); SCFAs, short-chain fatty acids.

and be taken up by the liver. A high butyrate supply is thought to be important for the health of the large bowel epithelium. In the presence of nitrogen (as ammonia from urea), carbohydrate in the large intestine provides the fuel for bacterial cell multiplication. But the production of acid lowers pH and may inhibit bacterial types, numbers and metabolism. For example, if lactulose (an indigestible disaccharide comprised of galactose and fructose) is consumed daily for a week, breath H_2 declines, indicating reduced hydrogen formation from colonic fermentation.

2.4   GLYCAEMIC RESPONSE TO CARBOHYDRATE-CONTAINING FOODS

After a meal containing carbohydrate, the plasma glucose rises, reaching a peak in about 15–45 minutes depending on the rate of digestion and absorption. The plasma glucose returns to the fasting concentration within two to three hours. Plasma insulin concentration mirrors that of glucose, stimulating both glucose oxidation and glycogen storage. Glucose oxidation is stimulated for up to six hours after the meal.

For many years it was assumed that all starchy foods were digested slowly giving rise to a flattened blood glucose and insulin response, but this assumption has been proven to be incorrect. Some starchy foods, including (cooked) potatoes, bread and many packaged breakfast cereals are digested and absorbed almost as quickly as an equivalent load of glucose. Many sugar-containing foods including fruit, ice cream, sweetened yoghurt, give low glycaemic responses. In general, carbohydrate-containing foods which are high in rapidly digestible starches, free glucose and/or oligosaccharides readily hydrolyzed to glucose (i.e. rich sources of rapidly available glucose) produce a high glycaemic response. On the other hand, foods which are rich in slowly digestible starches, fructose or contain substantial amounts of either insoluble fibre or fat produce a low glycaemic response.

In the early 1980s, the glycaemic index was introduced to express the relative ability of different foods to raise the level of glucose in the blood (Table 2.4). Many studies since then indicate that the glycaemic index concept is a useful tool in the dietary management of diabetes. Low glycaemic index foods improve blood glucose control and sometimes plasma lipids. The glycaemic and insulin response to sugars and starches is also relevant to sports performance, satiety and serotonin-related phenomena, such as sleepiness. When using the glycaemic index to give advice on choices of carbohydrate-containing foods it is important to bear in mind that some low glycaemic index foods may be high in fat.

The procedure for measuring the glycaemic index of a food is shown in Fig. 2.5.

2.5   METABOLIC FATE OF DIETARY CARBOHYDRATE

Absorption of carbohydrate produces a range of metabolic and hormonal responses that help to limit the rise in plasma glucose levels to within an acceptable range. Levels above 10 mmol/litre (and in some people even lower) will result in glycosuria (glucose in the urine) which is a waste of valuable energy. Insulin is the central hormone involved in the metabolism of carbohydrate and a relative or absolute deficiency of insulin leads to diabetes which is characterized by increased blood levels of glucose and glycosuria (see Chapter 20). Dietary carbohydrate has several related metabolic fates.

Table 2.4 Glycaemic index (GI) of foods (glucose = 100)

Breakfast cereals		Vegetables		Dairy foods	
All Bran	30	Beetroot	64	Milk whole (av)	27
Cocopops	77	Carrots	49	chocolate flavour	34
Cornflakes	77	Sweet corn	48	Ice cream (av)	61
Porridge (av)	50	Peas (green)	48	low fat	50
Muesli		Potato		Yoghurt flav, low fat	33
toasted*	43	baked (av)	85		
untoasted	56	new (av)	62	Beverages	
Rice Bubbles	89	French fries*	75	Apple juice	41
Weetbix	75	Sweet potato	48	Orange juice	57
				Soft drink, carbonated	68
Grains/Pasta		Legumes			
Rice		Baked Beans (av)	48	Snacks	
long grain white	50	Haricot beans (av)	38	Corn Chips	72
Calrose	83	Butter beans (av)	31	Popcorn	55
Basmati	59	Chickpeas (av)	33	Potato Crisps*	57
Noodles: instant	47	Kidney beans (av)	27		
Pasta: spaghetti (av)	41	Lentils (av)	28	Confectionery	
		Soya beans (av)	18	Chocolate*	49
Bread				Jelly beans	80
White bread (av)	70	Fruit		Life Savers	70
Wholemeal bread (av)	77	Apple (av)	36	Mars bars*	68
Heavy grain bread (av)	45	Apricot (dried)	43		
Rye: pumpernickel	50	Banana (av)	60	Sugars	
Rye: blackbread	76	Cherries	23	Honey	58
		Grapefruit	25	Fructose	20
Crackers/crispbread		Grapes	43	Glucose	100
Puffed crispbread	81	Kiwifruit	58	Lactose	57
Ryvita	69	Mango	51	Maltose	105
Watercracker	78	Orange (av)	43	Sucrose	59
		Papaya (paw paw)	56		
Sweet biscuits		Peach			
Arrowroot	69	canned in juice	30		
Shortbread	64	fresh	28		
Oatmeal	55	Pear (av)	36		
Shredded wheatmeal	62	Pineapple	66		
		Plum	24		
Cakes		Raisins	64		
Apple muffin*	44	Rockmelon	65		
Banana cake*	47	Sultanas	56		
Sponge cake	46	Watermelon	72		

* Foods with a high fat content. GI ranges: the figures form a continuum; but in general low GI foods may be those below 55; moderate between 55 and 70; and high more than 70; av, average.
Source: Foster-Powell K, Brand Miller J. International tables of glycemic index. *Am J Clin Nutr* 1995; **62** (suppl.): 871S–93S.

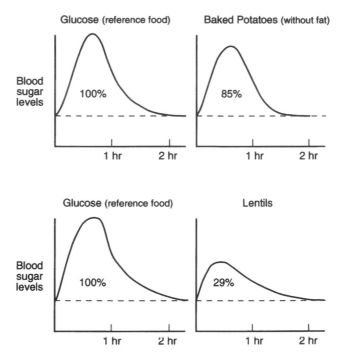

Fig. 2.5 Calculation of the glycaemic index of a food. The area under the blood glucose curve is calculated geometrically using the fasting level as baseline and expressed as a percentage of that seen after consumption of 50 g pure glucose. In practice, 8–12 people are tested and the mean of the group is the glycaemic index of the test food.

2.5.1 Oxidation in tissues

After its absorption from a meal containing carbohydrate glucose is transported into insulin-sensitive cells. In the mitochondria of these cells glucose is metabolized to pyruvate by the pathway of glycolysis (Fig. 2.6). Insulin is involved not only by enhancing glucose uptake into cells, but also by stimulating several steps in the glycolytic pathway. Glycolysis can occur in the absence of oxygen (anaerobic conditions) and under such conditions glucose is converted as far as lactate. However, in the presence of oxygen pyruvate is further metabolized to acetyl CoA which can enter the citric acid cycle for complete oxidation to carbon dioxide and water with liberation of free energy as ATP in the process of oxidative phosphorylation. In this way glucose is the major source of energy for many tissues.

2.5.2 Storage as glycogen

For several hours after a carbohydrate-containing meal, the amount of ingested carbohydrate far exceeds the energy needs of the tissues. The excess is converted to glycogen (glycogenesis) which is stored in liver and skeletal muscles for later use as an energy source. The process through which glycogen stores are drawn upon to replenish glucose

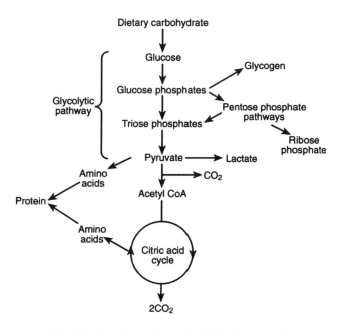

Fig. 2.6 Simplified overview of carbohydrate metabolism.

in the blood in the fasting state is known as glycogenolysis. The body's glycogen stores are relatively small (250–500 g in a 50–70 kg adult human), although the capacity to store more can be developed by sports training and diet. Most of the stored glycogen is released and oxidized within 12 hours.

2.5.3 Storage as triglyceride

In rats and mice the conversion of carbohydrate to fat is an important pathway in the liver and adipose tissue, but in humans this lipogenesis (the synthesis of fat from non-fat precursors such as glucose) is quantitatively unimportant. Fatty acids may be synthesized from acetyl CoA derived from carbohydrate. Triose phosphate (see Fig. 2.6) provides the glycerol moiety of triglycerides. The pentose phosphate pathway, which arises from intermediates of glycolysis, is a source of reducing equivalents for the biosynthesis of fatty acids.

In humans, even a very large amount of carbohydrate (500–700 g) does not induce a net gain in lipid. If overfeeding of carbohydrate continues for several days, glycogen stores become saturated (at about 1000 g) and net conversion of carbohydrate to fat occurs, but this represents an artificial situation, unlikely to occur outside the laboratory. In everyday life, a high intake of carbohydrate increases satiety and subsequently intake is decreased.

2.5.4 Conversion to amino acids

Conversion to amino acids is similarly a relatively unimportant fate of ingested carbohydrate, although pyruvate and intermediates of the citric acid cycle provide the carbon skeletons for the synthesis of amino acids.

2.5.5   Metabolism of fructose and galactose

When fructose reaches the liver, most is removed from the bloodstream and enters the glycolytic pathway. Fructose is more rapidly metabolized by the liver than glucose because it bypasses the first step in the glycolytic pathway. The formation of triglyceride is greater after fructose than after glucose feeding because of 'flooding' of the pathways in the liver. High intakes of fructose may lead to increased plasma levels of triglyceride and lactate. Because of the rapid rate of metabolism only very small amounts of fructose are detected in the blood even when measurements are made shortly after eating substantial amounts of fruit or large quantities of sucrose.

Galactose is rapidly converted to glucose in the liver and unless ethanol (which inhibits this conversion) is consumed simultaneously with galactose, only miniscule amounts are detectable in the plasma.

2.6   HEALTH ISSUES RELATING TO DIETARY CARBOHYDRATE

2.6.1   Lactose intolerance and inborn errors of carbohydrate metabolism

The inability to hydrolyze some forms of dietary carbohydrate is well recognized, especially with reference to lactose. The signs and symptoms of lactose intolerance include abdominal discomfort, borborygmi, flatulence and diarrhoea. In severe cases, the stools may contain lactose, or have a low pH due to colonic fermentation of the lactose to short-chain fatty acids. Hydrogen gas is a by-product of colonic fermentation of carbohydrate and some of it is absorbed into the portal vein and is excreted in the breath. Carbohydrate malabsorption can be detected by measuring breath hydrogen before and after giving a test dose of the carbohydrate. A biopsy of the small intestinal epithelium can be carried out to detect low lactase levels. Primary low lactase levels arise some time after weaning (two to three years) in over three-quarters of the world's human population (the exception being most Caucasians) and most of the animal kingdom, including dogs and cats.

Secondary lactase insufficiency can arise as a result of disease of the intestinal tract (e.g. protein-energy malnutrition, coeliac disease, intestinal infections and non-specific gastroenteritis). Most individuals with low lactase activity can still tolerate small amounts of milk (e.g. 100 ml, containing 5 g lactose) without symptoms. Fermented dairy products (e.g. commercial yoghurts) are better tolerated because the culture, viable *in vivo*, hydrolyzes lactose in the lumen.

A range of other inborn errors may occasionally affect metabolism of carbohydrates (see Table 2.5).

2.6.2   Minimum requirements

Although glucose is the most common source of energy available to cells (16 kJ/g or 4 kcal/g), it is essential only in a few organs: the brain, the kidney (medulla) and the red cells. The adult brain requires about 140 g glucose/day and the red cells about 40 g/day. In the absence of dietary carbohydrate, the body is able to synthesize glucose from lactic acid, certain amino acids and glycerol via gluconeogenesis. Gluconeogenesis

Table 2.5 Inborn errors of carbohydrate metabolism

Inborn error	Consequence
• Absence of fructokinase	• Prevents fructose breakdown, fructosuria
• Absence of fructose-l-phosphate aldolase	• Inhibition of glycogenolysis, hypoglycaemia
• Deficiency of galactokinase	• Galactose not phosphorylated, cataracts
• Deficiency of glucose-6-phosphate dehydrogenase	• May result in red cell haemolysis and anaemia

can supply about 2 mg/kg body weight per minute or 130 g/day. The difference between essential glucose requirements and gluconeogenic supply is therefore 50 g/day (180 minus 130 g). In the absence of a dietary source of carbohydrate, ketones are formed as a by-product of fatty acid oxidation. In prolonged fasting or starvation, the brain adapts to the shortfall of carbohydrate and oxidizes ketone bodies for the remainder of its energy needs. The ketotic state, however, is not desirable because judgement may be impaired and the fetus may be adversely affected. Thus, it could be said that the absolute minimum requirement for carbohydrate is about 50 g/day. In pregnancy and lactation, this figure should be probably doubled.

2.6.3 Beneficial effects of diets high in carbohydrates

High carbohydrate diets, especially those also high in dietary fibre, appear to be usually associated with low rates of obesity, perhaps because they are more satiating than high fat foods and perhaps because synthesis of fat from carbohydrate is not an important pathway in humans; excessive carbohydrate intake appears to be balanced by higher rates of carbohydrate oxidation. High carbohydrate diets are also usually recommended for people trying to achieve weight reduction.

Several strands of evidence suggest that diets high in dietary fibre may provide some protection against coronary heart disease. Levels of low density lipoprotein and other cardiovascular risk factors are reduced, especially when the diet is rich in soluble forms of dietary fibre (see Chapter 3). Diets high in carbohydrate and dietary fibre are invariably also low in fat, and this further reduces risk. Longitudinal studies have shown that those with the highest intake of dietary fibre have lower rates of coronary heart disease (CHD), but there is always a possibility that the high intake of dietary fibre is simply a surrogate for other dietary factors (e.g. a high intake of antioxidants) or other characteristics of a healthy lifestyle (e.g. not smoking, physical activity) which also protect against CHD. High carbohydrate diets which are not also high in dietary fibre may cause higher levels of fasting plasma triglyceride and reduced levels of high-density lipoprotein (HDL). This appears to be the case particularly, when diets which are extremely high in sucrose and fructose and saturated fats are fed in experimental situations. It is not clear whether this effect is a permanent one or temporary. However, this is of little practical relevance since diets very high in sucrose or fructose are not consumed outside the experimental situation.

Diets high in insoluble fibre (especially coarse wheat bran) speed up transit time through the gut, increase stool weight and relieve constipation. They are also associated with a reduced risk of diverticular disease and are of benefit in relieving at least some of the symptoms in those with established diverticulosis.

High intakes of resistant starch and non-starch polysaccharides may also reduce the risk of large bowel cancer. Fibre may bind the carcinogenic substances and speed their transit through the gut. Fibre also increases the amount of water in the faeces, thereby diluting the effect of any carcinogens. Fermentation of resistant starch and non-starch polysaccharides in the colon to short-chain fatty acids, especially butyrate, may also play an important role in maintaining the health of the colonic epithelial cell (see Chapter 19). The protective role of resistant starch and non-starch polysaccharide remains to be confirmed in clinical trials, and it is conceivable that the strong circumstantial evidence described here and the confirming epidemiological evidence is also explained by the fact that diets rich in fibre also contain plenty of fruit and vegetables which may have other anticancer effects (e.g. indole compounds in brassica vegetables).

There is some evidence that high cereal fibre diets protect against diabetes. Diets high in soluble fibre can help to improve glycaemic control as well as the dyslipidaemia of both insulin-dependent and non-insulin-dependent diabetes. While many factors determine the glycaemic response to foods and meals, the most practical way of achieving optimal glycaemic control is by recommending foods with a low glycaemic index (see Table 2.4).

2.6.4 Disadvantages of high carbohydrate diets

The most widely quoted deleterious effect of high carbohydrate diets is dental caries. Individual carbohydrate-rich foods have different cariogenic potential. Sucrose, glucose and fructose are amongst the most cariogenic, but starch is also fermentable by dental plaque bacteria. The potential to cause caries is greatly influenced by the mode and frequency of intake. Sticky foods (e.g. some confectionery and dried fruit) which have a long residence time next to the teeth are more likely to produce decay than sugar solutions such as soft drinks. Frequency of consumption is more important than amount eaten. Fluoride in some water supplies and many toothpastes has dramatically reduced the incidence of dental caries round the world. For this reason there is no longer a clear relationship between total sugar intake and the number of decayed, missing and filled teeth in children in developed countries (see Table 2.3).

Contrary to what was once believed it is now clear that intake of dietary sugars does not increase the risk of diabetes or coronary heart disease, although some authorities would argue that high intakes may predispose to obesity and so indirectly influence diabetes and CHD. While it is sensible to recommend a moderate intake of added sugars (<10–12% energy), it must be conceded that there is also no direct evidence linking intake of sucrose and other sugars to obesity. Most dietary recommendations for people with diabetes permit the inclusion of modest intakes of added sugars for those who are not overweight, provided the sugars are taken at meal times and incorporated as part of a dietary prescription which is high in dietary fibre (see Chapter 20).

Very high intakes of dietary fibre may have some adverse effects. Physical symptoms include loose stools, increased bowel frequency and flatulence. These 'inconvenient' symptoms may prevent widespread acceptance of high fibre diets, but are usually negligible if intake of fibre is gradually increased. There is also a possibility that high fibre diets may decrease bioavailability of minerals such as iron, calcium and zinc, but there is little evidence that deficiencies result in practice.

2.6.5 Dietary reference values for carbohydrate

Apart from the minimum requirements for carbohydrate described above in Section 2.6.2 there are few definitive recommendations regarding intake. Typically, energy from carbohydrate makes up the remainder when more precise recommendations have been given for intake of fat and protein. However, British Dietary Reference Values suggest population averages of 10% total energy for non-milk extrinsic sugars, 37% for starch and intrinsic and milk sugars, making 47% of energy for total carbohydrate. (The respective percentages of energy just from food are 11%, 39% and 50% since in adults alcohol provides on average 3% total energy.) The same source suggests a population average of 18 g/day of non-starch polysaccharide (equivalent to approximately 25 g of total dietary fibre) with the recommended individual minimum of 12 g (17 g total dietary fibre) and an individual maximum of 24 g (35 g total dietary fibre). Obviously, much higher intakes can be compatible with good health since in many parts of the world a far greater percentage of total energy is derived from carbohydrate. However, high carbohydrate, high fibre diets are not recommended for infants and young children since it may be difficult for them to obtain intakes of total energy sufficient for optimal growth from such diets.

FURTHER READING

1. Acheson KJ, Schutz Y, Bessard T, Amantharaman K, Flatt JP, Jequier E. Glycogen storage capacity and de novo lipogenesis during massive carbohydrate overfeeding in man. *Am J Clin Nutr* 1988; **48**: 240–7.
2. Asp NG. Nutritional classification and analysis of carbohydrates. *Am J Clin Nutr* 1994; **59** (suppl.): 679S–81S.
3. Green SM, Burley VJ, Blundell JE. Effect of fat- and sucrose-containing foods and the size of eating episodes and energy intake in lean males: potential for causing over-consumption. *Eur J Clin Nutr* 1994; **48**: 547–55.
4. Brand Miller J. The importance of glycemic index in diabetes. *Am J Clin Nutr* 1994; 59 (suppl.): 747S–52S.
5. Cummings JH, Roberfroid MB and members of the Paris Carbohydrate Group. A new look at dietary carbohydrate: chemistry, physiology and health. *Europ J Clin Nutr* 1997; **51**: 417–23.
6. Englyst HN, Kingman SM, Cummings JH. Classification and measurement of nutritionally important starch fractions. *Europ J Clin Nutr* 1992; **46** (suppl. 2): S33–S50.
7. Englyst HN, Veenstra J, Hudson GJ. Measurement of rapidly available glucose (RAG) in plant foods: a potential *in vitro* predictor of the glycaemic response. *Br J Nutr* 1996; **75**: 327–37.
8. Gibson SA. Consumption and sources of sugars in the diets of British school children: are high sugar diets nutritionally inferior? *J Nutr Dietet* 1993; **6**: 355–71.
9. Lissner L, Levitsky DA. Dietary fat and the regulation of energy intake in human subjects. *Am J Clin Nutr* 1987; **46**: 886–92.
10. Mann J. Diabetic dietary prescriptions. *BMJ* 1989; **298**: 1535–6.
11. Truswell AS. Food carbohydrates and plasma lipids—an update. *Am J Clin Nutr* 1994; **59** (suppl.): 710S–8S.

3

LIPIDS

Jim Mann and Murray Skeaff

Lipids are a group of compounds that dissolve in organic solvents such as petrol or chloroform, but are usually insoluble in water. The most obvious lipids are oils which are liquid at room temperature and fats which are solid at room temperature. Many people in Western countries regard fats and oils as foods which should be avoided as far as possible because of their perceived role in the development of obesity and coronary heart disease. However, in addition to enhancing the flavour and palatability of food, lipids make an important contribution to adequate nutrition. They are major sources of energy; some are essential nutrients because they cannot be synthesized in the body yet are required for a range of metabolic and physiological processes and to maintain the structural and functional integrity of all cell membranes. Lipids are also the only form in which the body can store energy for a prolonged period of time. These stored lipids in adipose tissue also serve to provide insulation, help to control body temperature, and afford some physical protection to internal organs. Lipids include the fat-soluble vitamins. Triacylglycerols, usually referred to as triglycerides, make up the bulk of dietary lipid with phospholipids and sterols making up nearly all the remainder.

3.1 NATURALLY OCCURRING DIETARY LIPIDS

Naturally occurring dietary lipids are derived from a wide variety of animal and plant sources including animal adipose tissue (the visible fat on meat, lard and suet); milk and products derived from milk fat (cream, butter, cheese and yoghurt); vegetable seeds, nuts, oils and products derived from them (e.g. margarines); eggs; fish oil and plant leaves. Many sources of dietary lipid are visible and obvious, others are less so, for example, those which are found in the muscle of lean meat, avocado, nuts and seeds, as well as those in processed or home prepared foods such as pies, cakes, biscuits and chocolates. In most Western countries, dietary lipid provides between 30–40% of total dietary energy. In Asian countries and throughout the developing world, the proportion of energy derived from dietary lipids is usually much lower.

3.1.1 Glycerides and fatty acids

Triglycerides make up about 95% of dietary lipids. A triglyceride molecule is formed from a molecule of glycerol (a 3-carbon alcohol) with three fatty acids attached (Fig. 3.1). Fatty acids consist of an even numbered chain of carbon atoms with hydrogens attached, a methyl group at one end and a carboxylic acid group at the other (Fig. 3.2). The carbon atoms were classically numbered from the carboxyl carbon

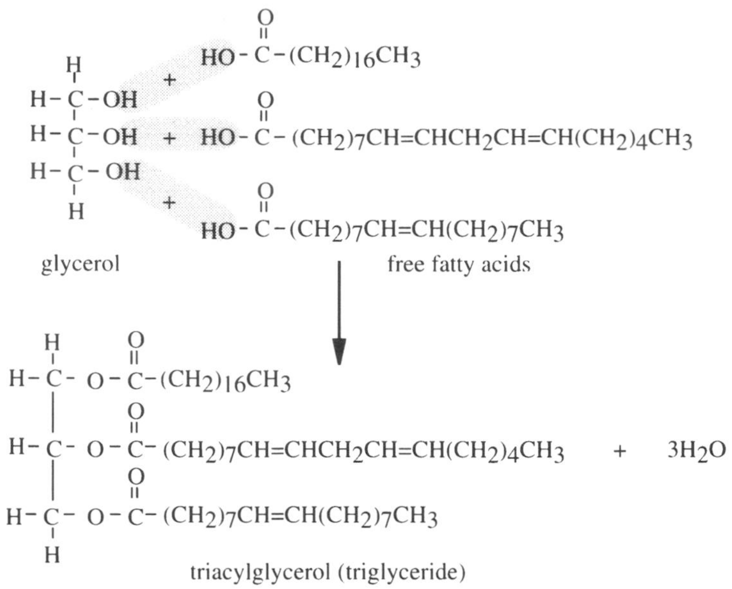

$$H-\underset{\underset{H}{|}}{\overset{\overset{H}{|}}{C}}-OH$$

$$+$$

$$HO-\overset{\overset{O}{\|}}{C}-(CH_2)_{16}CH_3$$

$$H-\underset{|}{\overset{|}{C}}-OH \quad + \quad HO-\overset{\overset{O}{\|}}{C}-(CH_2)_7CH=CHCH_2CH=CH(CH_2)_4CH_3$$

$$H-\underset{\underset{H}{|}}{\overset{|}{C}}-OH$$

$$+$$

$$HO-\overset{\overset{O}{\|}}{C}-(CH_2)_7CH=CH(CH_2)_7CH_3$$

glycerol   free fatty acids

$$H-\underset{|}{\overset{\overset{H}{|}}{C}}-O-\overset{\overset{O}{\|}}{C}-(CH_2)_{16}CH_3$$

$$H-\underset{|}{\overset{|}{C}}-O-\overset{\overset{O}{\|}}{C}-(CH_2)_7CH=CHCH_2CH=CH(CH_2)_4CH_3 \quad + \quad 3H_2O$$

$$H-\underset{\underset{H}{|}}{\overset{|}{C}}-O-\overset{\overset{O}{\|}}{C}-(CH_2)_7CH=CH(CH_2)_7CH_3$$

triacylglycerol (triglyceride)

Fig. 3.1 Formation of a triglyceride molecule.

(carbon number 1). The methyl end carbon is known as the *n* minus (*n*-) or omega (ω) carbon atom. The physical and biological properties of triglycerides are determined by the nature of the constituent fatty acids. They float on water and do not dissolve in it.

Saturated fatty acids are those in which carbon–carbon bonds are fully saturated with hydrogen atoms (i.e. 4 hydrogens per carbon–carbon bond). When 2 hydrogens are absent, the carbons form double bonds with each other and monounsaturated (single double bond) or polyunsaturated (two or more double bonds) fatty acids result. Double bonds in polyunsaturated fatty acids are always separated by one CH_2 (methylene group). Fatty acids can be described by their common name, their chemical name, their full or simplified chemical structure, or a shorthand notation in which the first number indicates the number of carbon atoms and the second the number of double bonds (Fig. 3.2). For monounsaturated and polyunsaturated fatty acids, a third descriptor indicates the position of the first double bond relative to and including the methyl end. Inserting a double bond in a saturated fatty acid reduces its melting point. For this reason fats (e.g. butter) containing a predominance of saturated fatty acids are usually solid at room temperature while oils (e.g. soybean oil) containing a predominance of polyunsaturated fatty acids are liquid at room temperature. The position of the unsaturated bonds in mono- and polyunsaturated fatty acids has a profound influence on their health effects and nutritional properties. The position of the first double bond relative to the methyl end indicates the 'family' to which the unsaturated fatty acid belongs. Polyunsaturated fatty acids in which the first double bond is three carbon atoms from the methyl end of the carbon chain are called *n*-3 or ω3 fatty acids and those in which the first double bond is next to the sixth carbon atom are *n*-6 or ω6 fatty acids. The third important family is the *n*-9 or ω9 group in which the first double bond is next to the ninth carbon atom

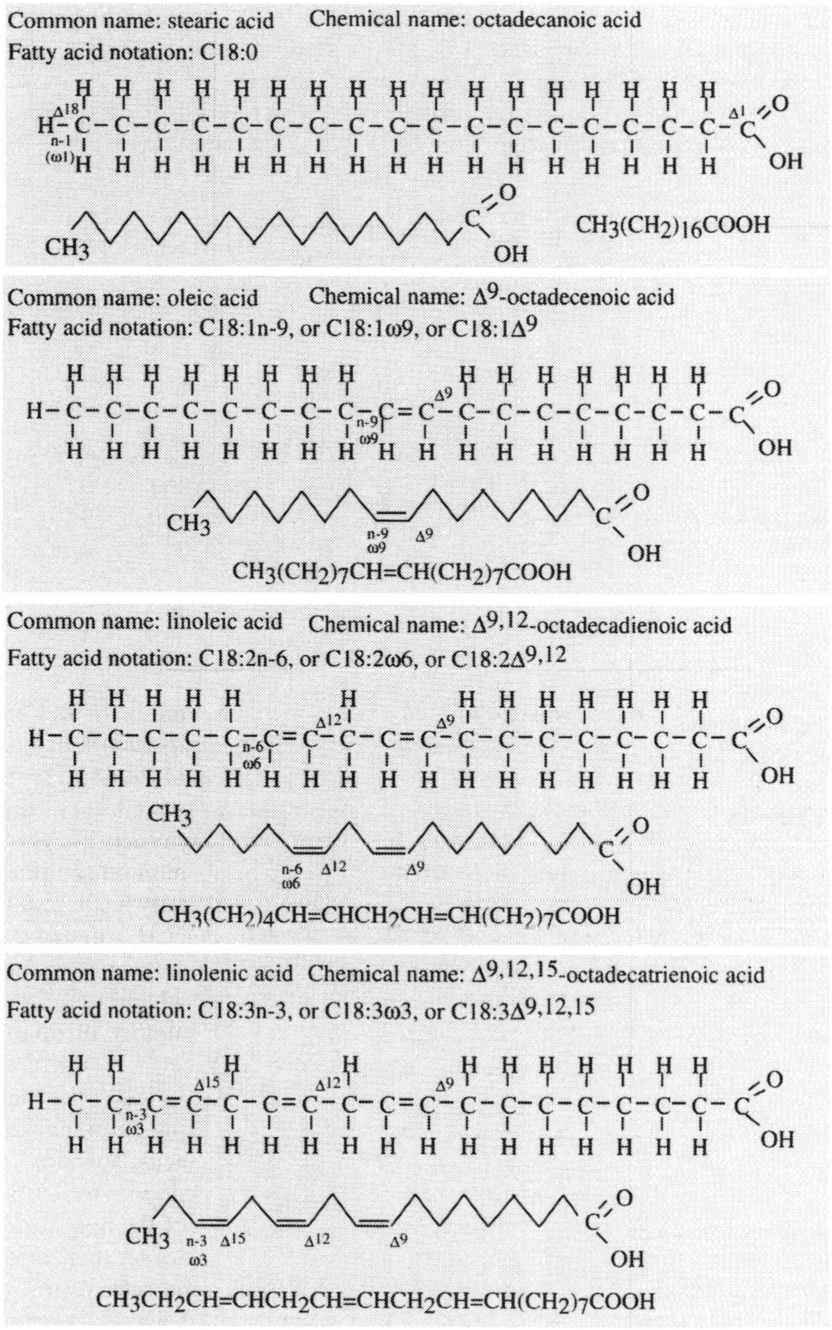
Common name: stearic acid Chemical name: octadecanoic acid
Fatty acid notation: C18:0
Δ18
n-1
(ω1)
Δ1
CH3(CH2)16COOH
Common name: oleic acid Chemical name: Δ9-octadecenoic acid
Fatty acid notation: C18:1n-9, or C18:1ω9, or C18:1Δ9
n-9
ω9
Δ9
CH3(CH2)7CH=CH(CH2)7COOH
Common name: linoleic acid Chemical name: Δ9,12-octadecadienoic acid
Fatty acid notation: C18:2n-6, or C18:2ω6, or C18:2Δ9,12
n-6
ω6
Δ12
Δ9
CH3(CH2)4CH=CHCH2CH=CH(CH2)7COOH
Common name: linolenic acid Chemical name: Δ9,12,15-octadecatrienoic acid
Fatty acid notation: C18:3n-3, or C18:3ω3, or C18:3Δ9,12,15
n-3
ω3
Δ15
Δ12
Δ9
CH3CH2CH=CHCH2CH=CHCH2CH=CH(CH2)7COOH

Fig. 3.2 Names and structures of some common fatty acids.

from the methyl end. Fatty acids are sometimes referred to as short (i.e. fewer than 8 carbons), medium (8–12 carbons), or long (14 or more carbons) chain fatty acids. A list of the fatty acids of nutritional interest is given in Table 3.1.

A single triglyceride molecule may contain either three identical fatty acids or more frequently a combination of different fatty acids. It is important to appreciate that while

Table 3.1   Fatty acid names and occurrence

Common Name	Nomenclature	Occurrence
Saturated		
Acetic	$2:0$	Vinegar
Butyric	$4:0$	Butter fat
Caproic	$6:0$	
Caprylic	$8:0$	Palm kernel oil
Capric	$10:0$	Butter fat, coconut oil
Lauric	$12:0$	Coconut oil
Myristic	$14:0$	Butter fat, coconut oil
Palmitic	$16:0$	Most plant and animal fats
Stearic	$18:0$	Most plant and animal fats
Arachidic	$20:0$	Peanuts
Behenic	$22:0$	Small amount in animal fats
Lignoceric	$24:0$	Plant cutin
Monounsaturated		
Palmitoleic	$16:1\omega7$	Fish and animal fats
Oleic	$18:1\omega9$	All plant and animal fats
cis-Vaccenic	$18:1\omega7$	Small amounts in animal fats
Eicosenoic	$20:1\omega9$	Rapeseed and animal fats
Gadoleic	$20:1\omega11$	Fish oils
Erucic	$22:1\omega9$	Rapeseed, animal tissue
Cetoleic	$22:1\omega13$	Fish oils
Nervonic	$24:1\omega9$	Animal tissue (brain)
Hexacosenoic	$26:1\omega9$	Minute amounts in animal tissues
Polyunsaturated		
Linoleic (LO)	$18:2\omega6$	Plant oils: cottonseed, sunflower, soybean, corn, safflower
α-Linolenic (LN)	$18:3\omega3$	Plant oils: soybean, mustard, walnut, linseed
γ-Linolenic (GLA)	$18:3\omega6$	Plant oils: evening primrose, borrage, blackcurrant
Dihommo-γ-linolenic acid (DGLA)	$20:3\omega6$	Small amounts in animal tissues
Arachidonic (AA)	$20:4\omega6$	Small amounts in animal tissues
Adrenic	$22:4\omega6$	Small amounts in animal tissues
Eicosapentaenoic acid (EPA)	$20:5\omega3$	Fish, fish oils
Docosapentaenoic (DPA)	$22:5\omega3$	Fish, fish oils, animal tissues (brain)
Docosahexaenoic (DHA)	$22:6\omega3$	Fish, fish oils, animal tissues (brain)

Table 3.2 Fat and cholesterol content of some common foods

Food item	Common serving size	Total fat (g)	SFA (g)	MFA (g)	PFA (g)	Chol (mg)
		per 100 g edible portion				
Trim milk *	1 cup (260 g)	0.4	0.3	0.1	0.0	4
Yoghurt	1 carton (150 g)	2.4	1.5	0.6	0.1	8
Cottage cheese	½ cup (120 g)	3.5	2.2	0.9	0.1	9
Whole milk	1 cup (260 g)	4.0	2.4	1.1	0.1	12
Ice cream	1 cup (143 g)	10.8	6.5	2.3	0.3	30
Cheddar cheese	1 × 2 cm cube (22 g)	35.2	22.3	8.4	0.8	107
Cream	1 tbsp (15 g)	40.0	24.9	10.1	1.3	104
Wholemeal toast	1 slice (22 g)	1.7	0.4	0.4	0.6	1
Toasted muesli	1 cup (110 g)	16.6	7.7	5.0	2.9	0
Egg	1 medium (49 g)	11.6	3.4	4.6	1.2	412
Baked potato	1 potato (90 g)	0.2	0.0	0.0	0.1	0
Potato crisps	1 packet (50 g)	33.4	14.3	13.8	3.8	1
Cauliflower	1 stem + flower (90 g)	0.2	0.0	0.0	0.1	0
Lentils	½ cup (100 g)	0.5	0.1	0.1	0.2	0
Peanuts	⅓ cup (50 g)	49.0	9.2	23.4	13.9	0
Cashew nuts	18 cashews (28 g)	51.0	8.3	25.4	15.1	0
Sole	1 fillet (51 g)	1.2	0.3	0.4	0.3	53
Mackerel	1 fillet (89 g)	2.9	0.8	0.8	0.9	53
Salmon (tinned)	½ cup (120 g)	8.2	2.0	3.1	2.1	90
Sausage	1 serving (79 g)	25.2	11.3	10.8	1.2	48
Beef blade steak (lean)	1 steak (216 g)	5.0	2.2	1.9	0.2	60
Beef mince	½ cup (130 g)	13.8	5.7	5.4	0.5	68
Chicken breast (lean, no skin)	1 breast (192 g)	5.5	1.7	2.5	0.6	66
Fried chicken	1 wing (37 g)	28.4	8.7	13.4	2.7	116
Pork loin steak (lean)	1 fillet (98 g)	2.3	0.9	0.9	0.2	68
Lamb midloin chop	1 chop (50 g)	5.7	2.5	2.0	0.2	66
Pizza	1 slice (57 g)	10.5	4.5	3.3	1.8	13
Hamburger	1 burger (204 g)	15.6	5.7	5.4	2.4	22
Muesli bar	1 bar (32 g)	19.4	9.1	7.2	1.9	1
Biscuit	1 biscuit (12 g)	30.0	19.2	6.2	1.2	98
Salad dressing	1 tbsp (16 g)	48.3	7.0	11.1	28.1	0
Palm oil	1 tbsp (14 g)	98.7	44.7	41.1	8.2	0
Olive oil	1 tbsp (14 g)	99.6	16.6	65.3	11.8	0
Sunflower seed oil	1 tbsp (14 g)	99.7	11.7	21.1	61.9	0

* Trim milk is fat-reduced (0.4%) with added skim milk solids.
SFA, saturated fatty acids; MFA, monounsaturated fatty acids; PFA, polyunsaturated fatty acids; Chol, cholesterol.
Source: New Zealand Food Composition Database (OCNZ95). Palmerston North: Crop and Food Research Institute.

Table 3.3 Fatty acid composition of plant and animal fats

Food item	4:0	6:0	8:0	10:0	12:0	14:0	16:0	18:0	16:1	18:1	18:2ω6	18:3ω3	20:4ω6	20:5ω3	22:6ω3	20:1ω11	22:1ω13	22:5ω3
										Percentage of total fatty acids								
Plant fats																		
Olive	–	–	–	–	–	–	12	2	1	72	11	1	–	–	–	–	–	–
Palm	–	–	–	–	0	1	42	4	0	43	8	0	–	–	–	–	–	–
Canola	–	–	–	–	–	–	5	1	2	56	24	10	–	–	–	–	–	–
Safflower	–	–	–	–	–	–	8	3	0	13	76	1	–	–	–	–	–	–
Sunflower	–	–	–	–	–	0	6	6	0	33	53	0	–	–	–	–	–	–
Avocado	–	–	–	–	–	–	12	–	3	75	9	0	0	–	–	–	–	–
Soybean	–	–	–	–	0	0	10	4	0	25	52	7	–	–	–	–	–	–
Coconut	–	–	8	7	48	16	9	2	–	7	2	–	–	–	–	–	–	–
Animal fats																		
Butter	4	2	1	3	3	11	28	16	1	26	1	2	–	–	–	–	–	–
Beef	–	–	–	–	–	3	28	13	7	43	2	1	1	–	–	–	–	–
Chicken	–	–	–	–	–	1	27	7	7	41	14	1	1	–	–	–	–	–
Lamb	–	–	–	–	–	6	25	22	1	40	3	3	–	–	–	–	–	–
Pork	–	–	–	–	2	27	13	4	41	8	1	1	–	–	–	–	–	
Salmon	–	–	–	–	–	5	19	4	6	23	1	1	1	8	11	8	5	3
Trout	–	–	–	–	–	2	37	13	5	17	1	–	–	3	11	2	2	2

Source: New Zealand Food Composition Database (OCNZ88).

one fatty acid, or class of fatty acids (e.g. saturated), might predominate in a particular food, most foods contain a wide range of fatty acids. Occasionally in naturally occurring glycerides, only one or two fatty acids are attached to a glycerol molecule. These are called monoacylglycerols (monoglycerides) and diacylglycerols (diglycerides). The major food sources of fatty acids and sources of triglycerides that contain them are shown in Table 3.2, and the detailed fatty acid composition of some fats and oils given in Table 3.3.

3.1.2 Phospholipids

Phospholipids comprise a relatively small proportion of total dietary lipid. The four major phospholipids comprise a diglyceride in which the third position of the glycerol molecule is occupied by a phosphoric acid residue to which one of four different base groups is attached (choline, inositol, serine, or ethanolamine). Along with sphingomyelin these four phospholipids comprise more than 95% of phospholipids found in the body and in foods. The structure of the most abundant phospholipid in nature, phosphatidyl-choline (also known as lecithin), is shown in Fig. 3.3. Phospholipids occur in virtually all animal and vegetable foods; liver, eggs, peanuts, soybeans and wheatgerm are very rich sources. The base group endows the phospholipid with a polar region soluble in water while the fatty acids constitute a non-polar region, insoluble in water. This

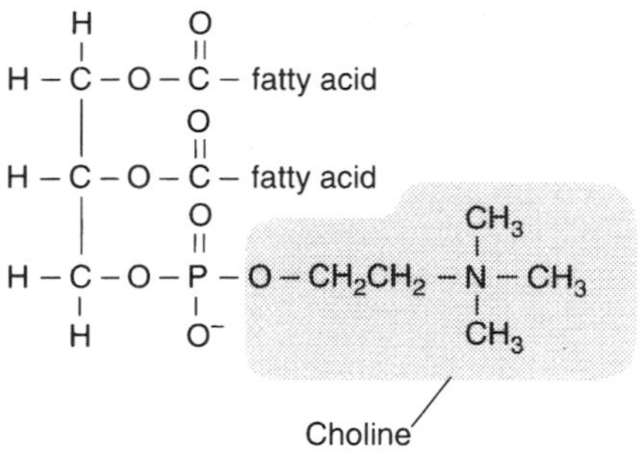

Fig. 3.3 Structure of phosphatidylcholine.

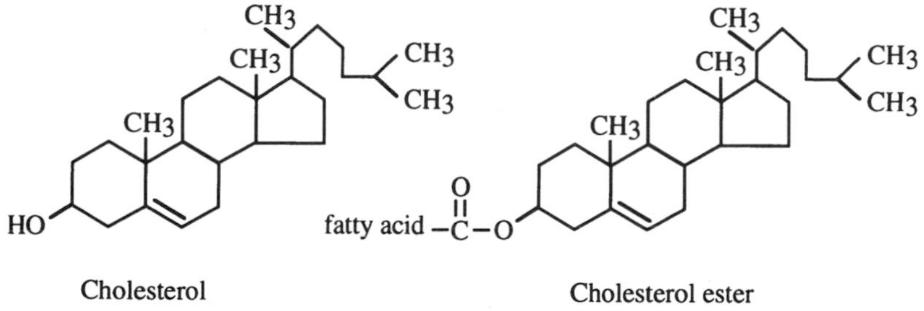

Cholesterol

Cholesterol ester

Fig. 3.4 Structure of cholesterol and cholesterol ester.

amphipathic nature—having both polar and non-polar characteristics—of the phospholipid enables it to act at the interface between aqueous and lipid media so they make excellent emulsifying agents. The structural integrity of all cell membranes and lipoproteins is dependent, among other factors, on the amphipathic nature of the constituent phospholipids. Phospholipids are also an important source of essential fatty acids.

3.1.3 Sterols

Sterols are also built up from carbon, hydrogen and oxygen, but in these lipid compounds, unlike triacylglycerols and phospholipids, the carbon, hydrogen and oxygen atoms are arranged in a series of four rings with a range of side chains. Cholesterol is the principal sterol of animal tissues and is found only in animal foods, especially eggs, meat, dairy products, fish and poultry. Cholesterol in food often has a fatty acid attached to it so it is cholesterol ester (Fig. 3.4). Approximate quantities of cholesterol in some common foods are given in Table 3.2. The major sterols of plants (group name phytosterols) are β-sitosterol, campesterol and stigmasterol. Cholesterol plays an important structural role in membranes and lipoproteins, and functions as the precursor of bile acids, steroid hormones, and vitamin D.

35

3.1.4 Other constituents of dietary fat

Dietary fats may also contain small quantities of other lipids including fatty alcohols, gangliosides, sulphatides and cerebrosides as well as vitamin E (tocopherols, tocotrienols), carotenoids (α- and β-carotene, lycopene, and xanthophylls) and vitamins A and D (see Chapters 11 and 14).

3.2 DIETARY FATS ALTERED DURING FOOD PROCESSING

The food industry incorporates fats and oils into margarines, biscuits, cakes, chocolates, pies, sauces and other manufactured food products. In addition to using naturally occurring lipids, food manufacturers use fats and oils which have been altered by the process of hydrogenation, adding hydrogen atoms to the double bonds in mono- or polyunsaturated fatty acids in order to increase the degree of saturation of the fatty acids in the oil (i.e. reduce the number of double bonds) and consequently increase the melting point of the fat. Through this process a polyunsaturated oil which is liquid can be converted into a fat that is solid at room temperature. Hydrogenation of oils is used by manufacturers to produce a fat consistency appropriate to the texture of the desired food. Margarines usually contain hydrogenated fats. Hydrogenation also changes the configuration of some of the remaining double bonds from the natural *cis*-configuration to a *trans*-configuration. *Cis* mono- and polyunsaturated fatty acids have the two hydrogen atoms attached to the carbons on the same side of the double bond and the molecule bends at the double bond. In *trans*-fatty acids the hydrogens are placed on opposite sides of the double bond and the molecule stays straight at the double bond (Fig. 3.5). *Trans*-unsaturated fatty acids behave biologically like saturated rather than like *cis*-unsaturated fatty acids. The bulk of *trans*-fatty acids in hydrogenated fats are monounsaturated (elaidic acid, C18:1n-9 *trans*, is the *trans* equivalent of oleic acid).

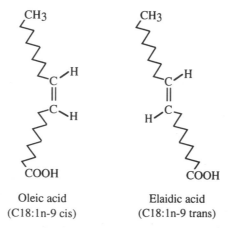

Oleic acid
(C18:1n-9 cis)

Elaidic acid
(C18:1n-9 trans)

Fig. 3.5   Structure of a *cis* and a *trans* monounsaturated fatty acid.

Small quantities of *trans*-fatty acids are found naturally in fats from ruminant animals (e.g. cow and sheep) but most of the dietary intake of *trans*-fatty acids is derived from margarine and other manufactured foods containing hydrogenated fats. Unfortunately, food tables do not routinely contain information about the relative proportions of *cis*- and *trans*-fatty acids so it is not possible at present to quantify the precise proportions of these different forms of unsaturated fatty acids. *Trans*-fatty acids have in the past made up 5–10% of fatty acids in soft margarines and are now being reduced by manufacturers, whereas hard margarines contain up to 40–50% of fatty acids in the *trans*-form.

3.3   DIGESTION, ABSORPTION AND TRANSPORT

3.3.1   Digestion (Fig. 3.6)

Triglycerides must be hydrolyzed to fatty acids and monoglycerides before they are absorbed. In children and adults, the process starts in the stomach where the churning action helps to create an emulsion. Fat entering the intestine is mixed with bile and further emulsified so that lipids are reduced to small bile acid-coated droplets which disperse in aqueous solutions and provide a sufficiently large surface area for the digestive enzymes to act. Bile acids facilitate the process of emulsification because they are amphipathic. Lipase enzymes secreted by the pancreas split by hydrolysis each triglyceride molecule, removing the two outer fatty acids, which can be absorbed with the remaining monoglyceride. Some monoglyceride (20%) is rearranged so that the lipase enzymes remove the third fatty acid. Phospholipids are hydrolyzed by a phospholipase and cholesterol ester by cholesterol ester hydrolase. In the newborn, the pancreatic secretion of lipases is low and fat digestion is augmented by lingual lipase secreted from the glands of the tongue and by a lipase present in human milk. The products of lipid digestion, along with other minor dietary lipids, such as fat-soluble vitamins, coalesce with bile acids into microscopic aggregates know as mixed micelles.

3.3.2   Absorption (Fig. 3.6)

Glycerol and fatty acids with a chain length of less than 12 carbon atoms can enter the portal vein system directly by diffusing across the enterocytes (cells lining the wall of the small intestine). On the other hand, monoglycerides, fatty acids, cholesterol, lysophospholipids, and other dietary lipids diffuse from the mixed micelles into the enterocytes of the small intestine where they are re-synthesized into triglycerides, phospholipids and cholesterol esters in preparation for their incorporation into chylomicrons. In general, absorption is efficient, with greater than 95% of dietary lipid absorbed (triglycerides, phospholipids, and fat-soluble vitamins). Cholesterol, other sterols and β-carotene are only partially absorbed (less than 30%).

Diseases which impair the secretion of bile (e.g. obstruction of the bile duct), reduce secretion of lipase enzymes from the pancreas (e.g. pancreatitis or cystic fibrosis), or damage the cell lining of the small intestine (e.g. coeliac disease) can lead to severe malabsorption of fat. Under such circumstances, medium-chain triglycerides can be better tolerated and are often used as part of the dietary treatment.

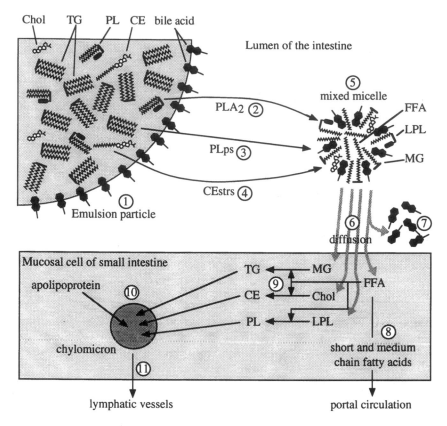

Fig. 3.6 Digestion and absorption of dietary lipids. (1) Dietary lipid leaves the stomach and enters the upper region of the small intestine where bile acids, released from the gallbladder, surround and coat droplets of fat to form emulsion particles. The emulsion particles provide the surface area for the pancreatic enzymes to degrade the dietary lipids. (2) Phospholipase A_2 (PLA$_2$) breaks down each phospholipid (PL) into a free fatty acid (FFA) and a lyso-phospholipid (LPL). (3) Pancreatic lipase (PLps) converts triglyceride (TG) into a monoglyceride (MG) and two free fatty acids. (4) Cholesterol esterase (CEtrs) splits cholesterol ester (CE) into free cholesterol (Chol) and a free fatty acid. (5) The products of lipid digestion coalesce with bile acids into mixed micelles. (6) The mixed micelles move close to the mucosal cell surface where the lipids diffuse down a concentration gradient into the mucosal cells. (7) Bile acids are not absorbed. (8) Short- and medium-chain fatty acids move immediately into the portal circulation where they are transported in the blood bound to albumin. (9) To maintain the concentration gradient necessary for lipid diffusion the breakdown products of lipid digestion are resynthesized into their parent lipids. (10) The lipids are combined with apolipoproteins, synthesized in the mucosal cells, to form chylomicrons. (11) Chylomicrons leave the mucosal cell via the lymphatic vessels.

3.3.3 Lipid transport (Fig. 3.7)

Since lipids are not soluble in water, it is necessary for them to be associated with specific proteins, the apolipoproteins, to make water-miscible complexes. Free fatty acids make up only about 2% of total plasma lipid and are transported in the blood as complexes

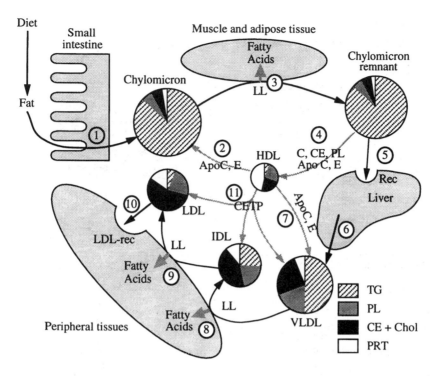

Fig. 3.7 Lipid transport and lipoprotein metabolism. (1) Chylomicrons transport recently ingested fats into the blood. (2) Upon entering the blood chylomicrons pick up apolipoproteins C and E (Apo C, E) from high-density lipoprotein (HDL). (3) Apolipoprotein C activates lipoprotein lipase (LL) on the walls of the capillaries causing triglyceride to be broken down to glycerol and three fatty acids. The fatty acids are taken up primarily by adipose and muscle tissue. (4) During breakdown of triglyceride (TG) some cholesterol (C), cholesterol ester (CE), and phospholipid (PL) along with Apo C and E pinch off to form HDL. (5) Following degradation of 70–80% of the chylomicron's TG, the resulting chylomicron remnant binds to receptors on the liver cells and is removed from the circulation. (6) Lipids synthesized in the liver and those delivered to the liver by chylomicron remnants are packaged into very low-density lipoproteins (VLDL) and secreted into the blood. (7) VLDL picks up Apo C and E from HDL. (8) LL, activated by Apo C, breaks down VLDL TG and the fatty acids are transferred to peripheral tissue (mainly muscle and adipose) resulting in the formation of intermediate-density lipoprotein (IDL). (9) Nearly all of the TG is removed from IDL producing a cholesterol-rich LDL. (10) Cholesterol is delivered to the tissue when LDL binds to LDL-receptors (LDL-rec) and is taken up into the tissues. (11) Cholesterol ester transfer protein redistributes cholesterol esters from HDL to VLDL, IDL, and LDL.

with albumin. The remainder of lipid in the plasma is carried as lipoprotein complexes (lipid + protein = lipoprotein). The structure of a lipoprotein is given in Fig. 3.8. They consist of a core of neutral lipid (triglyceride and cholesterol esters) surrounded by a single surface layer of polar lipid (phospholipid and cholesterol). Coiled chains of apolipoproteins extend over the surface. There are five classes of lipoproteins which are identified according to their density (Table 3.4) and five major groups of apolipoproteins (apo A, apo B, apo C, apo D and apo E) which play important roles in determining the

39

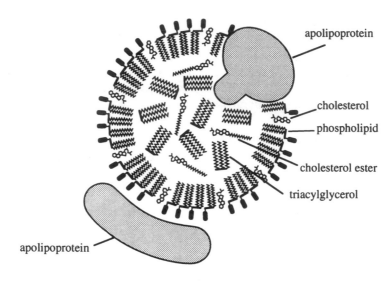

Fig. 3.8 Structure of a plasma lipoprotein.

Table 3.4 Composition of human plasma lipoproteins

Class	Density	Composition (weight %)		Percentage of total lipid (weight %)					Major apoproteins
		Protein	Lipid	TAG	PL	CE	Chol	FFA	
Chylomicrons[a]	<0.95	2	98	88	8	3	1	–	AI, AIV, B-48, Cs & E from HDL
Very low-density lipoprotein, (VLDL)[b]	0.95–1.006	10	90	56	20	15	8	1	B-100, Cs & E from HDL
Intermediate-density lipoprotein (IDL)[c]	1.006–1.019	11	89	29	26	34	9	1	B-100, E
Low-density lipoprotein (LDL)[c]	1.019–1.063	21	79	13	28	48	10	1	B-100
Lipoprotein(a) (Lp(a))[b]	1.05–1.12	31	69	11	29	48	11	1	B-100, apo(a)
High-density lipoprotein (HDL$_2$)[a]	1.063–1.125	33	68	16	43	31	10	–	As, Cs, E
High density lipoprotein (HDL$_3$)[b,c]	1.125–1.210	57	43	13	46	29	6	6	As, Cs, E
Albumin[b]	>1.281	99	1	–	–	–	–	100	Albumin

[a] Origin: intestine.
[b] Origin: liver.
[c] Origin: very low-density lipoprotein. TAG, triacylglycerol (triglyceride); PL, phospholipid; CE, cholesterol ester; Chol, cholesterol; FFA, free fatty acids.

Table 3.5 Functions of human plasma lipoproteins

Class	Function
Chylomicrons[a]	Transports dietary lipids from intestine to peripheral tissues and liver
Very low-density lipoprotein (VLDL)[b]	Transports lipids from liver to peripheral tissues
Intermediate-density lipoprotein (IDL)[c]	Precursor of LDL
Low-density lipoprotein (LDL)[c]	Transports cholesterol to peripheral tissues and liver
Lipoprotein(a) (Lp(a))[b]	?
High-density lipoprotein (HDL$_2$)[a] High-density lipoprotein (HDL$_3$)[b,c]	Removes cholesterol from tissues and transfers it to the liver or other lipoproteins
Albumin[b]	Transports free fatty acids from adipose tissue to peripheral tissues

[a] Origin: intestine. [b] Origin: liver. [c] Origin: very low-density lipoprotein.

functions of the lipoproteins. Each has distinct physiological roles (Table 3.5) and when present in inappropriate amounts (too high or too low) has different adverse health consequences.

Chylomicrons transport lipids of dietary origin so they consist predominantly of triglycerides. Chylomicrons are abundant in the blood after eating food, particularly fatty food, but are scarce in fasting blood. The fatty acid composition of the lipids in chylomicrons is largely determined by the composition of the meal just eaten. Chylomicrons leave the enterocytes of the small intestine and enter the bloodstream via lymph vessels. The enzyme lipoprotein lipase, located on the walls of capillary blood vessels, hydrolyzes the triglycerides allowing the free fatty acids to move into muscle or heart tissue where they can be used for energy, or into adipose tissue where they can be stored. During its short life in the circulation (15–30 minutes), more than 90% of the triglyceride in the chylomicron is removed. The resulting chylomicron remnant is cleared from the circulation by the liver. The fat-soluble vitamins (A, D, E, and K) are delivered to the liver as part of the chylomicron remnant.

Very low-density lipoproteins (VLDL) are large triglyceride-rich particles made in the liver. They function as a vehicle for delivery of fatty acids to the heart, muscles and adipose tissue, lipoprotein lipase again being needed for their liberation. Lipoprotein lipase in the heart has a much stronger affinity for triglyceride than that in the adipose tissue or muscle so when triglyceride concentration is low, triglyceride is preferentially taken up by heart tissue. Following removal of much of the triglyceride from VLDL the remaining remnant particles are intermediate-density lipoproteins (IDL) which are the precursors of low density lipoprotein.

Low-density lipoprotein (LDL) is the end product of VLDL metabolism and its lipid consists largely of cholesterol ester and cholesterol. Its surface has only one type of apolipoprotein, apo B100. LDL carries about 70% of all cholesterol in the plasma. LDL is taken up by the liver and other tissues by LDL receptors.

High-density lipoprotein (HDL) is synthesized and secreted both by the liver and intestine. A major function of HDL is to transfer apolipoprotein C and E to chylomicrons so that lipoprotein lipase can break down the triglycerides in the lipoproteins. HDL also plays a key role in the reverse transport of cholesterol (i.e. the transfer of cholesterol back from the tissues to the liver). HDL can be divided into two subfractions of different densities: HDL_2 and HDL_3.

Lipoprotein (a), (Lp(a)) is a complex of LDL with apolipoprotein (a).

3.3.4 Nutritional determinants of lipid and lipoprotein levels in blood

The fact that plasma lipid and lipoprotein levels are important predictors of coronary heart disease risk (discussed in Chapter 18) has led to a great deal of research into nutritional and other lifestyle factors which influence their concentration in the blood (Table 3.6).

The chylomicron count and the fatty acid composition of chylomicron lipid are principally determined by the amount and type of fat eaten in the preceding meal. VLDL levels tend to be low in lean individuals and those who have regular physical activity.

Table 3.6 Nutritional determinants of lipoprotein levels

Nutritional factor	VLDL	LDL	HDL	Comments
Obesity	↑	↑	↓	
Saturated fat				
Lauric (12:0)	–	↑	↑	
Myristic (14:0)	–	↑↑	↑	
Palmitic (16:0)	–	↑↑		
Stearic (18:0)	–	–	–	
Monounsaturated fat				
Oleic (18:1*cis*)	–	↓	↑	
Elaidic (18:1*trans*)	–	↑↑	↓	
Polyunsaturated fat (ω6)				HDL may ↓ if 18:2ω6 is
Linoleic (18:2ω6)	–	↓↓	(↑)	>10% of total energy
Polyunsaturated fat (ω3)				↑ in LDL if initial LDL
α-Linolenic (18:3ω3)	↓↓	(↑)	(↓)	is high
Eicosapentaenoic (20:5ω3)	↓↓	(↑)	(↓)	↓ in HDL if fed in large
Docosahexaenoic (22:6ω3)	↓↓	(↑)	(↓)	quantities

↑, ↓, increase or decrease; ↑↑, ↓↓, appreciable increase or decrease; VLDL, very low-density lipoproteins; LDL, low-density lipoproteins; HDL, high-density lipoproteins.

Obesity and an excessive intake of alcohol are associated with higher than average VLDL levels. An increased intake of carbohydrate is generally associated with an increase in VLDL as a result of increased hepatic synthesis of triglycerides, although adaptation may occur if the high carbohydrate intake is sustained over a prolonged period. Populations with habitual high carbohydrate intakes (e.g. Asians or Africans consuming their traditional diets) do not have particularly high plasma VLDL concentrations. Consumption of eicosapentaenoic (20:5ω3) and docosahexaenoic (22:6ω3) acids as fish or fish oils, lowers plasma VLDL levels. In routine clinical work plasma triglyceride rather than VLDL is measured since the bulk of triglyceride levels in blood taken from fasting (10–12 hours) individuals tend to parallel levels of VLDL.

Levels of LDL and total plasma cholesterol are determined by an interaction of genetic factors and dietary characteristics. High intakes of saturated fatty acids, especially myristic and palmitic acids, and *trans*-fatty acids (e.g. elaidic acid) are associated with raised LDL-cholesterol, while high intakes of linoleic acid, the major polyunsaturated acid in foods, as well as *cis*-monounsaturated fatty acids, tend to reduce cholesterol levels. The precise mechanism has not been established but high intakes of saturated fatty acids appear to decrease the removal of plasma LDL by LDL-receptors whereas mono- and polyunsaturated fatty acids are associated with increased LDL-receptor activity. Dietary cholesterol seems to be an important determinant of plasma total and LDL-cholesterol only when a high proportion of dietary lipid is saturated fatty acids (greater than 15% of energy) and cholesterol intake exceeds 300 mg/day. It is less clear whether dietary cholesterol is of great importance over the relatively low range of intakes now seen in many countries and when saturated fatty acid intake is reduced. Plant sterols (e.g. β-sitosterol) are very poorly absorbed and interfere with the absorption of cholesterol.

The ability of soluble forms of dietary fibre to reduce total and LDL-cholesterol is small by comparison with the effect of altering the nature of dietary fat. Dietary protein may also influence plasma lipids and lipoproteins: in particular soybean protein has some cholesterol-lowering properties. Vegetarians have lower levels of total and LDL-cholesterol in general than non-vegetarians but it is not clear which characteristic of the vegetarian diet principally accounts for this effect.

Dietary factors do not have much effect on HDL-cholesterol concentration. However, HDL-cholesterol can be slightly reduced by very high intakes of polyunsaturated fatty acids (e.g. when the dietary polyunsaturated fat : saturated fat ratio is greater than 1), or by increasing carbohydrate from more usual levels consumed (less than 45% of energy) in affluent societies to 60% or more of total energy, or by increasing *trans*-unsaturated fatty acids. The HDL-lowering effect of a high carbohydrate diet may be reduced or prevented if the carbohydrate is high in soluble forms of non-starch polysaccharide. HDL levels tend to be raised by diets relatively high in dietary cholesterol and saturated fatty acids, although this 'positive' effect is offset by the larger increases in LDL-cholesterol caused by such diets. Increasing *cis*-forms of monounsaturated fatty acids appears to be a dietary means of maintaining HDL levels when reducing saturated fat consumption. Most dietary studies have not included measurements of the subfractions of HDL. HDL-cholesterol is raised in people who take substantial amounts of alcohol (see Chapter 6).

3.4   Essentials of Lipid Metabolism

3.4.1   Biosynthesis of fatty acids

Saturated and monounsaturated fatty acids can be synthesized in the body from carbohydrate and protein. This process of lipogenesis occurs especially in a well-fed person whose diet contains a high proportion of carbohydrate in the presence of an adequate energy intake. Insulin stimulates the biosynthesis of fatty acids. Lipogenesis is reduced during energy restriction or when the diet is high in fat. Unsaturated fatty acids may be further elongated or desaturated by various enzyme systems (Fig. 3.9).

3.4.2   Essential fatty acids

Essential fatty acids are those that cannot be synthesized in the body and must be supplied in the diet to avoid deficiency symptoms. They include members of the ω6 (linoleic acid) and ω3 (α-linolenic acid) families of fatty acids. When the diet is deficient in linoleic acid, the most abundant unsaturated fatty acid in tissue, oleic acid, is desaturated and elongated to eicosatrienoic acid (20:3ω9) which is normally present in trace amounts. Increased plasma levels of this 20:3ω9 suggest a deficiency of essential fatty acids. Essential fatty acid deficiency is rare except in those with severe, untreated fat malabsorption or those suffering from famine. Symptoms include dry, cracked, scaly, and bleeding skin, exessive thirst due to high water loss from the skin, and impaired liver function resulting from the accumulation of lipid in the liver (i.e. fatty liver).

Linoleic acid and α-linolenic acid are not only required for the structural integrity of all cell membranes, they are also elongated and desaturated into longer chain, more polyunsaturated fatty acids that are the precursors to a group of hormone-like eicosanoid

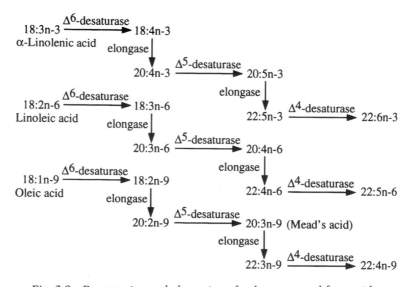

Fig. 3.9   Desaturation and elongation of polyunsaturated fatty acids.

compounds, prostaglandins, and leukotrienes (see Section 3.4.4). Linoleic acid ($18:2\omega6$) is converted to arachidonic acid ($20:4\omega6$) while α-linolenic acid ($18:3\omega3$) is converted to eicosapentaenoic ($20:5\omega3$) and docosahexaenoic ($22:6\omega3$) acids. A high ratio of linoleic to α-linolenic acid in the diet tends to reduce the amount of α-linolenic acid converted to eicosapentaenoic and docosahexaenoic acids.

There is some question as to whether the arachidonic, eicosapentaenoic, and docosahexaenoic acids incorporated into the body's tissues comes predominantly from endogenous desaturation and elongation of dietary essential fatty acids or is obtained from the diet as preformed fatty acids. Whatever the answer, the body appears to have a capacity to desaturate and elongate essential fatty acids because individuals following strict vegan diets (no animal foods) ingest plenty of linoleic and α-linolenic acids but only negligible amounts of arachidonic, eicosapentaenoic, and docosahexaenoic acids, yet have normal levels of these latter fatty acids in their blood.

3.4.3 Membrane structure

Unsaturated fatty acids in membrane lipids play an important role in maintaining fluidity. The critically important metabolic functions of membranes such as nutrient transport, receptor function, and ion channels are affected by interactions between proteins and lipids. For example, the phosphoinositide cycle, which determines the responses of many cells to hormones, neurotransmitters and cell growth factors and which controls processes of cell division, is influenced by the proportion of $\omega6$ to $\omega3$ fatty acids.

3.4.4 Eicosanoids

Eicosanoids are biologically active, oxygenated metabolites of arachidonic acid, eicosapentaenoic acid (EPA), or dihomo γ linolenic acid ($C20:3\omega6$). They are produced in virtually all cells in the body, act locally, have short life spans, and act as modulators of numerous physiological processes including reproduction, blood pressure, haemostasis, and inflammation. Eicosanoids are further categorized into prostaglandins/ thromboxanes and leukotrienes which are produced via the cyclooxygenase and lipoxygenase pathways, respectively (Fig. 3.10). Considerable recent interest has centred around the cardiovascular effects of eicosanoids, in particular the role they play in thrombosis (i.e. vessel blockage). Thromboxane A_2 (TxA_2), synthesized in platelets from arachidonic acid, stimulates vasoconstriction and platelet aggregation (i.e. clumping) while prostacyclin I_2 (PGI_2), produced from arachidonic acid in the endothelial cells of the vessel wall, has the opposing effects of stimulating vasodilation and inhibiting platelet aggregation. The balance of these two counteracting eicosanoids helps to determine the overall thrombotic tendency.

Research, initially based on the observation that the Inuit (Eskimo) people of Greenland have very low rates of coronary heart disease, led to the demonstration that a high dietary intake of EPA (usually in fish oil) can profoundly influence the balance of thromboxanes and prostacyclins. Such diets lead to the substitution of EPA for arachidonic acid in platelet membranes. TxA_2 production decreases, not only because of lower levels of platelet arachidonic acid, but also because the increased levels of EPA in

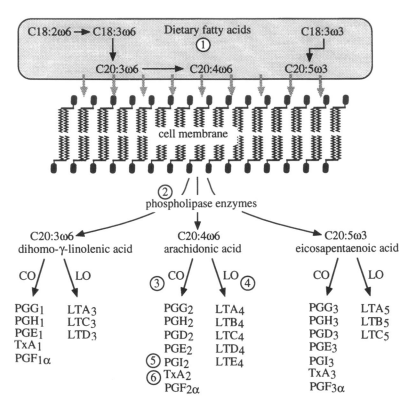

Fig. 3.10 Formation of eicosanoids. (1) Dihomo-γ-linolenic acid (DGLA), arachidonic acid (AA), and eicosapentaenoic (EPA) acid, obtained ready-made in the diet or via desaturation and elongation of their respective parent ω6 (linoleic acid) or ω3 (linolenic acid) essential fatty acids, are incorporated into the phospholipids of cell membranes. (2) When cells are stimulated by hormones or activating substances, phospholipase enzymes release DGLA, AA, and EPA into the interior of the cell. (3) Once released from the cell membranes DGLA, AA, and EPA can be converted via the cyclooxygenase pathway (CO) into prostaglandins (PG) and thromboxanes (Tx) of the 1, 2, and 3 series, respectively; (4) or via the lipoxygenase pathway (LO) to leukotrienes (LT) of the 3, 4, and 5 series, respectively. (5) In platelets, AA is converted primarily to the 2 series thromboxane (TxA$_2$) which stimulates platelet clumping and increases blood pressure. (6) In the endothelial cells lining arterial vessels, AA is converted into the 2 series prostacylin (PGI$_2$) which counters the action of TxA$_2$ by inhibiting platelet clumping and decreasing blood pressure.

platelets inhibit the conversion of arachidonic acid to TxA$_2$. On the other hand, PGI$_2$ production in the endothelial cells is only slightly reduced and there is a sharp rise in the production of PGI$_3$ from EPA which has equal vasodilatory and platelet-inhibiting properties. The overall changes in eicosanoid production contribute to reduce thrombotic risk.

Leukotrienes are believed to be important in several diseases involving inflammatory or hypersensitivity reactions including asthma, eczema, and rheumatoid arthritis. The effect of EPA consumption on leukotriene synthesis is to shift production from the more inflammatory 4 series leukotrienes, synthesized from arachidonic acid, to the less inflammatory 5 series leukotrienes synthesized from EPA. This metabolic effect helps to explain the improvements in some of the clinical symptoms experienced by rheumatoid arthritis sufferers who consume significant quantities of fish (i.e. EPA).

3.4.5 Effects of fatty acids on other metabolic processes

Fatty acids influence a range of other metabolic processes that have been less well studied in humans. Hydrolysis of some phospholipids results in the formation of biologically active compounds such as the platelet-activating agent (PAF) from 1-alkyl, 2-acyl phosphatidylcholine. Different polyunsaturated fatty acids in the precursor phospholipid can modify PAF formation. ω3-Fatty acids influence the production of cytokines, including the interleukins and tumour necrosis factors, which are involved in regulation of the immune system. An exciting area of current research is the study of the effects of fatty acids on the expression of genes encoding for enzymes that are involved in lipid metabolism, as well as the expression of genes involved in cell growth regulation.

3.4.6 Oxidation of fatty acids

Those fatty acids not incorporated into tissues or used for synthesis of eicosanoids are oxidized for energy. Oxidation of fatty acids occurs in the mitochondria of cells and involves a multiple step process by which the fatty acid is gradually broken down to molecules of acetyl CoA, which are available to enter the tricarboxylic acid cycle and so to generate energy. The rate of oxidation of fatty acids is highest at times of low energy intake and particularly during starvation. As the acetyl CoA splits off, ATP (adenosine triphosphate) is generated which is also a source of energy. Fatty acids of different chain lengths and degrees of saturation are oxidized via slightly different pathways but the ultimate purpose of each is the production of acetyl CoA and the generation of energy. Ketone bodies are produced during times of particularly rapid fatty acid oxidation during the process of ketogenesis. An absolute insulin deficiency such as is seen in severe uncontrolled insulin-dependent diabetes results in a very high rate of production of ketones and acidosis results because of accumulation of acetoacetic and β-OH butyric acids. In healthy individuals with a functioning pancreas, the ingestion of glucose stimulates insulin secretion and thereby prevents or abolishes ketosis. This can be achieved by as little as 50–100 g of glucose daily. In the normal fasting individual a modest increase in level of ketone bodies stimulates insulin secretion. The insulin inhibits further ketogenesis and enhances peripheral ketone body use so that ketone body levels do not rise above 6–8 mol/litre. (In severe diabetes levels may be twice as high as this.) In prolonged starvation there is further ketone body formation and a moderate degree of ketosis may result. However, ketoacidosis does not occur in the absence of insulin deficiency.

3.4.7 Lipid storage

Energy intake in excess of requirements is converted to fat for storage. Stored fat in adipose tissue provides the human body with a source of energy when energy supplies are not immediately available from ingested carbohydrate, fat or glycogen stores. Triacylglycerols are the main storage form of lipids and most stored lipids are found in adipose tissue. The lipid is stored as single droplets in cells called adipocytes which can expand as more fat needs to be stored. Most of the lipid in adipose tissue is derived from dietary lipid and the stored lipid reflects the composition of dietary fat. The triacylglycerol stores of adipose tissue are not static but are continually undergoing lipolysis and re-esterification.

3.4.8 Cholesterol synthesis and excretion

Cholesterol is present in tissues and in plasma lipoproteins as free cholesterol or combined with a fatty acid as cholesterol ester. About half the cholesterol in the body comes from synthesis and the remainder from the diet. It is synthesized in the body from acetyl CoA via a long metabolic pathway. Cholesterol synthesis is regulated near the beginning of the pathway, in the liver by the dietary cholesterol delivered by chylomicron remnants. In the tissues, a cholesterol balance is maintained between factors causing a gain of cholesterol (synthesis, uptake into cells, hydrolysis of stored cholesterol esters) and factors causing loss of cholesterol (steroid hormone synthesis, cholesterol ester formation, bile acid synthesis, and reverse transport via HDL). The specific binding sites and receptors for LDL play a crucial role in cholesterol balance since they constitute the principal means by which LDL-cholesterol enters the cells. These receptors are defective in familial hypercholesterolaemia (Chapter 18.1.4). Excess cholesterol is excreted from the liver in the bile either unchanged as cholesterol or converted to bile salts. A large proportion of the bile salts that are excreted from the liver into the gastrointestinal tract are absorbed back into the portal circulation and returned to the liver as part of the enterohepatic circulation, but some pass on to the colon and are excreted as faecal bile acids.

3.5 HEALTH EFFECTS OF DIETARY LIPIDS

Most fatty acids can be made in the body, except for the essential fatty acids (EFA), linoleic and α-linolenic acids, which must be obtained from the diet (see Section 3.4.2). The fact that specific deficiencies resulting from inadequate intakes of EFAs are very rare in adults, even in African and Asian countries where total dietary fat can provide as little as 10% total energy, suggests that the minimum requirement is low. Among adults, EFA deficiency has only been reported when linoleic acid (18:2ω6) intakes are less than 2–5 g/day or less than 1–2% of total energy. Most adult Western diets provide at least 10 g/day of EFA and healthy people have a substantial reserve in adipose tissues. Clinical manifestations of α-linolenic acid deficiency are rare in humans.

Among adults in Western countries the major health issues concerning intake of fat centre around the role of excessive dietary fat in coronary heart disease (Chapter 18), obesity (Chapter 16) and certain cancers (Chapter 19). There is concern too regarding the optimal balance of ω3 to ω6 fatty acids with regard to risk of thrombosis and consequent coronary heart disease risk as well as the effect this balance may have on inflammatory and immunological responses.

Human milk provides 6% of total energy as essential fatty acids (linoleic and α-linolenic acids); it also contains small amounts of preformed eicosapentaenoic, EPA ($20:5\omega3$) and docosahexaenoic acids, DHA ($22:6\omega3$). Commercial baby milk formulae contain comparable amounts of essential fatty acids but none of the longer-chain, more polyunsaturated fatty acids, EPA or DHA. Formula-fed infants have lower levels of EPA and DHA in their plasma and red cells in comparison to similar breast-fed infants. In premature infants, these reduced levels of EPA and DHA may be associated with impaired and delayed visual development (the retina and the brain have high contents of DHA).

Concern has been expressed that the desire to reduce total fat intake by some health conscious parents in affluent societies might result in a diet high in complex carbohydrate and dietary fibre and containing insufficient energy for growth and development in childhood. These wide-ranging issues need to be taken into account when making nutritional and dietary recommendations.

3.6 RECOMMENDATIONS CONCERNING FAT INTAKE

3.6.1 Minimum desirable intakes

In adults, it is necessary to ensure that dietary intake is adequate to meet energy needs and meet the requirements for EFAs and fat-soluble vitamins. Adequate intakes are particularly important during pregnancy and lactation. Thus, for most adults, dietary fat should provide at least 15% total energy, and 20% for women of reproductive age. British recommendations suggest that at least 1% of total daily energy should be derived from linoleic acid and 0.2% energy from α-linolenic acid. This level is rather arbitrary and is based on the amounts required to cure EFA deficiency. In view of the divergent and often opposing effects of the various eicosanoids derived from ω3 and ω6 fatty acids, other recommendations have concentrated on the balance of the fatty acids in the diet. It has been suggested that the ratio of linoleic to α-linolenic should be between $5:1$ and $10:1$ (the range in human milk) and that those eating diets with a ratio greater than $10:1$ should be encouraged to eat more ω3 rich food such as green leafy vegetables, legumes and fish. Particular attention must be paid to promoting adequate maternal intakes of EFAs throughout pregnancy and lactation to meet the needs of the fetus and young infant in laying down lipids in their growing brains (which have high contents of DHA and arachidonic acids).

For infants and young children, the amount and type of dietary fat are equally important. Breast milk fulfils all requirements (50–60% energy as fat, with appropriate balance of nutrients) and during weaning it is important to ensure that dietary fat intake does not fall too rapidly. At least until the age of two years, a child's diet should contain about 40% of energy from fat and provide similar levels of EFAs to breast milk. The inclusion in infant formulae of EPA and DHA in proportions similar to those found in breast milk would help this, but this suggestion has not been widely adopted by manufacturers.

It is necessary to also take into account associated substances, in particular several vitamins and antioxidants. These are considered in other chapters. In particular, vitamin

E (Chapter 13) in edible oils is required to stabilize the unsaturated fatty acids. Foods high in polyunsaturated fatty acids should contain at least 0.6 mg α-tocopherol equivalents per gram of polyunsaturated fatty acids. In countries where vitamin A deficiency is a public health problem, the use of red palm oil should be encouraged wherever it is available.

3.6.2   Upper limits of fat and oil intakes

In most Western countries, dietary recommendations concerning fat intake have focused primarily around desirable upper limits of intake. The strongest reason for reducing intake of total fat from the typical Western intake of 35–40% total energy is the widespread problem of obesity and the expectation that reducing fat intake to 30% or less of total energy will help to reduce the near epidemic proportions of this problem (Chapter 16). Reducing total fat may also reduce the frequency of some cancers (Chapter 19), but the evidence here is more tenuous and it may also be that the extent of fat reduction required to reduce cancer risk (to around 20% total energy) is unlikely to be achievable in most Western countries in the forseeable future. The case for reducing intake of saturated fatty acids in the expectation of reducing coronary heart disease rates is very strong. The debate concerning the acceptable upper limits of intake are likely to continue into the future. The use of high fat convenience foods is increasing in many countries and powerful vested commercial interests are involved. From a pragmatic point of view it seems appropriate for nutritional advice to focus on an appreciable reduction of saturated fatty acids. This should facilitate a reduction in total fat intake. These issues are discussed in some detail in Chapter 18.

FURTHER READING

1. Grundy SM, Denke MA. Dietary influences on serum lipids and lipoproteins. *J Lipid Res* 1990; **31**: 1149–72.
2. Gurr MI, Harwood JL. *Lipid biochemistry*, 4th ed. London: Chapman & Hall, 1991.
3. Tso P. Gastrointestinal digestion and absorption of lipid. *Advances Lipid Res* 1985; **21**: 143–86.
4. Vergroeson AJ, Crawford M (eds). *The role of fats in human nutrition*, 2nd ed. London: Academic Press, 1989.

4
PROTEIN
Alan Jackson

4.1 NORMAL GROWTH AND THE MAINTENANCE OF HEALTH

To maintain normal weight, function and health in adults and growth in childhood requires a constant intake of oxygen, water, energy and nutrients. In adults, this intake is matched by an equivalent loss of elements as carbon dioxide, water and solutes in urine, or solids in stool. In this way balance is achieved and body weight and composition are maintained relatively constant over long periods of time. In childhood, there is positive balance associated with the net deposition of new tissue. If intake is less than that needed for normal function then there is loss of weight and function is compromised to a point where it eventually impairs health; in childhood, growth is curtailed or stops.

Proteins are fundamental structural and functional elements within every cell and undergo extensive metabolic interaction. This widespread metabolic interaction is intimately linked to the metabolism of energy and other nutrients. Following water, protein and fat are the next most abundant chemical compounds in the body in normal health. All cells and tissues contain proteins. For an adult man who weighs 70 kg, about 16% will be protein (i.e. about 11 kg). A large proportion of this will be muscle, 43%, with substantial proportions being present in skin, 15%, and blood 16%. Half of the total is present in only four proteins; collagen, haemoglobin, myosin and actin, with collagen comprising about 25% of the overall total. Proteins fulfil a range of functions and the amount of protein does not, of itself, provide any indication of the importance or relevance of the function. Indeed, some of the most important functionally active proteins might only comprise a small proportion of the total present (e.g. peptide hormones such as insulin, growth factors, or cytokines). The biochemical activity of proteins is an attribute of their individual structure, shape and size. This in turn is determined by the sequence of amino acids within polypeptide chains, the characteristics of the individual amino acids (size, charge, hydrophobicity or hydrophilicity) and the environment which together determine the primary, secondary and tertiary structure of the protein. The tertiary structure of the protein determines the nature of the biochemical reactions in which the protein will engage.

Proteins taken in the diet are broken down in the upper gastrointestinal tract to amino acids in the processes of digestion and absorption. Absorbed amino acids contribute to the amino acid pool of the body, from which all proteins are synthesized. The proteins of the body exist in a 'dynamic state' as they are constantly turning over through the processes of protein synthesis and degradation (Fig. 4.1). On average the rates of synthesis and degradation are similar in adults, so that the amount of protein in the body remains more or less constant over long periods of time. During growth, protein

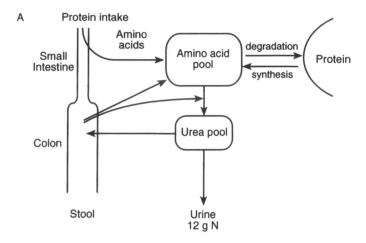

Fig. 4.1(A)   There is a dynamic interchange of protein, amino acids and nitrogen in the body which conceptually takes place through an amino acid pool. Amino acids are added to the pool from the degradation of body proteins and also from dietary protein, following digestion and absorption. There is the continuous breakdown of amino acids with energy being made available when the carbon skeleton is oxidized to water and CO_2. The amino group goes to the formation of urea. Although urea is an end-product of mammalian metabolism, a significant proportion of the nitrogen is salvaged for further metabolic interaction following hydrolysis of urea by the flora resident in the colon.

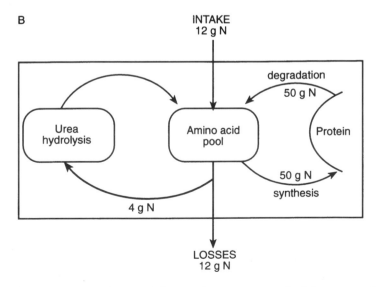

Fig. 4.1(B)   The quantitative relations of these exchanges in normal adults expressed as grams of (amino) nitrogen (N).

Box 4.1 The pattern of amino acids which form proteins give them very different shapes, chemical and physical properties, thereby enabling them to carry out a wide range of functions within the body

---

Structural

Body:	skeleton and supporting tissues, skin and epithelia
Tissue:	connective tissues and ground substance
Cell:	cellular architecture

Protective

Barrier:	non-specific defences/turnover keratins skin, tears, mucin
Inflammation:	acute phase response
Immune response:	cellular and humoral

Transport/Communication

Plasma proteins:	albumin, transferrin, apolipoproteins
Hormones:	insulin, glucagon, growth hormone
Cell membrane and receptors:	intracellular communications/second messenger

Enzymic

Extracellular:	digestive, clotting; haemoglobin and O_2, CO_2 transport; acid base
Metabolic pathways:	glycolysis, protein synthesis, citric acid cycle, urea cycle

---

synthesis exceeds protein degradation, so there is net deposition of protein. The process of turnover is obvious for some proteins (e.g. enzymes, skin or mucosa, digestive juices), but is also true for plasma proteins such as albumin or γ-globulins, and even structural proteins such as muscle and bone. There are many hundreds of proteins in the body, each of which is formed and degraded at a characteristic rate, which may vary from minutes to days or even months. Each protein fulfils a specific function, which might either be structural, protective, enzymatic, involved in transport or an aspect of cellular communication (Box 4.1).

4.2   PROTEIN STATUS OF THE BODY

There is no single way in which the protein status of an individual can be determined. Different approaches will provide information of different aspects. The amount of protein contained in the body cannot be measured directly during life. However, most of the nitrogen in the body is present as amino acids in protein, and most protein is present as lean tissue. The nitrogen content of the body can be determined by *in vivo* neutron activation analysis.

On the assumption that the protein content of tissues remains fairly constant, the determination of the lean body mass (which approximates the fat free mass), will also give an index of the total protein content (see Chapter 25). Indirect measures of lean body mass include assessment of total body water, total body potassium, underwater weighing or fat fold thickness. Organ and tissue size can be determined by imaging techniques. Muscle mass and changes in muscle content in clinical situations can be assessed from the urinary excretion of creatinine or the girth of limbs, such as the mid-upper arm circumference or thigh circumference. The determination of the concentration of amino acids in plasma or the albumin concentration have been used as indirect indices of body protein status. However, each of these can be difficult to interpret (see below).

The assessment of the function of the metabolically active tissues has been used as an index of protein status (e.g. muscle function tests, liver function tests, tests of immune function). The content of the body is not static, and therefore measurements of the rates at which proteins are formed and degraded in the body and the rate at which nitrogen flows to the end-products of metabolism provide one important approach to determining the mechanisms through which nitrogen equilibrium is maintained in health, positive balance achieved during growth, or negative balance brought about during wasting conditions.

4.3 PROTEINS, AMINO ACIDS AND OTHER NITROGEN-CONTAINING COMPOUNDS

The structure and function of all proteins is related to the amino acid composition; the number and order of linkages, folding, intra-chain linkages, and the interaction with other groups to induce chemical change (e.g. phosphorylation/dephosphorylation, oxidation and reduction of sulphydryl group). The amino acids are linked in chains through peptide bonds. The structure of individual amino acids and the patterns of their linkages give the unique properties to an individual protein. Proteins may have critical requirements for either a tight or loose association with micronutrients and this is particularly likely for enzymes which might require the presence of co-factors or prosthetic groups in close association with the active centres.

For each protein the amino acid composition is characteristic. For a protein to be synthesized requires that all the amino acids needed are available at the point of synthesis. If one amino acid is in short supply, this will limit the process of protein synthesis; such an amino acid is defined as the 'limiting amino acid'. There is no dietary requirement for protein *per se*, but dietary protein is important for the individual amino acids it contains. There are 20 amino acids required for protein synthesis and these are all 'metabolically essential'. Of the 20 amino acids found in protein, eight have to be provided preformed in the diet for adults and are identified as being 'indispensable' or 'essential' (lysine, threonine, methionine, phenylalanine, tryptophan, leucine, isoleucine, valine). The other amino acids do not have to be provided preformed in the diet, provided that they can be formed in the body from appropriate precursors in adequate amounts and are identified as being 'dispensable' or 'non-essential'. The non-essential amino acids are not necessarily of lesser biological importance. They have to be synthesized in adequate amounts endogenously. Their provision in the diet appears to spare additional quantities of other (essential) amino acids or sources of nitrogen which would be required for their synthesis. In early childhood a number of amino acids, which are not essential in adults cannot be formed in adequate amounts, either because the demand is high, the pathways for their formation are not matured or the rate of endogenous formation is not adequate or some combination. These amino acids have been identified as being conditionally

Box 4.2   There are 20 amino acids which are found as the constituents of proteins. All are 'essential' for metabolism, but not all have to be provided preformed in the diet, because they can be made in sufficient amounts from other metabolic precursors. If the situation arises where the formation in the body is not adequate to satisfy the metabolic needs, the amino acids become conditionally essential

Indispensable (essential) amino acids	Conditionally indispensable (essential) amino acids	Dispensable (non-essential) amino acids
Leucine (Leu)		Glutamic acid (Glu)
Isoleucine (Ile)		Alanine (Ala)
Valine (Val)		Aspartic acid (Asp)
Phenylalanine (Phe)	Tyrosine (Tyr)	
Threonine (Thr)	Glycine (Gly)	
	Serine (Ser)	
Methionine (Met)	Cysteine (Cys)	
Tryptophan (Trp)		
Lysine (Lys)		
	Arginine (Arg)	
	Glutamine (Gln)	
	Asparagine (Asn)	
	Proline (Pro)	
	Histidine (His)	

Box 4.3   Amino acids are the precursors for many other metabolic intermediates and products with structural and functional roles

Product/Function	Examples
Nucleotides	Formation of DNA, RNA, ATP, NAD
Energy transduction	ATP, NAD, creatine
Neurotransmitters	Serotonin, adrenaline, noradrenaline, acetylcholine
Membrane structures	Head groups of phospholipids: choline, ethanolamine
Porphyrin	Haem compounds, cytochromes
Cellular replication	Polyamines
Fat digestion	Taurine, glycine conjugated bile acids
Fat metabolism	Carnitine
Hormones	Thyroid, pituitary hormones

essential, because of the limited ability of their endogenous formation relative to the magnitude of the demand (arginine, histidine, cysteine, glycine, tyrosine, glutamine, proline). There may be disease situations during adult life whereby for one reason or another a particular amino acid, or group of amino acids, becomes conditionally essential.

Although most of the amino acids are found in proteins, some amino acids also have metabolic activities which are not directly related to the formation of proteins, or act as the precursors for other important metabolically active compounds (Box 4.3). Not all amino acids are found in proteins and there are metabolically important amino acids which play no direct part in the formation of proteins (e.g. citrulline). There is a relatively small pool of free amino acids in all tissues. This is the pool from which amino acids for protein formation are derived and to which amino acids coming from protein degradation contribute; therefore, the amino acid pools have a very high rate of turnover.

There are many other nitrogen-containing compounds which are neither proteins, polypeptides nor amino acids.

4.4 DIETARY PROTEINS, THE AMINO ACID POOL AND THE DYNAMIC STATE OF BODY PROTEINS

Before proteins taken in the diet can be utilized, they have to be broken down to the constituent amino acids through digestion. The catalytic breaking of the peptide bond is achieved through enzymes, which act initially in the acid environment of the stomach and the process is completed in the alkaline environment of the small intestine. A series of proteolytic enzymes selectively attack specific bonds (Table 4.1). The products of digestion are presented for absorption as individual amino acids, dipeptides or small oligopeptides. Absorption takes place in the small intestine as an energy-dependent

Table 4.1 Human protein digestion

Organ	Activation	Enzyme	Substrate	Product
Stomach	pH < 4	Pepsin	Whole protein	Very large polypeptides with C-terminal tyr, phe, trp, also leu, glu, gln
Pancreas	pH 7.5 enterokinase secreted by small intestinal mucosa	Endopeptidases	Bonds within peptide chain	
		Trypsin	Peptides	Peptide with basic amino acid at C-terminal, arg, lys
		Chymotrypsin	Peptides	Peptide with neutral amino acid at C-terminal
		Exopeptidases	C-terminal bonds	
		Carboxypeptidase	Successive amino acids at carboxy-terminal	Amino acids
		Aminopeptidase	Successive amino acids at amino terminal	Amino acids

Note: Enzymes that digest proteins are secreted as inactive precursors (e.g. pepsinogen, trypsinogen, chymotrypsinogen, etc.) and are activated under appropriate conditions by the removal of a small peptide from the parent molecule.

process through specific transporters. There is evidence for the absorption of small amounts of intact protein, which is unlikely to be of great nutritional significance but may be of potential importance in the development of allergies. The extent of absorption of whole proteins is not clear, nor whether this can take place through intact bowel, or requires mucosal lesions.

The absorptive capacity of the bowel for amino acids has to be greatly in excess of the dietary intake, because there is a considerable net daily secretion of proteins into the bowel. This protein is contained in secretions associated with digestion and the enzymes contained therein, mucins and sloughed cells. The amount varies, but estimates suggest a minimum of 70 g protein/day, and possibly up to 200–300 g protein/day. The amounts are thus at least as great as the dietary intake. Dietary amino acids mix with and are diluted by endogenous amino acids. There is further dilution of the dietary intake as the amino acids are taken up into the circulation and distributed to cells around the body.

4.5 PROTEIN TURNOVER

When dietary amino acids are labelled with either stable or radioactive isotopes, their fate in the body can be determined. As a matter of course there is retention of the labelled amino acids in the body, and the labelled amino acids can be recovered from the proteins of most tissues. This approach can be used as the basis for measuring the rate at which body proteins are synthesized and degraded. The relative rates of protein synthesis and

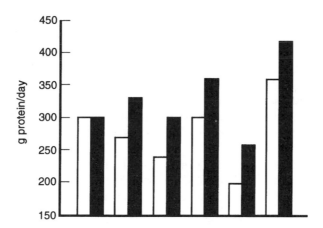

Fig. 4.2 Proteins in the body are constantly turning over (i.e. they are being synthesized and degraded). The net amount of protein is determined by the relative rates of synthesis and degradation, not the absolute rate. When the rate of protein synthesis (□) is equal to the rate of protein degradation (■) there is no change in the amount of protein (first column). Loss of protein and negative nitrogen balance will result when the relative rate of protein degradation exceeds the rate of protein synthesis. The five columns to the right show that this might be achieved either through a decrease in protein synthesis, an increase in protein degradation or any combination of the two, at either high or low absolute rates of protein synthesis and degradation.

degradation determine the overall nitrogen balance. For nitrogen balance to be achieved the rates of protein synthesis and protein degradation have to be equal. If synthesis exceeds degradation then nitrogen balance is positive and if degradation exceeds synthesis nitrogen balance is negative. The achievement of balance itself provides no information on the absolute rates of either process because overall balance is determined by the relative rates of synthesis and degradation. As shown in Fig. 4.2, negative nitrogen balance can result from a range of patterns of change in synthesis and degradation. As factors which act on or control synthesis are different from those affecting degradation, interventions which are designed to modify balance, or improve growth might act on one or the other process. On average, about 50% of protein synthesis takes place in the visceral tissues, with liver predominating (25%), and 50% takes place in the carcass, with muscle predominating (25%). The mass of liver is much less than the mass of muscle, so the intensity of turnover in liver (fractional turnover, 100%/day) is much greater than that in muscle (fractional turnover, 18%/day).

4.6   PROTEIN SYNTHESIS AND DEGRADATION

The dynamic state of proteins, constantly being synthesized and constantly being degraded, represents a major and fundamental aspect of the metabolic function of the body. Protein synthesis is an intracellular event and the amounts and pattern of proteins being formed in a cell at any time is determined by the factors which control genomic expression, the translation of the message and the control exerted upon the activity of the synthetic machinery on ribosomes. Protein degradation is also an intracellular event and is thought to take place through three major pathways, the calcium-protease, ATP-ubiquitin, or lysosomal pathways.

In normal adults about 4 g protein/kg body weight are synthesized each day; about 300 g protein/day in men and 250 g protein/day in women. In newborn infants the rate is about 12 g protein/kg, falling to about 6 g/kg by one year of age. Basal metabolic rate is closely related to the size, shape and body composition of an individual and the same is true for protein synthesis. In adults in a steady state, protein synthesis is matched by an equivalent rate of protein degradation, but in infancy and childhood, protein synthesis exceeds protein degradation because of the net tissue and protein deposition associated with growth.

Dietary intake and the metabolic behaviour of the body show a diurnal rhythmicity. Food is normally ingested during the daytime. There is a diurnal pattern of nitrogen excretion in urine, which is more marked on higher protein intakes, with increased excretion during daytime and reduced losses during the night. On average, over a 24-hour period, nitrogen equilibrium is maintained. However, as intake exceeds losses during the day and losses exceed intake during the night, there is a diurnal pattern of nitrogen balance, which is positive during the day and negative during the night. It is likely that nitrogen is retained in a number of forms during the day. There is evidence that protein deposition is most marked in the gastrointestinal tract, liver and other visceral tissues with lesser deposition in muscle. There are equivalent losses of these relatively labile pools of protein during the night. In situations of fasting or longer-term undernutrition, the early losses of protein appear to be from the liver and gastrointestinal tract, but after a short time the majority of the losses are borne by peripheral tissues such as muscle and skin.

Despite the diurnal swings in protein turnover, the effect of protein intake on the average whole body protein synthesis is relatively modest, provided the intake exceeds the minimal dietary requirement. Below the minimal dietary requirement, about 0.6 g/kg per day, there is a relative fall in protein synthesis during the fed period.

4.7 ENERGY COST OF PROTEIN TURNOVER

Both protein synthesis and protein degradation consume energy, 4 kJ/g of protein of average composition. Protein degradation takes place through ATP-dependent pathways, which are both lysosomal and non-lysosomal. At the level of the whole body the biochemical cost of peptide bond formation for protein synthesis is estimated to be about 15–20% of the resting energy expenditure. There are additional energy costs to the body if protein turnover is to be sustained, as processes such as transport of amino acids into cells require energy, etc. If the full energy costs of maintaining the system are included, then the physiological cost is probably in the region of 33% of resting energy expenditure.

There is a general interaction between the intake of dietary energy and nitrogen balance. Thus, although nitrogen balance and protein synthesis appear to be protected functions, modest increase in energy intake leads to positive nitrogen balance, and decreasing energy intake results in a transient negative nitrogen balance. In general, there is about 2 mg nitrogen retained or lost for a change in energy intake of 4 kJ (1 kcal).

In childhood, growth and net tissue deposition is a normal feature. During adulthood, the demands for net tissue formation occurs under three important circumstances: in women during pregnancy or lactation, or during recovery from some wasting condition.

4.8 GROWTH

Growth consists of a complex of processes and changes in the body. There is an increase in stature and size and the proportions of the individual tissues change resulting in changes in the composition of the body. These changes are related to the physiological maturation of function which is an orderly series of changes in time. Maturation of function underlies development in general and mental or intellectual development in particular. The orderly sequence of neurological maturation is directly linked into more complex behavioural changes which under normal circumstances involve social interaction and the development of patterns of behaviour that are identified as social development.

At the level of cells and tissues growth can be characterized as either an increase in the number of cells (hypertrophy), or an increase in the size of cells (hyperplasia) or a combination of the two processes (mixed hypertrophy and hyperplasia), which then leads to differentiation and specialization of function.

Net protein deposition is required for growth to take place so protein synthesis must exceed protein degradation. There is an increase in protein synthesis, but there is also an increase in protein degradation, so that overall about 1.5–2.0 g protein are synthesized for every 1 g of net deposition. The apparent inefficiency of the system might be accounted for by:

(i) a measure of flexibility to allow remodelling;

(ii) transcriptional and translational errors; and

(iii) wear and tear on the protein synthetic machinery.

4.9 Linear Growth

Linear growth is a function of the growth and development of the long bones, the deposition of a collagenous matrix (protein) within which the deposition of bone mineral crystals can take place. Ultimate adult height is determined by the genetic make up of an individual, but at every stage of development there àre factors which might operate to limit the extent to which this potential is achieved. Following an illness or deprivation there may be recovery in height gain when the adverse influence is removed, but there may be a loss of some of the capacity for achieving the full genetic potential.

The hormones, insulin, thyroid hormone, growth hormone and insulin-like growth factors (IGFs) have all been shown to modulate linear growth within physiological ranges. Calcification of bones is directly related to vitamin D hormones, parathormone and osteocalcin.

An adequate intake of energy is an absolute requirement for growth, but is not of itself sufficient to achieve optimal growth in height: an adequate intake of protein and other nutrients is also required. Human and animal studies have identified a specific need for dietary protein, which is thought to have a direct effect upon IGFs. Balance studies indicate the need for adequate calcium, phosphorus, zinc and other micronutrients.

Adverse influences, such as infection, inflammation, psychological and social factors might act either directly, or indirectly through nutritional effects. Activity is an important positive factor for the healthy development and calcification of bones.

Stunting, or linear growth retardation, is the major nutritional problem across the globe affecting the socially and economically disadvantaged within and between societies. There is clear evidence that stunted individuals have a higher death rate from a variety of causes and increased number of illnesses. Stunted individuals have below average physical work performance and impaired mental and intellectual function.

4.10 Protein Turnover in Muscle and Its Control

Muscle contains a large proportion of the protein in the body. Considerable interest has been shown in the growth of muscle which is commercially important for the livestock industry. Muscle is one tissue most affected by wasting, and being relatively accessible has been the subject of more detailed study *in vivo* in humans than any other tissue. The rate of muscle tissue deposition is determined by hormones, the availability of energy and nutrients, and muscle activity (stretch).

Protein turnover in muscle is responsive to the hormonal state. Adrenal corticosteroids produce a decrease in synthesis and an increase in degradation. Insulin and growth hormone have an overall anabolic (tissue-building) effect, mainly through stimulating protein synthesis. Thyroid hormones increase protein synthesis and degradation. At normal physiological levels they have a greater effect on synthesis than on degradation and thus exert a net anabolic effect. At hyperthyroid levels the increase in degradation exceeds the increase in synthesis, hence an overall catabolic effect. β-Adrenergic anabolic agents such as clenbuterol promote muscle growth by decreasing protein degradation.

People on bed-rest go into negative nitrogen balance and lose weight through wasting of muscle. Activity is required to maintain muscle mass and the pull of contracting muscles on bone serves to promote bone growth. Mechanical signals exert an effect on cellular function through direct effect on the intracellular cytoskeleton, through activated ion channels and through second messenger signal transduction processes. Prostaglandins have a direct effect on muscle protein synthesis and degradation, with $PGF_{2\alpha}$ stimulating synthesis and PGE_2 stimulating degradation. The activity of phospholipase A_2 (PLA_2) makes arachidonic acid available for the synthesis of $PGF_{2\alpha}$ (blocked by indomethacin). The activity of PLA_2 is enhanced by stretch (activation of calcium) or insulin (cyclic AMP), and inhibited by glucocorticoids. Lipopolysaccharide exerts an influence on the release of arachidonic acid under the action of PLA_2, with the formation of PGE_2, which increases protein degradation through increased proteolysis within the lysosomes.

Stress, trauma or surgery all induce a negative nitrogen balance in rats and humans. In wasted individuals or people on a low protein diet, a catabolic response, with negative nitrogen balance may not be evident. Those who do not show the response are more likely to die, giving the impression that the negative response is purposive and that under these circumstances the catabolic response is more important than conserving body protein.

4.11   INJURY AND TRAUMA

Injury and trauma are characterized by an inflammatory, or *acute-phase response*. This is a co-ordinated metabolic response by the body which appears to be designed to limit damage, remove foreign material and repair damaged tissue. Under the influence of cytokines there is a shift in the pattern of protein synthesis and degradation. Substrate from endogenous sources is made available to support the activity of the immune system. In muscle, protein synthesis falls and protein degradation might increase, resulting in net loss of protein from muscle with wasting. The amino acids made available by muscle wasting provide substrate for protein synthesis in liver and the immune system. In the liver there is a shift in the pattern of proteins synthesized, with a reduction in the formation of the usual secretory proteins, albumin, transferrin, retinol binding protein, etc., and an increase in the formation of the acute-phase reactants, C-reactive protein, α_1-acid glycoprotein, α_2-macroglobulin, etc. In combination with a loss of appetite, the changes in protein turnover in liver and muscle result in a negative nitrogen balance. There is usually an increase in protein degradation overall, and the intensity of the increase is determined by the magnitude of the trauma. Protein losses range from 5 g/day (or less) with uncomplicated elective surgery to more than 70 g/day with burn injury at the upper end of the scale. The dietary intake appears to have an important influence upon the extent to which protein synthesis can be maintained and hence the magnitude of the negative nitrogen balance and the severity of the consequent wasting.

4.12 Amino Acids

The habitual dietary intake of about 80 g protein/day in adults is only about a quarter of the protein being formed in the body each day. The minimal dietary requirement for protein, about 35 g protein in adult men, is approximately one-tenth of the protein being formed in the body each day.

The pattern and amounts of amino acids required to support protein synthesis is determined by the amount and pattern of proteins being formed. Although it has been presumed that the overall pattern is dominated by proteins of mixed composition similar to that seen in muscle, this is not necessarily true for all situations, especially some pathological states. For example, the amino acid pattern of collagen is rich in glycine and proline, but poor in leucine and the branched-chain amino acids. During growth, where the demands for collagen formation are increased, the balance of amino acids needed is therefore likely to be shifted towards the collagen pattern. During an inflammatory response increased synthesis occurs of the antioxidant glutathione and the zinc-binding protein metallothionein, which are particularly rich in cysteine. In animals with fur, the need for extensive keratin formation places a heavy demand upon sulphur-containing amino acids. The demand for the most appropriate pattern of amino acids can vary with different situations. The nature of the demand may change from one time to another, being determined by the physiological state: such as pregnancy, lactation or growth. or the pathological state, such as infection, the response to trauma or any other reason for an acute-phase response.

4.13 Amino Acid Turnover

The amino acid pool is the precursor pool from which all amino acids are drawn for protein synthesis and other special pathways. It is helpful to identify the pool for each amino acid individually and to consider the general factors which are of importance (see Fig. 4.3). For any amino acid there are three inflows to the pool and three outflows. The flows from the pool to protein synthesis and other metabolic pathways represent the metabolic demand for the amino acid. Flow to amino acid oxidation is determined either

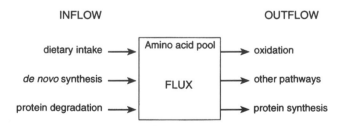

Fig. 4.3 The dynamic turnover of any amino acid in the body can be characterized by a model in which there is a single pool of an amino acid. Inflows to the pool are from three potential sources, protein degradation, the diet and *de novo* synthesis. There are three outflows from the pool, to protein synthesis, other metabolic pathways and to oxidation with the breakdown of the amino acid.

by the need to use amino acids as a source of energy, or as a degradative pathway for amino acids in excess of what can be used effectively at the time.
This demand has to be satisfied from:

(i) amino acids coming from protein degradation; *or*

(ii) *de novo* synthesis of amino acids; *or*

(iii) dietary amino acids.

First, it might be expected that in a steady state amino acids coming from protein would represent a perfect fit for the proteins which are being synthesized and hence there should be no general need for amino acids to be added to the system. However, this is not so. The amino acids released from protein degradation are different from those used in protein synthesis, because some amino acids are altered during the time they are part of a polypeptide chain. For example, amino acids might be methylated or carboxylated. These post-translational modifications relate to the structure and function of the mature protein. Lysine as part of a protein might be methylated to trimethyl-lysine. When the protein is degraded, the released trimethyl lysine is of no value in future protein synthesis, but it can act as a metabolic precursor for the synthesis of carnitine. Carnitine plays a fundamental role in fatty acid metabolism (Chapter 3). The endogenous formation of carnitine facilitates fatty acid oxidation and limits the need for a dietary source of carnitine, but an additional source of lysine is still needed for protein synthesis to be maintained. As lysine is an indispensable amino acid, and cannot be synthesized endogenously, lysine has to be obtained preformed from the diet.

4.14 AMINO ACID FORMATION AND OXIDATION

The *de novo* synthesis of an amino acid requires that its carbon skeleton can be made available from endogenous sources and this skeleton can then have an amino group effectively added in the right position. The sulphur moiety also has to be added for the sulphur amino acids. In mammalian metabolism there are some amino acids which are readily formed from other metabolic intermediates, for example transaminating amino acids: alanine, glutamic and aspartic acid derived from intermediates of the citric acid cycle, α-ketoglutarate, pyruvate, oxaloacetate. These amino acids are important in the movement of amino groups around the body and also in gluconeogenesis (e.g. the glucose–alanine cycle between the liver and the periphery), or renal gluconeogenesis from glutamine during fasting. Some dispensable amino acids derive directly from an indispensable amino acid (e.g. tyrosine from phenylalanine), and the endogenous formation of the amino acid is determined by the availability of the indispensable amino acid. Methionine and cysteine are amino acids which contain a sulphydryl group, with considerable chemical activity. Although methionine can be formed in the body from homocysteine, this is part of a cycle (*methionine cycle*) which generates methyl groups for metabolism and in which there is no net gain of methionine (Fig. 4.4). Homocysteine, has an alternative metabolic fate, towards the formation of cysteine. In this pathway the sulphydryl group derived from methionine is made available to a molecule of serine with the formation of cysteine: the carbon skeleton derived from methionine is subsequently

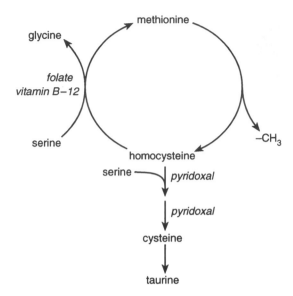

Fig. 4.4 *The methionine cycle*. Methionine has to be provided in the diet and like other amino acids is required for protein synthesis. In addition, it has a number of other important functions. Apart from acting as a signal for protein synthesis it is the precursor for cysteine and other reactions in which methyl groups are made available to metabolism. In donating its methyl group, methionine forms homocysteine which can be reformed to methionine using a single carbon group, derived either from serine or betaine (a breakdown product of choline). Homocysteine is a branch point in metabolism as it also has another important fate, the formation of cysteine and taurine. In these pathways the sulphydryl group is transferred to the carbon skeleton of serine. Thus, serine is used for the further metabolism of homocysteine, down either pathway. Increased amounts of homocysteine in the circulation are associated with increased risk of cardiovascular disease.

oxidized. Cysteine is the precursor for taurine which, with glycine, is required for the formation of bile salts from bile acids. Thus, cysteine can be formed in the body provided there is sufficient methionine and serine available. However, the pathway for cysteine formation has not fully matured in the newborn, making cysteine a conditionally essential amino acid at this time.

For some amino acids the pathway for their formation appears complex and tortuous involving a complex pathway shared between a number of tissues. The renal formation of arginine is an example (Fig. 4.5). Arginine is the precursor of nitric oxide which has important metabolic functions as a neurotransmitter, in maintaining peripheral vascular tone and one of several oxidative radicals formed during the oxidative burst of leucocytes. Arginine is also the direct precursor of urea, the main form in which nitrogen is excreted from the body. Arginine is formed in two main sites, kidney and liver. Arginine formed in kidney is available for the rest of the body, whereas arginine formed in liver is cleaved to urea and ornithine in the *urea cycle* (Fig. 4.6). In both locations the arginine is made from citrulline, but whereas in liver the citrulline is generated locally in the mitochondria, in kidney it is imported. The imported citrulline has been formed in the gastrointestinal tract, one of the end-products of the oxidation of glutamine. The glutamine itself has been generated in muscle from the branched-chain amino acids.

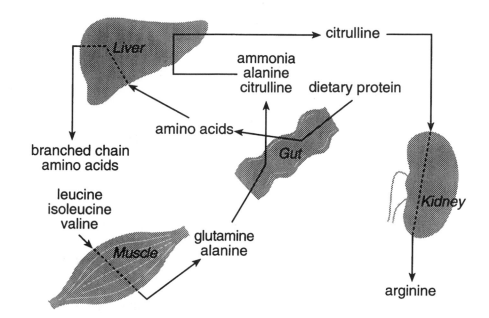

Fig. 4.5 There is a complex system of inter-organ co-operation for many aspects of amino acid metabolism, and the partitioning of different functions between organs is of critical importance for effective metabolic control. Arginine is formed in significant amounts in both liver and kidney, but that formed in the liver goes to urea formation in general, whereas that formed in the kidney is exported and available for the needs of the rest of the body in, for example, the generation of nitric oxide. Arginine is formed from citrulline in the kidney, with the citrulline being derived from the gastrointestinal tract, where its formation is linked to the utilization of glutamine. Glutamine itself is formed in large amounts in muscle, in part from the breakdown of the branched-chain amino acids, leucine, isoleucine and valine. The branched-chain amino acids coming from dietary protein are, as a group, handled in a special way: following absorption they tend to pass through the liver without being metabolized and are preferentially taken up by the muscles.

During the digestion and absorption of the amino acids taken in protein in a meal, most of the amino acids are first taken up by liver, but more of the branched-chain amino acids pass directly through the liver and are taken up preferentially by muscle, where they give rise to glutamine. This complex pattern of metabolic interchange enables control to be exerted, and in particular creates a mechanism through which two important sets of metabolic interaction of arginine are separated and therefore can be controlled independently.

There are other amino acids, such as glycine, which are required as the building blocks for more complex compounds in relatively large amounts: haemoglobin and other porphyrins, creatine, bile salts and glutathione, but the pathways which enable the formation of large quantities of the amino acid are not clear.

It has generally been considered that the carbon skeleton of the indispensable amino acids cannot be formed at all in the body. However, the possibility exists that the colonic bacteria synthesize these amino acids for their own use, and some may be made available to the host, although in small amounts.

MITOCHONDRION

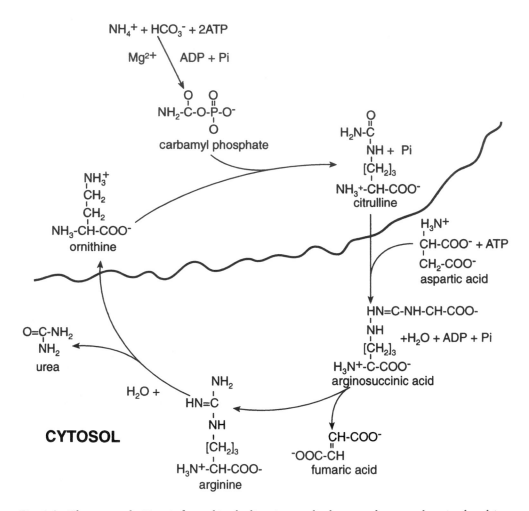

Fig. 4.6 *The urea cycle.* Urea is formed in the liver in a cyclical process between the mitochondrion and the cytosol. A molecule of ornithine and the synthesis of a molecule of carbamyl phosphate, from ammonia and CO_2, is the starting point with the ultimate formation of arginine which is hydrolyzed to reform orthinine and a molecule of urea. The cycle utilizes three molecules of ATP for each revolution.

In a number of inborn errors of metabolism, an enzyme involved in the oxidation of amino acids does not function normally and there is considerable accumulation of an amino acid or its breakdown products. The extent to which the body can tolerate an excess for any single amino acid might vary, but sustained, high increased levels of amino acids in the body almost invariably exert toxic effects. Therefore, the body goes to some lengths to maintain very low levels. The catabolic pathways for individual amino acids are active, although the activity may decrease on very low protein intakes. For the indispensable amino acids in particular, the amount of individual amino acids usually found in diets is in excess of the normal requirements. This may be the reason why the body has not selected to maintain the pathways for their formation. The dietary requirement for the indispensable amino acids determines the minimal physiological requirement for protein and has been used in the past for defining protein quality, protein requirements and the recommendations for protein for populations. For the dispensable amino acids the body is able to tolerate larger amounts of the amino acid, but also control can be exerted at two levels, the rate of formation and the rate of oxidation, making toxicity less likely. On a daily basis, for a person in balance an equivalent amount of protein, or amino acids is oxidized as is taken in the diet. Therefore, for a person consuming 80 g protein each day, an equivalent 80 g of amino acids will be oxidized to provide energy with the amino group going to the formation of urea. Thus, the proportion of total energy derived from protein each day is similar to the relative contribution of protein to the energy in the diet.

4.15 NITROGEN BALANCE

On average about 16% of protein is nitrogen, and therefore by measuring its nitrogen and multiplying by 6.25 the approximate protein content of a food or tissue can be obtained. Nitrogen balance identifies the overall relationship between the nitrogen removed from the environment for the body and the nitrogen returned to the environment. The intake is almost completely dietary, mainly as protein, but also in part as other nitrogen-containing compounds, such as nucleic acids, and creatine in meat and vitamins. Nitrogen can be lost from the body through a number of routes, but 85–90% is lost in urine and 5–10% in stool, with skin and hair or other losses making up the remainder. Nitrogen is lost as soluble molecules in urine as urea (85%), ammonia (5%), creatinine (5%), uric acids (2–5%), and traces of individual amino acids or proteins. There may be large losses of nitrogen through unusual routes in pathological situations (e.g. through the skin in burns, as haemorrhage or via fistulae).

The achievement of nitrogen balance in response to a change in either intake or losses is brought about largely by a change in the rate at which urea is excreted in the urine. A reduction in the dietary intake of protein is matched by an equivalent reduction in the urinary excretion in urea, which returns nitrogen equilibrium within three to five days. Faecal losses of nitrogen on habitual intakes are usually 1–2 g nitrogen/day, or about one-tenth of the intake. However, faecal nitrogen may increase on diets which are rich in dietary fibre. There is then a reduction in the excretion of urea in urine equivalent to the increase in faecal nitrogen. Increased cutaneous loss, through excessive sweating, exudation or burns, is associated with a proportionate decrease in urinary urea.

In a system that is constantly turning over, the retention of body protein is a necessary condition for maintaining the integrity of the tissues and tissue protein. Any limitation in the availability of energy or a specific nutrient will lead to a net loss of tissue, and to negative nitrogen balance through increased losses of nitrogen. Thus, the major control over the protein content of the body is established by modifications in the rate at which nitrogen is lost from the body. Balance is re-established by a change in the rate of nitrogen excretion, which for most part means a change in the rate at which urea is excreted. So, it is important to consider the factors which might control or influence the formation and excretion of urea.

4.16 UREA METABOLISM AND THE SALVAGE OF UREA NITROGEN

Urea is formed in the liver in a cyclical process on a molecule of ornithine (Fig. 4.6). Within the mitochondria carbamyl phosphate, from ammonia and carbon dioxide, condenses with ornithine to form citrulline. The citrulline passes to the cytosol where a further amino group is donated from aspartic acids with the eventual formation of arginine (which has three amino groups). It is hydrolyzed with the formation of urea and the regeneration of ornithine. Urea is lost to the body by excretion through the kidney. In the kidney urea fulfils an important physiological role in helping to generate and maintain the concentrating mechanism in the counter-current system of the loops of Henle. The rate of loss of urea through the kidney is influenced by the activity of the hormone, vasopressin, on the collecting ducts. On low protein diets, urea is reabsorbed from urine in the collecting duct of the kidney so nitrogen is potentially retained in the system. Normally, more urea is formed in the liver than is excreted in the kidney. About one-third of the urea formed passes to the colon where it is hydrolyzed by the resident microflora. About one-third of the nitrogen from urea released in this way is returned directly to urea formation, but the other two-thirds is incorporated into the nitrogen pool of the body presumably as amino acids. In other words urea-nitrogen has been salvaged.

In situations where the body is trying to economize on nitrogen the proportion of urea-nitrogen lost in the urine is decreased, and the proportion salvaged through the colon is increased. This happens when demand for nitrogen for protein synthesis increases, as in growth, or when the supply of nitrogen is reduced, as on a low protein diet. In situations of very rapid growth, in early infancy or during catch-up from wasting conditions, the salvage of urea-nitrogen may reach very high levels, compared with the dietary intake. In normal adults increased salvage is seen as the intake falls from habitual levels of intake (around 75–80 g protein/day) to a protein intake around the minimum requirement (about 35–40 g/day). On the lower protein intake balance is maintained by a reduction in the rate of urea excretion and an increase in urea-nitrogen salvage. Below this level of protein intake, nitrogen balance is not maintained, urea excretion increases and salvage falls. Thus a central part of adapting to low protein diets is an enhancement of the salvage of urea nitrogen. In this way nitrogen may be retained within the system in a functionally useful form.

The optimal intake of protein is likely to be that which provides appropriate amounts of the different amino acids to satisfy the needs of the system. There is no evidence that the ingestion of large amounts of protein of itself confers any benefit. Indeed, the system may be stressed by the need to catabolize the excess amino acids which cannot be directed to synthetic pathways and have to be excreted as end-products. High protein intakes increase renal blood flow and glomerular filtration rate. In individuals with compromised renal function this may increase the risk of further renal damage.

The two clinical situations in which control of protein intake and metabolism is of considerable importance are renal failure and hepatic failure. In hepatic failure, there is a limitation of the liver's ability to detoxify ammonia through the formation of urea. In renal failure the ability to excrete effectively the urea formed is impaired. In each situation reduction of the intake or modification of metabolism of protein or amino acids is an important part of treatment.

4.17   THE NATURE OF PROTEIN IN THE DIET

The majority of foods are made of cellular material and therefore in the natural state contain protein. Processing of foods may alter the amounts and relative proportions of some amino acids, for example, the Maillard reaction and browning reduces the available lysine. The pattern of amino acids in animal cells is similar to the pattern in human cells and therefore the match for animal protein foods is good. For plant materials there may be very different patterns of amino acids. This difference has in the past led to the concept of first and second class proteins, for animal and plant protein foods respectively. However, diets are hardly ever made up of single foods. In most diets, because different foods tend to complement each other in terms of the amino acid content, any potential imbalance is likely to be more apparent than real for most situations. Thus the mixture of amino acids provided in most diets matches the dietary requirements of normal humans fairly well.

4.18   HOW MUCH PROTEIN DO WE NEED?

The amount of dietary protein required to maintain nitrogen equilibrium in the absence of any gain or loss of weight is about 0.6–0.7 g/kg per day at all ages. If the intake of protein is reduced below this level, without any change in the intake of energy and other nutrients, then weight will be lost and nitrogen equilibrium will be established once again when the protein intake is back around 0.6 g/kg per day. However, there is an important interrelationship between energy intake and the level of dietary protein to maintain nitrogen equilibrium. If the energy intake is increased at the same time as the nitrogen intake is decreased, equilibrium might be established at lower levels of nitrogen intake without any loss of weight. The mechanisms through which this is achieved are not clear. For an adult male, who weighs 70 kg, with a total energy expenditure of 10 000 kJ/day and maintenance dietary protein requirement of 42 g/day the proportion of energy in the diet derived from protein would be 6.2%, and for a female of 60 kg expending 8000 kJ/day and requiring 0.6 g dietary protein/kg per day, would be 7.2%.

For individuals in positive nitrogen balance (i.e. during normal growth, pregnancy or lactation), protein intake needs to be above the maintenance level to achieve a positive balance. The magnitude of the increase can be directly related to the rate of and pattern of tissue deposition, and the 'quality' of the protein in the diet. Quality of protein is a statement about the pattern of amino acids in the tissue being deposited and the pattern of amino acids available from the diet and endogenous formation. There is the need for energy for the deposition of new tissue, and therefore a relationship can be drawn between the energy intake required and the protein required for tissue deposition (see below).

4.19   HOW MUCH PROTEIN DO WE EAT?

The amount of protein eaten each day is determined by the total food intake and the protein content of the food. In general, the proportion of energy derived from protein is between 11% and 15% of the total energy of the diet, which is generous for all normal purposes.

Figure 4.7 shows the estimated average amount of protein available to different populations around the world. There is a twofold difference overall between the technologically developed countries and the underdeveloped countries. The protein available from non-meat sources was very similar for all countries, around 50 g protein/head per day, varying by less than ± 10% for the extremes. In contrast, the protein available from meat sources varied by 10-fold between the extremes. Virtually all of the difference in protein availability between different countries was determined by the availability of meat protein. Within a population there are differences among individuals in the amount of protein taken on average. To a very large extent this will be determined by the total food intake. Figure 4.8 shows the relationship between protein intake and energy intake among a group of young women vegetarians. The proportion of energy derived from protein was similar for each individual. Those who were most active had the greatest intake of energy and the highest protein intake. Those who were relatively sedentary had a protein intake which approached the maintenance level.

In young children, energy expenditure per unit body weight is high, and therefore energy intake per unit body weight is high. In consequence, the dietary protein requirement for normal growth is relatively low, as a proportion of total energy. For example, for an infant weighing 10 kg at one year of age and growing at a normal rate, for an energy intake of 95 kcal/kg per day and a protein requirement of 1.5 g/kg per day, the proportion of total energy coming from protein would be 6.3%. The highest relative requirement for protein is in sedentary individuals. For example, for a 70-year-old

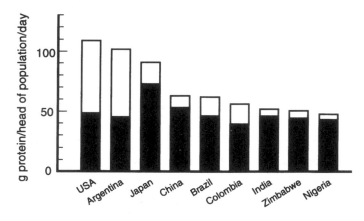

Fig. 4.7   The amount of protein available to the population can be assessed (g protein/head of population/day) and divided into meat protein (□) and non-meat protein (■). For countries of widely different characteristics the availability of non-meat protein falls within a narrow range (within ± 10%), whereas the availability of meat protein varies widely, over a 10-fold range.

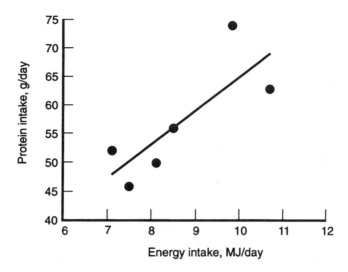

Fig. 4.8 Under most normal circumstances the total food intake of a person is determined by their energy expenditure which sets their energy requirement. The energy requirement consists of a reasonably fixed component, basal metabolic rate (BMR), and a variable component which is determined primarily by the level of physical activity. The protein content of most diets provides between 10% and 15% of dietary energy, and therefore the total protein intake is closely related to the total energy intake, and hence the level of physical activity. (mJ, megajoule.)

woman who weighs 80 kg, lying relatively immobile in bed, the proportion of total energy coming from protein would have to be 20%, which is not readily achievable on a normal diet.

4.20   DIETARY PROTEIN DEFICIENCY AND PROTEIN DEFICIENT STATES

For the diets consumed by most populations the intake of protein is adequate provided that the overall intake of food is not limited (e.g. by inactivity or unavailability). However, for some diets in which the density of protein to energy is low, and/or where the quality of amino acids is low, there may be situations related to relative inactivity when the ability to satisfy the protein intake is marginal.

Protein deficient states, where the content of protein in the body is reduced are relatively much more common. These are most likely to be the result of:

(a) an increase in demand (e.g. in infection or stress);

(b) an increase in losses (e.g. with haemorrhage, burns or diarrhoea); or

(c) a failure of the conservation systems (e.g. with impairment of urea salvage in the colon).

Protein energy malnutrition is described in Chapter 17.

In correcting the deficient state it is as important to remove the underlying cause, as it is to provide adequate amounts of protein or amino acids in the diet.

71

FURTHER READING

1. Barbul A. Arginine: biochemistry, physiology and therapeutic implications. *J Parent Ent Nutr* 1986; **10**: 227–38.
2. Grimble RF. Nutrition and cytokine action. *Nutr Res Rev* 1990; **3**: 193–210.
3. Grimble RF. Interaction between nutrients, pro-inflammatory cytokines and inflammation. *Clin Sci* 1996; **91**: 121–30.
4. Jackson AA, Wootton SA. The energy requirement of growth and catch-up growth. In Schurch B, Scrimshaw NS (eds). *Activity, energy expenditure and energy requirements of infants and children*. Lausanne: International Dietary Energy Consultative Group, 1990.
5. Jackson AA. Chronic malnutrition: protein metabolism. *Proc Nutr Soc* 1993; **52**: 1–10.
6. Jackson AA. Salvage of urea-nitrogen and protein requirements. *Proc Nutr Soc* 1995; **54**: 535–47.
7. Millward DJ, Bowtell JL, Pacy P, Rennie MJ. Physical activity, protein metabolism and protein requirements. *Proc Nutr Soc* 1994; **53**: 223–40.
8. Millward DJ. A protein-stat mechanism for regulation of lean body mass. *Nutr Res Rev* 1995; **8**: 93–120.
9. Waterlow JC, Schurch B. Causes and mechanisms of linear growth retardation. *Eur J Clin Nutr* 1994; **48** (suppl.): S210–11.
10. Waterlow JC. Whole-body protein turnover in humans—past, present and future. *Ann Rev Nutr* 1995; **15**: 57–92.

5

ENERGY

Joop van Raaij

Consideration of energy in nutrition is primarily focused on the chemical energy of food, the body's energy need to perform work, the body's energy stores, and the possibilities for adaptation.

The chemical energy from food is the only source of energy for humans. This form of energy may be used by the human body to perform mechanical work (muscular contraction), electrical work (maintaining ionic gradients across membranes) and chemical work (synthesis of new macromolecules). If ingested food energy is not used for doing work it will be stored as chemical energy (mainly as body fat). Adults who have a stable body weight are in energy balance, which means that for them the energy available from food equals needs of the body to perform work. In pregnant and lactating women and in children the energy available from food should also sustain adequate pregnancy weight gains, or allow sufficient milk production, or support adequate growth. There is still little known about the individual's capacities for adaptations in energy expenditure if energy balance deteriorates.

In this chapter the International System of Units (SI units) will be used. The SI unit of energy is the joule (J), which is the energy used when 1 kilogram (kg) is moved 1 metre (m) by a force of 1 newton (N). Since 1 joule is a very small amount of energy, in most uses in nutrition the kilojoule (kJ, i.e. 10^3 J) or the megajoule (MJ, i.e. 10^6 J) are more convenient. The adoption of SI units in human nutrition has been slow, and many texts still express energy in kilocalories (kcal). If the thermochemical calorie conversion factor is used, then 1 kcal $=$ 4.184 kJ.

5.1 ENERGY VALUE OF FOODS

5.1.1 Chemical energy

The chemical energy of any food is determined by measurement in the laboratory of the heat produced when its organic molecules are fully oxidized. This is done in a bomb calorimeter. A sample of the food is placed inside a water jacket in a thick steel case (the bomb). Oxygen is introduced and combustion is set off by an electric current. The heat produced in the water is measured with a thermocouple.

This total chemical energy of a food is the heat of combustion or the gross energy.

5.1.2 Metabolizable energy

Not all the chemical energy in food is available to the human that eats that food. First, not all food eaten is absorbed from the digestive tract. That part of the chemical energy of food that is actually absorbed (digestibility coefficient) is called *digestible energy*. Second, in the body (unlike the bomb calorimeter) amino acids (the form in which proteins are absorbed) are metabolized only as far as urea, not all the way to nitrogen oxides which would be more toxic. Urea still has chemical energy, nearly a quarter of the original chemical energy of a mixture of amino acids. For these two reasons the energy losses through faeces and urine need to be subtracted from the gross energy of a food to obtain the energy available to the body. This available energy is termed the *metabolizable* energy of the food.

5.1.3   Measurement versus calculation of metabolizable energy

Under experimental conditions the metabolizable energy that an individual obtains from their diet can be measured by bomb calorimetry on duplicate portions of the foods together with bomb calorimetry on samples of urine and faeces. These duplicate portions and samples should be collected over an adequate period of time (e.g. seven days). In Table 5.1 an example is given of measuring metabolizable energy of a daily diet.

In theory, the metabolizable energy intake of an individual can also be calculated accurately if the exact composition of the diet is known (amounts of various carbohydrates, fatty acids, amino acids, alcohol) and if for each of these nutrients metabolizable energy conversion factors are available. Usually, it is not done this way. Information on the composition of the diet is obtained by use of food composition tables (with their limitations) and the most common energy conversion factors used are the so-called Atwater factors (named after W.O. Atwater who one century ago carried out the studies from which these factors were derived). These are averages for categories of nutrients (starch, fat, protein, and alcohol) and based on absorption rates as observed for typical Western diets. In Table 5.2 an example is given of calculating the metabolizable energy of a daily diet using these Atwater factors.

Table 5.1   Example of measuring metabolizable energy of a daily diet

Subjects	
• young women	
Given	
• collection over 7 days	Bomb calorimetry*
• duplicate portions of diet	(a) 9900 kJ/day
• faeces	(b) 710 kJ/day
• urine	(c) 420 kJ/day
Derived	
• gross energy of food (a)	9900 kJ/day
• digestible energy ($a-b$)	9190 kJ/day
• digestibility coefficient $\left[\dfrac{100(a-b)}{a} \right]$	92.8%
Metabolizable energy ($a-b-c$)	8770 kJ/day

* See Chapter 24.2.5 for a description of this method.

Table 5.2 Example of calculating metabolizable energy of a daily diet

Subjects		
• young women		
Given		
• food records over 7 days		
• food composition table		
• Atwater factors:		
– carbohydrate	17 kJ/g (4 kcal/g)	
– fat	37 kJ/g (9 kcal/g)	
– protein	17 kJ/g (4 kcal/g)	
– alcohol	29 kJ/g (7 kcal/g)	
Derived		
• carbohydrate	245 g/day	4165 kJ/day
• fat	90 g/day	3330 kJ/day
• protein	75 g/day	1275 kJ/day
• alcohol	0 g/day	0 kJ/day
Metabolizable energy		8770 kJ/day

It should be noted that the energy values of foods as given in food composition tables are not gross chemical energy values but metabolizable energy values, usually derived from the chemical composition of foods multiplied by the Atwater factors.

5.2 DIRECT AND INDIRECT CALORIMETRY: MEASUREMENT OF ENERGY EXPENDITURE

The term 'metabolizable energy' refers to food and is in fact a theoretical concept since it indicates how much energy from the food may become available to the body if the food were to be oxidized. In reality, not all the ingested and absorbed food is immediately oxidized. Most nutrients will be stored for a shorter or longer period or might be incorporated into essential body structures. The term 'metabolized energy' refers to the actual oxidation of substrates within the body. In the short term (hours) the proportion of the mixture of carbohydrates, fatty acids and amino acids that is actually oxidized may not necessarily reflect the composition of the ingested meal, but in the long term (days) it will reflect the composition of the usual diet, unless the composition of the body has changed.

The amount of metabolized energy is also referred to as expended energy. The classic methods to study energy expenditure are based on direct and indirect calorimetry.

5.2.1 Direct calorimetry

Principle A direct calorimeter measures the heat production of a human subject over, say, 24 hours. This is a difficult and by no means routine experiment. The heat loss is

Table 5.3 Example of direct calorimetry used to measure energy expenditure over 24 hours

Subjects
- young women, sedentary activity pattern

Given
• sensible heat loss	6650 kJ
• evaporative heat loss	1540 kJ
• heat loss through faeces/urine	60 kJ
• performed mechanical work	520 kJ
• heat storage (assumed to be 0)	

Derived
- energy expenditure = heat loss + performed mechanical work = 8770 kJ

mainly sensible heat loss and evaporative heat loss. Direct calorimetry is based on the fact that all the energy liberated in the substrate oxidation will eventually be released as heat and as mechanical work performed in the outside environment. Direct calorimetry is time-consuming with each measurement taking several hours. If changes in body heat stores are not measured it has to be assumed that no heat is stored in or lost from the body. Energy expenditure may be calculated from heat loss, from changes in heat stores, and, if appropriate, from performed mechanical work. In Table 5.3 an example is given of deriving energy expenditure from data collected by direct calorimetry.

Equipment Room-sized chambers designed to detect heat loss have been built for human use. However, in practice, the construction and operation of such chambers is technically difficult and expensive. One more recent approach has been to use a water-cooled garment in which the subject can move more freely than in a calorimeter chamber, but measurements remain technically difficult. There are very few working direct calorimeter chambers across the world and unlikely to be any increase in their number. The heat exchanging body suit is said to be uncomfortable and there has been very little research reported of its use. Most measurements of energy expenditure are made by techniques other than direct calorimetry.

5.2.2 Indirect calorimetry

Principle Indirect calorimetry is the usual method of measuring energy expenditure. It is easier to carry out than direct calorimetry and provides information about the metabolic fuel that the body is using. It is based on measuring the respiratory gas exchange. The most used fuel in the body is glucose, from starch, sugars and glucogenic amino acids. The equation for its complete oxidation is:

$$C_6H_{12}O_6 + 6O_2 \rightarrow 6CO_2 + 6H_2O + heat$$

1 mole CHO $(180\,g) + (6 \times 22.4)l \rightarrow (6 \times 22.4)l + (6 \times 18)\,g + 2780\,kJ$.

(The heat produced from one gram-molecule of glucose has been measured by bomb calorimetry.) Hence,

$$1 \text{ litre of oxygen} = 2780 \div (6 \times 22.4) \text{ kJ} = 20.7 \text{ kJ}.$$

If the subject is metabolizing only carbohydrate, then for every litre of oxygen used in respiration 20.7 kJ of heat (or energy) is produced. Energy expenditure can be measured from the oxygen utilization.

If the body is using fat for energy, whether from the diet or from stored adipose tissue the equation is more complex because triglyceride molecules are larger and contain different fatty acids. A typical fatty acid molecule (e.g. palmitic acid, $C_{16}H_{34}O_2$), contains a lower proportion of oxygen than glucose. Fat metabolism requires more oxygen carbohydrate. Oxygen is used not only for production of carbon dioxide but also for oxidation of hydrogen to water.

The ratio of CO_2 production to the oxygen consumption is the *respiratory quotient* (RQ). For carbohydrates it is 1.00; when fat is being metabolized it approximates 0.70 (Table 5.4).

The energy production per litre of oxygen consumed is very similar whether carbohydrate, fat or protein is being used as the fuel. Consequently a value, of 20.3 kJ per litre of oxygen consumed, based on the mixture of energy-yielding nutrients in an average diet, can be used as a good approximation of the energy expenditure.

For greater accuracy from indirect calorimetry the actual energy equivalents per litre oxygen should be used for the various nutrients. This means that the composition of the mixture of carbohydrate, fat, and protein which is actually oxidized must be known (the metabolic mixture). This information can be obtained if in addition to oxygen consumption, carbon dioxide production and urinary nitrogen excretion are also measured. The oxidation equations for carbohydrate, protein and fat show that the molar ratio of carbon dioxide production to oxygen consumption (respiratory quotient, RQ) differs for each nutrient. Mean values of RQ are close to 0.7 for fat and 1.0 for carbohydrate, with protein having an intermediate value. So the value of the actual RQ can give us information about the composition of the metabolic mixture. However, this is not enough. Since amino acids are not completely oxidized, information on urinary nitrogen excretion is also needed.

Table 5.4 Energy yields per gram of substrate and per litre of oxygen consumed

1 gram of:	O_2 consumed (ml)	CO_2 produced (ml)	RQ	Energy or heat developed (kJ)	Energy per 1 litre O_2 (kJ)
Starch	830*	830	1.00	17.5	21.1
Fat	2020	1430	0.71	39.6	19.6
Protein	965	780	0.81	18.6	19.3

* 1 g starch produces on hydrolysis more than 1 g glucose for metabolism. The energy developed from starch is therefore greater than the energy developed from glucose (15.6 kJ). RQ, Respiratory quotient.
Source: Durnin JVGA, Passmore R. *Energy, work and leisure.* London: Heinemann, 1967; based on experiments by Zuntz (1897).

If oxygen consumption, carbon dioxide production and urinary excretion are all measured it is possible to estimate the oxidation rates for carbohydrates, fats and protein. In principle the first step is to estimate the protein oxidation. This is 6.25 times the urinary nitrogen excretion (because average dietary proteins weigh 6.25 × their nitrogen content). Taking the RQ for protein as 0.81 and data from metabolizable energy of pure protein, the oxygen consumption and CO_2 production due to protein oxidation can be calculated. These are subtracted from the measured (total) oxygen consumption and CO_2 production. The ratio of the remaining O_2 and CO_2 give the non-protein RQ. Oxidation of carbohydrates and fats can be calculated from the non-protein RQ, non-protein O_2 consumption and CO_2 production. Nomograms and several published formulae are available for this. Livesey and Elia (1988), however, point out that with fats the RQ ranges from 0.70 to 0.74 depending on the fatty acid pattern and with proteins including clinical nutrition products the RQ can range from 0.80 to 0.85.

For energy expenditure we have seen six different published equations, some of which have a long history. Differences between them in the coefficients for oxygen consumption and CO_2 production are small but the differences in coefficients for protein urinary nitrogen are larger. The equation recommended by Brockway (1987) is well reasoned:

$$\text{Energy expenditure (kJ)} = 16.58O_2 + 4.51CO_2 - 5.90N$$

If it is not practicable to measure urinary nitrogen, for example, in short experiments the equation can be simplified to:

$$kJ = 21V\,\Delta O_2$$

where V is the ventilation rate, and ΔO_2 is the difference in oxygen concentration between inspired and expired air. Table 5.5 gives an example deriving energy expenditure from data collected with indirect calorimetry.

Equipment   The classic method uses the Douglas bag (see Fig. 5.1). This is a large bag impermeable to gas, usually of 100 litre volume. The subject wears a nose clip and breathes out into the bag via a tube containing a valve which separates inspired from expired air. At the end of the experiment, which has to be short (up to 15 minutes) because of limited capacity of the bag, the volume of expired air is measured with a gas meter. The oxygen and CO_2 content of a sample of the expired air are analyzed. Oxygen consumption is calculated from the difference between oxygen in ambient (inspired) and expired air multiplied by the ventilation rate. This equipment is simple and inexpensive but cumbersome and may interfere with the subject's normal activity. The face mask may be uncomfortable.

For short duration measurements during exercise the Kofrani–Michaelis respirometer (KM) (see Fig. 5.1) had been more widely used since it measures expired air volume as it is produced, and therefore only a small sample of the expired air needs to be retained for subsequent gas analysis. The KM respirometer is no longer being manufactured, so a new generation of portable instruments have replaced it, such as the Oxylog and the Cosmed K2. The Oxylog incorporates both a volume meter and oxygen sensors, so there is no need for subsequent gas analysis. Electronic components calculate the oxygen consumed. The Cosmed K2 has a device for transmitting data to a radio receiver remote

Table 5.5 Example of indirect calorimetry

Subjects	
• young women	
Given	
• oxygen consumption 24 h (Vo_2):	435 l
• carbon dioxide production 24 h (Vco_2):	370 l
• urinary nitrogen excretion 24 h (N):	12 g
Respiratory quotient	
$= Vco_2$ (l) $\div Vo_2$ (l) $= 0.85$	
Metabolic mixture	
carbohydrate oxidation (g)	
$= 4.706\ Vco_2$ (l) $- 3.340\ Vo_2$ (l) $- 2.714$ N(g)	$= 256$ g
fat oxidation (g)	
$= 1.768\ Vo_2$ (l) $- 1.778\ Vco_2$ (l) $- 2021$ N(g)	$= 87$ g
Protein oxidation (g) $= 6.25$ N(g)	$= 75$ g
Energy expenditure (kJ)	
$= 16.489\ Vo_2$ (l) $+ 4.628\ Vco_2$ (l) $- 9.079$ N(g)	$= 8776$ kJ
Energy expenditure (kJ) (assuming 15 energy % from protein)	
$= 16.318\ Vo_2$ (l) $+ 4.602\ Vco_2$ (l)	$= 8801$ kJ
Energy expenditure (kJ) (assuming 20.3 kJ/litre oxygen)	
$= 20.3\ Vo_2$ (l)	$= 8831$ kJ

from the subject. The portable respirometers were developed for short-duration measurements at rest and during exercise in 'field' situations but can also be used in laboratory settings.

Ventilated hood systems (see Fig. 5.1) avoid the discomfort of a face mask, etc. With this equipment air flows at high rate over the subject's head which is in a perspex hood while they lie or sit quietly. Samples of air from inside the hood can be drawn directly to gas analysers. The system is suited to situations in which the subject's gas exchange is measured in the laboratory for periods of 30 minutes to 6 hours. In whole-body indirect calorimeters or respiration chambers the subject spends time, often 24 hours, in a small sealed room while it is ventilated with a constant supply of fresh air. The subject's respiratory gas exchanges are measured by continuous analysis of well-mixed samples of air from the chamber. From differences in oxygen and CO_2 content between the air going in and the air coming out the respiratory exchange is calculated and from this the energy expenditure of the subject. Subjects can carry out activities of a sedentary life inside the room—sitting, reading, watching TV, eating, a period of controlled exercise and sleeping. Typical equipment in a respiration chamber are a chair, desk, TV, video, radio, telephone, exercise equipment and folding bed. Food and drink are passed in through one airlock and urine and faeces out through another. The temperature of the room is controlled and excessive humidity avoided. There are respiration chambers at a number of nutrition research centres around the world.

To measure energy expenditure in hospital patients (which is increased in some diseases) a portable metabolic monitor, such as the Deltatrac™ II is used at the bedside. It operates on a similar principle to the ventilated hood.

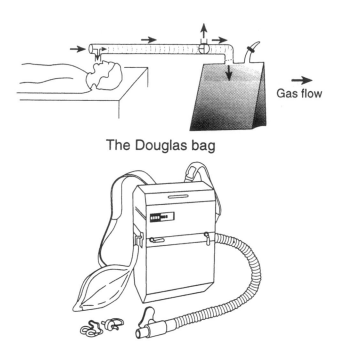

The Douglas bag

The Kofrani-Michaelis respirometer

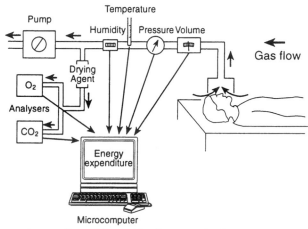

A ventilated hood indirect calorimeter

Fig. 5.1 Most commonly used devices for indirect calorimetry. *Source*: Garrow JS, James WPT (eds). *Human nutrition and dietetics*, 9th ed. Edinburgh: Churchill Livingstone, 1993.

5.3 THE BODY'S NEED FOR ENERGY

Energy expenditure in health is made up of three different components, each of which can be measured. These are: the energy required to maintain basal metabolism, the energy released as a result of the thermic effect of food, and the energy required for physical activity.

5.3.1 Basal metabolism

Definition   The energy needed to maintain basal metabolism is the amount required to sustain the basic essential metabolic processes involved in keeping the body alive and healthy and, where applicable, growing at an appropriate rate. The energy required to sustain basal metabolism is also known as the basal metabolic rate (BMR). In most individuals the BMR is the largest single component of 24-hour energy expenditure (50–70% of daily energy expenditure).

Experimental approach   The basal metabolic rate is measured under defined conditions. It is measured while the subjects are lying in bed or on a couch, immediately after awakening, in a state of physical and emotional relaxation, and in a thermoneutral environment. They should have fasted for the 12–14 hours immediately before the measurement, and heavy physical exercise should be avoided on the day before the measurement. Subjects should also be free from disease and not suffer from fever. If any of the conditions for BMR are not met, the energy expenditure should be termed the resting metabolic rate (RMR) of the subject.

BMR is most frequently measured using the Douglas bag or ventilated hood technique, or sometimes using portable respirometers. BMR is measured in kJ/min, but often extrapolated to 24 hours and then expressed as MJ/day.

Factors affecting basal metabolism   The BMR of a subject is influenced by many factors such as body size, body composition, age, sex, nutritional and physiological state.

Body size and body composition are major determinants of the BMR. For example, adipose tissue has a lower metabolic rate than other tissues. Therefore BMR is usually expressed per kg of body weight or, even better, per kg of fat-free mass. Age affects energy expenditure in the sense that BMR/kg of body weight declines from birth to old age. In children, an addition to the basal metabolism is required for growth. This is about 21 kJ/g of tissue gained and works out less than many parents suppose—only around 250 kJ/day or 3% of energy expenditure at age 10 years—but it fluctuates considerably. (Most of the relatively large energy intake in children is to match their high levels of physical activity.) The decline in metabolic rate after early adulthood is largely explained by the changes in body composition, usually a decline in fat-free mass and an increase in adipose tissue. The generally lower energy expenditure in women than men is partly because women are usually smaller, partly because a woman of the same weight as a man has more fat and less muscle and muscle has a higher metabolic rate than adipose tissue.

Sometimes it has been found that energy intakes above or below energy requirements may lead to an increase or decrease in BMR, over and above what would be expected from the change in body weight and body composition. Such changes in energy expenditure are sometimes called 'adaptive' since they act to offset the energy surplus or deficit (see below).

Extremes of climate can affect energy expenditure. It will be increased if heat production is needed to maintain body temperature in a cold climate. In everyday life situations cold-induced thermogenesis is, however, not an important factor of daily energy expenditure because of our clothing and the indoor environmental temperature. Conversely there are some reports that the BMR is reduced in hot climates. Whether genetic differences exist in energy expenditure is still unclear. Other factors which can affect BMR are hormonal state, pharmacological agents and disease (e.g. fever).

5.3.2 Thermic effect of food

Definition The thermic effect of food (TEF) is the stimulation of metabolism that occurs up to three to six hours after a meal as a result of the processing of the food in the stomach and intestine and of nutrients in the blood and body cells. The energy corresponding to the thermic effect of food includes the energy costs of the absorption, metabolism, and storage of nutrients within the body. The magnitude of the thermic effect of food over 24 hours is about 10% of the total daily energy expenditure.

This thermic effect of food was originally called the 'specific dynamic effect of food' because the stimulation of energy expenditure depends upon the composition of the diet. The thermic effect of food is also called postprandial thermogenesis (PPT) or diet-induced thermogenesis (DIT).

Experimental approach The thermic effect of food (TEF) or the thermic effect of a meal (TEM) is usually measured over three to six hours after ingestion of the meal with measuring conditions similar to those of measuring basal metabolic rate. The postprandial energy expenditure (in kJ/min) is continuously measured over this period and compared with the basal metabolic rate (in kJ/min) before eating the meal. The cumulative increase above basal metabolic rate is calculated as the thermic effect of food (expressed in kJ or as percentage of the energy content of the meal). The thermic effect of meals are usually measured using a ventilated hood system but sometimes also in respiration chambers. Figure 5.2 shows the principle of calculating the thermic effect of a meal (diet-induced thermogenesis).

Factors affecting thermic effect of food (TEF) The TEF is greater in response to protein ingestion than to the same energy intake in the form of carbohydrate or fat. There is some evidence that the magnitude of the thermic effect of food as a whole is genetically determined.

The thermic effect of food has been subdivided into two components: (1) obligatory thermogenesis and (2) facultative thermogenesis. The obligatory component is the unavoidable energy cost associated with absorption and transport of nutrients and the synthesis of protein, fat and carbohydrate required for the renewal of body tissues and the storage of energy. Facultative thermogenesis is thought to be partially mediated by 'futile' heat-releasing metabolic cycles and the activity of the nervous system. The magnitude of the facultative thermic effect of food seems to depend on several factors, including the energy content of the meal itself, how well-nourished a person is, and the composition of the diet they have been following, but in fact there is little conclusive evidence.

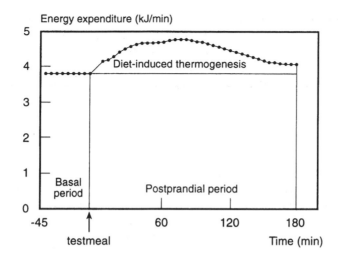

Fig. 5.2 The principle of calculating diet-induced thermogenesis.

5.3.3 Physical activity

Definition Energy expenditure for physical activity is the increase in metabolic rate above basal metabolic rate and the thermic effect of food. In affluent countries physical activity accounts for 20–40% of total energy expenditure in most individuals. The energy expended in physical activity depends on the nature and duration of the various activities carried out throughout the day.

Experimental approach The energy expenditure of standardized activities such as treadmill walking and cycling on a bicycle-ergometer is usually measured using the Douglas bag or the ventilated hood technique. Everyday-life or 'field' activities are usually measured using portable respirometers. The energy costs of activities are usually expressed in kJ/min, or as multiple of BMR (PAR, physical activity ratio). For example, if an individual's BMR is 4.5 kJ/min, and the energy cost for a task is estimated to be 3.0 times BMR (so, PAR-value is 3.0), then the estimated energy cost for that task will be 13.5 kJ/min. If energy costs are expressed in kJ/min they are usually inclusive of basal metabolism and thermic effect of food. If they are expressed as multiple of BMR they are usually also inclusive of the thermic effect of food.

Factors affecting energy costs for physical activity The energy cost of any particular activity varies between individuals, depending on the size of the subject, the speed of the activity, the time resting between movements, the skill with which the movements are made and the efficiency of the muscles.

In Table 5.6 an overview is given of application options of measures of energy intake and energy expenditure in nutritional research. Detailed examples can easily be found in the literature (see also Further reading at end of this chapter).

Table 5.6 Application of measures of energy intake and energy expenditure in nutritional research

Field of nutritional research
1. Metabolic and biological efficiency
2. Work efficiency and work capacity
3. Daily energy requirement

Measures of energy intake and energy expenditure
Digestibility [field 1]
Metabolizability [field 1]
24 h energy intake [field 3]
Basal metabolic rate [fields 1 and 3]
Thermic effect of meal [field 1]
Energy cost of standardized activity
• weight-bearing (e.g. treadmill) [field 2]
• non-weight-bearing (e.g. bicycle ergometer) [field 2]
Energy cost of common activities [field 3]
24 h energy expenditure [field 3], etc.

5.4 ESTIMATION OF TOTAL ENERGY NEEDS

A person's total energy needs comprise the energy required to maintain basal metabolism, the energy required for the thermic effect of food, and the energy required for activity. Over the years many methods have been developed to measure total energy expenditure. The classic methods based on direct or indirect calorimetry are the most accurate, but the major disadvantage of both methods is that the subjects cannot perform all of their habitual activities because of their confinement in a small chamber or the need for them to wear a cumbersome apparatus. To overcome the disadvantage and because the energy needed for activity is the most variable component in total energy needs, various 'field' methods have been developed to measure total energy expenditure under free-living conditions. These include factorial methods, food intake and energy balance methods, heart rate monitoring, registration of body motion, and the doubly labelled water technique.

5.4.1 Factorial methods

One factorial method for measuring total energy expenditure involves calculation of each of the three categories of energy need: (1) basal metabolic need, (2) thermic effect of food, and (3) activity need. The basal metabolic need is usually estimated from prediction equations based on body weight, age, sex, and sometimes also height. The thermic effect of food is taken to be 10% of the total energy expenditure. The energy required for activity can be derived from published values on energy cost of activities (exclusive of basal metabolism and influence of food) combined with a record of activities performed over a day or a number of days. If values for energy cost of activities are used which already include basal metabolic rate and the thermic effect of food (i.e. physical activity ratio, PAR), then the factorial approach is, of course, more simple.

Table 5.7   Example of modified factorial approach (FAO/WHO/UNU 1985)

Subjects: young housewives in affluent societies average BMR of 5520 kJ		
In bed at 1.0 × BMR	8 hour	1820 kJ
Occupational activities		
• extra housework at 2.7 × BMR	1 hour*	630 kJ
Discretionary activities		
• socially desirable and household tasks at 3.0 × BMR	2 hour	1380 kJ
• cardiovascular and muscular maintenance at 6 × BMR	$\frac{1}{3}$ hour	460 kJ
For residual time, energy needs at 1.4 × BMR	$12\frac{2}{3}$ hour	4040 kJ
Total = 1.51 × BMR		8330 kJ

* The remaining household activities are included in maintenance (= 1.4 × BMR).

A modified factorial approach (Table 5.7) is being introduced by the Food and Agriculture Organization (FAO) and the World Health Organization (WHO). In this approach the estimated BMR (derived from prediction equations) is multiplied by a so-called BMR-factor. This multiple of the BMR should be representative for the person's typical level of activity. In the modified approach the BMR-factor covers both the activity need and the thermic effect of food.

The main limitations of factorial methods concern the observations of activity. When individuals are going about their normal lives, there are likely to be significant errors in the reporting of time spent on each activity and how strenuously the activities were pursued. In addition, one should work with integrated energy indices (IEI) instead of with PAR values for activities. The term 'IEI' relates to the energy cost over the whole period of time allocated to a task. It therefore includes the time taken for pauses between the specific activity which characterizes work, household tasks or discretionary activities (e.g. pauses between episodes of dancing, digging, playing football).

5.4.2   Food intake and energy balance method

The food energy intake and energy balance method is based on comparison of total energy intake over several days with the amount of energy required for any observational change in body composition. If weight is gained some energy should be subtracted from observed energy intake, if weight is lost then some energy should be added to observed energy intake. The resulting figure can be considered as an estimate of total energy needs.

The accuracy of this procedure obviously depends on the accuracy of the food intake record (duration of trial, method used, problem of over- and under-reporting, failure to keep accurate food records, etc.) and the accuracy of measurements of change in body composition (duration of trial).

5.4.3   Heart rate monitoring

This method is based on the positive correlation between heart rate and oxygen consumption. Continuous monitoring of heart rate is easy to perform under free-living conditions with electronic portable equipment. Before undertaking such free-living studies, however, the relationship between an individual's heart rate and level of oxygen consumption must be calibrated in laboratory trials in which heart rate and oxygen consumption are both directly monitored while the subject undertakes a series of increasingly strenuous activities. It is necessary to use a number of different activities to establish this relationship, since heart rate and energy expenditure do not follow a simple linear relationship. A mathematical equation describing the relationship between heart rate and oxygen consumption can then be derived for each individual. This equation allows an approximate level of oxygen consumption to be predicted for any heart rate. Assuming a certain energy equivalent per litre of oxygen consumed, energy expenditure rates can then be estimated.

The correlation between heart rate and oxygen consumption is strong from a certain level of activity onwards. At lower rates of activity especially, other factors may confound the relationship, so for daily activity patterns classified as very light or light this heart rate monitoring method might be less appropriate. On the other hand, the method is inexpensive and non-restrictive to the subject and it can therefore be used in large numbers of subjects.

5.4.4 Registration of body movement

Various mechanical and electrical motion sensors have been developed for the recording of body movement in humans. Ankle- or waist-mounted pedometers are used to count the steps during walking or running. The number of steps in time is used as a measure of physical activity. Pedometers were designed for walking and running activities, but with another mechanical motion sensor, the actometer, it became possible to measure and quantify body movements. The major drawbacks of mechanical motion sensors are the low reliability and the complicated calibration of the instruments. Over the past two decades various types of electronic accelerometers have been introduced. These sensors measure both frequency and amplitude of accelerations produced during body movement. Due to the current knowledge in miniature computer technology there is also the opportunity to build very small and light instruments that can be worn for several days or weeks. The use of body-fixed accelerometers is an attractive and frequently applied method for the assessment of daily physical activity, but for translation of results to daily energy expenditure rates some more information is still needed.

5.4.5 Doubly labelled water techniques

The doubly labelled water technique is based on the fact that hydrogen atoms of body water leave the body via the usual routes of water loss—within urine, sweat and saliva, and as evaporated water—while the oxygen atoms of body water leave the body by the same routes but also via bicarbonate as carbon dioxide gas. Labelling a small proportion of body water molecules with the stable, non-radioactive isotopes ^2H and ^{18}O (heavy hydrogen and heavy oxygen) taken as a special drink of water, allows the respective fates of hydrogen and oxygen atoms in the water to be monitored: ^{18}O is lost at a faster rate than ^2H and the difference between the two disappearance rates in successive urine (or blood) samples is proportional to the subject's carbon dioxide production (see Fig. 5.3) over a period of one to three weeks. The composition of the diet should be estimated to

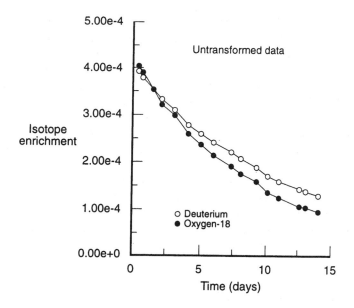

Fig. 5.3 Example of isotope disappearance curves from a typical adult subject (deuterium, ^{2}H). *Source*: Murgatroyd PR *et al. Int J Obesity* 1993; 17: 549–68.

give an estimate of RQ and hence, an estimate of the oxygen consumption. Subsequently, energy expenditure can be calculated by the traditional formulae for indirect calorimetry.

There are three main assumptions in the doubly labelled water method. One is an assumption about fractionation of the heavier isotope (e.g. when water evaporates via the lungs). A second assumption is that there is no net incorporation of ^{2}H into body tissues (as would occur if the subject gained weight). A third assumption is that the RQ can be adequately estimated for the whole one to three week experiment. This is usually obtained from the proportions of carbohydrate, fat and protein in the subject's diet (the 'food quotient').

The doubly labelled water method for the first time permits researchers to estimate objectively the energy expenditure of people going freely about their ordinary lives over about two weeks. It has given nutritionists new insights (e.g. that obese people under-report their energy intake). Disadvantages of doubly labelled water are that the ^{18}O isotope is very expensive and that a high-tech mass spectrometer and experienced operator are needed. It cannot be used to measure energy expenditure for shorter periods (e.g. 24 hours or the day-to-day variability of energy expenditure).

5.5 ADAPTATION IN ENERGY EXPENDITURE

5.5.1 Energy balance

Energy balance is usually defined as the difference between food energy intake (metabolizable energy) and energy expenditure (metabolized energy). If an individual is in a state of positive energy balance (i.e. if energy intake exceeds energy expenditure), body tissues will be deposited and body weight will increase. Likewise, in a state of negative energy balance body tissues will be mobilized and weight will decrease.

5.5.2 Adaptation in energy balance

If an individual with a stable body weight (and body composition) and an established daily activity pattern changes his/her habitual energy intake, he/she will get out of energy balance. The disturbance in energy balance will be partly compensated for by the altered contribution of dietary-induced thermogenesis. However, since thermogenesis amounts to about 10% of energy intake, only 10% of the disturbance will be met by the altered thermogenesis. In order to re-establish energy balance, 90% of the imbalance needs to be covered by other means. In principle, three types of adaptation in energy expenditure are conceivable: (1) biological adaptation, (2) social/behavioural adaptation, and (3) metabolic adaptation.

Biological adaptation means a change in body weight (or body composition). Suppose that the habitual intake of an individual has been reduced whereas their activity pattern remains unaltered. Then body weight will diminish, and so will the individual's basal metabolism and their energy cost for physical activity (a smaller body to be moved!). In this situation, body weight will decline until the reduced energy expenditure balances the new level of habitual intake.

Social/behavioural adaptation means a modification in activity pattern (including changes in pace of activities). An individual whose habitual intake has been reduced might achieve energy balance without losing weight if he/she reduces energy expenditure for physical activity by a lower activity pattern.

Metabolic adaptation includes mechanisms which might increase efficiency of energy metabolism. Little is known about metabolic adaptation, and many scientists doubt its existence. If metabolic adaptation really exists, it would mean that an individual whose habitual energy intake has been changed might re-establish energy balance without changes in body weight or in activity pattern.

It will be clear that with the various types of adaptation an individual may achieve energy balance at different levels of energy intake. In this respect adaptation can be considered as a process of moving from one energy balance level to another in response to fluctuations in energy intake.

5.5.3 Prices attached to adaptation

The various types of adaptation have a 'price'. In situations of reduced food intakes a new state of energy balance can be achieved by lowering body weight (biological adaptation). However, there will be a borderline for body weight under which a price is to be paid in terms of deterioration of health status or in terms of inability to maintain economically necessary and socially desirable physical activity. There will also be a borderline above which such prices are to be paid. This holds for all groups within the community. There will be borderlines for growth rates of infants and children, for weight gains over the period of pregnancy, for birth weights, for breast milk production, and so on, beyond which prices have to be paid in terms of economic and social function. The same is true for social/behavioural adaptations. Reducing levels of physical activity cannot continue without limit. A certain level (borderline) of physical activity will be needed for keeping good health and for allowing maintenance of economically necessary and socially desirable activity. Metabolic adaptation, if it exists, is the only type of adaptation which would be more or less without 'price'.

The World Health Organization has defined the energy requirement of an adult as the level of energy intake from food that will balance energy expenditure when the individual has a body size and composition, and level of physical activity, consistent with long-term good health; and that will allow for the maintenance of economically necessary and socially desirable physical activity. As noted before, an individual may achieve energy balance at different levels of energy intake. Whether a price has to be paid will depend upon how energy balance is re-established and upon the borderlines passed. Unfortunately, such borderlines have not been adequately mapped out. Until more is known about them, a definition of energy requirement as given by WHO is of limited use. More research about the borderlines of adaptation beyond which health status and level of economically and socially desirable physical activity are reduced warrants priority and is a big challenge for medical doctors, nutritionists, anthropologists, economists, and social scientists.

FURTHER READING

1. Brockway JM. Derivation of formulae used to calculate energy expenditure in man. Human Nutrition: *Clin Nutr* 1987; **41C**: 463–471.
2. FAO/WHO/UNO. *Energy and protein requirements*. Report of a joint expert consultation. Technical Report Series No. 724, Geneva: WHO, 1985.
3. Durnin JVGA, Passmore R. *Energy, work and leisure*. London: Heinemann, 1967.
4. Scrimshaw NS, Waterlow JC, Schürch B (eds). Energy and protein requirements. *Eur J Clin Nutr* 1996; **50** (suppl.): S1–S197.
5. James WPT, Schofield EC. *Human energy requirements. A manual for planners and nutritionists*. Oxford University Press, 1990.
6. Livesey G, Elia M. Estimation of energy expenditure, net carbohydrate utilization, and net fat oxidation and synthesis by indirect calorimetry: evaluation of errors with special reference to the detailed composition of fuels. *Am J Clin Nutr,* 1988; **47**: 608–28.
7. McNeil G. Energy. In: Garrow JS, James WPT (eds). *Human nutrition and dietetics*, 9th ed. Edinburgh and London: Churchill Livingstone, 1993: 24–37.
8. Murgatroyd PR, Shetty PS, Prentice AM. Techniques for the measurement of human energy expenditure: a practical guide. *Int J Obesity* 1993; **17**: 549–68.
9. Weir JB deV. New methods for calculating metabolic rate with special reference to protein metabolism. *J Physiol* 1949; **109**: 1–9.

$\mathbb{6}$

ALCOHOL

Stewart Truswell

Alcohol is the only substance that is both a nutrient and a drug affecting brain function. For chemists there are many alcohols but in day-to-day parlance, in the pub or bar, and in this chapter, 'alcohol' is used to mean ethyl alcohol (ethanol), C_2H_5OH. Other nutrients can have minor and subtle effects on brain function. A hungry person's behaviour can change after a satisfying meal without alcohol. Coffee contains the nutrient, niacin, but the mental stimulant in coffee is another substance, caffeine.

Alcohol is normally consumed not pure ('neat') but in aqueous solution in alcoholic beverages that were first developed thousands of years ago. Beer was drunk by the Sumerians and Babylonians, around 4000 BC and has been brewed in the Old World since. Wine is mentioned occasionally in the Old Testament (in Genesis 9, Noah planted a vineyard and got drunk), and was important in the life of classical Greece and Rome. It featured in Jesus' first miracle at the marriage feast in Cana and at his last supper, and passed into the central part of the Christian mass. Alcoholic beverages were also developed in prehistoric times in East Asia, e.g. sake fermented from rice, and in Africa beers from fermented millet or maize. Alcoholic beverages were thus independently discovered in different parts of the world by prehistoric sedentary agriculturalists who were growing barley, rice or grapes. But the indigenous peoples of Oceania (Polynesians and Australian Aborigines) and of America (American Indians) did not know alcohol until the arrival of the Europeans and had not established ways of using and controlling it.

From the basic fermented beverages alcohol can be concentrated by the process of distillation (which was brought to Europe by the Arabs). Brandy and whiskey first appeared in the fifteenth century.

6.1 PRODUCTION OF ALCOHOLIC BEVERAGES

Alcohol is produced by alcoholic fermentation of glucose. The specific enzymes are provided by certain yeasts, saccharomyces, which are unicellular fungi. The biochemical pathway first follows the usual nine steps of anaerobic glycolysis to pyruvate, as in animal metabolism (Chapter 2). Yeast contains the enzyme, pyruvate decarboxylase, not present in animals. This converts pyruvate to acetaldehyde, then alcohol dehydrogenase (working in the opposite direction from its role in humans) converts acetaldehyde to ethanol. The overall reaction is:

$$C_6H_{12}O_6 + \text{co-factors} + \text{ATP} \rightarrow 2C_2H_5OH + 2CO_2.$$

The co-factors include NADH, thiamin pyrophosphate and magnesium.

Grapes are unusual among fruits in containing a lot of sugar, nearly all glucose (around 16%), so providing an excellent substrate for alcoholic fermentation. Starch is a polymer of glucose. Before it can ferment to alcohol it has to be hydrolyzed to its constituent glucose units. Beers are made by malting the starch in barley. To do this the barley is spread out, wet and warm, and allowed to germinate for several days. Enzymes are generated in the sprouting grain that break down the stored starch into glucose. For *sake* a different process is used to break down the rice starch. It is first treated with a mould, *Aspergillus oryzae*, that grows on the rice and secretes an amylase to hydrolyze the starch.

Beer contains around 5% alcohol (unless alcohol-reduced), wines contain around 10% alcohol (unless fortified) and spirits are about 30% alcohol. Alcoholic beverages also contain variable amounts of unfermented sugars and dextrins (in beers), small amounts of alcohols other than ethyl (e.g. propyl alcohol), moderate amounts of potassium, almost no sodium, small amounts of riboflavin and niacin but no thiamin, and sometimes vitamin C, or they also contain a complex array of flavour compounds, colours (e.g. in red wines), phenolic compounds, a preservative (e.g. sodium metabisulphite), and sometimes additives. A standard drink (e.g. 1 pint of beer, see Table 6.3) provides 10 g of ethanol.

6.2   METABOLISM OF ALCOHOL

Ethanol is readily absorbed unchanged from the jejunum; it is one of the few substances that is also absorbed from the stomach. It is distributed throughout the total body water (moving easily through cell membranes), so that after having one drink its 10 g of alcohol is diluted in about 40 litres of water in an adult, giving a peak concentration of 0.025 g/dl in the blood and in the rest of body water. For comparison, the permitted limit of blood alcohol for driving in many countries is double this, 0.05 g/dl (11 mmol/l). Alcohol is nearly all metabolized in the liver but a small amount is already metabolized as it passes through the stomach wall (first pass metabolism). A small amount of alcohol passes unchanged into the urine and an even smaller (but diagnostically useful) amount is excreted in the breath.

There are three possible pathways for alcohol metabolism in man. The major pathway in most people starts with alcohol dehydrogenase (ADH), a zinc-containing enzyme in the cytoplasm of the liver (Box 6.1). ADH is the rate-limiting step in alcohol metabolism. ADH occurs in slightly different forms and some individuals have more active ADH than others. It may seem surprising that humans naturally possess this enzyme for dealing with beer and wine, to which our hunter–gatherer ancestors were not exposed. However, some alcohols are produced naturally by fermentation in the large intestine (e.g. small amounts of methyl alcohol from pectin), and they occur in over-ripe fruits. The next step

Box 6.1

$$CH_3CH_2OH + NAD \xrightarrow{\text{ADH}} CH_3CHO + NADH + H^+$$

Ethanol   Acetaldehyde

is conversion of acetaldehyde to acetate by aldehyde dehydrogenases (ALDH), which are present in the cytoplasm, mitochondria and microsomes (Box 6.2). In most people, there is no build up of acetaldehyde but nearly 50% of Chinese and Japanese people lack the mitochondrial ALDH, so after moderate intake of ethanol, their blood acetaldehyde increases. This causes facial flushing and headaches.

In long-term heavy drinkers the microsomal ethanol oxidizing system (MEOS) with cytochrome P450 becomes a second important route for alcohol metabolism. The microsomes proliferate (are induced) in heavy drinkers. As with ADH, ethanol is converted to acetaldehyde. A third minor pathway for conversion of ethanol to acetaldehyde is via catalase in peroxisomes.

On average, people can metabolize about 5 g of ethanol per hour (i.e. half a standard drink). The rate varies about twofold between individuals. Alcohol absorption can be slowed by having a meal, or even milk, in the stomach but there is no agent that increases the rate of alcohol metabolism. Smaller people are likely to have smaller livers and so

Box 6.2

$$CH_3CHO + NAD + H_2O \longrightarrow CH_3COOH + NADH + H^+$$

Acetaldehyde   ALDH   Acetic acid

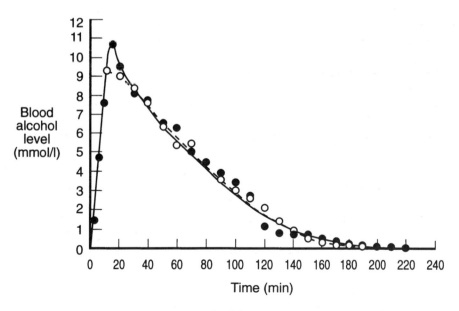

Fig. 6.1 Blood alcohol concentrations in a healthy young Caucasian man who took 0.3 g pure ethanol/kg body weight in orange juice, drunk rapidly and followed by a 4.4 MJ mixed meal. (○ and ● are duplicate determinations.) Ethanol was measured by gas chromatography.

93

metabolize less alcohol per hour. Women on average have smaller livers than men, a lower percentage of total body water (in which to distribute the alcohol) and also have less first pass gastric alcohol dehydrogenase, so that they are less tolerant of alcohol than men. East Asian people may suffer from headaches and flushing at quite low intakes of alcohol because of acetaldehyde accumulation. This may limit their intake.

A drug used to control alcohol addiction, disulfiram (Antabuse) antagonizes aldehyde dehydrogenase. People taking it experience unpleasant symptoms (headache, nausea, flushing) as a result of acetaldehyde accumulation when they have a drink.

6.3   EFFECT OF ALCOHOL ON THE BRAIN

Pharmacologists classify ethanol as a central nervous system depressant in the same group as general anaesthetics. With increasing levels of blood alcohol people pass through successive stages of alcohol intoxication (Table 6.1).

At the biochemical level alcohol affects a number of neurochemical processes simultaneously. Decreased levels of cyclic AMP and cyclic GMP, inhibition of voltage-sensitive calcium channels, increased intracellular calcium, increased GABA (γ-aminobutyric acid) activity and decreased glutamate have all been reported. Ethanol increases cell membrane fluidity.

Ingestion of alcohol has effects in other systems of the body. There is peripheral vasodilation and increased heart rate. The imbiber may feel warm but be losing more heat than usual. Alcohol inhibits hypothalamic osmoreceptors, hence there is pituitary antidiuretic hormone secretion so there is diuresis (an increased urine output) which can lead to dehydration, especially after drinking spirits.

Table 6.1   Successive stages of acute alcohol intoxication

Blood alcohol concentration (g/dl)	Stage	Effects
Up to 0.05	Feeling of well-being	Relaxed, talks a lot
0.05–0.08	Risky state	Judgement and finer movements affected
0.08–0.15	Dangerous state	Slow speech, balance affected, eyesight blurred, wants to fall asleep, likely to vomit, needs help to walk
0.2–0.4	Drunken stupor	Dead drunk, no bladder control, heavy breathing, unconscious (i.e. deep anaesthesia)
0.45–0.6	Death	Shock and death

6.4 ENERGY VALUE OF ETHANOL

The gross chemical energy of ethanol can be measured outside the body in a bomb calorimeter, and the value is between the energy value of carbohydrates and that of fat, about 30 kJ or 7.1 kcal/g.

However, in a metabolic ward, with food intakes strictly controlled Lieber (1992) replaced 50% of subjects' energy (calorie) intake by isocaloric amounts of ethanol (they had been accustomed to high alcohol intakes). Instead of gaining weight they lost weight. Free-living heavy drinkers are not usually overweight. It appears that above a certain intake ethanol provides less than 7 kcal/g. Alcohol increases the basal metabolic rate (thermogenesis) and it is thought that metabolism of alcohol by liver microsomes yields less energy than the ADH route.

In heavy drinkers, 10–30% (or more) of energy intake comes from alcohol, but alcoholic beverages contain no protein and very few micronutrients, that is, this nutrient-poor source of calories displaces other foods that normally provide essential nutrients. Appetite may be suppressed in heavy drinkers, either by alcoholic gastritis or by associated smoking. So alcohol dependency is an important cause of conditioned (or secondary) nutritional deficiency—the drinker may have access to enough foods and their nutrients but is not eating them. Nutrients that are typically depleted in alcoholics include thiamin, folate, niacin, and several inorganic nutrients (see below).

6.5 DIRECT CONSEQUENCES OF ALCOHOL INTAKE

6.5.1 Acute intoxication

Acute intoxication can lead to road and other accidents, or domestic and other violence. Intoxicated people can suffer a range of injuries. Occasionally people consume such a large dose of alcohol that they die with lethal blood levels. The breathalyzer was developed to reduce road traffic accidents. In many countries, a driver stopped at random by a police check who has a breathalyzer reading corresponding to a blood level of 0.05 g/dl has his driver's licence suspended. This measure has reduced traffic accidents and contributed to the decline of alcohol consumption in a number of developed countries.

6.5.2 Hangovers

The excess intake of alcohol the night before may not yet have all been cleared from the blood. Dehydration may be present from diuresis and, with some drinks (e.g. brandy), toxic effects of higher alcohols contribute to the symptoms.

6.5.3 Chronic alcoholism

Some people become dependent or addicted to alcohol and cannot face the world unless they have some alcohol in their blood throughout the day. Thus they maintain an intake of alcohol per day larger than their liver's capacity to metabolize it.

Box 6.3   Different patterns of alcohol consumption

> • The inexperienced drinker (e.g. an adolescent) who misjudges the dose and has an accident.
> • The person who doesn't drink during the week but drinks to excess and gets drunk on payday or Saturday night.
> • The person who enjoys a controlled 1 or 2 drinks most days.
> • The person who has too many drinks each day (most after work) but more or less maintains their (increasingly inefficient) usual life.
> • The person who goes on a binge or bender for weeks of heavy drinking.

6.5.4   Delirium tremens or alcohol withdrawal syndrome

This is the withdrawal syndrome in alcohol addicts, who have maintained some alcohol in their blood continuously for weeks or longer. Because of an accident or an illness they are abruptly removed from their alcohol supply and many experience severe agitation, tremors and hallucinations—not always pink elephants!

6.5.5   Binge drinkers

One pattern of alcohol excess is that a person starts drinking heavily and cannot stop. Consequently, as alcohol displaces much of the usual food intake there can be an acute deficiency of a micronutrient with the smallest reserve in the body, usually thiamin (see Wernicke–Korsakoff syndrome).

6.6   MEDICAL CONSEQUENCES OF EXCESS CONSUMPTION

6.6.1   Liver disease

Alcohol causes three types of liver damage. The least severe is fatty liver. Metabolism of large amounts of ethanol in the liver produce an increased ratio of NADH/NAD, this depresses the citric acid cycle and oxidation of fatty acids, and favours triglyceride synthesis in the liver cells. It used to be thought that the fatty liver was due to an associated nutritional deficiency but fatty liver has been observed (using needle biopsy of the liver) in volunteers who took a moderately large intake of alcohol but with all nutrients provided under strictly controlled conditions in hospital. The symptoms of fatty liver are not striking; on abdominal examination a doctor can feel that the liver is somewhat enlarged.

Alcoholic hepatitis   (inflammation of the liver) is more serious. This type is not caused by a virus but by prolonged excess alcohol intake. There is loss of appetite, fevers, tender liver, jaundice and elevation in the plasma of enzymes produced in the liver (e.g. aminotransferases (transaminases), glutamyl transpeptidase and alkaline phosphatase).

Alcoholic cirrhosis   may be associated with chronic alcoholism. When the liver has to metabolize large amounts of alcohol over a long time, membranes inside the cells become disordered; mitochondria show ballooning. In its fully developed form, irregular strands of fibrous tissue criss-cross the liver, replacing damaged liver parenchymal cells. These effects may be due to acetaldehyde or to free radical generation by neutrophil polymorph white cells in the liver. Cirrhosis seems to occur in people who have managed to consume large amounts of alcohol over many years but carry on a reasonably regular life and are able to eat and afford the alcohol. The amount of alcohol needed to cause cirrhosis is difficult to establish exactly because many people understate their alcohol consumption, especially heavy drinkers. It is greater than 40 g of ethanol in women and 50 g in men over years, usually much more.

6.6.2　Metabolic effects

Moderate regular drinkers who are apparently well tend to have increased plasma triglycerides (an overflow from the overproduction of fat in the liver). Plasma urate is raised because of reduced renal excretion probably due to increased blood lactate, which follows alcohol ingestion.

6.6.3　Fetal alcohol syndrome

Women who drink alcohol heavily during pregnancy can give birth to a baby with an unusual facial appearance (small eyes, absent philtrum, thin upper lip), prenatal and postnatal growth impairment, central nervous system dysfunction and often other physical abnormalities. Mothers of children with the fetal alcohol syndrome were heavy drinkers during their pregnancy and most were socially deprived. More moderate drinkers may have babies that are small for dates but otherwise normal. Some authorities insist that pregnant women should avoid all alcohol, but in a careful prospective study in Dundee, Scotland, Florey's group found that, after adjustment for the effect of smoking, social class and mother's size, there was no detectable effect on pregnancy of alcohol consumption below 100 g/week (i.e. one standard drink a day).

6.6.4　Wernicke–Korsakoff syndrome

In binge drinkers who consume large amounts of alcohol and virtually stop eating for three or more weeks, brain function can be affected by acute thiamin deficiency. Ethanol uses up thiamin for its metabolism, yet alcoholic beverages provide no thiamin; there is no rich food source of thiamin and body stores are very small (Chapter 12). In Wernicke's encephalopathy the patient is quietly confused—not an easy state to recognize in an alcoholic. The diagnostic feature, if the sufferer is brought to medical attention, is that the eyes cannot move properly (ophthalmoplegia). When Wernicke's encephalopathy is treated, the ophthalmoplegia and confusion clear but the patient may be left with a loss of recent memory, the inability to recall what has happened recently (Korsakoff's psychosis). It has been suggested that when an alcoholic has a partner who provides food, containing some thiamin, Wernicke's encephalopathy is less likely. The incidence has been high in Australia and as a preventive measure bread has been fortified with thiamin since 1991, as it already is in the United States, United Kingdom and most other developed countries. Korsakoff's psychosis can be permanent. It is one cause of alcohol-related brain damage. Wernicke's encephalopathy uncommonly occurs in people who have not taken alcohol (e.g. with persistent vomiting of pregnancy, hyperemesis gravidarum).

6.6.5   Other nutritional deficiencies in alcoholics

In societies with adequate food supply, vitamin deficiencies are rare but do occur in heavy drinkers. Chronic thiamin or other B-vitamin deficiency may be responsible for a peripheral neuropathy in the legs, with reduced function of the motor and sensory nerves and diminished ankle jerks. Folate metabolism is commonly impaired in alcoholics and megaloblastic anaemia may be seen. Vitamin A metabolism is abnormal where there is alcoholic liver disease: the liver does not store retinol normally or synthesize retinol-binding protein adequately. There can, consequently, be reduced plasma retinol and night blindness. Among inorganic nutrients, plasma magnesium and zinc can be subnormal in alcoholics.

6.6.6   Predisposition to some types of cancer

The risk of cancer of the mouth and pharynx is increased, especially when high alcohol intakes are combined with smoking. Other cancers associated with alcohol consumption are those of the oesophagus or liver (primary cancer of the liver is a complication of cirrhosis) and the rectum (in some beer drinkers).

6.6.7   Gastrointestinal complications

Chronic gastritis and gastric or duodenal ulcers may be associated with excessive alcohol consumption. Acute pancreatitis is a severe complication.

6.6.8   Hypertension

The prevalence of hypertension (raised arterial blood pressure) increases with usual alcohol intakes above 3 or 4 drinks per day. Prompt falls of moderately elevated blood pressures have been well documented in heavy drinkers admitted to hospital for detoxication. The mechanism for the hypertensive effect of chronic alcoholism is not yet clear. However, in acute intoxication the blood pressure tends to fall.

6.7   Alcohol and Coronary Heart Disease

Opposed to the deleterious effect of alcohol on blood pressure is its beneficial effect in reducing the risk of coronary heart disease, the commonest single cause of death in many countries. Over 20 large population studies, undertaken by leading epidemiologists in several countries, have all found that light to moderate alcohol consumption appears to protect against coronary heart disease (CHD). At post-mortem examination pathologists have long known to expect little or no atheroma in the arteries of people dying of alcoholic complications. But the discovery that light to moderate drinking is negatively associated with CHD emerged only in the 1980s. It was surprising to find a major health benefit of alcohol drinking.

The longest established mechanism for this protective effect (known since 1969) is that alcohol consumption increases plasma high-density lipoprotein (HDL) cholesterol which is a well-established protective factor for CHD (Chapter 18). There are two main fractions of HDL: less dense HDL_2 has a closer negative association with CHD than the more dense HDL_3. When subjects took moderate controlled amounts of alcohol in short-term experiments, only HDL_3 was increased, but in surveys of population samples HDL_2 cholesterol was also raised in people regularly consuming moderate amounts of alcohol (i.e. the HDL fractions appear to respond differently to long-term than to short-term alcohol intake). The increase of HDL cholesterol in moderate drinkers is not sufficient to fully explain their lower risk of CHD.

Two other mechanisms have been proposed. It seems likely that alcohol reduces the tendency to thrombosis. It is not possible to test this directly but alcohol reduces the aggregation of platelets on glass in response to collagen and ADP. A third mechanism is that polyphenolic compounds (e.g. quercetin) are present in wines, and they have antioxidant properties that may reduce oxidation of low-density lipoprotein (LDL) (Chapters 15 and 18). The evidence to support this is indirect. In one experiment subjects consumed 400 ml red wine/day for two weeks: their blood was taken, LDL extracted and shown *in vitro* to be less susceptible to oxidation (by copper) than at the start of the experiment. It has been suggested that the antioxidants in wine, especially red wine, might explain the French paradox (Box 6.4).

Box 6.4   The French paradox

- The death rate from coronary heart disease in France is apparently lower than in any other developed country (see Fig. 18.2).
- However, French diet is considered to be rich in fat. National consumption of butter and cheese are both high, and plasma cholesterols measured with standardized techniques by WHO monitoring (MONICA) centres are much the same in Strasbourg and Lille (France) as in Glasgow (Scotland), a city with a high rate of CHD; percent above 6.5 mmol/l, are 46%, 49% and 43% respectively.
- It is suggested that France's high alcohol consumption (highest in the world) and anti-oxidants in vegetables and fruits or red wine might explain this French paradox.
- Meanwhile, life expectancy at birth in 1993 was 77 years in Australia, Canada, Israel, Italy, Netherlands and Norway, the same as in France, and the French death rate from cirrhosis of the liver is about the highest in the world.

6.8   ALCOHOL AND ALL CAUSES DEATH RATE: THE J- OR U-SHAPED CURVE

Because of all the social and medical complications of excess alcohol intake we might expect a graph of total mortality against alcohol consumption to be a straight line upwards with the lowest rate in teetotallers. However, the results of at least 18 large prospective studies in seven different countries in men and women all show that the death rate in light to moderate drinkers is lower than in teetotallers.

Table 6.2   Relative risks of total mortality and mortality from coronary heart disease (CHD) in 276 802 men in the United States (aged 40–59 years at entry) in a 12-year follow-up

	Drinks per day							
	0	<1	1	2	3	4	5	6+
Total death rate	1.00	0.88	0.84	0.93	1.02	1.08	1.22	1.38
CHD death rate	1.00	0.86	0.79	0.80	0.83	0.74	0.85	0.92

Source: Boffeta P, Garfinkel L. Alcohol drinking and mortality among men enrolled in an American Cancer Society Prospective Study. *Epidemiology* 1990; 1: 342–8.

This lower death rate at light to moderate intakes is due to protection from CHD, which is the commonest single cause of death. With higher intakes the death rate climbs to exceed the teetotallers rate due to increasing rates of accidents, cirrhosis, hypertension, strokes, some cancers, etc. But note that nearly all prospective studies have studied people who were middle aged at entry.

Whether moderate alcohol consumption is good for health overall depends on people's age and risk of CHD. For example, Scragg (1995) estimates that alcohol was responsible for 20% of all deaths in 15 to 34-year-olds in New Zealand, mostly from road injuries. In contrast, it is estimated to have prevented 0.5% of all deaths among 35 to 64-year-olds and prevented 3.4% of all deaths among people over 65 years of age. Since young people can expect to live longer than older people the number of person-years lost among ages less than 35 years was greater than those saved in the older age group. Thus, advantageous effects of alcohol are not widely recommended as a beneficial public health measure.

6.9   RECOGNITION OF THE PROBLEM DRINKER

There are different types of alcohol abuse. An 'alcoholic' is a group term for any person whose drinking is leading to harm. This harm may be alcohol dependence or physical disease or social harm.

People drinking more than others or more than they feel they should are very likely to underestimate their alcohol intake when asked. The spouse or other family member may give a very different answer. Doctors are trained to suspect when someone is drinking too much and researchers use tactfully drafted questionnaires. Alcohol can be smelt on the breath and detected in the breath, blood or urine within hours of drinking. If a person has not been recently drinking there are changes in the blood which are suggestive of long-term excessive alcohol intake:

1. Increased red cell volume (mean corpuscular volume).

2. Increased γ-glutamyl transferase (GGT) activity.

3. Increased plasma (fasting) triglycerides (i.e. very low-density lipoproteins).

4. Increased plasma urate.

5. Increased plasma transaminases (aminotransferases).

6. Increased plasma carbohydrate-deficient transferrin.

These vary in sensitivity and specificity. Enzymes (2) and (5) and proteins (3) and (6) are produced in the liver. Increased urate is a result of increased plasma lactate. Increased red cell volume is sometimes due to folate depletion; its cause in most cases is not yet clear.

6.10   Is Alcoholism a Disease or the Top End of a Normal Distribution?

Alcoholism is a costly problem in most communities because of associated diseases, accidents, loss of earning, medical expenses and social misery. There are two philosophical approaches. One is the medical model which sees alcoholism as a disease which should be treated by the health professions. The other is the society model: the more alcohol sold and consumed, the larger will be the number of alcoholics. There are sections of society (e.g. some occupations, deprived minorities) who are at increased risk and there are social practices that contribute to alcohol abuse.

Ledermann (1956) put forward the hypothesis that in a homogeneous population the distribution of alcohol consumption is a logarithmic normal curve and that the number of people who drink a certain amount can be calculated if the average consumption is known (Fig. 6.2). This theory predicts that major complications of alcoholism in a country will be related to average national consumption. Governments rely on this principle in maintaining substantial taxes on alcohol, and other measures to reduce its free availability.

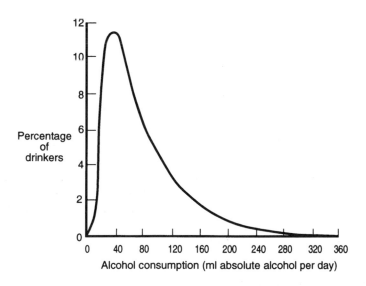

Fig. 6.2 Hypothetical curve proposed by Ledermann (1956). In a homogeneous population alcohol consumption is distributed in a logarithmic normal curve. *Source*: From British Medical Journal 1982.

6.11 GENETIC LIABILITY TO ALCOHOL DEPENDENCE?

Occurrence of alcoholism in families could be learnt behaviour rather than genetic. From comparing monozygotic with dizygotic twins the heritability of amount and frequency of alcohol drinking appears to be about 0.36 (i.e. one-third of the way along the scale from purely environmental to purely genetic). But studies on twins cannot completely exclude environmental effects. Adoption studies have shown that the sons of alcoholic fathers are four times more likely to become alcoholics than the sons of fathers who were not alcoholics. The search is on to find one or more variation of brain metabolism which makes people more likely to become alcohol-dependent. There have been several claims (e.g. abnormality of brain handling of dopamine or serotonin) but none has been convincingly confirmed.

6.12 RECOMMENDED INTAKES OF ALCOHOL

Nutritionists have been slow and reluctant to accept the accumulated evidence that there are some health benefits for older people of moderate alcohol intake, along with the undoubted costs of the many complications of excessive alcohol intake. The usual form in which alcohol is mentioned in national sets of dietary guidelines (Chapter 32) is drink alcohol in moderation, if at all.

Because women have lower rates of metabolizing alcohol, advice on safe drinking levels has to be different for men and women. Recommendations are expressed in standard drinks that contain 10 g of pure alcohol. In men, two to three standard drinks per day (20–30 g alcohol) (i.e. 140–210 g alcohol/week), are usually biologically safe, but no more than two drinks before driving and a minority of men should not take this

Table 6.3 Volume of various alcoholic beverages providing approximately 10 g ethanol

Type of drink	Usual % ethanol[a] v/v (by volume)	Vol. that provides approx. 10 g ethanol
Low alcohol beer	2–3%	568 ml = 1 (UK) pint = 20 oz
Average beer	4–5%	285 ml = $\frac{1}{2}$ (UK) pint = 10 oz
Average wine[b]	10%	120 ml = 4 oz
Fortified wine (e.g. sherry, port)	20%	60 ml = 2 oz
Spirits (e.g. whisky, gin, vodka, brandy)	40%	30 ml = 1 oz

[a] *Note:* (1) That these are approximations. The exact percentage of alcohol should be on the label of the bottle. (2) The specific gravity of ethanol is 0.790. To convert to g/100 ml multiply by 0.79 (or 0.8).
[b] Wine bottles usually contain 750 ml = $6\frac{1}{4}$ standard drinks.

much, or even any alcohol (e.g. people with liver disease, taking other sedative drugs, with a history of alcohol dependence). In women, the biologically safe intake is one to two drinks (10–20 g alcohol) per day (i.e. 70 to 140 g alcohol/week). As well as the same contraindications as in men, intake should be one drink or less in pregnancy or if a woman thinks she might be pregnant. Children should not take alcohol but in some cultures they are offered a small amount of wine with the family's main meal and some believe this can be a good training in moderation in consumption of alcohol. The quantities of various alcoholic beverages providing 10 g ethanol are shown in Table 6.3.

FURTHER READING

1. *Alcohol problems: ABC of alcohol; alcohol and alcoholism.* London: The British Medical Journal, 1982.
2. Boffeta P, Garfinkel L. Alcohol drinking and mortality among men enrolled in an American Cancer Society prospective study. *Epidemiology* 1990; **1**: 342–8.
3. Doll R, Peto R, Hall E, Wheatley K, Gray R. Mortality in relation to consumption of alcohol: 13 years' observations on male British doctors. *BMJ* 1994; **309**: 911–8.
4. Frezza M, di Padova C, Pozzato G, Terpin M, Baraona E, Lieber CS. High blood alcohol levels in women. The role of decreased gastric alcohol dehydrogenase activity and first-pass metabolism. *N Engl J Med* 1990; **322**: 95–9.
5. Holman CDJ, English DR, Milne E, Winter MG. Meta-analysis of alcohol and all-cause mortality: a validation of NH & MRC recommendations. *Med J Aust* 1996; **164**: 141–5.
6. Ledermann S. *Alcool, alcoolism, alcoolisation.* Paris: Presse Universitaires de France, 1956.
7. Lieber CS (ed.). *Medical and nutritional complications of alcoholism. Mechanisms and management.* New York and London: Plenum, 1992.
8. Norton R, Batey R, Dwyer T, MacMahon S. Alcohol consumption and the risk of alcohol related cirrhosis in women. *BMJ* 1987; **295**: 80–2.
9. Rimm EB, Klatsky A, Grobbee D, Stampfer MJ. Review of moderate alcohol consumption and reduced risk of coronary heart disease: is the effect due to beer, wine, or spirits? *BMJ* 1996; **312**: 731–6.
10. Sulaiman ND, Florey C du V, Taylor DJ, Ogston SA. Alcohol consumption in Dundee primigravidas and its effects on outcome of pregnancy. *BMJ* 1988; **296**: 1500–3.
11. Scragg R. A quantification of alcohol-related mortality in New Zealand. *Aust NZ J Med* 1995; **25**: 5–11.

Part II: Organic and inorganic essential nutrients

7

WATER, ELECTROLYTES AND ACID–BASE BALANCE

James Robinson

7.1 BODY WATER

7.1.1 Importance of water

In 1913, Lawrence Henderson explained how peculiar properties resulting from its hydrogen-bonded structure make water an essential constituent of all known forms of life. It is, remarkably, liquid in the range of 'ordinary' temperatures at which biochemical reactions can occur in solution or at active sites of enzymes in contact with water. Its high specific heat moderates temperature gradients; high latent heats allow efficient cooling by evaporation and protect against damage by frost. A dielectric constant large enough to reduce by 80 times forces between charges immersed in it makes water a superb solvent for ionic compounds. It is also a good solvent for most organic compounds (apart from fats and hydrocarbons) and even when the active sites of enzymes are in clefts which exclude water molecules, most reactants must arrive and most products move away in aqueous solution.

7.1.2 Amount and distribution in the body

The extent to which freely diffusible substances (e.g. ethanol, urea, isotopic forms of water) are diluted after being ingested or injected shows that adult persons contain about 35–45 litres of water, which makes up 50–70% of their body weight, depending on how fat they are. The fat-free tissues contain 60–80% of water by weight, but fat stored in fat cells contains none.

However, the body is not just a tracksuit-shaped bag, two-thirds full. The water is in a large number of smaller compartments—in cells, body cavities, blood vessels, etc. Dilution of solutes that do not cross cell membranes gives volumes outside the cells (in extracellular fluid, ECF) between 12 and 20 litres, the higher estimates being better than older ones based on test solutes that failed to diffuse completely into dense tissues. The volumes quoted are approximate. No two people are identical; different observers and methods yield results which are similar but not the same. Hence books do not all agree, but 42 litres for total body water (TBW), 23 litres intracellular (IC), and 19 litres extracellular (EC) water per 70 kg body weight are reasonable estimates. Of the ECF, 3.5 litres is plasma circulating in the blood vessels. The rest bathes the cells—an overcrowded

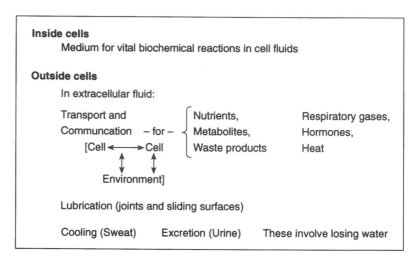

Fig. 7.1   Principal functions of water in the body.

and somewhat salty pond we carry with us for them to live in. In 1878, Claude Bernard called the ECF the 'internal environment' of the cells; it nourishes them, supplies their needs and takes away their waste products. The circulating blood keeps it stirred so that it can transport heat and substances in solution from one cell to others, and between cells inside the body and the external environment. The principal functions of water in the body are summarized in Fig. 7.1.

7.1.3   Body fluids

The fluids in the body are not pure water. Intracellular fluid (ICF) and extracellular fluid (ECF) are distinct solutions, with different things dissolved in them. The ECF is like a diluted sea water, containing mainly sodium salts, chiefly chloride, some bicarbonate, small but important concentrations of potassium, calcium and magnesium. The ICF contains mainly potassium salts, mostly organic phosphate and proteinate; small amounts of sodium, magnesium and bicarbonate; a little chloride and very little calcium (see Table 7.1). The cell membranes are somewhat permeable to sodium and potassium, hence cells must use a large part of the energy from their metabolism pumping out sodium that diffuses in and getting back potassium that leaks out. Even at rest, the cells are very busy! They use about 40 kg adenosine triphosphate (ATP) each day to supply the energy for maintenance; up to 0.5 kg per minute during maximal exertion!

The cell membranes are also permeable to water, so the total concentration (osmolarity) is the same in the cells and in the ECF. The concentration of sodium in the ECF is about 150 mmol/l, and the concentration of potassium in the cells is about 150 mmol/l of cell water. A very important consequence of this is that so long as osmolarity throughout the body water is kept constant (the kidneys and thirst together control this), the volume of ECF is fixed by the amount of sodium in it (litres of ECF = mmol of EC Na ÷ 150 mmol/l), and the volume of the cells is likewise fixed by the amount of intracellular potassium (mmol cell K/150 mmol/l).

Table 7.1 Muscle cell fluid and blood plasma as typical intracellular fluid (ICF) and extracellular fluid (ECF)

Muscle cell fluid (mmol/l water)				Plasma (mmol/l water)			
K^+	150	Org P^-	130	Na^+	150	Cl^-	110
Na^+	10	HCO_3^-	10	K^+	5	HCO_3^-	27
Mg^{2+}	10	Cl^-	5	Ca^{2+}	2	Org^-	5
Ca^{2+}	10^{-4}	$Prot^{17-}$	2	Mg^{2+}	1	$H_2PO_4^-$	2
						$Prot^{17-}$	1
Reaction:	pH 7.1			pH 7.4			
Osmolarity:	285 mosmol/l cell water			285 mosmol/l plasma water			

Note: Because only about 95% of plasma is water, laboratory results per litre of plasma are lower than these. Average cell fluid is only about 80% water.
Source: Modified with permission from Bray JJ, Cragg PA, Macknight ADC, Mills RG, Taylor DW. *Lecture notes on human physiology*. 3rd ed. Oxford: Blackwell, 1994.

Note that the kidneys, by adjusting the excretion of water to keep osmolarity constant in the body fluids, set the stage both for the amount of sodium in the ECF to determine its volume, and for the cells to determine their own volume by regulating the amount of potassium they contain. This assumes an adequate supply of water; the kidneys cannot make water but only regulate its loss.

7.1.4 Water balance

The fact that people keep very much the same weight implies that the amount of water in the body is kept constant, gains being balanced against losses. Weighing is therefore the best way to measure day-to-day changes in the amount of water in the body.

Regulation of water balance Loss of water makes body fluids more concentrated. All the cells lose water and shrink as osmotic pressure of the ECF rises. Special cells in the hypothalamus at the base of the brain respond to shrinking: (1) by sending messages which excite the sensation of thirst, and (2) by releasing into the blood an antidiuretic hormone (ADH) which allows the renal tubules to reabsorb water from dilute urine and return it to the blood. If gains of water exceed losses, cells swell, the thirst message is switched off, no more ADH is released and a flow of dilute urine, 'water diuresis', quickly gets rid of excess water. There are also nervous paths from receptors in the heart and large central blood vessels that stimulate thirst and release of ADH when the volume of blood shrinks, or stop the release of ADH when blood volume is restored.

Orders of magnitude of gains and losses of water

Intake

1. 'Solid' food, 1.0 l/day.
2. Metabolic water (oxidation of hydrogen in metabolites), 0.3 l/day.
3. Beverages, 1.0 l/day or more, voluntary intakes may be much more!

Output

Note. Most of these are unavoidable losses from the body.

1. *Evaporation* of vapour from skin and lung surfaces, which must be moist to remain flexible and to allow exchange of gases in solution. About 1.0 l/day at rest; much more from the lungs with increased ventilation during exercise, especially at high altitudes; more than 2.0 l/day above 6000 m. The first successful ascent of Mount Everest depended partly on allowing for the magnitude of this loss.

2. *Sweat*: up 15 l/day may be secreted by sweat glands to get rid of heat.

3. *Faeces*: normally 0.1 l/day; with choleraic diarrhoeas may reach 10 or 12 l/day.

4. *Urine*: at least as much water as can carry the day's soluble waste products in the most concentrated urine the kidneys can make. With normal kidneys, and urine four times as concentrated as plasma, this is about 0.6 l; it becomes 2.4 l if kidneys cannot make urine more concentrated than plasma, and may be more than 10 l in patients with diabetes insipidus who fail to produce ADH or whose kidneys do not respond to it.

Wild animals (at greater risk from predators when they stand still to drink or urinate) often seem to drink only enough to replace unavoidable losses. Many people drink more and rely on water diuresis to match output to their voluntary intake.

Both excesses and deficiencies of body water can occur, and may threaten life.

7.1.5   Deficiency of body water

Simple dehydration from loss of water may be caused by reduced intake or increased losses, or by a combination of both. Even when intake is zero, unavoidable losses continue, and they may be increased, for example, from skin and lungs by activity and fever, from the gut by diarrhoea or vomiting; the continuous aspiration of stomach contents to prevent vomiting can also make the mouth a channel of loss instead of intake.

If water is lost, first from the ECF, which is in contact with the external environment, and is not replaced, the osmolarity of all the body fluids and the concentration of sodium in the plasma increase. Osmotic pressure could be corrected by excreting sodium, but this does not happen in man. Instead, sodium disappears from the urine and is avidly retained in the body. Its concentration in sweat, intestinal and other secretions is also reduced as more aldosterone is secreted from the adrenal cortex in response to the lower volumes of plasma and ECF. This 'dehydration reaction' has survival value—the high osmotic pressure maintains thirst and the output of ADH, minimizing urinary loss and keeping up the search for water. Increased extracellular osmolarity also withdraws water from cells and helps to sustain the volumes of ECF and circulating blood which are essential to the search for water and take precedence over the regulation of osmolarity. In rats, rabbits, sheep and dogs, an initial increase in the excretion of sodium may precede the onset of this dehydration reaction.

Symptoms   The cardinal manifestation of primary deficiency of water is thirst, which can dominate what remains of a disordered consciousness ('My thirst was the tallest tree in a forest of pain', Admiral Byrd). Loss of 20% or more by American men in the desert may leave the dry skin cracking and oozing blood ('blood sweat') as the men become senseless automata scratching in the sand for water until they die, from respiratory failure. See Box 1 for information on effects of water loss in open country in New Zealand.

Fresh water may be as unavailable at sea as in deserts; the dry mouth, swollen tongue, and delirium with hallucinations were admirably described in 1798 by Samuel Taylor Coleridge, in *The Rime of the Ancient Mariner*.

> And every tongue through utter drought, Was withered at the root;
> We could not speak, no more than if We had been choked with soot.
> With throats unslaked, with black lips baked, We could not laugh nor wail;
> Through utter drought all dumb we stood! I bit my arm, I suck'd the blood,
> And cried, 'A sail! a sail!'

R.A. McCance, Professor of Experimental Medicine at Cambridge (England), during World War II was chairman of a subcommittee of the British Admiralty concerned with safeguarding the lives of hundreds of men cast adrift in lifeboats or rafts after their ships were sunk by enemy action. He studied volunteers in life rafts in temperate, arctic and tropical seas, and came to the firm conclusion that sea water could not be used to supplement limited supplies of fresh water. Reports of survivors showed that those who drank sea water became more delirious and were liable to disappear over the side. Sea water has a higher salt concentration than human kidneys can achieve; hence drinking it actually removes water from the body and makes dehydration worse. Any temporary improvement in circulation and feeling when water is withdrawn from cells is over-shadowed by shortened survival. It is of no ultimate advantage to feel better on Monday and die on Tuesday if it happens that your party is not going to be rescued until Wednesday.

Treatment   The remedy for primary water deficiency is water, as the predominant symptom of thirst indicates. It is important to realize that this kind of dehydration is not confined to oceans and deserts; it can even turn up in hospital wards if thirst fails or cannot be satisfied. Unconscious patients do not experience thirst; others may be too

---

Box 7.1   Survival without water in New Zealand

Amount of body water lost:

- 1–5% body weight: thirst; vague discomfort; economy of movement; no appetite; flushed skin; impatience; increased pulse rate; nausea.

- 6–10% body weight: dizziness; headache; laboured breathing; tingling in limbs; absence of saliva; blue body (cyanosis); indistinct speech; inability to walk.

- 11–12% body weight: delirium; twitching; swollen tongue; inability to swallow; deafness; dim vision; shrivelled skin; numb skin.

'A man can exist for days without food, but only for 2–5 days without water.'

Source: Hildreth B. *How to survive in the bush, on the coast, in the mountains of New Zealand*. Wellington, Government Printer, 1979.

confused or too weak to drink water set beside them. Alexander Leaf once remarked: 'These people are in great danger, for their osmostat is in their physician's head.' A full jug and glass on the bedside locker does not guarantee there is enough water in the patient.

Summing up   In primary dehydration from simple lack of water, the cells share the loss with the ECF; and hence arouse thirst, which normally indicates what is needed for treatment. Old people and their caregivers need to bear in mind that thirst, water diuresis and the response to ADH tend to become attenuated with advancing years; hence these people are increasingly at risk of dehydration, with the possibility of a vicious circle if chronically high osmolarity further impairs their awareness of thirst and the need for water.

7.1.6   Excess of body water

An excessive amount of water in the body is rarer than deficiency, for water diuresis protects agains excess, and normal kidneys can excrete water as fast as the gut can absorb it. But water diuresis can fail:

(1) *in anuria*: with absence of renal function the kidneys cannot respond to absence of ADH; and

(2) *with inappropriate release of ADH*: e.g. after trauma, including surgery, head injury, or antidiuretic substances from some tumours.

If patients in these conditions are given much more than about 1 litre per day, which they need to replace unavoidable losses, EC osmolarity and sodium concentration fall, so that water goes into cells, which swell. Weakness and cramps appear. Swelling of brain cells leads to water intoxication in which disturbances of consciousness and behaviour may progress to convulsions and death.

Low osmolarity and low plasma sodium concentration (hyponatremia) can occur without an excess of total body water (e.g. if the water, but not the salt, lost in profuse sweating is replaced). Muscle cramps are then the chief feature—once known as miners' cramps and stokers' cramps, common in English coal mines and ships. J.B.S. Haldane showed in 1928 that extra salt prevents or cures these cramps, and miners in hot mines commonly added salt to their beer.

7.2   SODIUM AND EXTRACELLULAR FLUID

7.2.1   Significance and functions of sodium

Salt has long been a valuable commodity and part of the fabric of human life and culture. We pay salaries, the *salarium* being the allowance for a Roman soldier to buy salt; and we still question whether a man is worth his salt. Salt mines are traditional sites of strenuous, unpleasant but essential labour. Some animals in arid regions trek vast distances to salt licks to get the sodium they need in order to excrete potassium from their high potassium vegetable diet.

Common salt is sodium chloride, NaCl; each gram contains 17.1 mmol of sodium, which is the principal cation in most extracellular fluids and is responsible for 95% of their osmolarity. Its concentration, regulated at 150 mmol/l in man and most animals, helps to stabilize the potassium/sodium ratio which determines the membrane potentials of most cells and the action potentials underlying the transmission of nerve impulses and the contraction of muscles. It is responsible for maintaining the volume (at 1 l for every 150 mmol, or 9 g NaCl) of the extracellular fluids that the cells live in.

7.2.2 Amount and distribution of sodium in the body

Adult persons contain about 5600 mmol of sodium (325 g NaCl). About half, 2800 mmol, is dissolved in the extracellular fluids, with 300 in cells and 2500 in bone mineral. Half of the sodium in the bones is exchangeable with isotopically labelled Na, the rest deeper and less accessible; hence classical analyses of dissolved bodies found more sodium than modern measurements based upon isotopic dilution during life.

7.2.3 Sodium balance

Intake

Diet: 70–250 mmol/day; very variable with habit, taste and custom.

1. Natural foods contain 0.1–3.0 mmol Na per 100 g; fruits 0.1 mmol/g; vegetables 0.3 mmol/g; meat, fish and eggs about 3.0 mmol/100 g.
2. Processed foods contain far more; bread around 20 mmol/100 g; cheese 30 mmol/ 100 g; salted butter 40 mmol/100 g; raw lean bacon as much as 80 mmol/100 g.

   People add widely varying amounts of salt in cooking or at the table. Nevertheless, discretionary salt taken is usually much lower than that obtained from manufactured and processed food products.

Output

1. *Faeces*: normally 5–10 mmol/day.
2. *Sweat*: 20–80 mmol/day; extremely variable, see 7.2.4 below.
3. *Urine*: variable; normally somewhat less than dietary intake.

   The kidneys are capable of excreting between 1 and 500 mmol/day; they normally keep the amount in the body constant by excreting the excess of intake over the sum of other losses. Homer Smith's one-time remark that the composition of the body depends 'not on what the mouth takes in but on what the kidneys keep' aptly sums up their control of sodium balance.

   The rate of excretion of sodium depends on the balance between glomerular filtration rate (GFR × [Na]) and tubular reabsorption. When blood and extracellular fluid (ECF) volumes fall, GFR is reduced by constriction of glomerular vessels, and reabsorption is increased by several factors. A major factor is aldosterone, secreted from the adrenal cortex. When blood pressure or volume is reduced and sympathetic nerves are activated, renin is released from the kidney; this is an enzyme which forms angiotensin-I from a precursor in the plasma. Another enzyme in blood and some tissues converts this to angiotensin-II which stimulates the adrenal cortex. When blood volume increases these conserving mechanisms are turned off, GFR increases, and renal nerves inhibit instead of promoting tubular reabsorption; reabsorption is also inhibited by a natriuretic peptide from the heart and by other hormones which keep being discovered!

7.2.4 Sodium depletion

Deficiency of sodium is not caused simply by a deficient intake, for the kidneys can make the urine almost salt-free. Abnormal losses causing depletion may be in:

1. *Sweat*, up to even 15 l/day. Sweat is hypotonic, but if its sodium concentration is 50 mmol/l, this takes as much salt as in 5 l of normal ECF, so that even after osmolarity is corrected by replacing water, the volume of the ECF will be reduced by 5 l.
2. *Intestinal fluid*. 10 l/day of intestinal secretions are normally reabsorbed; but with diarrhoea absorption is depressed and intestinal fluid secretion often increased; losses may reach 18 l/day in cholera, and the fluid lost is almost isotonic, equivalent to its own volume of ECF.
3. *Urine*. The kidneys normally act to guard the body's stores of sodium, but in Addison's disease the adrenal cortex fails to produce aldosterone, and the kidneys fail to conserve sodium. The kidneys may also lose sodium in some types of renal failure. Diuretic drugs, and osmotic diuresis (e.g. with the load of glucose and ketone acids in diabetes), may remove large amounts of sodium in the urine.

Provided that osmolarity is maintained, 1 litre of water is lost with every 150 mmol of sodium; the result used to be called 'dehydration secondary to loss of salt' but 'saline depletion' is a better description. It is important to realize that all the water that is lost comes from the extracellular fluid, which bears the brunt of the dehydration. Without loss from the cells, there are only weaker, non-osmotic, stimuli to release antidiuretic hormone (ADH), so that the urine may not be extremely scanty and concentrated; thirst is also less pronounced than after the loss of a similar amount of water without salt, but the threat to survival through the reductions in the volumes of blood and ECF is much more severe.

Symptoms   The cardinal manifestation is peripheral circulatory failure, which may be sudden and unexpected if premonitory signs are missed: dry mouth and tongue, shrunken skin lacking turgor, sunken eyes with low pressure, rapid weak pulse, low blood pressure. Packed cell volume (PCV), the concentrations of haemoglobin and plasma albumin, and blood viscosity all increase as the volume of plasma falls along with that of the ECF. When oxygen transport to tissues is badly impaired, cells swell taking up sodium and water; this further reduces the volume of ECF and may set up a vicious circle leading rapidly to a disastrous collapse of the circulation—a sort of 'medical shock'.

Treatment   Salt as well as water is required to treat this desperate state. Water given alone or by infusing glucose solutions will disappear into the cells with the risk of water intoxication. Isotonic saline supplies sodium and water in the proportions in which they are deficient.

7.2.5 Experimental human salt deficiency

R.A. McCance subjected himself and a few other healthy people to forced sweating for two hours each day while they ate a low salt diet and drank only distilled water. They lost about 1 kg/day for three or four days, while plasma sodium concentrations remained normal. After that the loss of sodium continued, but not the loss of weight; plasma sodium concentration fell and water moved into the cells. Their faces shrank; they lost appetite and sense of taste, and became very weak, weary and muddleheaded, with a general sense of exhaustion, little initiative, delayed excretion of water loads, and almost continuous muscle cramps. Many of McCance's symptoms resembled those of severe Addison's disease, though the adrenal glands were presumably overactive! They endured these miseries for a week or two, and then enjoyed a rapid cure by eating salty fried herrings and licking the salt out of the frypan. McCance's fascinating description in the third of his Goulstonian Lectures (*Lancet* 1936) is a precious medical and nutritional classic.

7.2.6 Excess of body sodium

An increased intake of salt does not usually increase the amount in the body, because the kidneys normally excrete the extra sodium and keep the volume of ECF constant. But they can be misdirected or malfunction, and retain too much sodium. Examples (with some contributary factors) include:

1. Congestive heart failure. Raised capillary pressure displaces fluid from plasma to interstitial spaces and the congested liver fails to destroy aldosterone normally.

2. Deficiency of plasma albumin (e.g. from loss in the urine in nephrotic syndromes), or from failure of production in hepatic failure or severe malnutrition, famine oedema. The lowered plasma volume reduces GFR and releases renin which stimulates secretion of aldosterone. But the plasma volume is not always low, indicating that there are other factors involved; these are incompletely understood.

3. Failure of the kidneys to respond to natriuretic hormones (hormones stimulating sodium loss) released when plasma volume increases.

Retained sodium first increases osmolarity in the ECF, provoking thirst and release of ADH. Water is taken in, and retained to accompany the retained salt. With normal osmoregulation, 1 litre of water is retained with each 150 mmol of sodium (9 g NaCl). If the extra saline is not held in the capillaries (e.g. if capillary pressure is raised or colloid osmotic pressure low from lack of albumin), it escapes into the tissues; hence blood volume is not expanded and signals to retain sodium are not turned off. The excess saline accumulates as ECF outside the circulation, body weight increases, and accumulation of more than 4 litres shows up as oedema.

Treatment   Extremely low salt diets are unpalatable, and attempts to restrict salt may be counter-productive by provoking increased secretion of aldosterone. Patients are more compliant when dietary salt intake is reduced less rigorously, and renal excretion is increased with diuretics which inhibit reabsorption of sodium by the renal tubules. See Table 7.2 for a summary of disturbances in the water content of the body.

Table 7.2 Summary of disturbances of the amount of water in the body

Disturbance	Cause	Osmotic pressure (Plasma [Na])	Volume change		Manifestation
Excess water	Water only	Reduced	ICF ↑	ECF ↑	Water intoxication
	Excess Na	Normal	ECF ↑		Oedema
Dehydration	Water loss	Increased	ICF ↓	ECF ↓	Thirst
	Na loss	Normal	ECF ↓		Circulatory failure

7.3 POTASSIUM

7.3.1 Significance and functions of potassium

According to a luminous phrase attributed to Wallace Fenn: 'Potassium is of the soil and not of the sea; it is of the cell and not of the sap.' Just as sodium belongs typically to seas and extracellular fluids, potassium is the predominant cation in the cells of both animals and plants. Its salts, mainly organic, are responsible for most of the osmolarity of animal cells and determine their volume. The cells' enzymes have evolved to require an environment rich in potassium. The hydrated potassium ion is smaller than that of sodium, and the cell membranes are much more permeable to it. Hence, the ratio of the intracellular (IC) to the extracellular (EC) concentration of potassium largely determines the resting potentials of cells and the transient action potentials which transmit messages and activate nerve cells and muscle fibres.

An increase in the small EC concentration of potassium lowers the concentration ratio of IC to EC potassium; this depolarizes membranes and blocks transmission, whereas a decrease in EC potassium concentration increases the ratio, hyperpolarizes membranes and raises the threshold for excitation. Consequently, the small concentration of potassium in the extracellular fluid is critically important; large (two- to threefold) increases or decreases can paralyse muscles and stop the heart.

The larger concentration of potassium in the cells is not so critical. Up to a third of body potassium can be lost without dramatic symptoms. A colleague in McCance's laboratory (Paul Fourman) depleted himself experimentally by ingesting ion exchange resins which prevented the absorption of potassium from his alimentary tract. He delayed analysing his stools until after a walking holiday, and then found that he had gone away without a fifth of his body's store of potassium. The IC and EC concentrations had presumably been reduced without dangerously disturbing the critical ratio. Had the cells suddenly recovered their lost potassium, the EC concentration would have fallen to zero and he would have died.

7.3.2 Amount and distribution in the body

An average human adult's body contains about 3800 mmol of potassium; most of this, about 3200 mmol, is in the cells. Indeed, a total body count of the natural isotope, ^{40}K, can yield an estimate of cell mass. About 300 mmol is contained in the skeleton, and only

80 mmol is in solution in the EC fluids. Hence if the cells increased their content by only 1.25% (40 mmol) at the expense of the ECF, the external concentration would be halved, with potentially serious consequences for neuromuscular and cardiac function.

7.3.3 Potassium balance

Intake

Diet: around 100 mmol/day.

1. Meat is animal muscle and vegetables contain plant cells, hence all foods contain potassium. No foods are exceptionally rich or poor, and there are no large differences between natural and processed foods, as there are for sodium.
2. Wholemeal flour, meats and fish supply 7–9 mmol/100 g.
3. Common vegetables, 5–9 mmol/100 g.
4. Milk, eggs and cheese 4–6 mmol/100 g.
5. Fruit 5–8 mmol/100 g; oranges 5 mmol/100 g, making orange juice a useful source of potassium.

The lowest values are for salted butter 0.5 mmol/100 g, and eating apples 0.3 mmol/100 g. Hence, ordinary mixed and vegetarian diets contain adequate amounts of potassium. It is difficult to devise a diet which is deficient.

Output

1. *Faeces*: about 10 mmol/day;
2. *Urine*: 90 mmol/day.

This can be varied widely to match alterations in intake. The kidneys hold the balance by adjusting the amount in the urine. They can excrete potassium rapidly if EC potassium concentration rises, and can conserve it when scarce, though not so avidly or so briskly as sodium. Their priority seems to be to keep the critically important concentration of potassium in the ECF within its normal range of 4–5 mmol/l.

7.3.4 Regulation of extracellular concentration

The most important factors are:

1. *Active uptake by cells.* This is maintained by ongoing metabolism and promoted by insulin. Potassium must be supplied to prevent a lethal fall in EC potassium concentration when patients with diabetic ketoacidosis treated with insulin and glucose begin to rebuild the severely depleted stores of glycogen and potassium in their muscles.
2. *Excretion by the kidneys.* The bulk of the potassium in the glomerular filtrate is reabsorbed from proximal tubules; what appears in the urine is mostly secreted by distal tubules. The rate of tubular secretion is increased by:
   - increased EC potassium concentration. This helps to avoid a dangerous increase in EC concentration when potassium escapes from cells; but the potassium is lost from the body in the process;

- aldosterone;
- faster flow through distal tubules; the secretory mechanism seems to set the concentration of potassium in the tubular fluid, so that the rate of loss is proportional to the flow;
- an increased concentration of sodium in distal tubular fluid, for potassium is secreted partly in exchange for reabsorbed sodium.

7.3.5 Potassium depletion

This implies a lack of potassium out of proportion to other body constituents. Small children and people who have lost weight are not considered potassium-depleted; their IC and EC concentrations are normal.

Deficiency of potassium is rarely caused by an inadequate intake alone; it requires also a failure of renal conservation, or abnormal losses, or both.

1. The alimentary tract can become a source of zero intake or even of loss through vomiting, aspiration of stomach contents, or diarrhoea, when lost fluid often contains more potassium than normal intestinal secretions. Abuse of purgatives can cause potassium depletion.

2. The kidneys may excrete instead of conserving potassium under the influence of adrenal steroids, diuretic drugs or acidosis. In diabetic ketoacidosis, deranged metabolism leads to loss of potassium from cells to ECF; increased renal excretion is driven by the high EC concentration and the osmotic diuresis provoked by large amounts of ketone acids and sodium in distal tubular fluid.

3. Most disturbances of acid–base balance increase the rate of excretion of potassium. Acidosis brings potassium out of cells, raising EC(K), so potassium removed from cells is excreted and lost. Alkalosis promotes uptake of potassium from plasma into cells including renal tubular cells, which pass it on into the urine. Thus, alkalosis as well as acidosis can deplete the body of potassium. Paradoxically, potassium depletion ultimately leaves distal tubular cells low in potassium so that they tend to secrete hydrogen ions instead of potassium, make the urine acid, and add extra bicarbonate to the plasma, thus creating a state of alkalosis in the plasma, while cells and urine are abnormally acid.

Symptoms   The symptoms of potassium deficiency are mild, vague and non-specific: fatigue, ill-defined malaise with weak skeletal, cardiac and intestinal muscles; the kidneys cannot concentrate the urine maximally. These are not obvious; there are no dramatic effects if cells and ECF lose potassium in proportion. Physicians must therefore anticipate when deficiency is likely to occur, and test for it. The electrocardiogram offers a readily available biological assay, using the patient's own heart, and may give an early warning to seek laboratory confirmation.

Treatment   After causes of loss have been removed, replacement is usually by the mouth; best as food. Infusions, when needed, must be slow and not concentrated, to avoid the danger of high EC potassium concentrations.

7.3.6 Excess of body potassium

Potassium is not stored in the body; there is no over-stocking of cells corresponding to oedema. Localized excesses in the form of high concentrations of potassium in ECF are dangerous, but these are rare in the absence of renal damage. The kidneys may fail to protect against excessive concentrations:

1. *In shock*; cells deprived of oxygen cannot retain potassium, and kidneys without adequate blood flow cannot excrete it.

2. *In crush injuries*; crushed muscles release potassium and also muscle haemoglobin which damages the kidneys by blocking the tubules.

3. *In anuria* (no production of urine) from any cause, excretion is impossible, and an increasing concentration of potassium in the plasma as cells break down may be a more pressing indication of the need for dialysis than a rising concentration of blood urea.

4. *In Addison's disease*, when adrenal cortical secretion is lacking, EC potassium concentration may be moderately increased without an increase in body potassium because the kidneys fail to conserve sodium but retain potassium.

7.4 ACID–BASE BALANCE

7.4.1 Regulation

The maintenance of acid–base balance implies keeping the body fluids 'blandly alkaline' (i.e. plasma and other ECFs at pH 7.35–7.45; cells about pH 7.1; note that pH 6.8 is neutral at body temperature). This alkalinity is essential for cells in 'irritable' tissues—nerves, muscles, and heart. It is achieved by:

1. controlling excretion of weakly acid carbon dioxide by the lungs (about 13 000 mmol/day); and

2. excretion of smaller amounts of non-volatile acid (hydrogen ions) or alkali (bicarbonate) by the kidneys.

The kidneys control the numerator, lungs the denominator of the Henderson–Hasselbalch Equation:

$$pH = 6.1 + \log = \frac{[HCO_3^-]}{0.03 P_{CO_2}} \quad \begin{array}{l} \leftarrow \text{kidneys} \\ \leftarrow \text{lungs and respiratory system} \end{array}$$

Normally, [bicarbonate] is kept near 24 mmol/l and partial pressure of carbon dioxide near 40 mmHg; hence pH must be $6.1 + \log(24/(0.03 \times 40)) = 6.1 + \log(24/1.2) = 6.1 + \log 20) = 6.1 + 1.3 = 7.4$.

Respiratory and renal diseases can disturb acid–base balance. Considering only dietary factors, it has been known for more than a hundred years that meat diets leave excess acid and vegetarian diets excess alkali in the body to be dealt with. Claude Bernard (1865) noticed that rabbits that happened to be starved produced acid urine instead of the usual alkaline urine characteristic of herbivorous animals. He deduced that starvation made them temporarily carnivorous, living on their own flesh, and found that he could make their urine alkaline or acid at will by giving them grass or meat to eat. He did the same with a horse.

7.4.2 Dietary considerations

Meat diets yield sulphuric acid from S-amino acids, and phosphoric acid from nucleo-proteins and phospholipids. Mixed diets leave about 70 mmol/day of hydrogen ions to be excreted. Food faddists may call sour fruits, etc. 'acid foods', but the organic acids they contain are either not absorbed or mostly oxidized to water and carbon dioxide. Most of this is breathed out, although a little remains in the body as bicarbonate; hence these acids taken in as potassium salts leave an excess of potassium bicarbonate which tends to make the blood more alkaline! Table 7.3 gives examples of food acids and their metabolic fates.

Hence these dietary acids pose no threat to the body's 'bland alkalinity'. Organic acids that can pose threats are:

1. Acetoacetic and other keto acids, particularly produced in diabetic ketoacidosis; smaller, less important amounts during fasting.
2. Lactic acid produced in severe muscular exercise or from tissues inadequately supplied with oxygen (e.g. in shock when blood pressure is very low).

7.4.3 The reaction of the urine

The reaction of the urine depends on the balance between the amounts of bicarbonate in the glomerular filtrate and of hydrogen ion secreted by the renal tubules. Since bicarbonate is formed as a by-product of the generation of hydrogen ions in the tubular cells, one mmol of bicarbonate is added to the plasma for each mmol of hydrogen ions secreted into the urine. The secreted hydrogen ion first destroys filtered bicarbonate, but effects its 'reabsorption' by replacing it mmol for mmol by new bicarbonate in the plasma. Further secreted hydrogen ions convert filtered buffers, especially phosphate, into their

Table 7.3 Acids in fruits and their metabolic fate

Food Source	Acid	Fate
Citrus, pineapples, tomatoes, summer fruits	Citric	Oxidized to CO_2 and H_2O
Apples, plums, tomatoes	Malic	Oxidized to CO_2 and H_2O
Cranberries, bilberries	Benzoic	Excreted as hippuric acid
Grapes	Tartaric	Not absorbed
Strawberries, rhubarb, spinach	Oxalic	Not absorbed; forms calcium oxalate in the gut

Source: Modified from Passmore R, Eastwood MA. *Davidson and Passmore's human nutrition and dietetics*, 8th ed. Edinburgh: Churchill Livingstone, 1988.

acid forms in acid urine. Hydrogen ions are also excreted as ammonium, and one mmol of additional bicarbonate is added to the plasma for every mmol of hydrogen ion excreted as acid buffer or ammonium. In alkalosis the concentration of bicarbonate in the plasma may be so high that there is more in the glomerular filtrate than the total rate of hydrogen ion secretion can cope with; the excess bicarbonate then escapes in alkaline urine, and lowers the concentration in the plasma.

FURTHER READING

1. Bray JJ, Cragg PA, Macknight ADC, Mills RG, Taylor DW. *Lecture notes on human physiology.* 3rd ed. Oxford: Blackwell Scientific Publications, 1994.
2. Passmore R, Eastwood MA. *Davidson and Passmore's human nutrition and dietetics.* 8th ed. Edinburgh: Churchill Livingstone, 1988.
3. Robinson JR. *Reflections on renal function.* 2nd ed. Oxford: Blackwell Scientific Publications, 1988.
4. Wrong O. Water and monovalent electrolytes. In: Garrow JS, James WPT (eds). *Human nutrition and dietetics.* 9th ed. Edinburgh: Churchill Livingstone, 1993: 146–61.

MAJOR MINERALS:
CALCIUM AND MAGNESIUM

8.1 CALCIUM

Ailsa Goulding

Calcium (Ca) is a remarkable and fascinating mineral. It is an essential constituent of all forms of life and is critically important for good health and human nutrition. The skeleton contains 99% of the body calcium and we need adequate dietary calcium and vitamin D to grow and keep healthy bones and teeth. Calcium is a divalent cation with an atomic weight of 40 (40 mg Ca = 1 mmol Ca). Calcium is the fifth most abundant element in our bodies. It is the main mineral in bone, being stored as hydroxyapatite, $Ca_{10}(OH)_2(PO_4)_6$. The skeleton protects the vital organs, and provides a 'bank' of mineral from which calcium and phosphorus may be continually withdrawn or deposited according to physiological need. The total body calcium content differs widely between individuals at all ages because some people grow better skeletons than others. This is partly due to genetic factors and partly to environmental and nutritional influences. In contrast, intracellular and extracellular calcium concentrations are tightly controlled within narrow limits. This is essential because interactions of calcium ions with proteins alter molecular activity. Ordered movement of ionic calcium plays a critical role in regulating muscle contraction, nerve conductivity, ion transport, enzyme activation, blood clotting, and the secretion of hormones and neurotransmitters.

Life without calcium is impossible and small variations in plasma calcium concentrations may have serious consequences. Hypocalcaemia and hypercalcaemia are common medical emergencies. Low blood calcium (hypocalcaemia) may cause seizures and tetany (musculoskeletal spasms and twitching, particularly in the fingers and face) and tingling and numbness due to increased neuromuscular activity. High blood calcium (hypercalcaemia) results in thirst, mild mental confusion and irritability, loss of appetite and general fatigue and weakness. Polyuria and constipation are common. When concentrations of calcium are high, calcium salts may precipitate in soft tissues and kidney stones may form.

8.1.1 Bone metabolism

There are two types of bone: dense cortical bone (80% of the skeleton) and spongy trabecular bone (20% of the skeleton). The skeleton undergoes constant renovation, rather like a building site. Old worn bits are being chiselled out or resorbed by multinucleate cells called osteoclasts, while new teams of cells called osteoblasts busily rebuild excavation holes with strong new bone. Bone cell activity affects biochemical markers: blood levels of alkaline phosphatase and osteocalcin reflect formation; urinary hydroxyproline, deoxypyridinoline and pyridinoline indicate resorption. Osteoblasts buried deep in bone mineral are called osteocytes; they seem to sense weight-bearing and may help to regulate bone remodelling responses to exercise. The different bone cells communicate actively. A complex, exquisitely sensitive 'internet' of chemical messages appears to control their differentiation and activity but we understand this bone language poorly. When the activity of the osteoblasts and osteoclasts is matched, or coupled, bone mass is stable. The amount of bone destroyed by osteoclasts is replaced by an equal amount of new bone. When bone remodelling becomes uncoupled, and resorption exceeds formation, bone is lost. Bone mass can be measured accurately *in vivo* using dual energy X-ray absorptiometry (DEXA scanning) or computerized tomography (CT scanning).

8.1.2 Bone disorders

Children with vitamin D deficiency develop rickets, and adults, osteomalacia (see Chapter 14.1). They do not calcify bone normally and their bones contain osteoid (unmineralized bone). Because this bone is weak, children with rickets often show bowed limbs. Rickets is still seen in developing countries but rarely in more affluent societies.

In developed countries the bone disease seen most often is osteoporosis. This is caused by substantial loss of bone. Although there is too little bone, what remains is normally calcified. Osteoporotic bones are thin and break easily, especially in the wrist, spine and hip. The thinner the bone density, the higher the risk of fractures.

8.1.3 Calcium stores

Bone stores When plump people are being weighed they sometimes say a little smugly 'I've got big bones'. However, bones are strong rather than weighty. The bones of an average adult constitute 14% of body weight, and bone mineral 4%. Men accumulate more skeletal calcium (1200 g) than women (1000 g). Approximately one-fifth of this (21%) is in the skull, half (51%) is in the arms and legs and the remainder (28%) is in the trunk (ribs 9%; pelvis 8%; spine 11%).

Peak bone mass The heaviest bone mass an individual achieves is called their peak bone mass (PBM). This is generally reached by 18–20 years of age. To achieve average PBM values men require a positive daily calcium gain of 160 mg, and women 130 mg, for every single day of the first 20 years of their lives! Ethnic, family and twin studies show that there are strong genetic influences on PBM. These may account for 80% of the variability in adult bone density. The variance in PBM is wide, with values ranging between 20% higher and 20% lower than the average. The variance does not change in the third and fourth decades of life, indicating that young adults with low density do not catch up bone density over time. Thus if a good PBM is not attained by the mid twenties, it is unlikely to be achieved at all.

Calcium in extraskeletal stores and body fluids   These stores are small (15 g): teeth (7 g), soft tissues (7 g), plasma and intracellular fluids (1 g). Cytoplasm concentrations are one thousand times lower than those in plasma. Breast milk contains a high level of calcium (350 mg/l or 8.8 mmol/l) and a lactating mother transfers around 260 mg daily to her baby. The plasma calcium concentration is 2.2–2.6 mmol/l (8.8–10.4 mg/dl): half of this is bound to protein (37% to albumin and 10% to globulin), 47% is free or ionized, and 6% is complexed to anions (phosphate, citrate, bicarbonate). The ionized calcium is biologically active: levels are regulated by the parathyroid vitamin D axis and calcitonin.

Control of plasma calcium   When ionized plasma calcium concentrations fall, parathyroid hormone (PTH) is secreted to increase calcium input from kidney, bone, and gut (Fig. 8.1). In the kidney PTH augments the tubular reabsorption of calcium, decreases tubular reabsorption of phosphate and bicarbonate, and stimulates conversion of $25(OH)D_3$ to $1,25(OH)_2D_3$ (calcitriol). In bone PTH promotes release of calcium and phosphate into blood. The effects of PTH on kidney and bone are direct and rapid

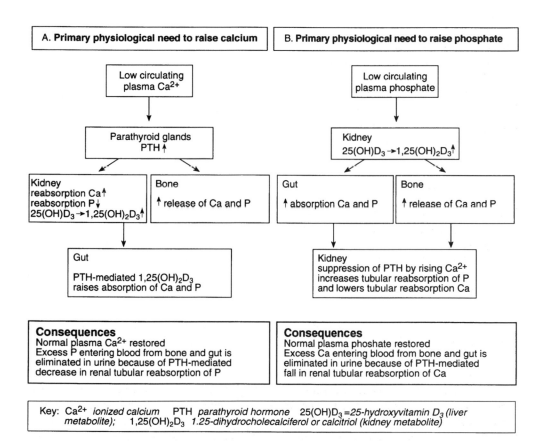

Fig. 8.1   Co-ordinated actions of parathyroid hormone and calcitriol in target organs regulate levels of calcium and phosphate in plasma.

125

and are assisted by $1,25(OH)_2D_3$; the ability of PTH to raise alimentary calcium and phosphate absorption, is mediated solely by calcitriol. When normal plasma calcium concentrations are restored PTH secretion decreases, the flow of calcium from bone diminishes, urinary calcium rises and $1,25(OH)_2D_3$ synthesis is shut off. The system is robust and PTH and calcitriol influence each other's synthesis. The role of vitamin D is discussed in Chapter 14.1.

Calcitonin, a hormone secreted by the thyroid gland, helps to fine-tune plasma calcium regulation. It lowers calcium by inhibiting bone resorption. It is secreted when ionized blood calcium levels rise above normal and probably helps to curb blood calcium fluctuations after meals. Calcitonin plays a smaller role in plasma calcium homeostasis than PTH and calcitriol, and patients who have had surgery on the thyroid gland maintain levels surprisingly well. In contrast, patients lacking either PTH or active vitamin D metabolites develop hypocalcaemia. Magnesium deficiency also causes hypo-calcaemia because magnesium is a co-factor for PTH secretion. Restoring magnesium corrects the problem in alcoholics and patients with steatorrhoea. Total plasma calcium rarely falls below 1.25 mmol/l (5 mg/dl) because calcium ions from bone mineral constantly exchange with extracellular fluid.

Obligatory losses of calcium · Significant amounts of calcium inevitably leak from the body. These are unavoidable dermal, faecal and renal losses of calcium, called obligatory losses. Dermal losses (epithelial cells and sweat) are generally less than 20 mg/day; faecal losses (unabsorbed digestive juice calcium) are 80–120 mg/day; while the obligatory urinary calcium loss varies between 40 and 200 mg/day, depending on how effectively calcium is reabsorbed from the glomerular filtrate. The tubules reabsorb more than 98% of the 10 000 mg calcium filtered daily by the glomeruli of the kidney. Dietary salt (NaCl), protein, and caffeine aggravate obligatory urinary calcium loss.

8.1.4 Calcium balance and absorption

If more calcium is retained than excreted a person is said to be in positive calcium balance. Negative calcium balance occurs if more calcium is excreted than ingested and zero calcium balance if the amount of calcium absorbed daily from food is matched exactly by the amounts of calcium lost in the faeces, urine, and from the skin (Fig. 8.2).

Alimentary calcium absorption This is not as efficient as renal tubular calcium reabsorption. Absorption is normally less than 70% (and usually less than 30%) of the calcium entering the gut. Net calcium absorption (the difference between calcium ingested by mouth and calcium excreted in the faeces) can be determined by traditional metabolic balance techniques. To avoid negative calcium balance, net absorption must fully offset calcium losses from the urine and skin. However, measurement of net calcium absorption considerably underestimates the total calcium absorbed from the intestine into blood, because some faecal calcium (endogenous faecal) is derived from calcium resecreted into the intestine in the digestive juices, rather than from unabsorbed food calcium. True alimentary calcium absorption (amount actually absorbed from the gut) is measured with radioisotopes or stable isotopes, ^{42}Ca and ^{44}Ca.

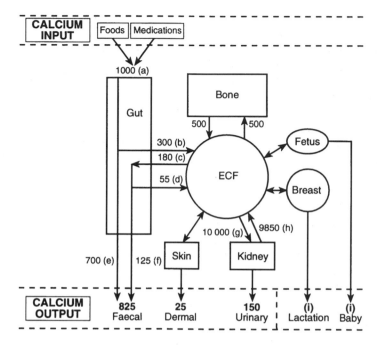

Fig. 8.2 Diagram of calcium fluxes (mg/day) of subject in calcium balance (input = output). ECF, extracellular fluid; a, total calcium ingested by mouth; b, dietary calcium absorbed; c, calcium in digestive secretions; d, reabsorbed endogenous calcium; e, unabsorbed dietary calcium; f, endogenous faecal calcium excretion; g, calcium load filtered at glomerulus; h, calcium reabsorbed from glomerular filtrate (>98%); i, losses only incurred in pregnancy (full-term baby has 25–30 g calcium) or lactation (160–300 mg/day in breast milk).

Factors affecting the bioavailability of calcium in the intestine   Variations in the efficiency of absorption are mainly determined by vitamin D metabolites and the rate of transit of gut contents through the intestine. Calcitriol improves calcium absorption (see Chapter 14.1). However, some is absorbed even in vitamin D deficient states, because some calcium is absorbed by passive concentration-dependent diffusion. The duodenum absorbs calcium most avidly, but larger quantities of calcium are absorbed by the ileum and jejunum because food spends longer there. Some calcium is also absorbed from the colon and surgical resection can impair absorption. Carbohydrates, such as lactose, improve calcium absorption by augmenting its passive diffusion across villous membranes. Diets rich in oxalate, fibre and phytic acid are reputed to depress alimentary absorption by complexing calcium in the gut. However, their overall effects seem small, possibly because bacterial breakdown of uronic acid and phytates in the colon frees calcium for absorption. Poor bioavailability of calcium from spinach is attributed to the high oxalate content. Dietary phosphorus increases the endogenous secretion of calcium into the gut. Lastly, calcium absorption diminishes in both sexes in the seventh decade of life because of lower renal synthesis of calcitriol and intestinal resistance to calcitriol, which contribute to the genesis of senile osteoporosis (see Section 8.1.6).

127

Factors influencing urinary calcium loss   Urinary excretion rises when the filtered load of calcium increases or the tubular reabsorption of calcium decreases. Acidifying agents, dietary sodium, protein and caffeine raise excretion. Phosphorus, alkaline agents (bicarbonate, citrate), and thiazide diuretics lower excretion. Variations in salt intake explain much of the day-to-day fluctuation in urinary calcium. One teaspoonful of salt (100 mmol NaCl) raises urinary calcium by 40 mg calcium/day, even on a low calcium intake. Purified sulphur-containing amino acids (methionine and cysteine) cause significant calciuria but phosphate in whole proteins mitigates their calciuric effect when consumed in foods. Vegetarians with an alkaline urine excrete less urinary calcium than meat-eaters, who have an acid urine.

8.1.5   Dietary calcium

Body calcium stores are built and maintained by extracting and retaining calcium from food. Dietary needs vary with gender, ethnicity, age, and the magnitude of obligatory

Table 8.1   United States recommendations for dietary allowances for calcium (RDA), and optimal calcium intake (NIH Consensus Statement)

Group	RDA 1989[a] (mg/day)	Optimal daily intake[b] (mg/day)
Infants		
birth–6 mths	400	400
6 mths–1 yr	600	600
Children		
1–5 yrs	800	800
6–10 yrs	800	800–1200
Adolescents/Young adults		
11–24 yrs	1200	1200–1500
Men		
25–65 yrs	800	1000
Over 65 yrs	800	1500
Women		
25–50 yrs	800	1000
Over 50 yrs (postmenopausal)		
On oestrogens	800	1000
Not on oestrogens	800	1500
Over 65 yrs	800	1500
Pregnant or lactating	1200	1200–1500

[a] National Research Council. *Recommended dietary allowances.* 10th ed. Washington DC: National Academy Press, 1989: 174–84.
[b] NIH Consensus Statement. *Optimal calcium intake.* JAMA 1994; 272: 1942–8.

calcium loss (Table 8.1). It is critically important at all stages of life to consume and absorb enough dietary calcium to satisfy physiological calcium needs because some bone will be mobilized to maintain blood calcium levels whenever losses of calcium exceed alimentary calcium absorption (Fig. 8.3).

Threshold concepts Few people consume too much calcium from natural foods. However, many eat too little: this may affect their skeletons detrimentally, especially in childhood when skeletal needs are high, and in later life (>65 years) when alimentary absorption of calcium deteriorates. There is a threshold intake for calcium below which skeletal calcium accumulation is a function of intake, and above which skeletal accumulation does not further increase, irrespective of further increases in intake. In other words 'enough' calcium is good, but 'extra' calcium will not increase bone formation.

Recommended nutrient intake There is considerable controversy over the optimal daily dietary intake of calcium for individuals to achieve peak bone mass (PBM), to maintain adult bone mass and to prevent loss of bone in later life. There may be ethnic and genetic differences in calcium requirements. Experts who argue for lower intakes point out that large sections of the population manage to grow and maintain bone on calcium intakes well below the current United States recommended dietary allowance (RDA) (Table 8.1). Many consider the even higher intakes recently advocated by the NIH Consensus Group in 1994 are extreme. It is disturbing to note that recommendations are continuing to climb. Many people find difficulty in consuming more than 1000 mg calcium daily from natural foods. Evidence of bone benefit from high dietary intakes in older adults seems insufficient to justify recommending calcium intakes exceeding the current United States RDA. Higher calcium intakes would require widespread use of food fortification or calcium supplementation by large sections of the

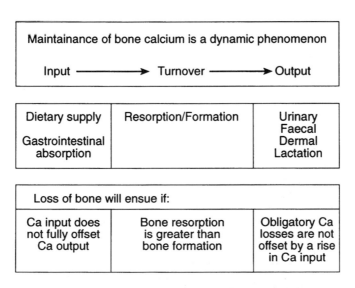

Fig. 8.3 Ways in which bone loss is caused.

population. A better way to boost the calcium economy would be to lower dietary salt intake. This will reduce obligatory loss of calcium and improve calcium balance. Moderate vitamin D supplementation may be useful in the housebound elderly.

Food sources of calcium   Foods vary greatly in their calcium content (Table 8.2). Milk has an especially high calcium content and in Western countries dairy products supply up to two-thirds of the total daily intake. Other excellent sources of calcium include cheeses, yoghurt, and soymilk substitutes. Good sources of calcium include milky dairy foods, nuts, canned fish with bones, leafy vegetables, and dried fruit. In some countries foods are fortified with mineral calcium supplements.

Dietary advice to increase calcium intake while following nutritional guidelines for lowering fat intake includes:

• have a serving of either yoghurt or milk daily for breakfast
• always have low fat milk available in the fridge
• choose low fat dairy products at the supermarket
• add cheese chunks or a sprinkling of nuts to salads/vegetables
• eat pieces of cheese, nuts or green vegetables as snacks
• add grated cheese or milk when serving soups and pasta
• use canned fish with bones in sandwich spreads
• try tofu chunks with salads and casseroles
• add a little skim milk powder to recipes when baking

Table 8.2   Calcium content of some common foods

Calcium sources	Serving size		mg Ca/serving
Excellent sources			
milk, whole	1 cup	250 ml	295
trim*, fat-reduced	1 cup	250 ml	375
soymilk	1 cup	250 ml	255
yoghurt	1 tub	150 g	180
cheddar cheese	1 slice	20 g	150
Good sources			
ice cream, vanilla	1 scoop	85 g	115
cottage cheese	½ cup	120 g	75
nuts, peanuts	½ cup	80 g	50
almonds/walnuts	10 nuts	12 g/50 g	30
canned sardines	½ can	50 g	270
canned salmon	½ cup	120 g	110
leeks/broccoli	1 cup	150 g	100
cabbage/spinach	1 cup	160 g	30–80
dried apricots	½ cup	70 g	65
dried figs	½ cup	100 g	290

* Trim milk, is fat-reduced (0.4%) with added skim milk solids.
Source: Burlingame BA, Milligan CC, Apimenika DE, Arthur JM. *Concise New Zealand food composition tables.* 2nd ed. Palmerston North, NZ: Institute for Crop and Food Research, 1994.

- serve vegetables in white sauces made with milk
- use yoghurt in place of cream with desserts

Satisfactory intake of calcium may be sustained life-long when individuals choose calcium-rich foods they like.

Calcium supplementation and food fortification   Individuals who find it difficult to eat enough calcium may benefit from mineral supplements. People with very low calorie intakes, milk allergies or symptomatic lactose malabsorption may need to consume foods fortified with calcium (soybean and citrus drinks, breakfast cereals) or take supplements. These are absorbed as well as food calcium.

Calcium intoxication   Ingestion of large amounts of alkaline calcium salts (more than 2.5 g Ca/day) can override the ability of the kidney to excrete unwanted calcium, causing hypercalcaemia and metastatic calcification of the cornea, kidneys and blood vessels. People consuming huge quantities of calcium carbonate in antacids are prone to this intoxication (milk alkali syndrome). Patients taking vitamin D, or its metabolites, may suffer similar symptoms. Large amounts of vitamin D are poisonous, and are used commercially to eliminate rodents!

8.1.6   Factors affecting bone growth and attrition

Normal growth   Both boys and girls display similar linear gains in calcium up to the age of about 10 years (Fig. 8.4). Their total body calcium then averages 400 g, indicating a daily increment of 110 mg over this period. Skeletal growth accelerates at puberty. Spinal density matures earlier in girls, who go through puberty earlier than boys. Total body calcium doubles in girls between the ages of 10 and 15 years (an average gain of 200 mg daily). Boys have two extra years of prepubertal bone gain before their pubertal growth spurt, when they deposit over 400 mg calcium daily in bone. Children do not

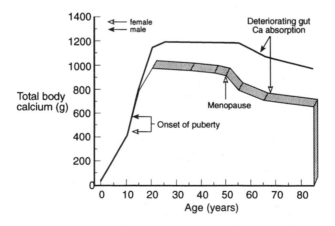

Fig. 8.4   Lifetime changes in total body calcium in men (upper curve) and women (lower curve).

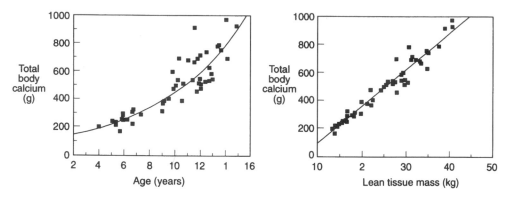

Fig. 8.5 Total body calcium changes in 50 growing girls aged 3–15 years, in relation to age (r = 0.92) and lean tissue mass (r = 0.97). Author's data.

have higher calcium absorption than adults. Obligatory losses are also high and there are concerns that many children consume too little calcium to meet their skeletal needs. In teenagers, bone mass can be increased by supplementation. However, the gain may be temporary and catch-up may occur in children who consume less calcium. It may just take children longer to attain their skeletal potential on moderate calcium intakes, than on very high intakes.

Environmental factors such as calcium intake, physical activity and sex steroid status influence bone accrual. Cigarette smoking and excess alcohol affect bone mass adversely whereas high physical activity, adequate dietary calcium, and sex steroids favour bone accrual. Regular moderate exercise should be recommended for youngsters. Children with good lean body mass have the best bone mass (Fig. 8.5). In teenagers with anorexia nervosa and athletic amenorrhoea, low oestrogen status causes poor PBM. Girls who recover from these conditions continue to show thin spinal bone years after plasma oestrogen levels have returned to normal.

Bone attrition Bone density declines after middle life. Falling levels of sex steroids cause trabecular loss while calcium deprivation speeds cortical loss. Effects of oestrogen deprivation are particularly sharp at menopause (Fig. 8.4). Bone losses are considerable: from youth to old age, women lose half their trabecular bone and a third of their cortical bone, while men lose a third of their trabecular bone and a fifth of their cortical bone. Low bone mass in the elderly may be due to poor PBM, to subsequent excessive loss of bone, or to both these factors. Bone density will fall below the fracture threshold at a younger age in people with low PBM than in those with high PBM. Variations in inheritance of polymorphisms of the vitamin D receptor (VDR) gene influence PBM and bone loss. (Adults with the bb genotype have better spinal and hip density and less fractures than those with the BB genotype.) People with different VDR genotypes may differ in their dietary calcium and vitamin D requirements.

Osteoporosis This is a serious and expensive public health problem, particularly in women. It causes significant pain and morbidity among elderly people (see Section 3.1.2). The incidence of osteoporotic fractures is expected to increase in future because people are living longer. In 1990, there were 1.66 million estimated hip fractures world-wide. By the year 2025, it is projected that there will be 1.16 million hip fractures in men and 2.78 million in women due to osteoporosis. At present, the best way to avoid osteoporotic fractures in later life is to grow a good skeleton, achieve optimal genetic skeletal mass, and then retain this as long as possible. Every effort should therefore be made to ensure life-long consumption, absorption and retention of sufficient calcium to do this.

8.1.7 Other possible health effects of calcium

Hypertension and pre-eclampsia may be influenced by dietary calcium. High intakes are considered protective. However, limited evidence for these relationships exists. Bowel cancer risk may be lowered among subjects consuming a high calcium diet. More conclusive evidence is required to support this contention which is based on epidemiological studies.

The consumption or absorption of other substances may be influenced by calcium intakes. Milk products contain considerable fat. However, fat-reduced dairy products are available for the cholesterol-conscious and those worried about obesity. There are concerns that high dietary calcium may lower iron absorption but eating citrus fruit, with its high vitamin C content, can prevent this. High levels of calcium also aggravate the inhibitory effect of phytic acid on zinc absorption. Calcium binds gut oxalate so supplements do not induce kidney stones. Calcium may lower absorption of tetracyclines.

Population subgroups with special nutritional needs and who are vulnerable to calcium deprivation should be targeted to improve calcium economy and safeguard bone health. Such groups include:

* people with habitually low dietary calcium intakes
* individuals with food allergies or lactose malabsorption
* adolescents building maximal bone
* girls with anorexia nervosa or athletic amenorrhoea
* the calorie-conscious (slimmers often avoid dairy foods)
* people with very low dietary energy intakes
* pregnant women (last trimester) and lactating women
* people with high intakes of common salt
* people with heavy alcohol consumption
* patients with malabsorption syndromes
* patients taking corticosteroid medication
* patients with renal disease
* the elderly
* people confined indoors who get no vitamin D from sunlight
* individuals with the BB vitamin D receptor genotype

FURTHER READING

1. Lee WT. Requirements of calcium: are there ethnic differences? *Asia Pacific J Clin Nutr* 1993; **2**: 183–90.
2. Matkovic V, Heaney RP. Calcium balance during human growth: evidence for threshold behaviour. *Am J Clin Nutr* 1992; **55**: 992–6.
3. Matkovic V, Jelic T, Wardlaw GM, Ilich JZ, Goel PK, Wright JK, *et al.* Timing of peak bone mass in caucasian females and its implication for the prevention of osteoporosis. *J Clin Invest* 1994; **93**: 799–808.
4. Morrison NA, Qi JC, Tokita A, Kelly PJ, Crofts L, Nguyen TV, *et al.* Prediction of bone density from vitamin D receptor alleles. *Nature* 1994; **367**: 284–7.
5. Nordin BEC. Calcium and Osteoporosis. *Nutrition* 1997; **13**: 664–86.

8.2 MAGNESIUM

Marion Robinson

Ever since McCollum observed a deficiency of magnesium in both rats and dogs in the early 1930s, magnesium has been an intriguing mineral. It has both physiological and biochemical functions and important interrelationships, especially with the cations calcium, potassium and sodium. Magnesium is also involved with second messengers, parathyroid hormone secretion, vitamin D metabolism and bone functions.

8.2.1 Distribution and functions

About 60–65% of the body content, 1 mole (25 g) of magnesium in an adult person, is found in the skeleton. Like calcium, it is an integral part of the inorganic structure of bones and teeth. Unlike calcium, magnesium is the major divalent cation in the cells, accounting for most of the remaining magnesium with 27% in the muscles and 7% in the other cells. Intracellular magnesium is involved in energy metabolism, acting mainly as a metal activator or co-factor for enzymes requiring adenosine triphosphate (ATP), in the replication of DNA and the synthesis of RNA and protein; it appears to be essential for all phosphate transferring systems. Several magnesium-activated enzymes are in-hibited by calcium while in others magnesium can be replaced by manganese.

The remaining 1% of the body content of magnesium is in the extracellular fluids; the plasma concentration is about one mmol/litre of which, as with calcium, about one-third is protein-bound. Magnesium and calcium have somewhat similar effects on the excitability of muscle and nerve cells, but calcium has a further important function in signalling, which requires its concentration in the cells to be kept extremely low.

8.2.2 Metabolism

Magnesium is absorbed primarily from the small intestine, both by a facilitated process and by simple diffusion. Absorption can vary widely and on average about 40–60% dietary intake is absorbed. Excretion is mainly through the kidneys, and increases with dietary intake. The kidney is extremely efficient in conserving magnesium; when the intake decreases, the urine can become almost magnesium-free. The intestinal and renal conservation and excretory mechanisms in normal individuals permit homeostasis over a wide range of intakes.

8.2.3 Dietary sources of magnesium

Magnesium is present like potassium in both animal and plant cells and is also the mineral in chlorophyll. Green vegetables, cereals, legumes and animal products are all good sources. Unlike for calcium, dairy products tend to be low in magnesium, with cow's milk containing 120 mg Mg/l (5 mmol/l) compared with 1200 mg Ca/l (30 mmol/l). The calcium, phosphate and protein in meat and other animal products reduce the bioavailability of magnesium from these sources. Average magnesium intake is about 320 mg/day (13 mmol/day) for males and 230 mg/day (10 mmol/day) for females.

8.2.4 Magnesium deficiency

Since magnesium is the second most abundant cation in cells after potassium, dietary deficiency is unlikely to occur in people eating a normal varied diet. Shils found it difficult to produce magnesium deficiency experimentally in his classical studies of the 1960s using human volunteers. These studies showed the interrelationships between magnesium and the other principal cations calcium, potassium and sodium. The plasma concentration of magnesium decreased progressively as did serum potassium and calcium, whereas the serum sodium remained normal even though sodium was being retained (Table 8.3). Functional effects, including personality changes, abnormal neuromuscular function and gastrointestinal symptoms, were restored to normal only by repletion of magnesium. Plasma magnesium returned rapidly to normal levels but there was a time delay before serum calcium regained baseline concentration.

Low levels of magnesium may occur in malabsorption, as part of the syndrome of malnutrition regardless of the cause, in people taking diuretics, and occasionally in other chronic conditions (e.g. inadequately controlled diabetes). Magnesium depletion may increase the risk of cardiac arrythmias and cardiac arrest. A low level of magnesium intake has been suggested as a risk factor in coronary heart disease but the evidence is unimpressive.

Table 8.3 Magnesium depletion and accompanying changes

	Blood chemistry	Metabolic balances
Magnesium	plasma Mg ↓	Mg negative
Potassium	serum K ↓	K negative
Calcium	serum Ca ↓	Ca positive
Sodium	serum Na no change	Na positive

8.2.5 Magnesium excess

Large dietary intakes of magnesium appear unharmful to humans with normal renal function; hypermagnesaemia is almost impossible to achieve from food sources alone. Large amounts of some magnesium salts (Epsom salts) have a cathartic effect.

8.2.6 Magnesium status

Serum magnesium concentration is the most frequently used index of magnesium status. Plasma is not used because anticoagulants may be contaminated with magnesium.

8.2.7 Recommended nutrient intakes (RNIs)

These are based upon an estimated requirement of 4.5 mg/kg per day for Australian children, adolescents and adults: 320 mg/day (13 mmol/day) for men and 270 mg/day (11 mmol/day) for women. The United Kingdom, RNIs are almost identical at 300 mg/day and 270 mg/day for men and women, respectively.

FURTHER READING

1. Bray JJ, Cragg PA, Macknight ADC, Mills RG, Taylor DW. *Lecture notes on human physiology.* 3rd ed. Oxford: Blackwell Scientific Publications, 1994.
2. Committee of Medical Aspects of Food Policy (COMA). Magnesium. In: *Dietary reference values for food and energy and nutrients for the United Kingdom.* Report 41, Health and Social Subjects, Department of Health. London: HMSO, 1991: 146–9.
3. Dreosti IE. Magnesium. In: Truswell AS (ed.). *Recommended nutrient intakes: Australian papers.* Sydney: Australian Professional Publications, 1990: 234–43.
4. Shils ME. Experimental production of magnesium deficiency in man. *Ann NY Acad Sci* 1969; **162**: 847–55.
5. Shils ME. Magnesium. In: Ziegler EE and Filer LJ (eds.). *Present knowledge of nutrition.* 7th ed. Washington DC: ILSI, 1996: 256–64.

9
IRON

Patrick MacPhail

Iron deficiency is the most frequently encountered nutritional deficiency in humans. It has been estimated that 500–600 million people suffer from iron deficiency anaemia. Many more have depleted iron stores and are at risk for the development of anaemia. Paradoxically, iron overload is also a major clinical problem in some populations. Genetic (HLA-linked) haemochromatosis affects 1 in 300 people in populations of northern European origin. In rural Sub-Saharan Africa, up to 25% of the adult population are iron overloaded while in parts of Asia and the Mediterranean there is a high prevalence of iron overload secondary to thalassaemia major. Both iron deficiency and iron overload have serious consequences and are major causes of human morbidity.

Iron owes its importance in biology to its remarkable reactivity. Of paramount importance is the reversible one-electron oxidation–reduction reaction that allows iron to shuttle between ferrous (Fe^{2+}) and ferric forms (Fe^{3+}). This reaction is exploited by most iron-dependent enzyme systems involving electron transport, oxygen carriage and iron transport across cell membranes. It is also responsible for the toxicity seen in acute and chronic iron overload. These contradictory properties are managed by highly specialized and conserved proteins involved in the storage and transport of iron and in regulating the concentration of intracellular iron.

9.1 BASIC IRON METABOLISM

The total body iron content is about 50 mg/kg. Over 60% is in the haemoglobin of red blood cells and about 25% is in the form of stores, mainly in the liver. The remainder is distributed between myoglobin in muscles (8%) and in enzymes (5%). A very small amount (about 3 mg) is in transit in the circulation bound to the plasma transport protein, transferrin.

9.1.1 Iron absorption

The mechanism by which iron is absorbed from the gut is not clearly understood. Four phases are recognized. In the *luminal phase*, food iron is solubilized, largely by acid secreted by the stomach, and is presented to the duodenum and upper jejunum where most iron absorption takes place. Factors which maintain the solubility of iron in the face of rising pH, such as valency (ferrous iron is better absorbed), mucin secreted by the cells lining the gut (mucosa) and chelators (ascorbic acid), appear to be important in this phase. The second phase, *mucosal uptake*, depends on iron binding to the brush border of the mucosal cell and transport of iron into the cell. The amount of iron crossing the cell membrane is dependent on the concentration of iron in the lumen of the gut but the role and existence of a number of putative iron-binding proteins remains uncertain. In the third *intracellular phase*, iron either enters a storage compartment in the storage protein ferritin or is transported directly to the opposite side of the mucosal cell and released. It has been suggested that ferritin plays a regulatory role, directing iron either to stores or to release. The bulk of recent evidence indicates that changes in intracellular ferritin are dependent on changes in intracellular iron and not the other way around. In *the last phase*, iron is released from the mucosal cell into the portal circulation where it is bound to the transport protein, transferrin. Both iron uptake and release by the mucosal cell appear to be inversely related to the amount of iron stored in the body.

9.1.2 Internal iron exchange

Once released from the mucosal cell iron enters the portal circulation where it is bound to the transport protein, transferrin (Fig. 9.1). Normally, transferrin is about 30% saturated with iron and most of the absorbed iron is transported directly to the bone marrow where it is incorporated in haemoglobin. The mechanism of uptake by the young red cells, and all active cells, involves a specific transferrin receptor expressed on the surface of the cell. The iron–transferrin–receptor complex is taken into the cell where the iron is released from transferrin. The transferrin–receptor complex, now devoid of iron, is cycled back to the cell surface where the transferrin is released back into the circulation. At the end of its life span the red cell is engulfed by cells of the reticuloendothelial system (RES), located mainly in the liver and spleen. The iron is separated from haem and either stored in ferritin or as haemosiderin, both in the RES and in hepatocytes, or released back into the circulation where it is again picked up by transferrin.

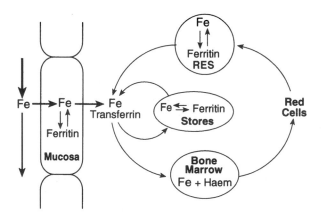

Fig. 9.1   The iron circuit. Iron is absorbed from the lumen of the small intestine (left), passes through the mucosal cell into the circulation where it is bound to transferrin and is redistributed to tissues. Most goes to the bone marrow for the production of heamoglobin in red cells. The red cells are eventually engulfed by cells of the reticuloendothelial system (RES) where iron may be stored in ferritin or redistributed back to the circulation.

It should be noted that the cycle is never reversed. There is normally only one way in and there is no way out except through blood loss or, in pregnancy, to the fetus. In reality, a small amount of iron is lost, mainly through loss of blood and surface cells of the gut, urinary tract and skin. In men this amounts to about 1 mg/day. The loss is relatively easily balanced by iron absorption. In women, additional losses through menstruation (0.5 mg Fe/day), and the cost of pregnancy (2 mg Fe/day) and lactation (0.5 mg Fe/day) make it more difficult to balance the loss through iron absorption.

9.2 IRON BALANCE

Iron requirements must be balanced by iron supply if iron deficiency or iron overload are to be avoided. Several factors combine to influence iron balance (Fig. 9.2). Obligatory iron losses, the requirements of growth and pregnancy as well as pathological losses due to excessive menstrual and other bleeding must be balanced against iron supply. Iron supply is influenced by the amount and the type of iron in food and the combination of various inhibitors and promoters of iron bioavailability. These requirements are buffered by iron available in stores. In addition, the body has the ability to modulate iron

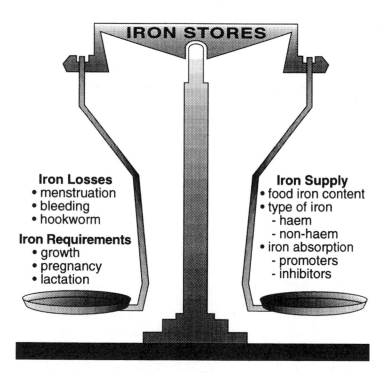

Fig. 9.2 Iron balance. Iron losses and requirements for growth (left) are balanced by iron supplied in the diet (right). Surplus iron is stored and can be drawn upon to supplement increased losses or requirements.

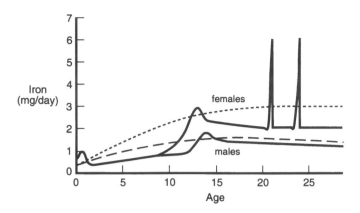

Fig. 9.3 Iron requirements for males and females vary during life. A Western diet, rich in meat and iron promoters (---) is able to meet iron requirements of the majority of females at all ages except in infancy, at the peak of the pubertal growth spurt and onset of menstruation and during pregnancies. In contrast, a cereal-based diet, without meat or iron promoters and with excess inhibitors of iron absorption (– – –) is not able to meet the requirements of most childbearing women and some men.

absorption according to its needs. Iron absorption is inversely related to body iron stores with more iron being absorbed by iron-deficient individuals than by iron-replete and iron-overloaded individuals. Furthermore, an increased rate of blood formation (erythropoiesis) with increased demand for iron enhances iron absorption. The body's iron requirements and the ability of the diet to meet the demand vary during life (Fig. 9.3). In infancy, during the pre-adolescent growth spurt and in women during reproductive life, particularly in pregnancy, the iron requirements may exceed the iron supply making iron deficiency more common during these periods. Individuals consuming a diet of low iron bioavailability are even more at risk.

9.3 IRON IN FOOD

Iron supply is greatly influenced by the composition of the diet. Two broad categories of iron are present in food: (1) Haem iron, derived mainly from haemoglobin and myoglobin in meat and fish, and (2) non-haem iron in the form of iron salts, iron in other proteins and iron derived from processing or storage methods. Haem iron enters the mucosal cells by a different mechanism and is better absorbed than non-haem iron. It is also less influenced by the body iron status, and is not affected by other constituents in the diet.

Non-haem iron compounds are found in a wide variety of foods of both plant and animal origin. The iron is present as metalloproteins (e.g. ferritin, haemosiderin, lactoferrin), soluble iron, iron bound to phytates in plants and contaminant iron such as ferric oxides and hydroxides introduced in the preparation and storage of food and by contamination from soil. The bioavailability of these forms of non-haem iron, unlike haem iron, is influenced by other constituents of the diet. Forms of iron that are similarly affected are said to enter a 'common pool'. The importance of this concept is that fortificant iron, added to food, will be subjected to the same inhibitory and promotive influences as the intrinsic food iron and will therefore have similar bioavailability. This concept, however, does not hold true for all forms of added iron. For example, most ferric salts, contaminant or added as fortificants, do not enter the common pool and have very low bioavailability.

9.4 PROMOTERS AND INHIBITORS OF IRON ABSORPTION

The relative concentrations of promoters and inhibitors of iron absorption in foods are responsible for the wide range of iron bioavailablity that has been demonstrated in foods (Table 9.1). The most important promoters of non-haem iron absorption are ascorbic acid (vitamin C) and meat. Other organic acids (e.g. citric acid) and some spices have also been shown to enhance iron absorption. The major inhibitors of non-haem iron absorption are phytate and polyphenols, common constituents of unrefined cereals and some vegetables.

Ascorbic acid is thought to enhance iron absorption by converting ferric to ferrous iron and by chelating iron in the lumen of the gut. This keeps iron in a more soluble and absorbable form and prevents binding to inhibitory ligands. It follows that the bioavailability of non-haem iron from foods with significant ascorbic acid content is relatively high. Moreover, the addition of ascorbic acid to meals of low bioavailability with potent inhibitors increases non-haem iron absorption.

The factor in meat responsible for enhancing non-haem iron absorption has not been identified. The enhancing effect is not shared by proteins derived from plants and other animal proteins such as milk, cheese or eggs. For example, substitution of beef for egg albumin as a source of protein in a test meal resulted in a fivefold increase in iron absorption. Present evidence suggests that peptides rich in the amino acid, cysteine, may play a role in the enhancement of non-haem iron absorption.

Polyphenols, commonly found in some vegetables (e.g. spinach), in some grains (e.g. red sorghum) and certain spices (e.g. oregano) are potent inhibitors of non-haem iron absorption. There is a strong inverse relationship between the concentration of polyphenols in foods and the absorption of iron from them. Many of the foods with low iron bioavailability listed in Table 9.1 are rich in polyphenols. Among the best known polyphenols is tannin, found in tea and other beverages (e.g. coffee, red wine), which has a profound inhibitory effect on iron absorption. Polyphenols also form strongly coloured compounds with iron which is a major problem in food fortification. This phenomenon can be illustrated by dropping a few crystals of ferrous sulphate into a cup of tea.

Phytates, found mainly in the husks of grains, are also major inhibitors of non-haem iron absorption. In this regard non-haem iron absorption is significantly less from non-polished rice than from polished rice, while increasing the bran content of a meal produces a dose-related depression in iron bioavailability. Both meat and ascorbic acid are able to counteract this inhibitory effect.

Calcium has been shown to inhibit absorption of both haem and non-haem iron. The effect is said to occur with calcium intakes up to approximately 300 mg/meal. High doses of certain other inorganic elements (e.g. zinc, manganese, copper) also interfere with

Table 9.1 Relative bioavailability of non-haem iron in foods

Food	Bioavailability		
	Low	Medium	High
Cereals	Maize Oatmeal Rice Sorghum Whole wheat flour	Cornflour White flour	
Fruits	Apple Avocado Banana Grape Peach Pear Plum Rhubarb Strawberry	Cantaloupe Mango Pineapple	Guava Lemon Orange Pawpaw Tomato
Vegetables	Aubergine Legumes Soyflour Isolated soy protein Lupin	Carrot Potato	Beetroot Broccoli Cabbage Cauliflower Pumpkin Turnip
Beverages	Tea Coffee	Red wine	White wine
Nuts	Almonds Brazil Coconut Peanut Walnut		
Animal proteins	Cheese Egg Milk		Fish Meat Poultry Breast milk

non-haem iron absorption; normally, dietary sources alone are unlikely to be high enough to have any adverse effect.

9.5 RECOMMENDED DIETARY INTAKES

The concept of a recommended dietary intake of iron is difficult to reconcile with the wide range of bioavailability (Table 9.1). The total iron content of a diet is a meaningless, although commonly employed, measure of its nutritional adequacy and may provide a false sense of nutritional security. For example, foods with high iron content due to large quantities of contaminant iron, or inappropriate fortificant iron, may be nutritionally worthless because of the low bioavailability of the iron. On the other hand, haem iron, making up only 10–15% of the total ingested iron, may account for a third of the iron actually absorbed. Similarly, the iron absorbed from a meal containing non-haem iron may be doubled if the meal is taken with a glass of orange juice (30 mg ascorbic acid) or reduced to a third if taken with tea. However, it is possible to divide diets into low, intermediate, and high iron bioavailability. These correspond to iron absorptions of about 5%, 10%, and 15% in subjects with depleted iron stores.

A diet of low bioavailability (<5%) with a high inhibitor content, negligible amounts of enhancers and little haem iron is based largely on unrefined cereals and legumes. Such diets are typical of many developing countries and supply about 0.7 mg of absorbed iron daily which is insufficient to meet the needs of most women, growing children and some men. A diet of intermediate bioavailability (~10%) includes limited amounts of foods which promote iron absorption and supplies enough absorbed iron (~1.5 mg) to meet the needs of 50% of women. A diet of high iron bioavailability (>15%) contains generous amounts of food rich in promoters and haem iron. The inhibitor content is low as cereals are often highly refined. Such diets, typical of many developed countries, supply sufficient iron (>2.1 mg daily) for most adults but still cannot match the daily amounts of absorbed iron required in the second half of pregnancy (5 mg daily).

The Food and Agriculture Organization/World Health Organization (FAO/WHO) recommendations (Table 9.2), based on estimates which apply to the 95th percentile of

Table 9.2 FAO/WHO recommended daily iron intake for individuals consuming diets of low, intermediate and high iron bioavailability. Requirements are given for absorbed iron

Group	Age (yrs)	Requirements of absorbed iron (μg/kg/day)	Recommended intake (mg/day)		
			Low (5%)	Intermediate (10%)	High (15%)
Children	0.25–1	120	21	11	7
	1–2	56	12	6	4
	2–6	44	14	7	5
	6–12	40	23	12	8
Boys	12–16	34	36	18	12
Girls	12–16	40	40	20	13
Adult men		18	23	11	8
Adult women					
menstruating		43	48	24	16
postmenopausal		18	19	9	6
lactating		24	26	13	9

Source: Report of a Joint FAO/WHO/Consultation. Requirements of vitamin A, iron, folate and vitamin B-12. FAO Food and Nutrition Series No. 23. Rome: FAO, 1988.

the population, are an attempt to take variations in bioavailability and requirements into account. Estimates of basal requirements of absorbed iron to prevent clinical signs of deficiency were corrected for individuals consuming diets of low, medium and high bioavailability of iron to give the recommended dietary iron intakes shown in Table 9.2. Values for the United States Recommended Dietary Allowances (RDAs) and the United Kingdom Dietary Reference Values (DRVs) for iron can be found in the reference list for Chapter 33 (pp. 536 and 537).

9.6 IRON DEFICIENCY

In the past, iron deficiency was thought to be due largely to abnormal loss of iron rather than insufficient iron supply. Credence for this view was given by the obvious effects of pathological blood loss and the high prevalence of iron deficiency in the developing world where hookworm infestation is endemic. However, it is now apparent that the poor bioavailability of iron in largely unrefined cereal-based diets is the major cause of iron deficiency in most developing countries. The impact of such diets is obviously enhanced when pathological blood loss or increased physiological iron demand is also present. These factors explain the geographical and gender variation in the prevalence of iron deficiency anaemia, which is reportedly most common in Asia where 58% of women and 32% of men are estimated to be anaemic. This should be compared to the prevalence in Europe and North America where only 10% of females and 3% of males are anaemic. The preponderance of anaemic females can be explained by increased physiological loss of iron in menstruation and pregnancy and to their lower food, and therefore iron, intake.

The development of iron deficiency is characterized by sequential changes in the amount of iron in the various iron compartments of the body (Fig. 9.4). In the first stage, iron stores become depleted but there is enough iron to meet the needs of red cell production. When iron stores are exhausted, the amount of iron in the circulation starts to fall and red cell production becomes compromised (iron deficient erthropoiesis). In

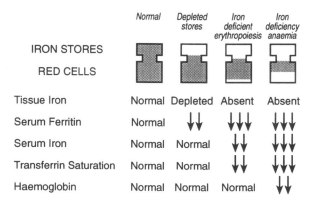

Fig. 9.4 The measurement of iron status and the stages of iron depletion. As iron in each of the body compartments is depleted (moving from left to right) different measurements of iron status become abnormal. No single biochemical index can assess all stages.

the final stage of exhausted iron stores, the amount of iron in the circulation is very low, red cell production is drastically reduced and microcytic hypochromic anaemia develops. The point at which the function of iron-containing enzymes becomes impaired is uncertain but probably depends on the rate of renewal of the enzymes and the growth of the tissues involved.

Iron deficiency has been associated with a number of pathological consequences of which anaemia is the most obvious. Severe anaemia is associated with weakness, impaired effort tolerance and eventually heart failure. There is no doubt that even mild iron deficiency anaemia limits work performance, and studies in Indonesia and Sri Lanka have linked it to reduced productivity. There is evidence from animal experiments that both the anaemia and tissue iron depletion are important. In children, iron deficiency is associated with impaired psychomotor development which is not reversed by subsequent iron therapy. In pregnancy, the weight of evidence suggests that iron deficiency anaemia is associated with prematurity, low birth weight and increased perinatal mortality. Changes in the gastrointestinal tract (atrophy of the mucosa of mouth, oesophagus and stomach) and the skin and nails (spoon-shaped nails) are well described but are infrequent. Other less well-recognized abnormalities include inability to adapt to cold and impaired immunity.

9.7 IRON OVERLOAD

Excessive amounts of iron may accumulate in the body and result in organ damage. The *acute* ingestion of a large amount of bioavailable iron, usually in the form of ferrous sulphate tablets, will exceed both the ability of the mucosa to control iron absorption and the capacity of transferrin to bind iron in the circulation. The acute iron toxicity that results is thought to be due to the generation of free radicals by free iron both in the gut and in the circulation. Most of the victims are children who mistakenly take their mothers' sugar-coated iron tablets. They develop severe abdominal pain, vomiting, metabolic acidosis and cardiovascular collapse. Severe poisoning has been described after the ingestion of 600 mg of iron, and death after 1 g.

Chronic iron overload develops insidiously and is seen mainly in three situations:

1. In genetic (HLA-linked) haemochromatosis there is an inherited defect, but as yet unknown, which appears to be at the level of iron release from the mucosal cell and from the reticuloendothelial system (RES) (see Fig. 9.1). The result is that iron floods the circulation and excessive iron is deposited over years in the liver, heart, pancreas and other organs. The damage to these organs is again thought to be due to free radicals and can result in liver cirrhosis, liver cancer, heart failure, arthritis and endocrine disease (diabetes and impotence). Removal of iron by repeated bleeding is an effective treatment. Recently, a gene (HFE) has been identified in the HLA region of chromosome six. Over 80% of patients with genetic haemochromatosis have been shown to be homozygous for a single base mutation of this gene. The gene appears to code for a protein similar to the human leucocyte antigen (HLA) class I proteins and is probably involved in regulating iron transport across the cell membrane.

2. African dietary iron overload is caused by the ingestion over many years, of large amounts of highly bioavailable iron in low alcohol beer brewed traditionally in iron pots.

Recent evidence suggests that there is also a genetic predisposition, but the nature of the genetic defect has yet to be demonstrated. Although the distribution of iron among the tissues in African iron overload differs from that seen in haemochromatosis the toxic effects are probably similar.

3. Secondary iron overload occurs in the so-called 'iron-loading anaemias' of which thalassaemia major is the most common. Excessive amounts of iron are absorbed over a relatively short period because of the increased turnover of red cells. In addition, repeated blood transfusions add to the iron burden. The iron overload occurs more rapidly and most victims die from iron-induced heart failure. A similar syndrome is seen in patients with bone marrow failure, kept alive by repeated blood transfusions.

It has been suggested that levels of body iron in the usually accepted normal range may be toxic. One hypothesis suggests that the increased incidence of coronary heart disease in men compared to women and in developed compared to underdeveloped countries could be explained by differences in iron status. It seems more likely that iron, in this instance, is a surrogate marker of overnutrition. Work from Finland showing that increased serum ferritin (a marker of iron stores) is a risk factor for acute myocardial infarction revived the debate. The proposed mechanism links iron to modification of low-density lipoproteins that increase its atherogenic potential. However, no other evidence has emerged to support this finding and the lower than normal risk of myocardial infarction in patients with haemochromatosis and its rarity in subjects with African iron overload, do not support the hypothesis.

9.8 ASSESSMENT OF IRON STATUS

Iron deficiency anaemia develops in three stages: (1) iron depletion, (2) iron-deficient erythropoiesis, and (3) iron deficiency anaemia, as shown in Fig. 9.4. No single biochemical index can assess all three stages.

- During *iron depletion* the amount of storage iron in the liver and in the reticuloendothelial cells of the spleen and bone marrow is progressively reduced, and can be detected by a parallel fall in serum ferritin concentration. The serum ferritin concentration falls below 12 μg/l (12 ng/ml) when the iron stores are exhausted. Iron depletion is the only cause of a serum ferritin below this level. Other measurements of iron status are normal at this stage.

- In *iron-deficient erythropoiesis* iron stores are exhausted (serum ferritin < 12 μg/l), and iron supply to the marrow is insufficient to meet the needs of haemoglobin production. This stage is detected by a low serum iron concentration and a transferrin saturation below 16%, although the haemoglobin concentration is still within the normal range. Transferrin saturation is derived from the serum iron and the total iron binding capacity (TIBC) as shown below:

$$\text{Transferrin saturation (\%)} = \frac{\text{Serum iron } (\mu\text{mol/l})}{\text{Serum TIBC } (\mu\text{mol/l})} \times 100\%$$

- In *iron deficiency anaemia*, the supply of iron to the marrow is so reduced that the concentration of haemoglobin falls below normal. The 'cut-off' value below which anaemia is diagnosed varies according to age and gender (below 110 g/l in children younger than six years and in pregnant women; below 120 g/l in women and adolescents under 15 years and below 130 g/l in adult men). There are obviously many other causes of anaemia other than iron deficiency (e.g. vitamin B_{12} and folate deficiency, chronic infection and intrinsic diseases of the bone marrow). The diagnosis of anaemia due to iron deficiency therefore requires that other measurements of iron status are also in the iron deficient range (serum ferritin <12 µg/l and transferrin saturation <16%). In addition, in established iron deficiency anaemia, the red cells become small (microcytosis) and pale (hypochromia). These changes can be detected by examination of a blood film or by a fall in the mean cell volume (MCV) below 85 fl and in the mean cell haemoglobin (MCH) below 27 pg.

- The serum ferritin concentration and the transferrin saturation are subject to variation due to causes other than iron status. For example, the serum iron concentration, and hence the transferrin saturation, exhibits marked diurnal (within day) variation and is depressed in infection, while the serum ferritin concentration is elevated by inflammation and tissue damage. Other tests can be employed that circumvent these problems. The production of haem is dependent on the supply of iron to the marrow. When iron supply is restricted, protoporphyrin, a precursor of haem, accumulates in red cells. This *free erythrocyte protoporphyrin* (FEP) is not subject to diurnal variation and provides the same information as the transferrin saturation. In addition, the FEP can be measured very easily on a single drop of blood using a simple instrument called a haematofluorometer. A transferrin saturation lower than 16% is associated with an FEP greater than 70 µg/dl (1.24 µmol/l) red cells. The FEP is, however, also elevated in lead poisoning and in inflammation. In this situation the serum ferritin concentration is usually elevated as well. Tissue iron depletion can also be measured by the concentration of *transferrin receptor* in plasma or serum. The expression of transferrin receptors on the surface of all cells is determined by the level of intracellular iron. In cellular iron depletion the concentration of soluble transferrin receptor in the plasma rises but, unlike the serum ferritin concentration, the level is not affected by inflammation. This test has only recently been developed and is expensive.

- The diagnosis of *iron overload* is also measured by a combination of measurements of iron status. A raised serum ferritin concentration (>400 µg/l) and transferrin saturation greater than 60% are highly suggestive of iron overload (e.g. hereditary haemochromatosis). However, high levels of serum ferritin may also be due to inflammation or tissue damage. In this situation, depression of serum iron concentration by inflammation may mask the presence of iron overload.

Diagnosis of iron deficiency and iron deficiency anaemia

Iron deficiency in populations with a high prevalence of chronic infection is difficult to diagnose because the transferrin saturation may be depressed and serum ferritin concentration elevated because of the presence of inflammation. The diagnosis of iron deficiency anaemia in this situation is best made by the combination of a low haemoglobin and an elevated serum transferrin receptor concentration. In the absence of inflammation, the combination of anaemia and two other measurements of iron deficiency makes a diagnosis of iron deficiency anaemia highly probable. In practice, a serum ferritin concentration of less than 12 μg/l, even in the presence of inflammation, is diagnostic of iron deficiency.

9.9 Treatment and Prevention of Iron Deficiency

Iron deficiency anaemia is best treated by the oral administration of ferrous iron salts. The cheapest and most effective is ferrous sulphate which is usually given in a dose of two tablets (100 mg iron) three times a day. The increase in haemoglobin concentration that can be expected with optimal doses of ferrous sulphate is about 2 g/l per day. Gastrointestinal side effects of oral iron therapy are common which has lead to a plethora of different oral iron compounds being available. Most differ in their formulation in an attempt to limit side effects, the most popular being slow release preparations. None has been shown convincingly to be better than ferrous sulphate and all will correct iron deficiency in time. The addition of ascorbic acid, while enhancing food iron availability, does little to improve therapeutic efficacy and probably increases the side effects. In individuals intolerant of oral iron therapy it is possible to give iron by intramuscular or intravenous injection.

It is theoretically possible to prevent iron deficiency by manipulation of the diet. This is well illustrated by the low prevalence of iron deficiency in industrialized countries where the diet is rich in haem iron and in promoters of non-haem iron absorption. However, this approach is sometimes impractical in developing countries where the diets are cereal-based and the problem of iron deficiency is greatest. An alternative is to fortify foods with iron or with iron plus a promoter of iron absorption. Unfortunately, iron fortification is fraught with practical difficulties. The major dilemma is the fact that the most bioavailable iron compounds are also the most soluble and the most reactive, leading to unacceptable changes in taste and colour of the food vehicle. Insoluble salts, such as ferric orthophosphate, and elemental iron powders produce no changes in food but are poorly absorbed. Recent experimental work has shown that the chelate, ferric EDTA, escapes the effects of inhibitors, particularly phytate, and in this setting is better absorbed than ferrous sulphate. It also produces little change in the colour of the food vehicle. Field trials, carried out systematically in iron-deficient populations, have shown ferric EDTA to be an effective fortificant. In one study, the prevalence of iron deficiency in women was reduced from 22% to 5% over a two-year period. No harmful effects of the EDTA itself, which is widely used in the food industry as an antioxidant, have been detected.

Despite these limitations, fortification of food with iron is commonplace in the industrialized world. Paradoxically, fortification programmes have often been carried out in a haphazard way with little attention being paid to the bioavailability of the fortificant or the efficacy of the programme. Iron used to fortify wheat flour contributes about 40% of the dietary intake in Sweden, 20% in the United States and 10% in the United Kingdom. Although there has been a decline in the prevalence of iron deficiency since iron fortification programmes were introduced their efficacy remains to be proved. This was highlighted by recent evidence showing that the elemental iron powder used to fortify flour in Sweden has a very low bioavailability. In contrast, iron fortification of infant formulas and infant cereals has been shown to be effective in combatting iron deficiency in this target group. In 1989, the United States Committee of Nutrition recommended that all infant formulas should be fortified with iron. In most cases, ferrous sulphate has been used to fortify milk and soy-based products. The bioavailability of the iron in these preparations is greatly enhanced by the addition of ascorbic acid.

In the developing world, iron fortification programmes face additional problems. Foods are seldom centrally processed, making fortification a difficult logistical problem. Furthermore, the diets are largely cereal-based and lack natural promoters of iron absorption which means that the added iron will be poorly absorbed. Attempts to overcome this problem have included the use of combinations of iron orthophosphate and ascorbic acid to fortify salt in India, the use of haem iron derived from slaughtered animals to fortify infant cereals and flour products in Chile and, more recently, the use of ferric EDTA. Although this latter compound is currently about six times more expensive than ferrous sulphate it is two to three times better absorbed from cereal-based meals. Ferric EDTA has recently been approved by the United Nations Joint Expert Committee on Food Additives (JECFA) as an iron fortificant which may herald better use of this promising chelate.

FURTHER READING

1. Bothwell TH, Charlton RW, Cook JD, Finch CA. *Iron metabolism in man.* Oxford: Blackwell Scientific Publications, 1979.
2. Brock JH, Halliday JW, Pippard MJ, Powell LW (eds). *Iron metabolism in health and disease.* London: WB Saunders, 1994.
3. Fomon SJ, Zlotkin S (eds). *Nutritional anaemias.* Nestlé Nutrition Workshop Series, Volume 30. Raven Press, 1992.
4. Food and Agriculture Organization of the United Nations. *Requirements of vitamin A, iron, folate and vitamin B_{12}.* Report of a Joint FAO/WHO Expert Consultation. FAO Food and Nutrition Series, No 23. Rome: FAO, 1988.
5. Lynch SR, Bothwell TH, Hurrell RF, MacPhail AP. *Iron EDTA for food fortification.* Report of the International Nutritional Anemia Consultative Group (INACG). Washington: The Nutrition Foundation, 1993.

10

TRACE ELEMENTS

Trace elements occur in the body in very small or 'trace' amounts (i.e. mg or μg/kg body weight); they generally constitute less than 0.01% of the body mass. They are considered essential when a deficient intake produces an impairment in biological function, and when supplementation with physiological levels of that element reverses the impaired function or prevents an impairment.

Trace elements differ in their properties and biological functions; many act primarily by forming metallo-enzymes. Deficiencies of trace elements produce multiple and diverse clinical signs and symptoms; only some have been explained in biochemical terms. Trace element deficiencies may arise from inadequate dietary intakes, and/or decreased bio-availability, or may be associated with disease states in which decreased absorption, excessive excretion, and/or excessive utilization occur.

10.1 ZINC

Samir Samman

10.1.1   Historical perspective

The essentiality of zinc was first recognized in microorganisms and plants in 1869 and 1926, respectively. Experimental deficiency was demonstrated in laboratory animals but the likelihood of deficiency in humans was considered remote because of the ubiquitous nature of zinc in the food supply and the relative difficulty in creating zinc-deficient animal models. Zinc deficiency was first recognized in humans in the Middle East in 1958.

10.1.2   Chemistry

Zinc is one of the IIB series of metals with a molecular weight of 65.4. It exists mostly in the divalent state which has a highly concentrated charge. It is the most common catalytic metal ion in the cytoplasm of cells. It is a good Lewis acid and does not undergo redox reactions. The most abundant stable isotopes are ^{64}Zn and ^{66}Zn.

10.1.3   Distribution

Adult humans contain between 1.2–2.3 g of zinc which is distributed in all tissues. Tissue concentration is high in the choroid of the eye and the prostate gland but most of the body zinc is in bones and muscles. In liver cells, zinc is associated with all subcellular fractions. The plasma concentration of zinc is approximately 98 μg/dl (15 μmol/l) of which a third is bound to α_2-macroglobulin and the rest to albumin. However, only 10–20% of the zinc in blood is found in the plasma, the rest is in red blood cells associated mainly with carbonic anhydrase. The red cell membrane contains some zinc. Semen has 100-fold the zinc concentration of plasma.

10.1.4 Functions

Zinc is a constituent of a large number of mammalian enzymes (more than 150) where it functions at the active site or as a structural component or both. Carbonic anhydrase was the first zinc-dependent enzyme to be discovered; other enzymes include: carboxypeptidase, alkaline phosphatase, transferases, ligases, lyases, isomerases, DNA/RNA polymerase, reverse transcriptase and superoxide dismutase. Therefore, zinc is important in a number of major metabolic processes including protein and nucleic acid synthesis. Zinc is essential for the synthesis and action of insulin. It also helps to stabilize the proinsulin and insulin hexamers by forming complexes with them.

Zinc 'fingers' have been identified in the human genome and are thought to outnumber the zinc-dependent enzymes. The proteins, which may contain up to 30 'fingers', have been identified as sequence-specific DNA-binding proteins which interact with DNA and act as transcriptional mediators. Zinc also plays a role in stabilizing macromolecules and cellular membranes and can function as a site-specific antioxidant. It can bind to or be in close proximity to thiol groups of proteins and reduce their reactivity.

10.1.5 Absorption and excretion

Zinc is absorbed mainly from the duodenum although some is absorbed lower down the small intestine. The mode of absorption involves both saturable and passive mechanisms. Unlike the absorption of calcium and some vitamins, zinc absorption is unaffected by age.

The exact site of absorption depends on the form of zinc and the presence or absence of other dietary components which may form complexes with zinc or impact on intestinal transit time. Absorption is increased by a number of dietary factors which include: the presence of amino acids (particularly histidine); lactose; and low dietary iron. Zinc absorption is reduced by low intakes of protein and high intakes of phytate. The latter effect is exacerbated by high intakes of calcium in humans. Supplementation with large doses of non-haem iron (equivalent to those given to pregnant women) can reduce the bioavailability of zinc; haem iron has no effect. Earlier studies suggested that citrate and picolinate enhanced zinc absorption but recent information de-emphasizes their role. Once absorbed, zinc is transported to the liver bound to albumin.

The major route of zinc excretion is by the intestine followed by the kidneys and the skin. Faecal zinc originates from unabsorbed dietary sources as well as endogenous excretion, arising from zinc excreted into the intestine along with the digestive juices. Both absorption and excretion of zinc can be manipulated to maintain homeostasis; smaller amounts of zinc are excreted in the urine or shed in skin cells. In addition, sexual activity in males contributes to zinc losses; each ejaculate is said to contain up to 0.5 mg of zinc, or approximately 5% of the dietary intake. Seminal zinc is thought to be derived from secretions of the prostate gland. Although conservation of zinc occurs during experimental zinc deficiency, the amount of zinc in ejaculates remains relatively high and hence contributes to a significant loss of body zinc, particularly when zinc intakes are chronically low. Hence, the role of zinc in men is analogous to iron in women because it is lost as part of normal sexual function.

10.1.6 Deficiency

Zinc deficiency was first described in male adolescents in Iran and Egypt. The original observations were made on a 21-year-old male subject who resembled a 10-year-old boy. This patient ate mainly bread as well as a considerable amount of clay. In other cases, the subjects had hookworm infections and ate mostly unleavened bread and beans. Further investigations identified zinc as the limiting nutrient responsible for numerous symptoms including growth retardation, hypogonadism and delayed sexual maturation. Other manifestations of zinc deficiency which have been reported subsequently include diverse forms of skin lesions, impaired wound healing, hypogeusia, behavioural disturbances, night blindness and immune deficiency. These features do not always occur together and seem to depend on the setting. For instance, in patients on total parenteral nutrition (without zinc supplements) there is mental confusion, depression, eczema and alopecia whereas in young children, zinc deficiency is expressed as a reduction in appetite, hypogeusia and poor growth.

Night blindness, a significant symptom of vitamin A deficiency in developing countries, can be induced by zinc deficiency because of the reduced activity of retinol dehydrogenase, a zinc-dependent enzyme responsible for the conversion of retinol to retinaldehyde. Also, zinc deficiency may be partly responsible for the increased prevalence of diarrhoea in developing countries. Zinc supplementation of infants and young children with acute diarrhoea results in reductions in the duration and severity of diarrhoea. Zinc deficiency has been observed in association with protein-energy deficiency malnutrition in infants with marasmus and during their recovery. Zinc supplements supplied to malnourished children during recovery were found to promote weight gain and lean tissue synthesis. Anorexia nervosa resembles marasmus; nevertheless, the role of zinc in anorexia nervosa is unclear. It is likely that zinc deficiency develops in some anorexic patients arising from an inadequate diet which sustains the disorder and prevents adequate weight gain. However, zinc does not appear to play a causal role in anorexia nervosa.

In pregnant women, plasma zinc concentrations are consistently lower than those of non-pregnant women. Although this can be attributed partly to physiological changes unrelated to zinc depletion, nevertheless, zinc intakes of pregnant women are often below the recommended intake. However, in pregnancy, adaptations such as increased absorption and reduced endogenous losses of zinc may help meet the zinc requirements. Supplementation with zinc may improve certain measures of pregnancy outcome such as birth weight and head circumference.

Biochemical abnormalities of zinc deficiency include a reduction in: plasma and hair zinc concentrations, protein synthesis, activity of metalloproteins, resistance to infection, collagen synthesis and platelet aggregation. In view of the large number of zinc finger proteins and the interaction between zinc and DNA, it has been hypothesized that zinc primarily restricts gene expression rather than the enzyme activities.

Conditions which predispose to zinc deficiency are related to:

* a decreased intake which is associated with an eating disorder;
* decreased absorption and/or bioavailability arising from high intakes of inhibitors (e.g. phytate) as reported in the first cases of human zinc deficiency;
* decreased utilization secondary to other conditions such as alcoholism;
* increased losses in conditions such as diarrhoea and excessive vomiting which may also be associated with an eating disorder;
* increased requirements associated with growth, pregnancy and lactation. The latter is recognized by a small increase in the recommended dietary intakes.

10.1.7 Bioavailability and food sources

It is well recognized that a number of factors can influence the bioavailability of zinc. The extent to which humans can adapt to foods with low bioavailability of zinc by increasing absorption is not fully understood and is confounded by the interactions with other nutrients and antinutrients. Current methods used for studying zinc bioavailability in humans include conventional metabolic balance studies and radioisotopic and stable isotope techniques. Use of radioactive isotopes is limited by ethical considerations such as long radioactive half-lives and the amount of radiation exposure to subjects. Use of stable isotopes may circumvent this issue but the technique requires costly isotopes and instrumentation and demanding analytical procedures.

Zinc is available widely in the food supply but its bioavailability from different foods is highly variable. Zinc in animal products, crustacea and molluscs is more readily absorbed than from plant foods. Rich sources of zinc include oysters, red meat and liver. Unrefined cereal grains and legumes are rich in phytate which reduces zinc absorption. The zinc content of refined cereals is lower than unrefined cereals but because a large part of the phytic acid present in the bran has been removed during the refining, the bioavailability of zinc is enhanced. The molar ratio of phytate:zinc has been used as a predictor of zinc bioavailability in foods and diets; ratios greater than 15 have been associated with suboptimal zinc status. Also, the phytate × calcium:zinc in the diet has been suggested as a marker of zinc bioavailability; however, there are limited data on the phytate content of foods. Hence, the consumption of high amounts of calcium from dairy products in the presence of high phytate intakes may increase the risk of zinc deficiency in at risk groups such as lacto-ovo-vegetarians.

The absorption of zinc from breast milk is high even in cases of the genetic disorder of zinc absorption (acrodermatitis enteropathica). The fractional absorption of zinc from breast milk in healthy exclusively breast-fed infants is approximately 54%.

10.1.8 Recommended intakes

The recommended dietary intakes for zinc (mg/day) for adult males and females and the suggested allowances for pregnancy and lactation are shown in Table 10.1. Both the basal and normative requirement estimates assuming moderate availability for dietary zinc set by the World Health Organization (WHO), 1996, are included.

Table 10.1 Recommended dietary intakes of zinc for adults (mg/day) (WHO 1996)

Group	UK	USA	WHO*	
			Basal	Normative
Males	9.5	15	5.7	9.4
Females	7.0	12	4.0	6.5
Pregnant	No increment	+3	1st tri +0.6	+0.8
			2nd tri +1.7	+2.8
			3rd tri +4.0	+6.8
Lactating	+2.5–6	+4–7	+2.6–5.1	+3.1–6.2

* Moderate availability; tri, trimester.

10.1.9 Assessment of zinc status

Plasma zinc concentrations provide a limited amount of information about zinc status. Zinc from the plasma is taken up by the liver in response to cytokines released during stress and infection, hence plasma zinc values fall. In addition, plasma zinc concentrations fall in pregnancy, with injuries, and in diseases such as atherosclerosis, liver cirrhosis and pernicious anaemia.

Plasma zinc also undergoes diurnal variation with a U-shaped response curve over a 24-hour period. Peak concentrations are found in the mornings and trough concentrations in the mid evening. The diurnal rhythm parallels that of plasma-ionized calcium. Hence, blood samples for plasma zinc should be taken under carefully controlled conditions, standardized with respect to time of day as well as position of the subject during blood collection, fasted or fed state, and length of time prior to separation of the plasma; all these factors influence plasma zinc concentration. Despite its limitations, the concentration of zinc in plasma is the most commonly used diagnostic indicator and the balance of evidence shows that the concentration falls in deficiency and rises in sufficiency (or supplementation). The zinc concentration of other accessible tissues such as red blood cells and platelets remains unchanged during controlled zinc deficiency and supplementation trials. Leucocyte and neutrophil zinc concentrations have been shown to be affected by zinc status in some studies but not others and their potential usefulness requires further investigation.

Although urine is readily accessible, collection of a 24-hour urine sample is awkward, inconvenient and susceptible to environmental contamination by exogenous sources of the trace metal as well as endogenous sources such as seminal fluid. Well-controlled studies have indicated that urine is not a good biomarker as its excretion is only sensitive to extreme changes in zinc status. Also, there are no established criteria for interpreting urinary zinc levels. Hair is also readily accessible, non-invasive, stable and requires no special storage conditions. Zinc concentrations in hair are higher than that of plasma, facilitating analysis. Studies have shown that provided standardized conditions are used for the sampling, washing, and analysis, hair zinc concentrations during infancy and childhood reflect chronic suboptimal zinc status in the absence of very severe protein-energy malnutrition, provided seasonal variations are controlled.

The activity of some metallo-enzymes is depressed during nutritional zinc deficiency whereas others remain unaffected. Alkaline phosphatase activity in erythrocyte membranes appears to be sensitive to zinc depletion and repletion and thus may be a valid index of zinc status. This enzyme, along with the metal-binding protein, metallothionein, are potentially suitable markers which deserve further investigation.

Although frank zinc deficiency can be identified, marginal zinc status is difficult to measure. Despite the extensive research in this field, little applied information has been obtained. It is recognized that the currently available biochemical tests for zinc status are not ideal; they are neither sensitive nor specific. The only sure way to diagnose zinc deficiency is by a positive response of mild clinical signs such as impaired growth, anorexia, reduced taste acuity, impaired immunocompetence to zinc supplementation.

10.1.10 Toxicity

Acute toxicity of zinc as a result of ingesting doses greater than 25 mg, results in a metallic taste in the mouth, nausea and gastric distress. Such cases may be induced by deliberate supplementation (self-medication), occupational hazards, or by food poisoning (e.g. preparation of acid food in galvanized containers). Rapid infusion of intravenous feeding solutions containing zinc can cause similar symptoms. Very large doses of zinc may cause death.

Chronic toxicity of zinc results from the long-term consumption of moderately high amounts of zinc. In such circumstances, risk of coronary heart disease is increased as a result of an increase in the low-density lipoprotein cholesterol concentration and a decrease in high-density lipoprotein in serum. The major adverse effect of chronic zinc toxicity, however, is due to the antagonistic interaction between zinc and copper absorption. Zinc induces the synthesis of metallothionein, a sulphur-rich protein which binds copper with a high affinity. In chronic zinc toxicity, copper status is reduced resulting in a decrease in copper-related functions including a reduction in copper metallo-enzyme activity, copper deficiency and anaemia. Reduction of copper absorption is advantageous under some circumstances. It is required in the treatment of patients with Wilson's disease; in these cases zinc supplementation is part of the management strategy.

FURTHER READING

1. Prasad AS. Discovery and importance of zinc in human nutrition. *Fed Proc* 1984; **43**: 2829–34.
2. Swanson CA, King JC. Zinc and pregnancy outcome. *Am J Clin Nutr* 1987; **46**: 763–71.
3. Aggett PJ. The assessment of zinc status: a personal view. *Proc Nutr Soc* 1991; 9–17.
4. Tamura T, Goldenberg RL. Zinc nutriture and pregnancy outcome. *Nutr Res* 1996; **16**: 139–81.
5. Thompson RPH. Assessment of zinc status. *Proc Nutr Soc* 1991; **50**: 19–28.
6. World Health Organization. Trace elements in human nutrition and health. Geneva: WHO, 1996: 72–104.

10.2 COPPER

Samir Samman

10.2.1 Historical perspective

The essential role of copper was realized in 1926 and soon after it was shown that it is required for the synthesis of haemoglobin in rats. In 1931, it was demonstrated that copper-supplemented infants with anaemia had accelerated haemoglobin synthesis when treated with iron.

10.2.2 Chemistry

Copper is one of the IB series of metals with a molecular weight of 63.5. It is one of the most effective cations for binding to organic molecules. It is commonly used in biological reactions that involve electron transfer. The most abundant stable isotopes are ^{63}Cu and ^{65}Cu.

10.2.3 Distribution

Adult humans contain about 100 mg copper which is distributed in concentrations of about 1.5 µg/g in the skin, skeletal muscle, bone marrow, liver and brain. Studies in animals suggest that the copper content may decrease with age. Approximately 10% of the total body copper pool is in the blood; small amounts exist in the red blood cells. The plasma copper concentration is approximately 95.3 µg/dl (15 µmol/l) (similar to zinc), up to 90% of this is associated with caeruloplasmin. Other copper proteins include many of the oxidases, metallothionein, α-fetoglobulin, superoxide dismutase and trans-cuprein. A distinguishing feature of copper proteins and enzymes is that the majority of the former are extracellular.

10.2.4 Functions

Copper has diverse functions including erythropoiesis, connective tissue synthesis (via lysyl oxidase), oxidative phosphorylation, thermogenesis and superoxide dismutation. As well as transporting copper, caeruloplasmin is one of the acute phase proteins and via its ferroxidase activity, catalyses the oxidation of ferrous iron. This latter reaction is essential for the mobilization of iron as a complex with transferrin. It is believed to be the mechanism by which copper is able to regulate the homeostasis of iron.

10.2.5 Absorption and excretion

Copper is absorbed by an active transport process initially then mostly by carrier-mediated diffusion from the stomach and duodenum. As absorption has been shown to control homeostasis, the efficiency increases in cases of deficiency. Absorbed copper is transported by albumin to the liver, where it is transferred to caeruloplasmin. Copper is excreted mainly via the gastrointestinal tract. Less is excreted in the urine and from the skin.

10.2.6 Bioavailability and food sources

Absorption is enhanced by organic nutrients such as amino acids and, in particular, histidine. Conversely, absorption is inhibited by excesses of other divalent cations such as zinc and iron. Studies in animals suggest that vitamin C may have an adverse effect on copper absorption but the results of trials in humans are not conclusive. Phytic acid and dietary fibre do not inhibit copper absorption.

Copper has a wide distribution in the food supply. Richest food sources are oysters, other shellfish, liver, kidney, followed by nuts, high protein cereals, and dried fruits and legumes. The concentration of copper in the water supply tends to be variable; copper pipes may contribute substantially to the intake of copper from drinking water.

10.2.7 Deficiency

Copper deficiency is relatively rare. It has been observed in protein-energy malnutrition, in patients on long-term copper-free total parenteral nutrition, and in premature infants. Symptoms include anaemia, neutropenia, skeletal demineralization, decreased skin tone, connective tissue aneurysms, hypothermia, neurological symptoms and depigmented hair. Conditions which are predisposing to copper deficiency are, in principle, similar to those described for zinc.

Defects in copper metabolism have been identified. Menkes' disease was established as a copper-related disorder following the recognition by Australian researchers that patients with the disease have 'kinky' hair similar to the kinks in the wool of sheep grazing on copper-deficient soils. Such changes in the hair together with low concentrations of copper and caeruloplasmin in plasma are characteristic features of the disease. Intestinal absorption of copper is impaired.

Patients who lack plasma caeruloplasmin, a condition termed 'acaeruloplasminaemia', have been identified. Recent findings in these patients have confirmed the essential role of this copper protein in iron metabolism. Symptoms associated with acaeruloplasminaemia include decreased copper and iron in plasma, increased iron concentrations in tissues and impaired copper absorption.

10.2.8 Recommended dietary intakes

The World Health Organization (1996) has set lower limits (mg/day) of the safe ranges of population mean intakes of dietary copper to meet both basal and normative requirement estimates. For pregnant and non-pregnant adults, basal and normative requirement estimates are 1.01 and 1.15 mg/day, respectively. No increase is recommended during pregnancy because of the enhanced copper retention. During lactation an additional amount of 0.1 mg is recommended to compensate, in part, for the level of copper in breast milk.

10.2.9 Assessment of copper status

Frank copper deficiency can be determined by measuring plasma copper concentrations, plasma caeruloplasmin (either as a concentration or an enzymatic activity) or the activities of copper-dependent enzymes such as superoxide dismutase. The haematocrit decreases and microcytic hypochromic anaemia occurs in frank copper deficiency. The assessment of marginal deficiency remains a challenge.

10.2.10 Toxicity

Acute copper toxicity has been reported as a result of accidental ingestion of large doses of copper or in industrial accidents. The symptoms induced by small doses include vomiting and nausea; large doses induce hepatic necrosis and haemolytic anaemia. Chronic toxicity is relatively rare. Wilson's disease is a rare familial copper-storage disease in which the copper concentrations of tissues increase as a result of insufficient ceruloplasmin. Patients usually present with neurological symptoms and liver disease.

FURTHER READING

1. Danks DM, Campbell PE, Stevens BJ, Mayne V, Cartwright E. Menke's kinky hair syndrome. An inherited defect in copper absorption with widespread effects. *Pediatrics* 1972; **50**: 188–201.
2. Milne DB. Assessment of copper nutritional status. *Clin Chem* 1994; **40**: 1479–84.
3. World Health Organization. Trace elements in human nutrition and health. Geneva: WHO, 1996: 123–43.

10.3 IODINE

Christine Thomson

Iodine was one of the earliest trace elements to be identified as essential. In the first half of the nineteenth century, the incidence of goitre was linked with low iodine content of food and drinking water. In the 1920s, iodine was shown to be an integral component of the thyroid hormone, thyroxine, required for normal growth and metabolism, and later in 1952, of triiodothyronine.

10.3.1 Chemical structure and functions of iodine

Iodine functions as an integral part of the thyroid hormones, the prohormone, thyroxine (T_4), and the more potent active form 3,5,3′-triiodothyronine (T_3) which is the key regulator of important cell processes. The thyroid hormones are required for normal growth and development of individual tissues such as the central nervous system and maturation of the whole body, and also for energy production and oxygen consumption in cells, thereby maintaining the body's metabolic rate.

If thyroid hormone secretion is inadequate, the basal metabolic rate is reduced and the general level of activity of the individual is decreased (hypothyroidism). The regulation of thyroid hormone synthesis, release and action is a complex process involving the thyroid, the pituitary, the brain and peripheral tissues. The hypothalamus regulates the plasma concentrations of the thyroid hormones by controlling the release of the pituitary's thyroid-stimulating hormone (TSH) through a feedback mechanism related to the level of T_4 in the blood. If blood T_4 falls, the secretion of TSH is increased which enhances both thyroid activities and the output of T_4 into the circulation. If the level of circulating T_4 hormone is not maintained because of severe iodine deficiency, TSH remains elevated and both these measures are used for diagnosis of hypothyroidism due to iodine deficiency.

10.3.2 Body content

Iodine occurs in the tissues in both inorganic (iodide) or organically bound forms. The adult human body contains about 15–50 mg iodine, of which 70–80% is in the thyroid gland which has a remarkable concentrating power for iodine, and the remainder is mainly in the circulating blood.

10.3.3 Metabolism

The metabolism of iodine is closely linked to thyroid function, since the only known function for iodine is in the synthesis of thyroid hormones. Iodine is an anionic trace element which is rapidly absorbed in the form of iodide. It is converted to iodine in the thyroid gland, and bound to tyrosine residues from which the hormones T_3 and T_4 are formed. Inorganic iodine is readily excreted in the urine. Since faecal output and losses from the skin are small, 24-hour urinary excretion of iodine reflects the dietary intake and hence may be used for estimating the intake.

10.3.4 Deficiency

Iodine deficiency is the world's greatest single cause of preventable brain damage and mental retardation. The term 'iodine deficiency disorders' (IDD) refers to the wide spectrum of effects of iodine deficiency on growth and development. Goitre, a swelling of the thyroid gland, is the most obvious and familiar feature of iodine deficiency (Fig. 10.1). However, other effects are seen at all stages of development, but especially during the fetal and neonatal periods.

A major effect of fetal iodine deficiency in areas where endemic goitre exists and iodine deficiency is severe, is endemic cretinism. In general, cretins are mentally defective with other physical abnormalities. Clinical manifestations may differ with geographical location, and two quite distinct syndromes have been observed. In myxoedematous cretinism, hypothyroidism is present during fetal and early postnatal development and results in stunted growth and mental deficiency. In the nervous or neurological type of cretinism, mental retardation is present as well as hearing and speech defects and characteristic disorders of stance and gait, while hypothyroidism is absent. This syndrome appears to result from iodine deficiency of the mother during fetal development.

The major cause of IDD is inadequate dietary intake of iodine from foods grown in soils from which iodine has been leached by glaciation, high rainfall or flooding. Goitre is usually seen where the intake is less than 50 µg/day and cretinism with intakes of 30 µg/day or less by the mother. However, thyroid function may also be impaired after exposure to antithyroid compounds in foods and drugs called 'goitrogens'. The aetiology

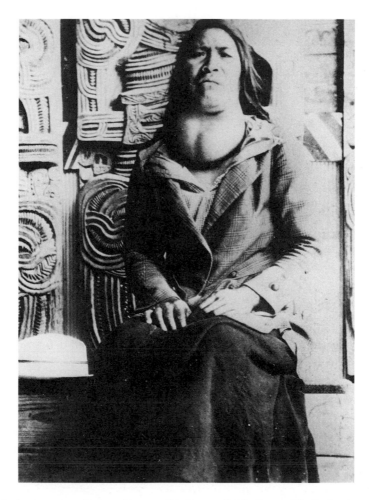

Fig. 10.1 Endemic goitre. *Source*: Hercus CE, Benson WN, Carter CL. Endemic goitre in New Zealand, and its relation to the soil-iodine. *J Hygiene* 1925; **24**: 321–402.

of myxoedematous and nervous cretinism may be influenced by the simultaneous occurrence of selenium deficiency along with iodine deficiency in some areas, because of the role of selenium as part of the enzyme type I iodothyronine 5'-deiodinase in thyroid hormone metabolism.

10.3.5 Measures to prevent iodine deficiency

Iodization of salt has been the major method for combating iodine deficiency since the 1920s when it was first successfully used in Switzerland. Since then, introduction of iodized salt in a number of other countries including New Zealand has resulted in the elimination of goitre in these regions. However, the success of iodization depends on whether all salt is iodized, as acceptability of iodized salt may be a problem in some countries. In Asia, where millions of people are affected there are major difficulties in producing, monitoring and distributing iodized salt.

Iodized oil by injection has been used in the prevention of endemic goitre in South America, Zaire and China. A single intramuscular injection of iodized oil given to girls and young women can correct severe iodine deficiency for a period of over four years.

Iodine deficiency is recognized as a major international public health problem because of the large populations at risk due to their iodine-deficient environments, characterized primarily by iodine-deficient soil. An estimated 400 million people in Asia alone are affected by disorders resulting from severe iodine deficiency. Endemic cretinism affects up to 10% of the populations living in severely iodine-deficient areas in India, Indonesia and China. Cretinism is also prevalent in Papua New Guinea, Africa and South America. The International Council for the Control of Iodine Deficiency Disorders (ICCIDD), formed in 1986, is working closely with other international organizations to develop national programmes to prevent and control iodine deficiency disorders. A Global Action Plan to eliminate IDD as a major public health problem by the year 2000 has now been adopted by the United Nations system (see Chapter 37).

10.3.6 Assessment of iodine status

The assessment of nutritional status of iodine is important in relation to a population or group living in an area or region that is suspected to be iodine deficient (Table 10.2). The methods recommended are:

- The goitre rate, including the rate of palpable (examined using the thumbs) or visible (when head tilted back or in normal position) goitre, classified according to acceptable criteria.
- Urinary iodine excretion: 24-hour excretion of iodine reflects dietary intake and hence may be used for estimating the intake. However, the 24-hour urine is difficult to collect in the field situation. Determination of the iodine status of a population can be determined from iodine concentration in casual urine samples from a group of approximately 40 subjects.
- The level of serum thyroxine or TSH provides an indirect measure of iodine nutritional status.

Table 10.2 Grades of severity of iodine deficiency disorders (IDD)

	Mild IDD	Moderate IDD	Severe IDD
Prevalence of goitre % (total)	5–19	20–29	> 30
Cretinism	0	0	0–5
Daily urine iodine (μg/day)	50–100	25–49	< 25
Median urine iodine (μg/dl)	3.5–5.0	2.0–3.4	0–1.9
Prevalence of neonatal TSH > 50 μU/ml (day 5 of life)	< 1%	1–5%	> 5%

Source: Clugston GA, Hetzel BS. Iodine. In: Shils ME, Olson JA, Shike M (eds). *Modern nutrition in health and disease*, 8th ed. Philadelphia, PA: Lea & Febiger 1994, Vol 1: 252–62.

10.3.7 Dietary intakes

Normal iodine intake is 100–150 µg/day. Foods of marine origin: sea fish and shell fish, seameal (custard made of ground seaweed) and seaweeds are rich in iodine, reflecting the greater iodine concentration of sea water compared to fresh water. The iodine content of plants and animals depends on the environment in which they grow. Vegetables, fruit and cereals grown on soils with low iodine content are poor sources of iodine.

In recent years, iodine contamination in dairy products and bread has made a major contribution to the daily intake. The use of iodophors as sanitizers in the dairy industry has resulted in variable but considerable amounts of residual iodine in milk, cheese and other milk products. The use of these compounds, however, is declining in New Zealand and Australia. The addition of iodate as a bread improver was adopted by Tasmania as an iodine supplement, but iodates are not permitted in New Zealand. Other adventitious sources of iodine include kelp tablets and drugs, beverages or foods containing the iodine-containing colouring, erythrosine.

10.3.8 Interactions

The utilization of absorbed iodine is influenced by goitrogens which interfere with the biosynthesis of the hormones. Goitrogens are found in vegetables of the genus brassica: cabbage, turnip, swede, brussel sprouts, broccoli and in some staple foods such as cassava, maize, lima beans used in developing countries. Most goitrogens are inactivated by heat, but not when milk is pasteurized.

10.3.9 Requirement and recommended dietary intakes

Recommended dietary intakes of iodine are based on the estimate of requirement for the prevention of goitre of about 1–2 µg/kg body weight plus a 100% margin of safety. Intakes between 50 µg and 1000 µg are considered safe. Table 10.3 gives recommended daily intakes for iodine.

10.3.10 Toxicity

Daily intakes of 2000 µg iodine should be regarded as excessive or potentially harmful. Such intakes are unlikely to be obtained from normal diets of natural foods except where they are exceptionally high in marine fish or seaweed, or where foods are contaminated with iodine from iodophors or other adventitious sources.

Table 10.3 Recommended dietary intakes of iodine (µg/day)

Group	UK		USA RDA	WHO* (1996) RI(PR)	European PRI
	LNRI	RNI			
Men and women	70	140	150	120–150	130
Pregnant women	–	–	175	175	–
Lactating women	–	–	200	175	–

* World Health Organization (1996).
LNRI, lower reference nutrient intake; RNI, reference nutrient intake; RI(PR), recommended intakes (population requirements) ≡ normative requirement estimates; PRI, population reference intake.

Excess intakes of iodide can cause enlargement of the thyroid gland, just as deficiency can. Iodine-induced thyrotoxicosis (Jod–Basedow) following the iodization programmes has been described particularly in women over 40 years of age who had always been living in a low iodine environment.

FURTHER READING

1. Clugston GA, Hetzel BS. Iodine. In: Shils ME, Olson JA, Shike M (eds). 8th ed. *Modern nutrition in health and disease*. Philadelphia, PA: Lea & Febiger 1994; Vol 1: 252–62.
2. Hetzel BS, Maberly GF. Iodine. In: Mertz W (ed.). 5th ed. *Trace elements in human and animal nutrition*. New York: Academic Press 1987; Vol 2: 139–208.
3. Hetzel BS, Dunn JT. The iodine deficiency disorders: their nature and prevention. *Ann Rev Nutr* 1989; **9**: 21–38.
4. *Global prevalence of iodine deficiency disorders*. WHO, UNICEF, ICCIDD. 1993.
5. World Health Organization. *Trace elements in human nutrition and health*. Geneva: WHO, 1996: 49–71.

10.4 SELENIUM

Christine Thomson

Selenium first attracted interest in the 1930s as a toxic trace element that caused loss of hair and blind staggers in livestock consuming high-selenium plants in South Dakota. In 1957, selenium was shown to be essential for animals when traces of this mineral prevented liver necrosis in vitamin E-deficient rats, and later to prevent a variety of economically important diseases such as white muscle disease in cattle and sheep, hepatosis dietetica in swine and exudative diathesis in poultry. The demonstration in 1973 of a biochemical function for selenium as a constituent of the seleno-enzyme, glutathione peroxidase (GSHPx), helped to explain the interrelationship between selenium and vitamin E. The importance of selenium in human nutrition was highlighted in reports in 1979 of selenium deficiency in a patient in New Zealand on total parenteral nutrition and of the selenium-responsive condition Keshan disease in China. Considerable research during the last two decades has provided information on the metabolism and importance of selenium in human nutrition leading to the recent establishment of recommended dietary intakes.

10.4.1 Functions of selenium

Selenium exerts its biological effect as a constituent of several selenoproteins. The following have been purified and studied:

- Glutathione peroxidases (GSHPx)
  - cytosolic, cellular
  - plasma
  - phospholipid hydroperoxide
  - gastrointestinal

- Selenoprotein P
- Iodothyronine 5'-deiodinase
- Sperm capsule selenoprotein
- Selenoprotein W
- 58, 56 and 14 kDa Se-binding protein

The first of these to be characterized was GSHPx which consists of four identical subunits, each containing one selenocysteine at the active site. Activity of this enzyme can be reduced to less than 1% in tissues of selenium-deficient animals. GSHPx, present in three different forms, in cells (including erythrocytes), plasma and the gastrointestinal tract, may function *in vivo* to remove hydrogen peroxide, thereby preventing the initiation of peroxidation of membranes and oxidative damage. However, the significance of this function in the body is uncertain, and it seems likely that the oxidant defence role for selenium is exerted more through other selenoproteins. GSHPx may have more specific functions in arachidonic acid metabolism in platelets, microbiocidal activity in leucocytes, and the immune response mechanism or perhaps as a storage protein.

Another selenium-containing enzyme, phospholipid hydroperoxide GSHPx, is different from the classic GSHPx in that it can metabolize fatty acid hydroperoxides that are esterified in phospholipids in cell membranes. This enzyme can inhibit microsomal lipid peroxidation and thus may account for some of the antioxidant activities of selenium.

In addition, a plasma protein designated selenoprotein P with no GSHPx activity has been purified and characterized from rat and human plasma. Selenoprotein-P is a glycoprotein containing selenium as selenocysteine, and its concentration in rat plasma falls to less than 10% of control in selenium deficiency. Its function is unknown, but it may have an oxidant defence, or transport role.

The most recently discovered selenoprotein is the type I iodothyronine 5'-deiodinase which catalyses the conversion of thyroxine (T_4) to its active metabolite, triiodothyronine (T_3), in the liver and kidney. Selenium deficiency results in an increase in levels of plasma T_4 and a corresponding decrease in levels of more active T_3. Thus, selenium plays a crucial role in metabolism of thyroid hormones which are essential for growth and development.

Several selenium-containing enzymes have been identified in microorganisms and other selenoproteins have been found in animal tissues, suggesting further functions for selenium. These include a mitochondrial selenoprotein in sperm, selenoprotein W in rat muscle and a 14 kDa and 56/58 kDa selenium-binding protein. Furthermore, selenium has strong interactions with heavy metals such as cadmium, silver and mercury and may protect against toxic effects of these metals. The most recent exciting development in the search for functions for selenium is the observation that selenium deficiency may accelerate viral evolution, which may help to clarify the aetiology of Keshan disease.

10.4.2 Metabolism of selenium

Selenoamino acids are the main dietary forms of selenium, with selenium replacing sulphur in selenomethionine in plants and selenocysteine in animals. Inorganic forms of selenium are used in experimental diets and as supplements. The metabolism of selenium, including absorption, transport, distribution, excretion, retention and transformation to the active form, is dependent on the chemical form and amount ingested, and on interacting dietary factors. There is considerable species variation in selenium metabolism.

Absorption   Selenium is absorbed mainly from the duodenum. Selenomethionine and methionine share the same active transport mechanism, but little is known about the transport of selenocysteine. Absorption of inorganic forms such as selenite and selenate is via a passive mechanism. Absorption of selenium is generally high in human subjects, probably about 80% from food; selenomethionine appears to be better absorbed than selenite. Absorption is unaffected by selenium status, suggesting that there is no homeostatic regulation of absorption.

Transport   Little is known about the transport of selenium in the body although it appears to be transported bound to plasma proteins, albumin in mice and β-lipoproteins in humans. Selenoprotein P has also been suggested as a transport protein, but there is little evidence at present for this function.

Metabolism and distribution   An outline of selenium metabolism is shown in Fig. 10.2. Selenium in animal tissues occurs in association with protein, and is present in two main compartments or forms. The first is selenocysteine which is present as the active form of selenium in selenoproteins. The second is selenomethionine which is incorporated in

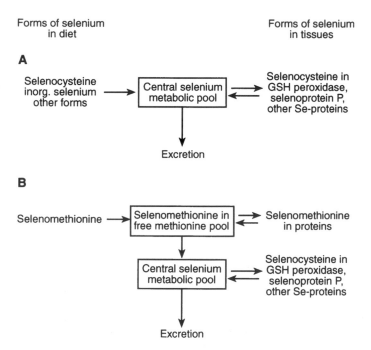

Fig. 10.2   Tissue selenium form and concentration as affected by dietary form. (A, selenocysteine; B, selenomethione.) *Source*: Levander OA, Burk RF. Selenium. In: Shils ME, Olson JA, Shike M, Malver PA (eds). 8th ed. *Modern nutrition in health and disease*. Philadelphia, PA: Lea & Febiger, 1994.

place of methionine in a variety of proteins, unregulated by the selenium status of the animal.

Selenium levels in tissues are influenced by dietary intake, which is reflected in the wide variation in blood selenium concentrations of residents of countries with differing soil selenium levels (Fig. 10.3). Retention of selenium is also influenced by the form administered, with selenomethionine much more effective in raising blood selenium levels than sodium selenite or selenate. The non-specific incorporation of seleno-methionine into protein contributes to tissue selenium which is not available for synthesis of functional forms of selenium until it is catabolized. Selenate is reduced to selenite then selenide, and in this oxidation state (-2) is introduced into selenocysteine. The selenium from inorganic forms or from catabolism of selenoamino acids is incorporated into serine to form selenocysteine which is then incorporated into the active site of selenoproteins.

Excretion   Urine is the principal route of selenium excretion, followed by faeces in which it is mainly unabsorbed selenium. Homeostasis of selenium is achieved by regulation of its excretion. Daily urinary excretion is closely associated with plasma selenium and dietary intake. Measurement of plasma renal clearance of selenium which expresses its rate of excretion in the urine in terms of the amount contained per unit volume of plasma, shows that kidneys of residents of the low selenium country, New Zealand, excrete selenium more sparingly than those of North Americans, and Chinese from low selenium areas have even lower renal clearances. This indicates possible adaptation to low selenium status.

Trimethylselenonium ion is only one of several urinary metabolites identified, but appears to be a minor metabolite in humans. Small losses of selenium occur through the skin, hair, or at high intakes, in expired air as volatile dimethylselenide.

Bioavailability   As well as absorption, utilization of a nutrient also includes transform-ation to a biochemically active form which for selenium is assessed by monitoring changes

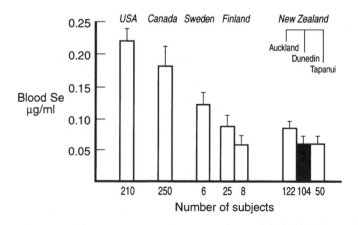

Fig. 10.3   Blood selenium levels reported in healthy adults in various countries. ($0.1\,\mu g\,Se/ml =$ $1.27\,\mu mol\,Se/l$). *Source*: Thomson CD, Robinson MF. *Am J Clin Nutr* 1980; **33**: 303–23.

in tissue GSHPx. Animal studies show a wide variation in the bioavailability of selenium from different foods. In rats, the bioavailability from mushrooms, tuna, wheat, beef kidney and Brazil nuts is 5%, 57%, 83%, 97% and 124%, respectively in comparison to sodium selenite. Human studies also show differences among various forms such as selenate, wheat and yeast, but this also depends upon the criterion of measurement used for bioavailability indicating the need to consider several variables including short-term changes in GSHPx activity, long-term retention of tissue selenium, and metabolic conversion to biologically active forms.

10.4.3 Deficiency

Interaction between selenium and vitamin E is observed in the aetiology of many deficiency diseases in animals and pure selenium deficiency is in fact rare. Thus, selenium deficiency may only occur when a low selenium status is linked with an additional stress such as chemical exposure or increased oxidant stress due to vitamin E deficiency. Although residents in some low selenium areas have low blood selenium, GSHPx activity and selenoprotein levels, there is little evidence that these are suboptimal or have resulted in noticeable oxidative damage or changes in other oxidative defence mechanisms. Moreover, people have not shown noticeably improved health when GSHPx activity is saturated by selenium supplementation. Whether any of the newer functions of selenium are suboptimal in persons with low selenium status has yet to be investigated.

Selenium responsive diseases in humans   Keshan disease, an endemic cardiomyopathy occurring in low selenium areas of China, was reported in 1979 to be responsive to supplementation with sodium selenite. The disease is associated with low selenium intake and low blood and hair levels, and affects mainly children and women of childbearing age. It is probably the only case of naturally occurring selenium deficiency. Because some features of Keshan disease (e.g. seasonal variation) cannot be explained solely on the basis of very low selenium status, Chinese researchers have suggested that some other factors may be involved such as virus, mineral imbalance or environmental toxins. Another disease that has been associated with poor selenium status in China is Kashin–Beck disease, an endemic osteoarthritis that occurs during pre-adolescent or adolescent years, but again other aetiologic factors are probably involved.

Selenium deficiency has been associated with long-term intravenous nutrition, because of the low levels of selenium in the fluids. Clinical symptoms of cardiomyopathy, muscle pain and muscular weakness are responsive to selenium supplementation, but are not seen in all patients with extremely low selenium status, indicating that there may be other interacting factors. Furthermore, children on very low selenium synthetic diets for inborn errors of metabolism, such as phenylketonuria, do not develop selenium-deficiency syndromes.

Anecdotal reports from New Zealand farmers in low selenium areas where sheep have selenium-responsive muscular dystrophy indicate their conviction that selenium relieves their own muscular aches and pains, although double-blind trials have failed to give a clear-cut answer.

Selenium and chronic disease   Many attempts have been made to link poor selenium status with diseases such as cancer and cardiovascular disease. Evidence from experimental animal studies suggest that selenium is protective against tumorigenesis at high levels of intake. Some early epidemiological studies in humans have suggested an association between low selenium status and some forms of cancer, but this has not been confirmed by others, and the low selenium/high cancer risk hypothesis is still not proven. Similarly, although a large case-control study in Finland suggested selenium was an independent risk factor for myocardial infarction in a low selenium population, evaluation of prospective epidemiological studies has failed to provide sufficient evidence to implicate selenium deficiency in most aspects of cardiovascular disease. However, selenium may have some role in protection against thrombosis and low-density lipoprotein-oxidation, in particular, in individuals such as smokers at risk from increased oxidant stress, which warrants further investigation. Further studies to clarify any possible role for selenium in these degenerative diseases are required.

10.4.4   Assessment of selenium status

Blood selenium concentration is generally considered a useful measure of both selenium status and intake, but other tissues are often assessed as well. Plasma selenium reflects short-term status and erythrocyte selenium long-term status; toenails are often used but selenium-containing shampoos restrict the use of hair. The close relationship between blood or red cell GSHPx activity and selenium concentrations (Fig. 10.4) is useful for assessment in people with relatively low status, but not once the saturating activity of the enzyme is reached at blood selenium concentrations above 100 ng/ml (1.27 µmol/l). The growing emphasis on functional rather than static indices poses difficulties for selenium because it is not always clear whether selenium is involved directly or as a limiting factor (e.g. platelet aggregation and ethane/pentane production). The situation is

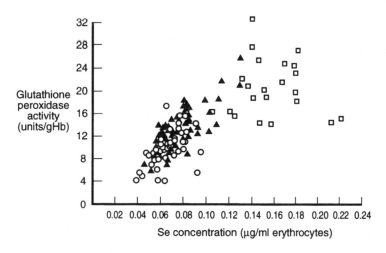

Fig. 10.4   Relationship between selenium concentration of erythrocytes (µg/ml erythrocytes) and glutathione peroxidase (GSHPx) activity for Otago patients (○); Otago blood donors (▲); and overseas subjects (□). (To convert µg Se/ml to µmol/l, multiply by 12.66.) *Source*: Rea HM, Thomson CD, Campbell DR, Robinson MF. *Br J Nutr* 1979; 42: 201–8.

further complicated by the large number of interacting factors. Furthermore, because selenium is present in biological materials in extremely low concentrations and is a volatile element, analysis is difficult.

10.4.5 Dietary intake

Food is the major source of selenium, with drinking water contributing little. Dietary intake varies with the geographical source of the foods and eating habits of the people. Plant food concentrations reflect selenium content of soils and its availability for uptake, as plants do not require selenium for growth; cereals and grains grown in soils poor or rich in selenium may vary over 100-fold in selenium content. Animal foods vary less. Fish and organ meats are the richest sources followed by muscle meats, cereals and grains, dairy products, with fruits and vegetables mostly poor sources. Average daily dietary intakes vary considerably depending on the levels of selenium in soils (Table 10.4) ranging from 10 μg to 20 μg selenium in the low soil-selenium areas of China where Keshan disease is endemic, about 30–60 μg in New Zealand, and up to over 200 μg in seleniferous areas in Venezuela. In 1985, selenium was added to fertilizers in Finland as a way of increasing selenium intake throughout the population and the daily intake rose from 40 μg to close to 100 μg/day, resulting in an increase in serum selenium in a group of healthy individuals from 65–70 ng/ml in 1985 to 120 ng/ml in 1989–91. In New Zealand intakes are increasing due to an increase in importation of Australian wheat, and selenium status is rising accordingly.

10.4.6 Requirements and recommended dietary intakes

Many countries have recently proposed recommended dietary intakes based upon estimates of requirements from Chinese intakes for endemic and non-endemic Keshan disease areas, as well as intakes at which saturation of plasma GSHPx activity occurred. The recommended dietary intake (RDI) for Australia was the first set in the world in 1986 and may have been cautiously on the high side at 85 μg and 70 μg selenium for

Table 10.4 Daily dietary intakes and whole blood values of selenium

Country	Selenium intake (μg/day)	Blood selenium (ng/ml)
China (Keshan area)	9–11	10–20
New Zealand (before 1990)	28–32	50–100
Finland (1985)	30	50–100
(1989–90)	100	120
Great Britain	60	80–320
USA	62–216	150–400
Venezuela (Caracas)	218	350
China (seleniferous area)	5000	3200

Source: Adapted from Dreosti I. Truswell A, Dreosti I, English R, Rutishauser I, Palmer N (eds). *Recommended nutrient intakes Australian Papers*. Sydney: Australian Professional Publications, 1990: 275–93.

Table 10.5 Recommended dietary intakes of selenium for adults (µg/day)

Group	Australia RDI	USA RDA	Canada RNI	UK		WHO* NR	European PRI
				LNRI	RNI		
Men	85	70	50	40	75	40	55
Women	70	55	50	40	60	30	55

*World Health Organization (1996).
RDI, recommended dietary intake; RDA, recommended dietary allowance; RNI, reference nutrient intake; LNRI, lower reference nutrient intake; NR, normative requirement estimate; PRI, population reference intake.

Australian men and women, respectively. Others, including recommended intakes of the United States, the United Kingdom and European countries, are summarized in Table 10.5. Each set of recommended intakes can be met from habitual diets in each country. Whether optimal health depends upon saturation of GSHPx activity has yet to be resolved; if not, recommended intakes may approach those in countries with naturally low selenium status such as New Zealand.

10.4.7 Toxicity

The margin between an adequate and toxic intake of selenium is quite narrow. Overexposure or selenosis may occur from consuming high selenium foods grown in seleniferous areas in Venezuela and some areas of China. The most common sign of poisoning is loss of hair and nails, but lesions of the skin, nervous system and teeth may also be involved. People following long-term liberal megadosing can also attain an undesirably high selenium status. Threshold toxicity intakes have yet to be established. Sensitive biochemical techniques are lacking for selenium toxicity, which is at present diagnosed from hair loss and nail changes.

FURTHER READING

1. Arthur JR, Beckett GJ. Newer metabolic roles for selenium. *Proc Nutr Soc* 1994; **53**: 615–24.
2. Dreosti I. Selenium. In: Truswell A, Dreosti I, English R, Rutishauser I, Palmer N (eds). *Recommended nutrient intakes*, Australian Papers. Sydney: Australian Professional Publications, 1990: 275–93.
3. Robinson MF, Thomson CD. The role of selenium in the diet. *Nutr Abstracts Rev* 1983; **53**: 3–26.
4. Robinson MF. Selenium in human nutrition in New Zealand. *Nutr Rev* 1989; **47**: 99–107.
5. World Health Organization. *Trace elements in human nutrition and health.* Geneva: WHO, 1996: 105–22.

10.5 FLUORINE

Marion Robinson

Even though the beneficial effects of fluorine (F) in the form of fluoride for dental health are well recognized, fluorine has yet to become accepted as an essential trace element.

From many studies of United States children, Dean (1942) showed an inverse relation between the natural fluoride concentration of United States communal water supplies in the range of 0–2 ppm F (parts per million, μg/g) and the prevalence of dental caries (Fig. 10.5). Earlier, a direct asssociation had been found between the fluoride content of water supplies (0–6 ppm F) and the occurrence of dental fluorosis or mottled enamel, developmental defects of tooth enamel, from barely noticeable white flecks affecting a small percentage of the enamel to brown-stained or pitted enamel, in the most severe cases (Fig. 10.6). Figures 10.5 and 10.6 show little increase in benefit above 1 ppm F, while fluorosis only became significant above 1 ppm F. This concentration therefore offered maximal protection against dental caries with minimal risk of dental fluorosis. Moreover, in communities, as in New Zealand, where the natural water supplies were unusually low, less than 0.3 ppm F, addition of fluoride or fluoridation of the water supply to achieve 1 ppm F was followed by a remarkable decline in prevalence of dental decay, up to 60%. Indeed, the impact of fluoridation of water supplies and more recently of toothpastes containing fluoride has been hailed as a remarkably cost-effective triumph of public health.

10.5.1　Function

Most of the calcium, phosphate and other minerals in bones and teeth exist as hydroxyapatite crystals with some fluoride being incorporated as the more acid-resistant fluorapatite. The role of fluoride in bone mineralization is still not clear; but it protects teeth against dental caries. Dental decay occurs when minerals from the tooth enamel

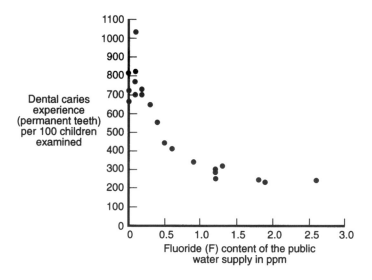

Fig. 10.5　Relation between the amount of dental caries (permanent teeth) observed in 7257 selected 12 to 14-year-old white schoolchildren of 21 United States cities of 4 states, and the fluoride (F) content of the public water supply. *Source*: Dean, Arnold, Ivove. *Pub Health Rep* 1942; 57: 1177.

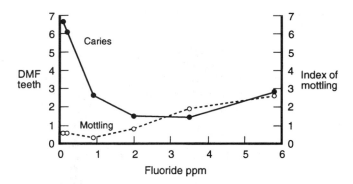

Fig. 10.6 Caries and enamel mottling according to fluoride level in drinking water. United Kingdom children aged 12–14 years (DMF, decayed, missing and filled teeth). *Source*: From Forrest (1956), British Dental Journal, BMJ Publishing Group.

dissolve under the influence of organic acids formed by dental plaque bacteria acting upon fermentable carbohydrates taken into the mouth. Fluoride interacts at different stages of the tooth–plaque–saliva system. It has an antibacterial effect in the plaque; it inhibits demineralization of the tooth and enhances remineralization, giving a surface crystal structure which is much more resistant to caries. The post-eruptive surface or topical role of fluoride to decrease dental decay, is now regarded as more important than the pre-eruptive systemic function of incorporation of fluoride into the structure of the enamel. The dental benefits of fluoride are therefore not confined to the developmental stage; they continue throughout life; hence fluoride is needed life-long for optimal protection against caries.

10.5.2 Metabolism of fluorine

The fluoride ion occurs in water, and both ionic and non-ionic or bound forms of fluorine occur in food and beverages. Ionic fluorine is rapidly and almost completely absorbed, whereas organic or protein bound forms are less well absorbed (about 75%) and inorganic bone fluorine as in bonemeal even less (<50%). There is a transitory rise in plasma fluoride immediately following fluorine ingestion, after which it returns to about 0.1 ppm F. Some fluoride is taken up by the bones and retained for a long time; but most is rapidly excreted in the urine, with small amounts in sweat and faeces. The urinary output gives a good indication of the daily fluorine intake, whereas the bone fluorine content reflects the long-term intake. There is minimal transfer of fluoride across the placenta. Fluoride content of breast milk is little affected by small supplements of fluoride, such as 1.5 mg/day.

10.5.3 Sources of fluoride

Dietary sources Beverages are the principal sources of fluoride and their contribution depends on the fluoride concentration of the water supply. Tea leaves are also major sources and hence tea infusions (about 1–2 ppm F) depending on the water fluoride content and strength of the infusion. Thus, beverages can give as little as 0.2 mg/day for non-tea drinkers drinking unfluoridated or low fluoride water, up to 2–4 mg/day or even up to 12 mg/day for liberal drinkers of strong tea prepared with fluoridated water.

Foods contain traces of fluoride, contributing for an adult about 0.5 mg/day; plant foods (1 ppm F) generally contain more fluoride than animal foods (0.1 ppm F) apart from marine fish (2–5 ppm F). The fluoride content of processed food comes mainly from the fluoride content of the water used in processing in the home or commercially. Fluoride content of infant formulas reflects the processing of the powdered formula and also the water used to make it up. Milk formulas usually contain more fluoride than human milk, and this needs to be monitored as does the fluoride content of infants' solid foods.

Non-dietary sources These include: fluoride tablets given mainly to children exposed to low fluoride water during the formation and maturation of teeth; fluoride toothpastes or dentifrices; and mouth rinses or topical fluoride applications, the painting of fluoride solutions on teeth by dentists.

10.5.4 Effects of high intakes

The range between exposure to too little and too much fluorine is not wide, with dental fluorosis occurring when too much is ingested while teeth are forming during the first eight years of life; this can happen from too liberal use of fluoride tablets and/or fluoride toothpastes which can contain as much as 1000 ppm fluoride. Young children are at risk if they regularly swallow large amounts, but toothpastes of lower fluoride content (400 ppm F) are now available for them.

The skeleton is affected by chronic high levels of fluoride intake as from using drinking water of 4–12 ppm fluoride. This may cause dense bones and joint abnormalities; skeletal fluorosis occurs in India, China and South Africa.

Large doses of fluoride have been used in the treatment of osteoporosis, but the bone quality tends to be poor, fractures may increase, and there are doubts about the safety of such treatment.

10.5.5 Fluoride and dental health

There is evidence that dental health is improving even in areas with low fluoride water supplies, and the marked difference in caries prevalence between fluoridated and non-fluoridated (low fluoride) areas has narrowed considerably. This most probably is related to the widespread introduction of fluoride toothpaste and other routine topical fluoride applications, as well as an increase in fluorine in the food chain. Some workers claim that much of the decline is independent of fluoride, but evidence strongly endorses the major role fluorine plays in preventing dental decay throughout life. The real issue has now become in what form fluorine is to be used in naturally low fluorine areas. Water fluoridation has the great advantage of reaching all members of the community, particularly those with poor dental health who otherwise might not seek the benefits of fluorine, whereas the use of fluoride toothpaste depends upon individual initiative. A combination of both is probably desirable throughout life for optimal protection against caries. It is estimated that the lifetime benefit for the average New Zealander drinking fluoridated water is the prevention of a total of 2.4–12.0 decayed, missing or filled teeth.

10.5.6 Recommended dietary intake

Although a physiological requirement for fluorine has yet to be established, most national and international health organizations recommend a water supply in the range 0.7–1.0 ppm F for temperate climates, using the average local maximum temperature as a predictor of water intake; the lower concentrations are for warmer climates, when more beverages are drunk. In addition, the United States (1989) has suggested a range of 'safe and adequate' intakes for adults of 1.5–4.0 mg/day, with much less for children, 1.5–2.5 mg/day, and for infants 0.1–1.0 mg/day during the first year of life.

10.5.7 Risks of water fluoridation

It is widely agreed that fluoridation of drinking water to a level of 1 ppm F has no known adverse health effects. There is no good evidence that fluoridated water is associated with allergic reactions and hypersensitivity, sudden infant death syndrome, stomach and intestinal problems, birth defects and Down syndrome, genetic mutations, or repetitive strain injury. The issue of fractures remains unresolved; if there is an increased risk of hip fractures, it is likely to be very slight. No association of cancer with exposure to fluoridated water was found in New Zealand or in other countries. The association suggested by Yiamouyiannis and Burk (1975) lacked plausibility in that no latency period was evident; the cancer mortality rate was described as increasing as soon as fluoridation was introduced, although cancer latency periods are nearly always at least five years (See Doll and Kinlen, 1977; Smith, 1980). Furthermore, there is little good evidence for the hypothesis that fluoride causes osteosarcoma in humans at levels associated with water fluoridation.

FURTHER READING

1. Brown RH. Fluoride and the prevention of dental caries. Part 1: The role of fluoride in the decline of caries. *NZ Dent J* 1988; **84**: 103–8.
2. Brown RH. Fluoride and the prevention of dental caries. Part 2: The case for water fluoridation. *NZ Dent J* 1989; **85**: 8–10.
3. Featherstone JDB. The mechanism of dental decay. *Nutr Today* 1987; **22**: 10–16.
4. New Zealand Public Health Commission. *Water fluoridation in New Zealand.* Wellington: Public Health Commission, 1994.
5. New Zealand Public Health Commission. *Fluoride and oral health.* Wellington: Public Health Commission, 1995.
6. Rao GS. Dietary intake and bioavailability of fluoride. *Ann Rev Nutr* 1984; **4**: 115–36.
7. Yiamouyiannis J, Burk D. Fluoridation and cancer. *Congressional Record* 1975; **121**: 7172–6.
8. Doll R, Kinlen L. Fluoridation of water and cancer mortality in the USA. *Lancet* 1977; **1**: 1300–2.
9. Smith AH. An examination of the relationship between fluoridation of water and cancer mortality in 20 large US cities. *NZ Med J* 1980; **91**: 413–6.
10. Forrest JR. Caries incidence and enamel defects in areas with different levels of fluoride in the drinking water. *Br Dent J* 1956; **100**: 195–200.

10.6 ULTRATRACE ELEMENTS

Rosalind Gibson

The ultratrace elements consist of more than 14 trace elements with estimated dietary requirements in humans of less than $1\,\mu g/g$ dry diet. They include arsenic, boron, bromine, cadmium, chromium, fluorine, lead, lithium, molybdenum, manganese, nickel, selenium, silicon, and possibly vanadium. Little is known about the chemical forms or bioavailability of most of the ultratrace elements in foods. However, because of their low estimated requirement, risk of dietary-induced deficiencies in humans is probably small. In animals, deficiencies have been induced by interactions of the ultratrace elements with certain forms of nutritional, hormonal, physiological and metabolic stress. Of the ultratrace elements, only arsenic, boron, chromium, molybdenum, nickel, selenium and silicon meet the criteria of essentiality noted at the beginning of this chapter. Selenium and fluorine have been considered earlier in Sections 10.4 and 10.5; the remainder are discussed briefly below.

Arsenic deprivation, generally manifested by impaired growth and abnormal reproduction, has been described in five animal species (i.e. rats, pigs, goats, chickens and hamsters). However, to date, the essentiality of arsenic for humans and its precise biochemical role have not been established. It may function as a methylated compound; the extent, severity and direction of the signs of arsenic deprivation are affected by dietary manipulations which alter methyl-group metabolism. Dietary intakes of arsenic typically range from $10\,\mu g$ to $20\,\mu g/day$ ($0.1–0.4\,\mu mol/day$). Major food sources are seafoods. They contain arsenobetaine, the non-toxic organic form which is readily absorbed and excreted. Inorganic arsenic is very toxic. A provisional maximum tolerable daily intake of $2\,\mu g/kg$ body weight for inorganic arsenic has been set by WHO/FAO Joint Committee on Food Additives.

Boron is essential in certain animals. In chickens deprived of both boron and cholecalciferol, growth is depressed and alkaline phosphatase activity enhanced. Some evidence suggests that boron is essential in humans. In an experimental study in postmenopausal women, increases in urinary calcium and magnesium excretion and decreases in serum 17β-oestradiol and testosterone occurred during boron depletion. These effects were reversed after boron supplementation. Average daily intakes of boron range from $0.5\,mg$ to $3.1\,mg/day$ ($0.05–0.29\,mmol/day$); richest food sources are plant-based, notably fruits, leafy vegetables, nuts and legumes. Toxicity of boron is low when it is administered orally.

Chromium is essential in humans. It potentiates the action of insulin in carbohydrate, lipid and protein metabolism, and may also have a role in gene expression. A chromium-responsive deficiency syndrome has been reported in some patients receiving long-term total parenteral nutrition (TPN). Clinical manifestations of deficiency included impaired glucose tolerance, hyperglycaemia, relative insulin resistance, peripheral or central neuropathy. Marginal nutritional deficiency states, confirmed by improved glucose tolerance after chromium supplementation, have also been described in malnourished children, in some studies of mild diabetics, and in middle aged subjects with impaired glucose tolerance. Dietary intakes of chromium (as trivalent chromium) in adults range from 13 µg to 61 µg/day (0.25–1.17 µmol/day), depending on age, country and gender. Food sources rich in chromium include brewers' yeast, nuts, prunes, asparagus, mushrooms, beer and wine; meat, fresh fruit and vegetables and cheeses are good sources, whereas refined cereals are poor sources. Trivalent chromium is poorly absorbed (approx 0.5%). No toxic effects of CrIII have been observed but chronic occupational exposure to hexavalent chromium can cause renal and hepatic necrosis.

Manganese deficiency has been described in several animal species. Abnormalities include growth failure, skeletal abnormalities, poor reproductive performance, impaired glucose tolerance, and abnormal connective tissue synthesis. Manganese is a constituent of three metallo-enzymes (i.e. arginase, pyruvate carboxylase, and manganese-superoxide dismutase), and activates a large number of enzymes (e.g. hydrolases, kinases, decarboxylases) most specifically, glycosyl transferases involved in mucopolysaccharide synthesis. No cases of naturally occurring manganese deficiency or toxicity in humans induced by diet alone have ever been documented. In experimentally induced manganese deficiency in humans, an itchy erythematous rash, *Milaria crystallina*, was the only clinical feature, although increases in serum calcium, phosphorus, and alkaline phosphatase and decreases in serum cholesterol and high-density lipoprotein (HDL) were also documented. Plant-based foods, especially whole grain cereals and legumes, are the richest food sources of manganese; flesh foods and dairy products are poor sources. Tea is also rich in manganese. Dietary intakes for omnivorous adults range from 2.2 mg to 2.8 mg/day (0.04–0.05 mmol/day); vegetarians have higher intakes. Cases of manganese toxicity have been described in miners exposed to manganese ores.

Molybdenum is essential in humans. A patient maintained on total parenteral nutrition (TPN) low in molybdenum for 18 months developed amino acid intolerance, irritability, disorientation, and eventually coma. Disturbances in sulphur metabolism and uric acid production also occurred which were reversed after addition of 300 µg/day of molybdenum to the TPN infusate. Molybdenum acts as a co-factor in the enzymes xanthine oxidase/dehydrogenase, aldehyde oxidase and sulphite oxidase which are involved in the metabolism of DNA and sulphites. A defect in molybdenum co-factor synthesis has been described in sulphite oxidase and xanthine oxidase deficiencies; the former genetic defect results in mental disturbances similar to those observed in the TPN patient. In an experimental depletion–repletion study, molybdenum-responsive functional changes (e.g. change in xanthine oxidase activity) were documented in adults fed 25 µg/day molybdenum (0.26 µmol/day) for 102 days. Major food sources of molybdenum are milk, beans, bread and cereals. Dietary intakes of molybdenum vary widely (i.e. 44–460 µg/day; 0.46–4.8 µmol/day). Dietary molybdenum is well absorbed but molybdenum toxicity is not a problem in humans.

Nickel is essential for several animal species and birds; features of deficiency are impaired growth and haemopoiesis. Whether nickel is essential for humans is currently unknown. Although the precise biochemical role for nickel has not been established, it is probably a component of several metallo-enzymes. Some evidence suggests that nickel may have a physiological role related to vitamin B_{12} metabolism. Intakes of nickel from diets based on animal foods and fats can be less than 60 μg/day (1 μmol/day); chocolate, nuts, dried beans, peas and grains are rich sources of nickel. Risk of nickel toxicity from diet alone is low.

Silicon is essential for the normal development of the skeleton and connective tissues in chickens and rats, probably via its role in bone and cartilage biosynthesis. The role of silicon in humans has not yet been clarified. Plant-based foods such as unrefined cereals and root vegetables are rich sources of silicon; animal foods are poor sources. Reported dietary intakes of silicon vary widely from 29 mg/day (1 mmol/day) in Finland to 1.2 g/day (43 mmol/day) in the United Kingdom. Absorption of silica varies; dietary silica is poorly absorbed, but when it is, in the form of silicic acid in foods and beverages, absorption is high. Toxicity of silicon taken orally is low.

FURTHER READING

1. Anon. Manganese deficiency in humans: fact or fiction. *Nutr Rev* 1988; **46**: 348–52.
2. Nielsen FH. Nutritional significance of the ultratrace elements. *Nutr Rev* 1988; **46**: 337–41.
3. Nielsen F. Other trace elements. In: Ziegler EE, Filer LJ, Jr (eds.). *Present knowledge in nutrition*. International Life Sciences Institute Nutrition Foundation, 7th ed. Washington, DC. 1996: 353–77.

11

VITAMIN A AND
CAROTENOIDS

Clive E. West

11.1 HISTORY

Hippocrates (*c.* 466–377 BC), the father of medicine, wrote that liver could cure night blindness. Snell demonstrated in 1880 that cod liver oil was effective in curing not only night blindness but also Bitôt's spots. Then Gowland Hopkins, the father of biochemistry in Britain, reported in 1912 that young rats on diets of pure protein, starch, sugar, lard and salts did not grow and died prematurely. McCollum and Davis, in Wisconsin, reported in the same year that there was an essential fat-soluble factor in butter, egg yolk and cod liver oil which promoted the growth of rats. Osborne and Mendel reported similar results. McCollum and Davis gave the name 'Fat-soluble factor A' to this food component to distinguish it from 'Water-soluble factor B' found in whey, yeast and rice polishings.

In 1920, Rosenheim and Drummond, reported that the vitamin A activity of plant foods was related to their content of carotene, a pigment isolated from carrots 100 years earlier. The ultimate proof that carotene was the precursor of vitamin A came from Thomas Moore in Cambridge, whose monograph (Moore 1957) on vitamin A is a classic.

11.2 UNITS, TERMINOLOGY, NOMENCLATURE AND CHEMICAL STRUCTURE

Vitamin A activity can be obtained from two classes of compounds (Fig. 11.1): preformed vitamin A, that is, retinol and related compounds (usually with 20 carbon atoms), and some carotenoids (β-carotene and a few related carotenoids, usually with 40 carbon atoms).

All-*trans* retinal (aldehyde form) is almost as active as all-*trans* retinol (vitamin A_1), 3-dehydroretinol (vitamin A_2) has 40% of the activity (Fig. 11.1). Retinoic acid is involved in regulation at the level of the gene and can support a number of functions, including growth but not others, notably vision. Historically, vitamin A activity is expressed in terms of the international unit (IU). This is equivalent to 0.300 μg or 0.0010473 μmoles of all-*trans*-retinol. For retinyl esters such as retinyl acetate and retinyl palmitate, the number of μmoles is the same but the weight is more. Thus IU is still used for labelling purposes because of this constant equivalence between IU and μmoles.

The carotenoids are pigments in plants, usually yellow or red. There are over 600 of them but only a small number have potential vitamin A activity. β-Carotene is the most

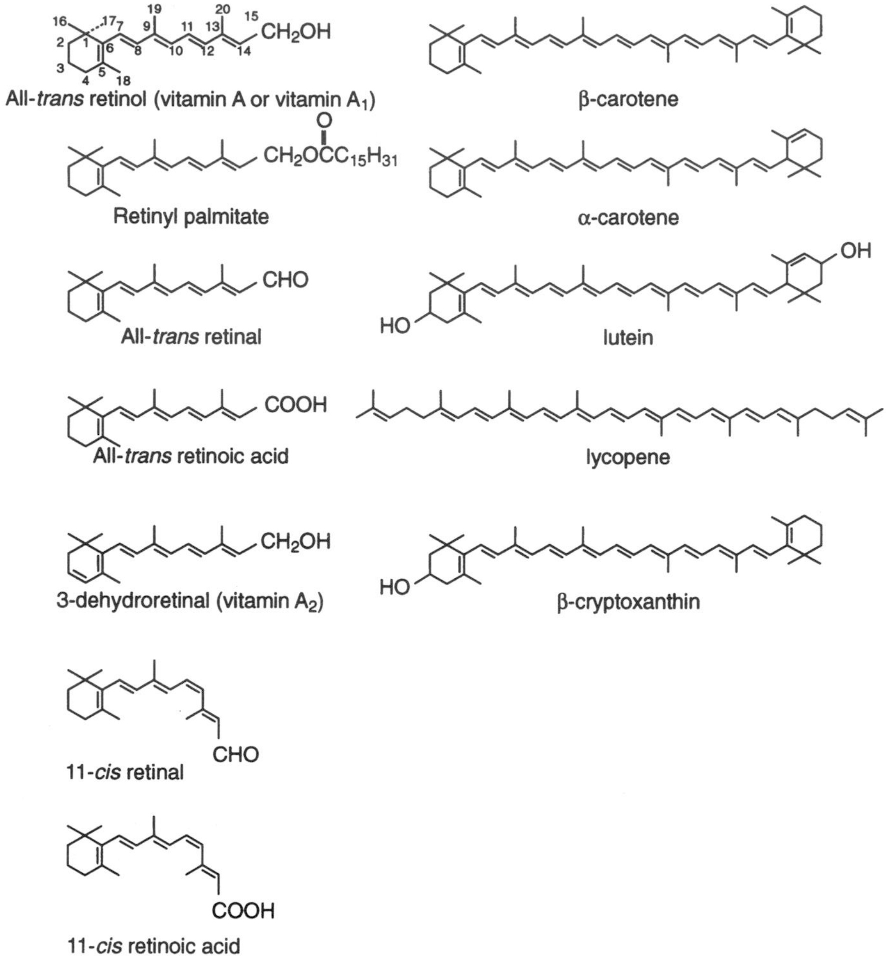

Fig. 11.1 Structures of common retinoids and carotenoids.

potent. Its molecule can be split in the middle by a specific 15,15'-dioxygenase in the gut or liver to form two molecules of retinol (see Fig. 11.2). α-Carotene and β-cryptoxanthin (Fig. 11.1) are also vitamin A precursors but only have half the activity. The ring at one end of these molecules is the same as in retinol, but not at the other end.

Since it was found that 0.6 μg of pure β-carotene had the same activity as 0.3 μg of retinol, one IU of β-carotene was defined as 0.6 μg. However, subsequent experiments carried out by Hume and Krebs in the World War II demonstrated that 2.4 μg of pure β-carotene in oil or 6 μg of β-carotene in food had the same vitamin A activity as one μg of retinol. The term 'retinol equivalent' (RE) was later introduced: this is the vitamin A activity equivalent to 1 μg of all-trans-retinol or 6 μg of β-carotene. Since the other

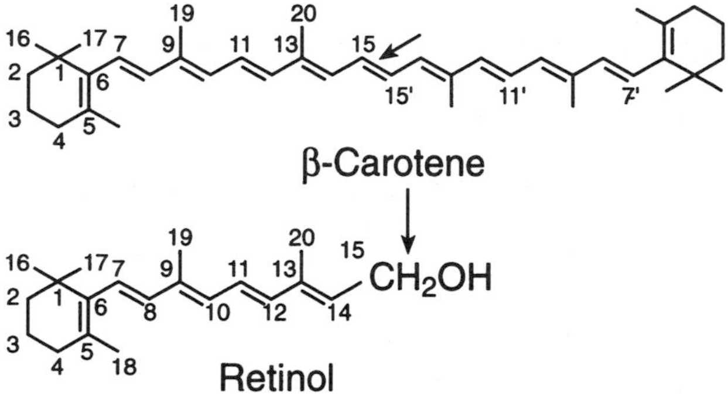

Fig. 11.2 Formation of retinol from β-carotene.

provitamin A carotenoids have half the activity of β-carotene, 1 RE of these is 12 μg. This simplistic equivalence has recently been brought into question as discussed later.

11.3 FUNCTIONS: PHYSIOLOGY, BIOCHEMISTRY, MOLECULAR BIOLOGY

Retinol is presented to target cells bound to plasma retinol-binding protein (plasma holo-RBP); and is then bound to a specific cell surface receptor from which the retinol is transferred into the cytoplasm of the cell where it is bound to cellular retinol-binding proteins. Inside the cell, retinol is involved in various biochemical/physiological processes. Those functions which only retinol can perfom are: vision at low light intensities; synthesis of 'active sulphate'; and reproduction. Functions in which retinoic acid can also participate include: involvement in cellular differentiation; involvement in morphogenesis; synthesis of glycoproteins; gene expression; immunity; growth, and prevention of cancer and heart disease.

11.3.1 Involvement of vitamin A in vision at low light intensities

The retina of the human eye contains two types of light receptor cells, the rods and the cones. The rods are used for seeing at low intensities of light (shades of grey) whereas colour vision is located in the cones. The outer segments of the rod cells contain many stacked, disc-like membrane vesicles which serve as light receptors. About half of the protein in the membrane of the vesicles consists of the light-absorbing lipoprotein complex, rhodopsin, containing the protein opsin, ethanolamine-containing phospholipid and the vitamin A derivative, 11-*cis*-retinal which is bound to interphotoreceptor retinol-binding protein (IRBP). When rhodopsin is exposed to light, the 11-*cis*-retinal is transformed to all-*trans*-retinal and this is accompanied by a change in the conformation of the protein through prelumirhodopsin to metarhodopsin. This interacts with G-protein (transducin) which ultimately leads to the activation of a phosphodiesterase that cleaves cyclic guanosine monophosphate (c-GMP) to guanosine monophosphate (GMP). These changes in cytostolic c-GMP and GMP lead to the closing of the sodium channel of the rod's outer segment. Membrane hyperpolarization is then transmitted as an electrical signal to the optic nerve. Ultimately, there is regeneration of opsin and the release of all-*trans* retinal which is still bound to IRBP. This is then isomerized to 11-*cis*-retinal which combines with opsin to commence the cycle again. As the rhodopsin system is involved in the perception of light at low light intensities, vitamin A deficiency produces night blindness. Vitamin A is also involved in the visual process in cone cells but the process has been more difficult to study biochemically.

11.3.2 Involvement of vitamin A in the synthesis of 'active sulphate'

The key component in sulphate transfer reactions is adenosine 3'-phosphate-5'-phosphosulphate (PAPS), which requires vitamin A for its synthesis. As PAPS is involved in the synthesis of mucopolysaccharides, deficiency of vitamim A produces the effects shown in Box 11.1.

Box 11.1   Effects produced by vitamin A deficiency

- Changes in the conjunctival–corneal epithelium result in reduced wettability of the eye surface.
- Changes in the tear ducts result in reduced tear production also contributing to dryness (xerosis) of the eye surface.
- Reduced production of mucous cells and of mucus in the respiratory tract and other mucous membranes, increases their susceptibility to infection.
- Changes in the taste buds result in reduced ability to taste (thus depressing appetite).
- Changes in the skin give rise to follicular keratitis; seen more in adults than in children.
- Changes in the ground substance of bone, cartilage and teeth results in defective formation of these tissues during growth.

11.3.3 Involvement of vitamin A in reproduction

Vitamin A deficiency results in infertility in males, involving the production of abnormal sperm, while in females low rates of conception and increased rates of stillbirths are seen. Retinal is probably a co-factor for enzymes involved in steroid hormone synthesis.

11.3.4 Involvement in cellular differentiation

Retinol transferred into the cytoplasm is bound to cellular retinol-binding protein (CRBP). The all-*trans*-retinol is oxidized to all-*trans*-retinoic acid which is transferred to cellular retinoic acid-binding protein (CRABP). It is also isomerized to 9-*cis*-retinol and subsequently to 9-*cis*-retinoic acid. Both all-*trans*-retinoic acid and 9-*cis*-retinoic acid are transferred on CRABP to the nucleus. Here, all-*trans* retinoic acid becomes bound to one or more of the three retinoic acid receptor proteins (RAR) while 9-*cis*-retinoic acid becomes bound to one or more of the three retinoid X-receptors (RXR). In the activation of the retinoic acid-responsive genes, RXR linked to RAR, or to nuclear receptors for other hormones binds to the response element and initiates transcription. The retinoid response element comprises a direct repeat (DR) of 6 DNA bases (AGGTCA or related sequence) separated by 1–5 nucleotides (designated DR1–DR5). DR1 elements preferentially bind RXR homodimers while DR2 and DR5 elements prefer RXR/RAR heterodimers. Because 9-*cis*-retinoic acid binds to RXR, which forms dimers with a variety of receptors, it seems to play a general role in cell differentiation. In contrast, all-*trans*-retinoic acid, which binds to RAR and only forms a heterodimer with RXR, seems to have more specific effects. Like the cytosolic retinoid-binding proteins, the nuclear retinoic acid receptor proteins appear in different cells and at different times in development.

11.3.5   Involvement of retinoids in morphogenesis

Embryological development is controlled, at least in part, by retinoids, particularly all-*trans*-retinoic acid. Both deficiency and excess have adverse effects. Implants containing all-*trans*-retinoic acid placed in the anterior part of a developing chick limb bud mimic the activity of the naturally occurring zone of polarizing activity. Digit duplication in the chick limb bud depends on the concentration of all-*trans*-retinoic acid. Chickens raised on vitamin A-deficient diets have an abnormal number of digits and treatment of laboratory animals with retinoic acid or large doses of vitamin A in early pregnancy also leads to malformations. This highlights the need for neither too little nor too much vitamin A in women of reproductive age.

11.3.6   Involvement of vitamin A and other retinoids
in the synthesis of glycoproteins

Retinol and other retinoids are involved in the 'glycosyl transfer reaction'. Hence, vitamin A deficiency results in reduced synthesis of thyroxine-binding globulin, γ-globulins, transferrin, α_2-macroglobulins and cell-surface glycoproteins. There is reduced adhesion between cells.

11.3.7   Involvement of vitamin A deficiency in host defence

Deficiency of vitamin A is associated with increased susceptibility to infection and increased rates of morbidity especially from respiratory diseases.

The ability of epithelia to act as an effective first line of defence against infection is impaired because of reduced mucin production and reduced cell-to-cell adhesion. In vitamin A deficiency mucus-producing goblet cells in the respiratory, gastrointestinal, conjunctival and genitourinary tracts are replaced by keratin-producing cells. After entering the body via epithelial surfaces, microbes spread to other tissues. Such spread is facilitated by the circulatory system and hindered by the non-specific activity of macrophages, monocytes and antimicrobial substances. In the macrophage component of non-specific immunity, vitamin A deficiency reduces bactericidal activity involving oxygen-dependent killing and reduces production of the bactericidal substance lysozyme which in tears provides protection for the ocular surface.

Vitamin A deficiency impairs various aspects of cell-mediated immunity and both systemic and mucosal humoral immunity. For cell-mediated immunity this involves: reduced size of thymus; reduced number of circulating T lymphocytes; impaired mitogen (phytohaemagglutinin)-induced proliferation; and reduced cytotoxic T lymphocyte activity.

11.3.8   Growth

Vitamin A influences growth by modulating the growth of bones through remodelling. The vitamin is necessary for the activity of cells in the epiphyseal cartilage which must undergo a normal cycle of growth, maturation and degeneration to permit normal bone growth. Although bone resorption is retarded, there is no defect in the normal bone calcification process.

11.3.9   Nutritional anaemia

Vitamin A deficiency can contribute to nutritional anaemia but the mechanisms involved are not yet clear. Iron absorption is not affected.

11.4   Absorption and Distribution, Transport (Fig. 11.3)

11.4.1   Digestion

Vitamin A and its precursors are ingested in a food matrix. The protein of this matrix is to a large extent broken down by proteolysis in the stomach, releasing the vitamin A and some of the carotenoids present in foods. However, much of the carotenoids in plant foods are present in more complex matrices, containing cellulose and lignin which are resistant to digestion. The released vitamin A and carotenoids aggregate with lipids into globules and pass into the upper part of the small intestine. Here, pancreatic lipase and other esterases hydrolyze lipids (triglycerides, etc.) and retinyl esters, and esters of carotenoids. With bile salts micelles are formed.

11.4.2   Absorption

As much as 90% of the retinol, but very little retinyl ester, is absorbed into the epithelial cells of the small intestine, probably by a carrier-mediated process at low concentrations. The absorption of β-carotene and other hydrocarbon carotenoids, which occurs by passive diffusion, appears to be as efficient as that of retinol at low concentrations but falls off at higher concentrations. In the epithelial cells, retinol is esterified while some of the β-carotene and other provitamin A carotenoids are split by the cytosolic enzyme 15,15'-dioxygenase to retinal which is subsequently oxidized to retinol.

11.4.3   Transport from the gut

Retinyl esters and carotenoids are transported from the gut in association with triglyceride in the core of chylomicrons via the lymphatics which drain into the jugular vein. The

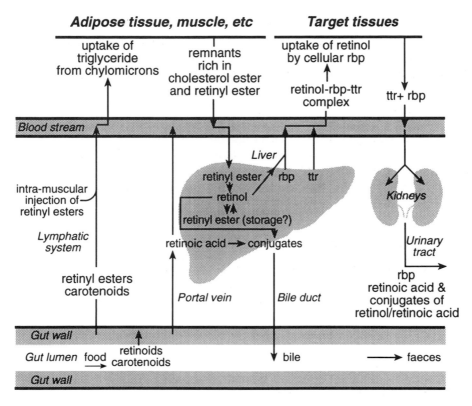

Fig. 11.3 Schematic representation of vitamin A metabolism; rbp, retinol-binding protein; ttr, transthyretin.

chylomicrons first lose most of their triglyceride in extrahepatic tissues and the resultant chylomicron remnants (rich in cholesterol esters, retinyl esters and carotenoids) are removed from the circulation almost entirely by liver parenchymal cells (the largest and most abundant cells in the liver). The retinyl esters are hydrolyzed in the parenchymal cells, then much of the retinol is transferred to the stellate cells (which comprise 7% of the cell numbers but only 2% of the cell volume of the liver). This transfer process involves plasma retinol-binding protein (RBP). Most of the retinol stored in liver is found in the stellate cells in the form of retinyl ester (>90% retinyl palmitate). Before release from the liver, retinol is transferred back to the parenchymal cells by a similar process. More than 80% of vitamin A in the body is stored in the liver with some stored in the kidney. Thus, the gold standard for vitamin A status is the liver content of vitamin A. Generally, the vitamin A content of the body increases with age. An average 70 kg adequately nourished man with a liver weighing 1800 g, would have 150–300 mg of stored vitamin A.

Of the total vitamin A absorbed, 10–40% is metabolized by oxidation or conjugation in the liver. The oxidized metabolites are generally excreted in urine while the conjugated products are secreted into the bile then excreted in the faeces.

11.4.4   Release of vitamin A from the liver and uptake by target tissues

Retinol is released from the liver bound to plasma retinol-binding protein (RBP), (molecular weight 21 000) which has one specific binding site for retinol. When RBP does not carry retinol, it is referred to as apo-RBP and when it does, it is holo-RBP. Holo-RBP released from the liver is bound to another protein, transthyretin (TTR) or thyroxine-binding prealbumin so there is a 1 : 1 : 1 complex of retinol, RBP and TTR. TTR is a tetramer with a molecular weight of about 55 000 and has a binding site for one RBP molecule. But despite its name, TTR is not the main carrier of thyroxine in plasma. (Instead it is thyroxine-binding globulin.) All unesterified retinol present in plasma is carried in the retinol–RBP–TTR complex.

The binding of retinol to RBP confers a number of physiological advantages:

* solubilization of water-insoluble retinol for transport from liver to target tissues;
* protection of retinol from oxidative damage during transport in plasma;
* regulation of retinol mobilization from liver and hence delivery to target tissues;
* delivery of retinol to specific sites on the surface of target cells.

Holo RBP is taken up by specific cell surface receptors. Once the retinol has been transferred inside the cell, the apo RBP is released from the receptor and can be recycled. As apo RBP has a molecular weight of 21 000, some of it is excreted by the kidney. Retinol within the cell becomes bound to cellular retinol-binding protein, CRBP.

Carotenoids are transported mainly in low-density lipoproteins. Although most of the conversion of β-carotene to retinal occurs during absorption, about 20% of the conversion probably takes place in other tissues, particularly the liver.

11.5   Factors Affecting Metabolism of Vitamin A

Synthesis of RBP is under close control; the plasma retinol is fairly constant over a wide range of hepatic vitamin A storage. However, adequate synthesis of RBP is related to the capacity of the liver to synthesize 'export' proteins, including serum albumin. Concentration is reduced when a subject has inadequate intake of protein which supplies the precursors and of other nutrients, especially zinc, essential for protein synthesis. Liver function including RBP synthesis is impaired in alcohol-induced cirrhosis, acute viral infections such as measles, and chronic viral hepatitis infections. The acute phase response to infection results in decreased transcription of the messenger RNA for RBP. At extremely high levels of vitamin A in the liver, plasma retinol increases but much of this is retinyl esters, so high fasting levels of retinyl esters can be used to diagnose chronic vitamin A toxicity. Excretion of vitamin A metabolites in urine is increased in fever resulting from measles, pneumonia and sepsis. The amount of retinol lost in urine, which is bound to RBP, can be as high as 1000 μg retinol per day. Increased faecal loss occurs in diarrhoea.

11.6   Experimental Deficiency in Animals

Experimental vitamin A deficiency has been produced in a wide variety of animals. Initially, this resulted in the discovery of vitamin A and of many of its functions. The rat is not always the most suitable model for studying vitamin A metabolism as it converts practically all of the provitamin carotenoids absorbed to retinol. Yellow-fat animals such as the rhesus monkey, mouse, domestic fowl, and the bovine absorb part of the ingested β-carotene intact while some white-fat animals such as sheep, goat, pig, dog, rat, guinea pig, and other monkeys, convert any β-carotene absorbed to retinol. Other white-fat animals such as the recessive white canary and cats have little or no ability to absorb β-carotene.

One useful model is the chicken. It has been possible to produce chicks with marginal vitamin A deficiency by restricting the supply of vitamin A to the hen and to infect chickens with Newcastle disease virus which is similar to human measles. Infection with Newcastle disease virus results in increased rates of morbidity in the marginally vitamin A-deficient chickens and a fall in plasma retinol levels.

11.7 RISK GROUPS FOR HUMAN DEFICIENCY

For many years, the emphasis on vitamin A deficiency was directed towards ocular signs which are grouped together under the term 'xerophthalmia' (meaning dry eyes). Using such criteria, Sommer and colleagues estimated that over 40 million children under the age of six years have mild or moderate xerophthalmia, that about 1% of these children go blind annually, and that half to three-quarters of them (perhaps about a quarter of a million children) die within one year. Children at high risk of xerophthalmia are found in Africa, Latin America and Asia (over half of them in India).

When vitamin A was first discovered, its importance for growth and strengthening defence against infection and preventing death were recognized. Since the 1980s these aspects have again come to the fore, especially interaction with measles. The group at highest risk is children beyond the weaning age (six months to six years). Pregnant and lactating women are also affected, with about a third of such women of lower to middle social class having marginal serum retinol in countries such as Indonesia. Some of the anaemia in women of childbearing age could be attributable to vitamin A deficiency. Another group at particular risk are displaced persons and those on inadequate food aid. Depending on the criteria used, the number of people with vitamin A deficiency in the world could be of the order of 500 million.

11.8 EXPERIMENTAL HUMAN DEFICIENCY

The best known experimental study was the 'Sheffield experiment' carried out during the World War II by Hume and Krebs to establish the human requirement. On the basis of studying four subjects (conscientious objectors who chose to be experimental subjects rather than join the army), they concluded that 750 μg of retinol or 1800 μg β-carotene were required to maintain adequate vitamin A levels. About 25 years later, Sauberlich's group concluded from their depletion experiments that 1200 μg of retinol or 2400 μg of β-carotene were required to maintain adequate vitamin A levels. Subsequent studies have resulted in recommended vitamin A intakes between these values. The experimental studies with humans, which sometimes extended up to two years (because of liver stores), noticed night blindness and skin changes such as follicular hyperkeratosis. Anaemia

187

which was refractory to medicinal iron but responsive to vitamin A was also observed. Because of the irreversible eye changes and possible risk of death, experimental vitamin A depletion can be hazardous.

11.9 FEATURES OF DEFICIENCY DISEASE

When vitamin A was discovered, most emphasis was placed on its ability to promote growth and to combat infection in laboratory animals. Hence, it was given the name 'anti-infection vitamin'. However, for a long time, much of this earlier work was forgotten and the principal role of vitamin A was regarded as preventing changes to the eye.

11.9.1 Changes to the eye

When vitamin A status is marginal, subjects become less able to see in dim light because of the low level of vitamin A in the rods of the retina. This is night blindness which is described by a specific word in many languages in areas in Asia, Africa and Latin America where vitamin A deficiency is a problem. Night blindness is correlated with low serum levels of vitamin A and thus is a useful tool in assessing vitamin A status.

With prolonged or more severe vitamin A deficiency, changes in the conjunctiva and cornea develop and a system of classifying these changes, collectively referred to as 'xerophthalmia', has been adopted by the World Health Organization (WHO) (see Box 11.2 and Fig. 11.4).

Box 11.2 Effects of vitamin A deficiencies on the eye

- *Conjunctival xerosis* (X1A) consists of one or more patches of dry, non-wettable conjunctiva which has been described as 'emerging like sand banks at a receding tide at the sea-shore' when a child ceases to cry. The condition is due to the non-wettability of the conjunctival surface.

- *Bitôt's spots* (X1B) are no more than an extension of the same process as in X1A. A Bitôt's spot usually has the form of a small plaque with a silvery grey colour, and a foamy surface: it is quite superficial and raised above the general level of the conjunctiva.

- *Corneal xerosis* (X2) is an extension of conjunctival xerosis to the cornea. The corneal surface also begins to lose its transparent appearance.

- *Corneal ulceration* (X3A) usually first occurs at the edge of cornea and are characteristically small holes, 1–3 mm in diameter, with steep sides. If vitamin A treatment is initiated at this stage, the effect will quite often be reversed and some sight will be retained.

- *More extensive corneal ulceration* (X3B) may develop and larger defects appear which result in blindness. In Africa, children with measles quite often develop X3B quickly without the appearance of the intermediate stages.

- *Corneal scars* (XS) result from the healing of the irreversible changes mentioned above. If the cornea ruptures and the contents of the cornea escape, a shrunken eyeball results.

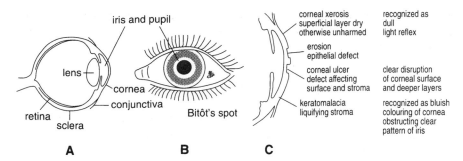

Fig. 11.4   Diagram of the eye (A, cross-section; B, front view) and the localization of the various eye lesions due to vitamin A deficiency with special reference to the localization of corneal defects (C).

11.9.2   Changes to other epithelial tissues

Vitamin A deficiency affects epithelial tissues other than the eye. For example, skin keratinization blocks the sebaceous glands with horny plugs which produces follicular hyperkeratosis. This is seen particularly in adults but the condition does not seem specific for vitamin A deficiency. Vitamin A deficiency also affects the epithelial lining of the respiratory, gastrointestinal, and genitourinary tracts. The relationship of vitamin A to immunity is discussed above (Section 11.3.7).

11.9.3   Morbidity and mortality

About 70 years ago, Green and Mellanby showed that when animals are raised on a diet lacking in vitamin A, practically all die with some infective lesions. The work of Sommer and colleagues in Indonesia showed that the death rate among children with mild xerophthalmia (night blindness and Bitôt's spots) was on average four times higher than that of children without xerophthalmia. It was found in a prospective longitudinal study that children with mild vitamin A deficiency developed respiratory disease twice and diarrhoea three times as frequently as non-xerophthalmic controls. Vitamin A supplementation reduces the severity rather than the incidence of diarrhoea and measles. In a meta-analysis of all trials of the effect of vitamin A supplementation, the mean reduction in death rate was found to be 23%. There is also evidence that vitamin A reduces the transfer of HIV from mothers to children.

11.9.4   Nutritional anaemia

Vitamin A deficiency can also contribute to nutritional anaemia. In a placebo-controlled field trial of anaemic pregnant women in West Java, Indonesia, vitamin A supplementation alone resulted in a significant increase in haemoglobin ($+4\,g/l$), iron alone increased haemoglobin, while supplementation with both vitamin A and iron had an additive effect. Similar results have been reported in children.

11.10   BIOCHEMICAL TESTS FOR VITAMIN A STATUS

Of all the biochemical tests proposed for measuring vitamin A status, the concentration of retinol in serum or plasma remains the most common and useful. Values below 10 μg/dl (0.3 μmol/l) indicate deficiency and below 20 μg/dl (0.7 μmol/l) are marginal.

The most accurate way to assess vitamin A status is to measure the concentration of vitamin A stored in the liver. However, it is usually not easy to obtain either biopsy or post-mortem samples of liver, the organ in which most vitamin A is stored. Estimates of body stores can be made by measuring the dilution of retinol with stable isotopes such as deuterium or ^{13}C but such techniques can only be used for research purposes. The concentration of retinol in breast milk is sometimes used as a measure of vitamin A status of lactating women and also as a surrogate measure of vitamin A status of the breast-fed child.

The concentration of vitamin A can be measured by UV absorption, fluorometrically, or colorimetrically after reaction with Lewis acids (antimony trichloride or trifluoroacetic acid) or by high pressure liquid chromatography (HPLC). Colorimetry was the most commonly used method but it suffers from interference from other compounds and the values often increase on storage. HPLC is now the preferred method and is becoming increasingly available in laboratories in countries where vitamin A deficiency is a problem. Serum β-carotene values can indicate β-carotene intake but not necessarily vitamin A status.

Since retinol is carried in plasma on retinol-binding protein (RBP), vitamin A status can also be evaluated by measuring the concentration of RBP in serum immunologically. As RBP exists in serum as both holo- and apo-RBP, methods which do not take this into account overestimate the concentration of RBP and this can lead to considerable errors especially when the concentration of RBP is low.

Because serum concentrations of vitamin A do not show body stores of retinol, indirect methods of measuring liver vitamin A stores have been sought. One of these is the relative dose response (RDR) test developed by Underwood from experiments in animals. The basis of the RDR test is that in deficiency more of a small dose of vitamin A goes into the plasma on RBP than normal.

A small oral dose of retinyl palmitate (450 μg or 1.6 μmoles) is given and the per cent increase of plasma retinol at five hours ($A_5 - A_0/A_5$) as percentage is the RDR. An increase greater than 15% indicates vitamin A deficiency. One problem with this method is that it is dependent to some extent on protein status and it requires two blood samples. The modified relative dose response (MRDR) uses 3-dehydroretinol and requires just one sample at five hours.

11.11   INTERACTIONS WITH OTHER NUTRIENTS

Adequate protein is important in digestion and release of retinol from the liver as holo-RBP; fat is important in absorption and transport from the gut; vitamin E protects vitamin A from oxidation. Zinc is involved in the synthesis of holo-RBP; it is also important in the molecular genetic aspects of cellular differentiation because of the zinc finger structure of DNA-binding proteins.

11.12 INTERACTIONS WITH DRUGS

A number of drugs can impair vitamin A absorption. Mineral oil dissolves carotenoids and retinol which are then carried down the intestine and excreted in the faeces. Neomycin decreases vitamin A absorption by inactivating bile salts. Cholestyramine decreases vitamin A absorption by adsorbing bile salts. In alcoholics, inhibition of the conversion of retinol to retinal (involving alcohol dehydrogenase) by alcohol can result in sterility in males and night blindness. Impaired RBP synthesis also compromises vitamin A status in alcoholics.

11.13 PHARMACEUTICAL USES

The term 'retinoids' is used for a group of chemical compounds similar to retinol, some of which are naturally occurring, whereas others have been synthesized in the search for new therapeutic agents. Retinoids influence proliferation and differentiation of the skin epidermis, inhibit keratinization, reduce production of sebum, and influence the immune response especially cell-mediated immunity. These properties have been used in therapy particularly for skin disorders. Such conditions include acne, seborrhoea (overproduction of sebum), certain keratinizing dermatoses, psoriasis (areas covered by profuse silvery scales especially on the elbows, knees, scalp and trunk of the body). Although it is highly effective, 13-*cis* retinoic acid is teratogenic (can cause fetal malformations) at high oral doses and can cause skin irritation when applied topically. Use of retinoids in women of childbearing age is therefore subject to strict control. There has been much effort to synthesize new retinoids for use in the treatment of not only skin conditions but also cancer. Some conjugated forms such as retinoyl-β-glucuronide and hydroxyphenyl retinamide retain their therapeutic actions with less or no toxicity. Topical all-*trans* retinoic acid can also reduce wrinkling and hyperpigmentation caused by photo-ageing.

A number of cancers (not the most common forms) have been successfully treated with retinoids. Some forms of skin cancer (mycosis fungoides) have been treated with large oral doses of vitamin A while all-*trans*-retinoic acid has been used effectively for treating acute promyelocytic leukaemia.

Carotenoids also have a limited use in therapy. Ingestion of one of them, canthaxanthin, has been used to promote tanning in patients with erythropoietic protoporphyria (a rare light-sensitive disease) in order to prevent blistering from the damaging effects of exposure to light.

11.14 FOOD SOURCES OF VITAMIN A AND CAROTENOIDS

In Western countries, the predominant source of vitamin A activity in the diet is preformed vitamin A (all-*trans* retinol) in animal products such as milk, butter, cheese, egg yolk, liver and some fatty fish. Liver is the richest source of retinol among common foods. Vitamin A is added to margarine to produce similar levels to those in butter. In addition to the preformed vitamin, vitamin A can also be derived from provitamin A compounds like β-carotene produced by plants. The main sources of provitamin A are dark-green leafy vegetables and some (not all) yellow- and orange-coloured fruits and vegetables.

In most tropical countries, where consumption of animal products is often low, the main sources of vitamin A activity in the diet are the carotenes, particularly β-carotene. Red palm oil is rich in β- and α-carotenes, as are carrots. Papayas are rich in β-carotene and β-cryptoxanthin.

11.15 BIOAVAILABILITY AND BIOCONVERSION

Absorption of retinol is generally probably more than 80% while that of carotenes is lower and affected by various factors. In addition, the bioconversion of carotenoids is influenced by a variety of factors. With pure β-carotene dissolved in oil, 2 µg of β-carotene in the diet results in the formation of 1 µg of retinol and the conversion factor of six to one is based on the lower bioavailability of β-carotene from plant sources.

However, work by de Pee *et al.* has shown that the bioavailability of provitamin A from dark-green leafy vegetables is less than previously thought. The factors which probably have an effect on the bioavailability of dietary carotenoids and their bioconversion to retinol have been incorporated into the mnemonic SLAMENGHI: *S*pecies of carotenoid; molecular *L*inkage; *A*mount of carotene consumed in a meal; *M*atrix in which the carotenoid is incorporated; *E*ffectors of bioavailability and bioconversion; *N*utrient status of the host; *G*enetic factors; *H*ost-related factors; and *I*nteractions between the other factors. The matrix in which the carotenoid is incorporated is possibly the most important factor. Carotenoids are present in chloroplasts in the leaves of dark-green leafy vegetables, which are not readily digested in the body, and in carrots they are in crystal form also in cells which are not readily broken down. In fruits, however, the carotenoids are contained within readily digestible cell walls in oil droplets from which they should be readily absorbed. Gastrointestinal infections and parasites can cause maldigestion, malabsorption and excessive loss of gut epithelium, possibly often reducing carotene bioavailability by more than half.

11.16 RECOMMENDED INTAKE

Recommendations for requirements for vitamin A from carotenoids are based on the assumption that 6 µg of β-carotene or 12 µg of other provitamin A carotenoids such as α-carotene each give rise to 1 µg of vitamin A (see Sections 11.2 and 11.8). On this basis, vitamin A activity is nowadays usually expressed in retinol equivalents (RE) with 1 RE = 6 µg β-carotene = 12 µg other provitamin A carotenoids. However, it is known that the rate of conversion depends on a number of factors including carotene intake.

The requirements for vitamin A recommended by FAO/WHO are shown in Table 11.1 together with those for the United Kingdom and United States.

11.17 TOXIC EFFECTS

Early reports of vitamin A toxicity came from explorers who had to resort to eating livers of polar bears or seals which are extremely rich in vitamin A. Acute toxicity arises when

Table 11.1 Recommended intake of vitamin A (µg retinol equivalents per day)

Group	Age (yrs)	FAO/WHO* (1988) (safe level of intake)	USA (1989) RDA	UK (1991) RNI
Both sexes	<1.0	350	375	350
	1–3	400	400	400
	4–6	400	500	500
	7–10	400	700	500
Males	11–12	500	1000	600
	13–15	600	1000	600
	Adult (>15)	600	1000	700
Females	11–12	500	800	600
	13–15	600	800	600
	Adult (>15)	500	800	600
	Pregnancy	+100	+0	+100
	Lactation	+350	+500	+350

*FAO, Food and Agriculture Organization; WHO, World Health Organization.
RDA, recommended dietary allowance; RNI, reference nutrient intake.

more than 200 mg (0.7 mmol or 666 000 IU) is ingested by adults or more than half this dose is ingested by children. This can produce vomiting, headache, blurred or double vision, vertigo, unco-ordinated muscle movements, increased cerebrospinal pressure, and skin exfoliation. Deaths have occurred. Chronic toxicity is induced by consuming for a month or more at least 10 times the recommended daily allowance, that is 10 mg (35 µmol or 33 300 IU) for an adult. A wide range of symptoms have been reported including headache, bone and muscle pain, ataxia, visual impairment, skin disorders, alopecia, liver toxicity and hyperlipidaemia.

However, the most serious toxicity problem with vitamin A is the teratogenic effect occurring during the first trimester of pregnancy. The effect is probably produced by peak concentrations of all-*trans*-retinoic acid and 9-*cis*-retinoic acid. Spontaneous abortion or fetal abnormalities including those of the cranium (microcephaly), face (hairlip), heart, kidney, thymus, and central nervous system (deafness and reduced learning ability) can occur. Thus, women who are pregnant or could become pregnant should not be exposed to retinoid therapy such as for the treatment of skin conditions. In addition, their daily intakes of vitamin A (retinol) should not exceed 3 mg (10 000 IU or 10.5 µmol). The usual source of high intake is from supplements and concern has also been expressed about high intakes from eating liver.

Ingestion of large amounts of carotenoids (e.g. from tomato juice, carrot juice or red palm oil), does not lead to toxic levels of retinol but can lead to increased plasma carotene (hypercarotenaemia) and yellow coloration of the skin, especially on the palms of the hands, soles of the feet and in the nasolabial folds. This is seen in Yoruba people in the coastal area of Nigeria consuming red palm oil. When the fat of breast milk of women in the area is separated by centrifugation it is often quite red. Accumulation of carotenoids can be distinguished from jaundice because the sclerae of the eyes are not yellow in hypercarotenaemia. It is generally agreed that there is no risk of toxicity of carotenoids from foods, although prolonged high doses from pharmaceutical preparations, especially in smokers, cannot be recommended.

11.18   Measures to Prevent Disease

The control of vitamin A deficiency in the world is now given top priority by national governments and international agencies. In a series of meetings (World Summit for Children in New York, 1990; Ending Hidden Hunger Conference in Ottawa, 1991; and the International Conference on Nutrition in Rome, 1992), practically all national governments pledged their countries to virtually eliminate vitamin A deficiency by the year 2000. There are four main approaches to controlling vitamin A deficiency:

(1) promoting better use of available foods;

(2) massive dosing and supplementation;

(3) fortification and enrichment; and

(4) public health and other indirect measures.

11.18.1   Using available foods

Many nutrient deficiencies would disappear if enough food was available to all members of the population to allow them to eat sufficient food in a balanced diet. As far as vitamin A is concerned, this means consuming enough retinol and/or provitamin A carotenoids (taking into account bioavailability). Up until recently, it was generally thought that dark-green leafy vegetables could provide sufficient provitamin A to meet the body's needs for this vitamin. However, there are now doubts whether this is the case. Therefore, where vitamin A deficiency is a problem, more emphasis will have to be given to provitamin A sources with a higher bioavailability or to retinol. It may be possible to increase carotenoid bioavailability by methods of food preparation but more work needs to be done in this area. Fruits such as mangos and papayas, yellow/orange varieties of vegetables such as pumpkin, sweet potato and plantain, milk and dairy products, eggs and the livers of animals and fish can all contribute significantly to vitamin A status. However, such foods are often not available, expensive or culturally unacceptable. Education is a very slow process and often it is necessary to overcome prejudices, which are part of the culture including the religion. Therefore, it is often necessary to go to supplementation and fortification. This is not surprising, because in Western countries resort has been made to these methods for controlling vitamin A deficiency.

11.18.2   Massive dosing and supplementation

Massive dosing involves giving a single large dose of a nutrient by mouth or by injection to provide sufficient to last an extended period of time. Vitamin A dissolved in oil (200 000 IU or 60 mg of vitamin A for people over the age of 12 months, and half the dose for children aged 6–12 months), is given in the form of capsules or as a liquid and provides sufficient vitamin A for a period of four to six months. Such a dose cannot be

Box 11.3   Policies for massive vitamin A programmes

1. Medical therapeutic dosing provided to patients presenting with xerophthalmia, measles or severe malnutrition.

2. Targeted prophylactic dosing directed at sections of the population at particular risk including:

    those under 5 years and mothers immediately postpartum, or refugees, or those receiving food aid because of drought, war or other reasons.

3. When deficiency is widespread in a population, massive dosing is sometimes extended to the whole population.

given to women of childbearing age because of the teratogenic risk to possible unborn children. The three separate policies used in massive vitamin A dosing programmes are listed in Box 11.3.

Since it is not safe to give more than 10 000 IU (3 mg) of vitamin A to women who might become pregnant, supplementation with small doses (1 mg daily) is used for women of childbearing age.

11.18.3   Fortification and enrichment

Fortification is the addition of vitamin A to a food which contains no vitamin A, whereas in enrichment, the food contains some vitamin A but the community is judged to need more. Margarine is a substitute for butter and in most Western countries and in many developing countries vitamin A is added during manufacture so that it is equivalent to the best summer butter, usually 200 IU (600 RE) per 100 g. In addition, all dried skim milk powder (DSM) exported for food aid programmes from the European Union, United States, Canada, Australia and New Zealand is enriched with 2000 RE per 100 g of DSM. The resulting milk powder when reconstituted makes milk containing the same amount of vitamin A as in fresh whole milk. Perhaps the most successful fortification in developing countries has been the addition of vitamin A to sugar in Guatemala at the rate of 1500 RE per 100 g of sugar, thus supplying about 300 RE per day to children.

11.18.4   Public health and other indirect methods

For controlling vitamin A deficiency, the most important public health method is immunization, especially against measles. Other indirect methods include increasing income and improving housing, sanitation and education to decrease the chance of infection which reduces utilization of vitamin A by the body.

FURTHER READING

1. Bauernfeind JC (ed.). *Vitamin A deficiency and its control*. Orlando: Academic Press. Inc. xviii + 530, 1986.

2. Beaton GH, Martorell R, Aronson KJ, *et al. Effectiveness of vitamin A supplementation in the control of young child morbidity and mortality in developing countries*. United Nations: ACC/SCN State of the Art Series: Nutrition Policy Discussion Paper No 13, 1993.
3. de Pee S, West CE, Muhilal, Karyadi D, Hautvast JGAJ. Lack of improvement in vitamin A status with increased consumption of dark-green leafy vegetables. *Lancet* 1995; **346**: 75–81.
4. de Pee S, West CE. Dietary carotenoids and their role in combating vitamin A deficiency: a review of the literature. *Europ J Clin Nutr* 1996; **50** (suppl.): S38–S53.
5. FAO/WHO. *Requirements of vitamin A, iron, folate and vitamin B-12*. FAO Food and Nutrition Series No 23. Report of a joint FAO/WHO Expert Consultation. Rome: FAO, 1988: 1107.
6. Moore T. *Vitamin A*. New York: Elsevier, 1957.
7. Sommer A, West KP, Jr. *Vitamin A deficiency: health, survival and vision*. Oxford University Press, 1996: xiii + 438.
8. Sporn MB, Roberts AB, Goodman DS (eds.). *The retinoids: biology, chemistry and medicine*. 2nd edn. New York: Raven Press, 1994: xvii + 679.
9. Underwood BA, Olson JA (eds.). *A brief guide to current methods of assessing vitamin A status*. Washington, DC: International Vitamin A Consultative Group, International Life Sciences Institute-Nutrition Foundation, 1993.
10. West CE, Rombout JHWM, Sijtsma SR, van der Zijpp AJ. Vitamin A and the immune response. *Proc Nutr Soc* 1991; **50**: 249–60.
11. World Health Organization. *Control of vitamin A deficiency and xerophthalmia*. Report of a Joint WHO/USAID/Helen Keller International/IVACG Meeting. Geneva: WHO, 1982 (WHO Technical Report Series, No 672).

THE B VITAMINS

Stewart Truswell and Robyn Milne

12.1 THIAMIN*

Eijkman, a Dutch medical officer stationed in Java discovered around 1897 that a polyneuritis resembling beri beri could be produced in chickens fed on polished rice. Subsequently he and his successor Grijns showed that this polyneuritis could be cured with rice bran or polishings. This contained B_1, the first of the vitamins to be identified, but it was not until 1936 that R.R. Williams finally elucidated the unusual structure and synthesized thiamin.

12.1.1 Functions

Thiamin (Fig. 12.1) as the diphosphate (or 'pyrophosphate'), thiamin pyrophosphate (TPP) is a coenzyme for the following major decarboxylation steps in carbohydrate metabolism:

1. Pyruvate → acetyl CoA (pyruvate dehydrogenase complex) at the entry to the citric acid cycle. Hence, in thiamin deficiency pyruvate and lactate accumulate.
2. α-Ketoglutarate → succinyl CoA (α-ketoglutarate dehydrogenase), half-way round the citric acid cycle.
3. Transketolase reactions in the hexose monophosphate shunt, alternative pathway for oxidation of glucose. Hence, in thiamin deficiency oxidation of glucose is impaired with no alternative route.
4. The second step in catabolism of the branched-chain amino acids, leucine, isoleucine and valine.

12.1.2 Absorption and metabolism

Thiamin is readily absorbed by active transport at low concentrations in the small intestine and by passive diffusion at high concentrations. Total body content is only 25 to 30 mg, mostly in the form of thiamin pyrophosphate in the tissues. There is another coenzyme form, thiamin triphosphate in the brain. Thiamin is excreted both unchanged and as metabolites in the urine. It has a relatively high turnover rate in the body; there

---

*We follow the spelling of the International Union of Nutritional Sciences (no final 'e'). The pharmaceutical sciences still spell it 'thiamine'.

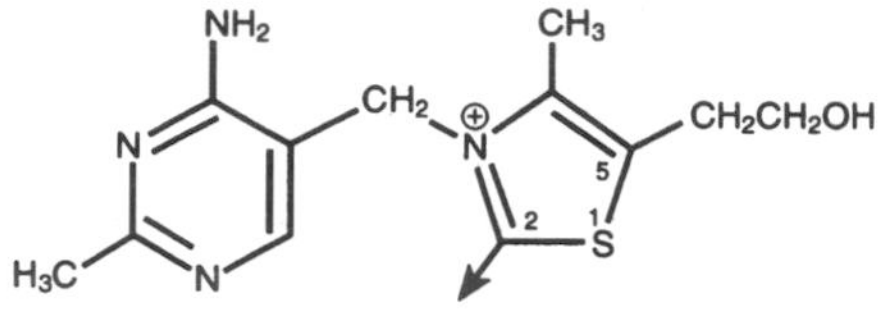

Fig. 12.1   Structure of thiamin.

is really no store anywhere in the body. On a diet lacking in thiamin, signs of deficiency can occur after 25 to 30 days.

12.1.3   Deficiency: animals

Pigeons and chickens are more susceptible than mammals. The characteristic effect is head retraction, called opisthotonus, from neurological dysfunction. In experimental mammals there is inco-ordination of muscle movements, progressing to paralyses, convulsions and death. The brain is dependent on glucose oxidation for its energy but the decrease in its pyruvate dehydrogenase and α-ketoglutarate dehydrogenase activities does not seem sufficient to explain the severe neurological dysfunction. Reduced formation of the neurotransmitter, acetylcholine (because acetyl CoA is not being formed), and a role of thiamin triphosphate in nerve transmission are other possible mechanisms.

Loss of appetite, cardiac enlargement, oedema, increased pyruvate and lactate are also seen.

12.1.4   Deficiency: humans

There are two distinct major deficiency diseases, beri beri and Wernicke–Korsakoff syndrome. They do not usually occur together.

Beri beri is now rare in the countries where it was originally described—Japan, Indonesia and Malaysia (the name comes from the Singhalese language of Sri Lanka). In Western countries occasional cases are seen in alcoholics. In acute beri beri there is a high output cardiac failure, with warm extremities, bounding pulse, oedema and cardiac enlargement. These features may be the result of intense vasodilatation from accumulation of pyruvate and lactate in blood and tissues. There are few electrocardiographic abnormalities. Response to thiamin treatment is prompt, with diuresis and usually a full recovery. In chronic beri beri the peripheral nerves are affected, rather than the cardiovascular system. There is inability to lift the foot up (foot drop), loss of sensation in the feet and absent ankle jerk reflexes.

Wernicke's encephalopathy is usually seen in people who have been drinking alcohol heavily for some weeks and eaten very little. Alcohol requires thiamin for its metabolism and alcoholic beverages do not contain it. Occasional cases are seen in people on a prolonged fast (such as hunger strikers) or with persistent vomiting (as in Wernicke's first described case). Cases occurred in malnourished soldiers in Japanese prisoner-of-war camps in World War II. Clinically, there is a state of quiet confusion, lowered level of consciousness and inco-ordination (fairly non-specific signs in an alcoholic). The characteristic feature is paralysis of one or more of the external movements of the eyes (ophthalmoplegia). This, and the lowered consciousness, respond to injection of thiamin within two days, but if treatment is delayed the memory may never recover. The memory disorder that is a sequel of Wernicke's encephalopathy is called Korsakoff's psychosis after the Russian psychologist who first described it. There is an inability to retain new memories and sometimes confabulation.

In people who die of Wernicke–Korsakoff syndrome lesions are found in the mamillary bodies, mid brain and cerebellum. It is not clear why one deficient person develops beri beri and another develops Wernicke–Korsakoff syndrome and why the two diseases seldom coincide. Possibly, the cardiac disease occurs in people who use their muscles for heavy work and so accumulate large amounts of pyruvate, producing vasodilatation and increasing cardiac work, while encephalopathy is the first manifestation in inactive people.

12.1.5   Biochemical test

Red cell transketolase activity, with and without thiamin pyrophosphate (TPP) added *in vitro*, is a good test. But heparinized whole blood must be used, it must be analysed fresh (or specially preserved) and the test will be normal if thiamin treatment has been already started. If the transketolase activity is increased more than 30% in the test tube with added TPP, this indicates at least some degree of biochemical thiamin deficiency. In Wernicke's encephalopathy this 'TPP effect' can be higher than this, around 70%, or even 100%. (Note: in this test, reported as 'TPP effect', high values are abnormal.)

12.1.6   Interactions: nutrients

The requirement for thiamin is proportional to the intake of carbohydrates + alcohol + protein. In homogeneous societies, where proportions of fat and carbohydrate do not greatly differ, the thiamin requirement is proportional to the total energy intake.

There is a danger that patients presenting with Wernicke's encephalopathy might be given an intravenous infusion of glucose solution because they have been vomiting and are dehydrated. This extra intravenous load of glucose is likely to aggravate or precipitate Wernicke's encephalopathy.

12.1.7   Food sources

There are no rich food sources of thiamin. The best sources in descending order are wheatgerm, whole wheat and products, yeast and yeast extracts, pulses, nuts, pork, duck, oatmeal, fortified breakfast cereals, cod's roe and other meats. In many industrial countries (United Kingdom, United States, etc.) bread flour is enriched with thiamin. Australia introduced mandatory fortification of bread flour with thiamin in 1991 as a measure intended to reduce that country's relatively high rate of Wernicke–Korsakoff syndrome. Thiamin is readily destroyed by heat and by sulphite and by thiaminase (present in raw fish).

The recommended dietary intake of thiamin is 0.4 mg per 1000 kcal (0.1 mg/kJ), (i.e. about 1.0 mg per day in adults). The toxicity of thiamin is very low.

12.2 RIBOFLAVIN

Vitamin B was originally considered to have two components, heat labile B_1 (=thiamin) and heat stable B_2. In the 1930s, it was discovered that a yellow growth factor in this latter fraction is distinct from the pellagra-preventing substance (niacin).

12.2.1 Structure

Riboflavin or 7,8-dimethyl-10-(1'D-ribityl)isoalloxazine, comprises an alloxazine ring connected to a ribose alcohol—the ribityl side chain is required for full vitamin activity. It is a yellow-green fluorescent compound.

12.2.2 Functions

Riboflavin (Fig. 12.2) is part of two important coenzymes, flavin mononucleotide (FMN) and flavin adenine dinucleotide (FAD) which are oxidizing agents. They participate in flavoproteins in the oxidation chain in mitochondria. They are also cofactors for several enzymes, e.g. NAD dehydrogenase, xanthine oxidase, L-amino acid oxidase, glutathione reductase, L-gulonolactone oxidase.

12.2.3 Absorption, metabolism

Absorption is by a specialized carrier system in the proximal small intestine, which is saturated at levels above 25 mg. The vitamin is transported as free riboflavin and FMN or bound to plasma albumin. The body contains only about 1 g of riboflavin, mostly found in the muscle as FAD. Riboflavin is excreted primarily in urine; urinary excretion tends to reflect dietary intake.

12.2.4 Deficiency: animals

The most common effects in animals are cessation of growth, dermatitis, hyperkeratosis, alopecia and vascularization of the cornea. Abortion or skeletal malformations of the fetus may occur. In some species, anaemia, fatty liver and neurological changes have also been reported.

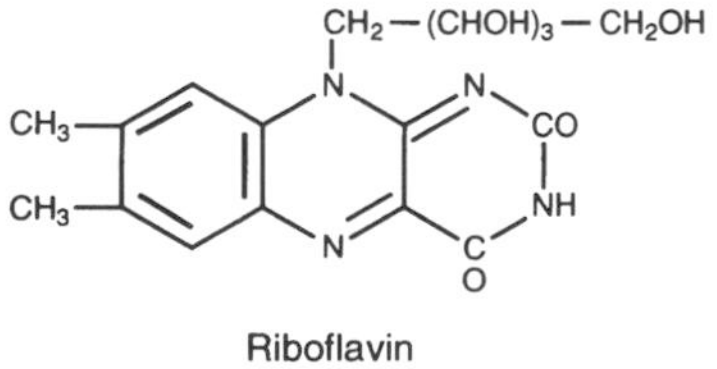

Riboflavin

Fig. 12.2 Structure of riboflavin. Ribitol is the alcohol form of the 5-carbon sugar, ribose. In FMN two phosphates are attached to the end of the ribitol. In FAD this is extended further with adenylate (ribose-adenine).

12.2.5 Deficiency: humans

The clinical symptoms of deficiency: angular stomatitis, cheilosis, atrophy of the tongue papillae, nasolabial dyssebacea and anaemia, are surprisingly minor, presumably due to the body's ability to conserve riboflavin, and the high affinity of the coenzymes for their respective enzymes. Riboflavin deficiency (ariboflavinosis) is most commonly seen alongside other nutrient deficiencies (e.g. pellagra).

12.2.6 Biochemical tests

1. Erythrocyte glutathione reductase activity (EGRA) coefficient. FAD is co-factor for this enzyme and its activity correlates with riboflavin status.

$$\text{The activity coefficient (or FAD effect)} = \frac{\text{EGRA with added FAD } in \ vitro}{\text{EGRA without FAD } in \ vitro}$$

Values of <1.2 are considered to be acceptable, but values of $1.3-1.7$ indicate inadequate riboflavin status. However, some doubts have been raised about the validity of the FAD effect, as it is elevated during exercise and pregnancy.

2. Measurement of urinary excretion of riboflavin:

| sufficient riboflavin status | 120 µg riboflavin/day |
| deficiency | < 40 µg riboflavin/day. |

12.2.7 Interactions: drugs

Phenothiazine derivatives (e.g. chlorpromazine) and tricyclic antidepressants have similar structures and can interfere with riboflavin metabolism. Reduced riboflavin status is observed in alcoholics, but is due more to decreased dietary absorption and intake, than to a direct effect of alcohol.

12.2.8 Food sources

Riboflavin is present in most foods although the best sources are milk and milk products, eggs, liver, kidney, yeast extracts and fortified breakfast cereals. Dairy products contribute significantly to riboflavin intake in Western diets. However, riboflavin is unstable in ultraviolet light, and after milk has been exposed to sunlight for four hours, up to 70% of riboflavin is lost.

The recommended dietary intake for adults is about 1.5 mg/day. The requirement is less in people with small energy intakes and more in those with large energy intakes.

12.2.9 Toxic effects

The toxicity is very low. The gastrointestinal tract cannot absorb more than about 20–25 mg of riboflavin in a single dose.

12.3 NIACIN

Niacin (Fig. 12.3) is a generic term for the related compounds that have activity as pellagra-preventing vitamins; the two that occur in foods are nicotinic acid (pyridine 3-carboxylic acid) and its amide, nicotinamide. They have apparently equal vitamin activity. Nicotinic acid is a fairly simple chemical (molecular weight 123) that was known long before its nutritional role was established. It was first isolated as an oxidation product of the natural alkaloid, nicotine, from which its name is derived. But nicotinic acid and amide have very different physiological properties from nicotine (which is α-N-methyl-d-β-pyridyl pyrrolidine).

12.3.1 Functions

Nicotinamide is part of the coenzymes nicotinamide–adenine dinucleotide (NAD) and nicotinamide–adenine–dinucleotide phosphate (NADP), the pyridine nucleotides. NAD has the structure: adenine–ribose–PO_4–PO_4–ribose–nicotinamide. It plays a central role in metabolism: it functions as the first hydrogen receptor in the electron chain during oxidative phosphorylation in the mitochondria. The pyridine ring of the nicotinamide is the part of the molecule that takes up a hydrogen ($NAD^+ = NADH$).

NADP has an extra PO_4 (phosphate) branching off the ribose adjacent to adenine. It has a more specialized function as hydrogen donor in fatty acid synthesis.

12.3.2 Absorption and metabolism

Nicotinic acid or its amide are water-soluble and well absorbed from the small intestine and transported in solution in the plasma. Stores of niacin and its coenzymes are only small and early features of pellagra can occur in human subjects after some 45 days of depletion.

12.3.3 Synthesis from tryptophan

A special feature of niacin is that in most conditions only about half of what is in the body is absorbed as preformed nicotinic acid or amide from the diet. About the same amount is synthesized in the liver from tryptophan, the indole amino acid, in a sequence of seven enzyme steps down the kynurenine pathway.

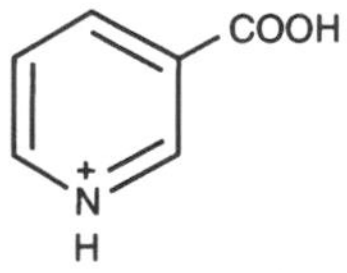

Nicotinic acid

Fig. 12.3 Structure of nicotinic acid (niacin). Nicotinamide is the corresponding amide, with $CONH_2$ in the side chain.

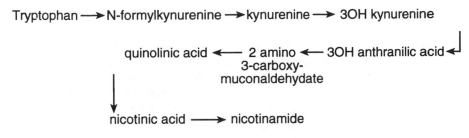

Fig. 12.4 Tryptophan → nicotinamide.

Most tryptophan in the body is used for protein synthesis—it is the least abundant in foods of all the essential amino acids—some also goes to serotonin. Normally, $\frac{1}{60}$th of the dietary tryptophan intake is converted in the liver to niacin (i.e. 60 mg tryptophan ≡ 1 mg niacin). The first enzyme in the kynurenine pathway, hepatic tryptophan oxygenase, is under hormonal control and the amount of niacin formed appears to be increased in pregnancy. It is down-regulated when the protein intake is inadequate (see Fig. 12.4).

12.3.4 Deficiency: animals

The classic animal model for pellagra is 'black tongue' in dogs. Puppies lose their appetite and have inflamed gums, dark tongue and diarrhoea with blood. Elvehjem's group at Wisconsin tested different fractions of liver for their ability to cure black tongue and in 1937 found the 'pellagra-peventing factor' was nicotinamide.

12.3.5 Deficiency: humans

There is one deficiency disease, *pellagra* (the name means 'sour skin' in Italian). There is inflammation of the skin where it is exposed to sunlight, resembling severe sunburn but the affected skin is sharply demarcated. The skin lesions progress to pigmentation, cracking and peeling. Often the skin of the neck is involved (Casal's collar) (See Fig. 12.5). Students are taught that pellagra is the disease of three Ds: dermatitis, diarrhoea and delirium or dementia. As well as diarrhoea there is likely to be an inflamed tongue (glossitis). In mild chronic cases mental symptoms (the third 'D') are not prominent. It is hard to explain the clinical manifestations by the known biochemical functions of niacin. Because some niacin is formed from tryptophan, pellagra can be cured by giving either niacin or a generous intake of easily assimilated protein.

Pellagra appeared in Europe after maize was introduced as a cereal crop from the new world after 1500, but the Mayas, Aztecs and original north Americans do not seem to have suffered from pellagra.

The niacin in cereals is in a complex, 'niacytin', which humans cannot absorb, so that although it appears in food tables (because the complex is split during extraction) it is not biologically available. If peasants eat a diet predominantly of maize, with few other foods their niacin has to come from tryptophan in the protein of the cereal. But the protein of maize is deficient in tryptophan, unlike other cereals, so little or no niacin can

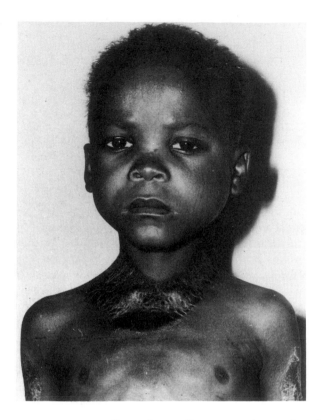

Fig. 12.5   A patient suffering from pellagra. Note the Casal's collar.

be made in the body via the kynurenine pathway. All cereals are low in lysine but maize
has less tryptophan than wheat and rice. In pre-Columbian America the ground maize
was steeped in warm lime water (calcium hydroxide), which liberates the niacin (making
it biologically available), and then made into tortillas, flat cakes—as it still is today in
Mexico and Guatemala.

Pellagra is rare in developed countries. It occurs in parts of Africa.

12.3.6   Biochemical tests

1. Urinary N'-methylnicotinamide (and/or its 2-pyridone) is the best known test but tests
   that require a 24-hour urine are inconvenient.
2. Red cell NAD concentration.
3. Fasting plasma tryptophan.

12.3.7   Interactions: nutrients

The most important is that tryptophan and hence dietary proteins (except in maize)
provide niacin. Tryptophan makes up about 1% of mixed dietary proteins so 6 g protein

($\rightarrow 60$ mg tryptophan)$\equiv 1$ mg niacin and a protein intake of 70 g/day is equivalent to about 12 mg niacin. The niacin requirement is thought to be proportional to the energy expenditure or energy intake.

Two of the enzymes in the kynurenine pathway are vitamin B_6-dependent so that vitamin B_6 deficiency is likely to reduce niacin synthesis from tryptophan.

12.3.8 Food sources

Good sources of preformed niacin, in descending order are liver and kidney (the richest sources), other meat, poultry, fish, brewer's yeast and yeast extracts, peanuts, bran, pulses, wholemeal wheat and (surprisingly) there is some niacin in coffee, including instant coffee. Other foods that are rich in protein provide tryptophan. If food tables give values for milligram niacin equivalents (NE), this is preformed niacin (mg) + [tryptophan $\div$ 60]. The British food tables (McCance and Widdowson) have separate columns for 'nicotinic acid' and for 'potential nicotinic acid from tryptophan, mg tryptophan $\div$ 60'. From this one can see, for example, that 100 g fresh whole cow's milk provides 0.08 mg preformed niacin but 0.80 mg potential niacin from tryptophan.

The recommended dietary intake for niacin in adults, expressed as niacin equivalents is 6.6 mg NE per 1000 kcal (1.6 mg NE per 1000 kJ); in absolute numbers about 13 mg in women and 17 mg in men.

12.3.9 Pharmacological doses

Well above the nutrient dose, nicotinic acid (but not the amide) produces cutaneous flushing from histamine release, at doses of 100 mg/day or more; it has been used for chillblains. At doses of 3 g/day or more (200 × the RDI) it inhibits lipolysis in adipose tissue and lowers plasma cholesterol and triglyceride. It is in the pharmacopoeia as a second line drug for combined hyperlipidaemia (i.e. high plasma cholesterol plus raised triglycerides). Side effects, as well as flushing, include gastric irritation, impaired glucose tolerance and disturbed liver function tests.

12.4 Vitamin B_6

12.4.1 Structure

Vitamin B_6 (Fig. 12.6) occurs in nature in three forms: pyridoxine, pyridoxal and pyridoxamine which are interconvertible within the body. Each form (vitamer) also occurs as a phosphorylated compound: the principal one in the body is pyridoxal 5'-phosphate (PLP). Vitamin B_6 activity is dependent on the 5-hydroxylmethyl group.

12.4.2 Functions

PLP is the major coenzyme form in the body. It functions in practically all the reactions involved in amino acid metabolism, including:

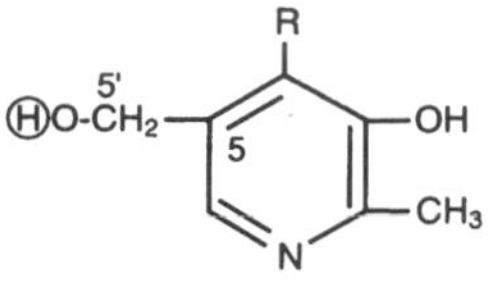

Vitamin B$_6$

Fig. 12.6 Structure of vitamin B$_6$. In pyridoxine, R = CH$_2$OH; in pyridoxal, R = CHO; in pyridoxamine, R = CH$_2$NH$_2$. In coenzyme forms, phosphate replaces the ringed H.

1. Transamination, and synthesis of non-essential amino acids.
2. Decarboxylations:
   (a) formation of neurotransmitters adrenalin, noradrenalin, serotonin and γ-amino butyric acid (GABA),
   (b) formation of δ-aminolaevulinic acid, which is the first step in porphyrin synthesis, making haemoglobin,
   (c) synthesis of sphingomyelin and phosphatidyl choline (lecithin),
   (d) synthesis of taurine, a conjugator of bile acids and important in eye and brain function.
3. Kynureninase: for the conversion of tryptophan to niacin. When this reaction is impaired, xanthurenic acid (major metabolite of 3(OH) kynurenine) accumulates in the urine, which is used as biochemical marker for B$_6$ status.
4. Deamination of serine and threonine.
5. Metabolism of sulphur-containing amino acids.

However, the role of vitamin B$_6$ is not restricted to protein metabolism; PLP is associated with glycogen phosphorylase which releases glucose from glycogen stores. Over half of total body B$_6$ is associated with glycogen phosphorylase enzyme in the muscles. PLP may also have a role in modulating steroid hormone receptors.

12.4.3 Absorption and metabolism

In the small intestine vitamin B$_6$ is absorbed by passive diffusion, mainly in the unphosphorylated form. The different forms of the vitamin are rapidly converted to pyridoxal in the intestinal cell, by the FMN-requiring enzyme, pyridoxal phosphate oxidase. Pyridoxal is transported in the circulation largely bound to albumin and haemoglobin, and after diffusion into the cell, pyridoxal is rephosphorylated by pyridoxal kinase, which maintains it within the cell.

The total body content of vitamin B$_6$ is estimated to be between 20 and 150 mg in adults. Most of this (90%) is tightly bound in tissues. Vitamin B$_6$ in the liver, brain, kidney, spleen and muscle is bound to protein which protects it from hydrolysis.

The major metabolite of vitamin B$_6$ is 4-pyridoxic acid, which is inactive as a vitamin and excreted in the urine.

12.4.4 Deficiency: animal studies

Dermatological and neurological changes are commonly observed in animals when vitamin B_6 is deficient. In rats, impaired growth, muscular weakness, irritability, dermatitis, anaemia, fatty liver, impaired immune function, hypertension and insulin insufficiency have all been observed. Neurological changes include convulsions.

12.4.5 Deficiency: humans

The symptoms of deficiency in humans are general weakness, sleeplessness, peripheral neuropathy, personality changes, dermatitis, cheilosis and glossitis (as in riboflavin deficiency), anaemia and impaired immunity. Deficiency on its own is rare, it is most often seen with deficiencies of other vitamins, or with protein deficiency. In 1953, a minor epidemic of convulsions in infants in the United States was traced to a milk formula which contained no vitamin B_6 because of a manufacturing error. Convulsions in pyridoxine deficiency are probably due to impaired synthesis of γ-aminobutyric acid (GABA), the major inhibitory neurotransmitter.

12.4.6 Deficiency: secondary

A number of inborn errors of amino acid metabolism respond to supranutritional doses of pyridoxine. Homocysteinaemia, a condition which may increase the risk for vascular disease, responds to supplements of folate, vitamin B_{12} and sometimes B_6.

Vitamin B_6 deficiency is common (80–100%) in chronic alcoholics, who may have impaired absorption. Acetaldehyde (oxidation product of ethanol) can inhibit the conversion of pyridoxine to PLP.

Pregnant women have a decrease in plasma PLP levels. It is unclear whether this indicates a deficiency or is a normal physiological change.

12.4.7 Biochemical tests

- Measurement of plasma pyridoxal phosphate. Normal levels are above about $10\,\mu g/ml$ (50 nmol/l).
- Increased urinary xanthurenic acid after a load of the amino acid, tryptophan.
- Activity of erythrocyte alanine aminotransferase, with and without *in vitro* PLP.
- Urinary 4-pyridoxic acid.

12.4.8 Interactions: other nutrients

High protein intakes increase metabolic demand for vitamin B_6.

12.4.9 Interactions: drugs

Isoniazid (used to treat tuberculosis), increases urinary excretion of vitamin B_6. Cycloserine, penicillamine, L-dopa and hydralazine are vitamin B_6 antagonists. Some biochemical indices of vitamin B_6 state may be abnormal in a proportion of women taking oral contraceptives, but these are indirect indices (e.g. alanine aminotransferase).

12.4.10   Food sources

The vitamin is distributed in a wide range of unprocessed (or lightly processed) foods. Major food sources in the Western diet are meats, whole grain products, vegetables and nuts. Refined cereal products such as white bread and white rice are not significant sources of vitamin B_6 due to milling losses.

The recommended dietary intake is 0.02 mg vitamin B_6 per gram of protein intake which works out to 1.5–2.0 mg/day in average adults.

12.4.11   Toxic effects

Vitamin B_6 toxicity was first reported in women taking supplements of very large doses of pyridoxine (2000–6000 mg/day). These supplements were taken for premenstrual syndrome or carpal tunnel syndrome and the women developed peripheral neuropathy and lost sensation in their feet. Intakes of supplements down to 200 mg/day (100 × RDI) have been associated with neuropathy.

12.5   BIOTIN

12.5.1   Functions

Biotin is a coenzyme for several carboxylase enzymes: pyruvate carboxylase (formation of oxaloacetate for the TCA (tricarbolic acid) cycle), acetyl CoA (coenzyme A) carboxylase (fatty acid synthesis), propionyl CoA carboxylase (catabolism of odd-chain fatty acids and some amino acids) and 3-methylcrotonyl CoA carboxylase (catabolism of the ketogenic amino acid leucine).

12.5.2   Deficiency: animals and humans

Biotin deficiency is very rare as biotin is found in a wide range of foods, and bacterial production in the large intestine appears to supplement dietary intake. Deficiency can, however, be produced when animals or humans eat large amounts of uncooked egg white, which contains avidin. This binds biotin in the gut, preventing absorption. Avidin is destroyed by heating. 'Egg white injury' (i.e. biotin deficiency) impairs lipid and energy metabolism in animals. It produces seborrhoeic dermatitis, alopecia and paralysis of the hind limbs in rats and mice.

In humans, cases of biotin deficiency have been associated with a scaly dermatitis (altered fatty acid metabolism may contribute to this skin condition), glossitis, anorexia, depression and hypercholesterolaemia. Biotin deficiency has been reported in patients on total parenteral nutrition whose infusions did not contain biotin.

12.6   PANTOTHENIC ACID

Coenzymes often contain unusual structures—unusual in the sense that higher animals have lost the ability to form them and they must be supplied in the diet. For coenzyme A it is pantothenic acid.

12.6.1 Functions

Pantothenic acid is part of coenzyme A (CoA) and of acyl carrier protein (ACP). CoA and ACP are both carriers of acyl groups. Acetyl-CoA participates in the tricarboxylic acid cycle (TCA) in the disposal of carbohydrates and ketogenic amino acids. CoA is also involved in the synthesis of lipids: fatty acids, glycerides, cholesterol, ketone bodies and sphingosine. ACP is involved in chain elongation during fatty acid synthesis.

Pantothenic acid is transported primarily in the CoA form by red cells in the blood, and is taken up into cells by a specific carrier protein. The highest concentrations of the vitamin are found in the liver, adrenals, kidney, brain, heart and testes. Most is in the CoA form.

All tissues are able to synthesize CoA from pantothenic acid. ACP is synthesized from a 4-phosphopantotheine residue transferred from CoA. These metabolically active forms can be degraded to free pantothenic acid, which is the major form of excretion in the urine. Urinary pantothenic acid reflects dietary intake, ranging from 2 mg to 7 mg/day in adults.

12.6.2 Deficiency: animals

In most species, pantothenic acid deficiency is associated with dermatitis, changes to hair or feathers, anaemia, infertility, irritability, ataxia, paralysis, convulsions and even death. In rats, a condition called 'bloody whiskers' is caused by release of protoporphyrin via the nose and tear ducts.

12.6.3 Deficiency: humans

Spontaneous human deficiency has never been described. As pantothenic acid is so widely distributed in foods, any dietary deficiency in humans is usually associated with other nutrient deficiencies. The word 'pantothen' means 'from everywhere' (Greek), but highly refined foods do not contain pantothenic acid.

Subjects given the antagonist ω-methylpantothenic acid, developed a deficiency with symptoms of depression, fatigue, insomnia, vomiting, muscle weakness, and a burning sensation in the feet. Changes in glucose tolerance, an increase in insulin sensitivity, postural hypotension, and decreased antibody production were also noted.

During World War II, malnourished prisoners of war in the Far East developed 'burning feet syndrome' which appeared to respond to large doses of Ca-pantothenate.

There is no official recommended daily intake but about 4 mg/day are required and must be provided in total parenteral nutrition.

12.7 FOLATE

Folate is used as the generic name for compounds chemically related to pteroyl glutamic acid, folic acid. Deficiency of folate is quite common in hospital patients, secondary to diseases, especially intestinal, neoplastic and haematological. Requirements are notably increased in pregnancy. The word 'folic' is from the Latin 'folia' (leaf), coined in 1941 for an early preparation of this vitamin from spinach leaves.

12.7.1   Structure

Folic acid (pteroyl glutamic acid) is the primary vitamin from the chemical point of view, and it is the pharmaceutical form because of its stability. But it is rare in foods and in the body. Most folates are in the reduced form, tetrahydrofolate (THF); they also have 1-carbon components (methyl or formyl) attached to nitrogen atom 5 or 10, or bridging between them (5,10-methylenetetrahydrofolate) (Fig. 12.7). In addition, they have up to 7 glutamic acid residues (instead of 1) in a row (at the right in Fig. 12.7).

12.7.2   Functions

Tetrahydrofolate plays an essential role in 1-carbon transfers in the body. It receives 1-carbon radicals from e.g. serine, glycine, histidine and tryptophan, and donates them at two steps in purine synthesis and one important step in pyrimidine synthesis: insertion of the methyl group in deoxyuridylic acid to form thymidylic acid, the characteristic nucleotide of DNA. (The folate derivative involved here is 5,10-methylene THF.)

5-Methyl THF co-operates with vitamin B_{12} in the action of methionine synthase, which adds a methyl group to homocysteine and forms methionine and THF (from which 5,10-methylene THF can be formed). When vitamin B_{12} is deficient, folate is trapped as the 5-methyl compound and 5,10-methylene THF is not available to form thymidylate for DNA synthesis (Fig. 12.8).

12.7.3   Absorption and metabolism

It was formerly thought that the polyglutamyl forms ('conjugated' folate) are not as well absorbed as folic acid with only 1–3 glutamates ('free' folate) but folate with 7 glutamates is nearly as well absorbed as pteroyl monoglutamate because there are conjugases in gastric and pancreatic juice and in the small intestinal epithelial cells. These split off the extra glutamates. More than half of folates in foods are in polyglutamyl form; after absorption, most folates in the plasma are in the monoglutamyl form. In the blood, red cells contain 30–50 times more folate than plasma. There is a small store of folate in the liver, mostly in polyglutamate form. Total body folate has been estimated at about 6–10 mg.

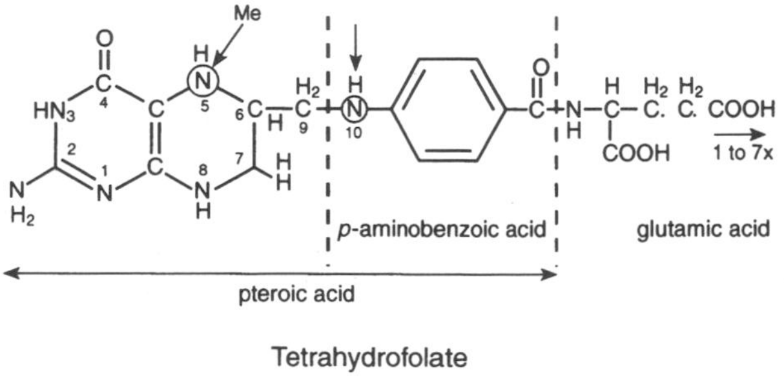

Fig. 12.7   Structure of folic acid. Tetrahydrofolate (pteroyl glutamic acid) monoglutamate.

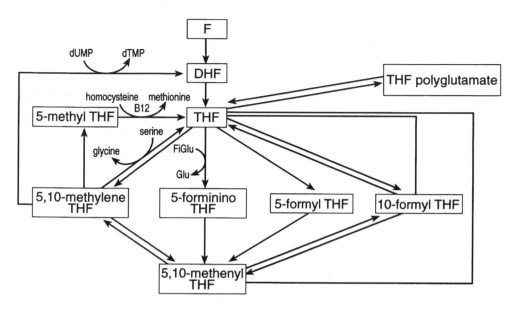

Fig. 12.8 Folate metabolism. Note that 5-methyltetrahydrofolate can only return to the pool for other functions if there is enough vitamin B_{12} for the homocysteine → methionine reaction, which takes up the methyl group. In the reaction of dUMP → dTMP, dTMP is thymidylate, one of the four essential bases of DNA. If there is insufficient 5,10-methylenetetrahydrofolate (the specific co-factor) DNA synthesis is reduced or stops. F = folate, DHF = dihydrofolate, THF = tetrahydrofolate.

12.7.4 Deficiency: animals

Chicks show reduced growth, anaemia and impaired feather growth. In guinea-pigs there is a low white blood cell count and growth failure.

12.7.5 Deficiency: humans

Folate is the final antimegaloblastic substance. In deficiency, the basic abnormality is reduced ability of cells to double their nuclear DNA, in order to divide, because of impaired synthesis of thymidylate.

There is megaloblastic anaemia (cells are enlarged, their nuclei large but with reduced density of chromatin) and similar changes in leucocytes, platelets and epithelial cells; there is also infertility and may be diarrhoea.

Pure dietary deficiency is seen occasionally. In a previously healthy physician (Victor Herbert) experimental depletion resulted in anaemia after 125 days, with biochemical and histological changes before this. But when there is increased cell proliferation or interference with folate metabolism features of deficiency appear earlier. Secondary deficiency is common in late pregnancy, in alcoholics, in haemolytic anaemias, uraemia, intensive hospital therapy and people with malabsorption.

12.7.6   Interactions: nutrients

Vitamin B_{12} (see below). Vitamin C in foods reduces loss of folate in cooking. Several drugs interfere with folate metabolism, most of them by antagonizing dihydrofolate reductase (which converts 2H folate to 4H folate, i.e. THF): methotrexate, aminopterin, amethopterin (used for chemotherapy for cancer) pyrimethamine (antimalarial), co-trimoxazole (antibacterial).

Folate is important at both ends of pregnancy. In late pregnancy some degree of megaloblastic anaemia is common and women are often given tablets of folic acid plus iron to prevent or treat this. This anaemia can sometimes first be noticed in the early weeks after childbirth.

Folic acid supplements have more recently been found to reduce the risk of a serious fetal malformation, neural tube defect, if taken around the time of conception. The neural tube closes at days 24–28 after conception and the extra folate must be taken before this (i.e. before the woman may be sure she is pregnant). In the Medical Research Council (UK) trial, women who had previously had a baby affected by neural tube defect agreed to take one of four different nutritional supplements periconceptionally. It was found that those taking supplements containing folic acid had 70% fewer deformed babies. From studies of serum folate of women who were subsequently found to have an abnormal baby it appears that neural tube defect is not caused by a deficiency but by a need for extra folate in some women at this time of embryonic development.

The recommended dietary intake for folate is 200 µg (0.2 mg) per day for adults. In late pregnancy 400 µg prevents the megaloblastic anaemia and it is estimated that 400 µg periconceptionally will prevent most cases of neural tube defect. This is approximately double the usual intake from food and is the reason for several countries encouraging folate enrichment of staple foods that contain some folate naturally.

12.7.7   Biochemical tests

Serum folate reflects recent intake. The normal level is above 3 ng/ml (7 nmol/l). Red cell folate gives a better idea of cellular status. It is normally above 100 ng/ml (225 nmol/l).

12.7.8   Food sources

Although the name comes from Latin 'folia' (leaf), and it does occur in leafy vegetables (spinach, broccoli, cabbage, lettuce) it also occurs in other foods: liver, kidney, beans, beetroot, bran, peanuts, yeast extract, avocadoes, bananas, wholemeal bread, eggs, some fish. There is even a little folate in beer and tea. In the United Kingdom and United States many breakfast cereals and some breads are now fortified with extra folic acid.

Analysis of folate in foods is difficult because of the multiple compounds. Early analyses used microbiological assay but human cells may not respond to different folate compounds in the same way as bacteria. Some recent methods are based on the major peaks on HDLC. Folate is destroyed in foods by prolonged boiling.

12.7.9   Toxicity

The main concern is that if someone with vitamin B_{12} deficiency (pernicious anaemia) is treated with a fairly high (supranutritional) dose of folic acid (5 mg/day) the anaemia may improve but the biochemical basis for the neurological symptoms of vitamin B_{12} deficiency is not corrected, so correct biochemical diagnosis is essential before anyone is treated for anaemia with folic acid. Otherwise, the toxicity of folic acid is low.

12.8   VITAMIN B_{12}

Early this century it was postulated that human gastric juice contained an 'intrinsic factor' which combined with an 'extrinsic factor' in animal protein foods (such as raw liver) and the combination would cure a type of anaemia that was until then untreatable, pernicious anaemia. In the late 1940s the extrinsic factor vitamin B_{12} was identified and human intrinsic factor was isolated in the 1960s.

12.8.1   Structure

Vitamin B_{12}, or cobalamin, is a red compound made up of a corrinoid ring (4 pyrrole rings) containing an atom of cobalt. This structure is complex and only synthesized by bacteria. There are a range of naturally occurring corrinoids but not all have vitamin B_{12} activity. The term 'vitamin B_{12}' is used here as a generic term for all active cobalamins in humans. Vitamin B_{12} has the largest molecule of the vitamins, with a molecular weight of 1355. The structure of vitamin B_{12} is large and three-dimensional—to view it, refer to a good textbook of biochemistry.

12.8.2   Functions

The coenzyme forms of vitamin B_{12} are methylcobalamin and deoxyadenosylcobalamin. Only two B_{12}-dependent enzymes have been identified in humans: methylmalonyl-CoA mutase (which requires deoxyadenosylcobalamin) and methionine synthetase (which requires methylcobalamin).

Methylmalonyl-CoA mutase is involved in the conversion of methylmalonyl-CoA to succinyl-CoA in the catabolism of propionate, in the mitochondria.

Methionine synthetase, found in the cytosol, transfers a methyl group from the donor 5-methyl-THFA (a form of folate) to homocysteine to produce methionine.

Homocysteinaemia, a condition which may increase the risk for vascular disease, responds to supplements of vitamins B_{12}, B_6, and folate.

12.8.3   Absorption and metabolism

Vitamin B_{12} is absorbed by an efficient active transport system involving 'intrinsic factor' (IF), a specific binding glycoprotein secreted by the gastric parietal cells. The IF-B_{12} complex binds to specific receptors in the mucosal brush border of the terminal ileum, to facilitate B_{12} uptake. At higher intakes, vitamin B_{12} is taken up by passive diffusion, but only about 1% is absorbed. In the plasma, B_{12} is transported by a specific binding protein, transcobalamin II (TC_{II}). Bone marrow cells and reticulocytes contain TC_{II}–B_{12} receptors. Other transcobalamins TC_I and TC_{III} appear to have more of a storage function.

213

The total body store is estimated to range from 1 to 5 mg, enough for 5 or more years! Most is found in the liver. Only about 0.2% of total body stores (2–5 µg) are excreted daily. Up to 5 µg/day of vitamin B_{12} is secreted in bile into the intestine, but most of this (65–75%) is reabsorbed. Urinary cobalamin is very low with most probably coming from the cells in the kidney.

12.8.4 Deficiency: animals

The most common signs of deficiency in animals are lack of growth and reduced food intake. Alterations in lipid metabolism occur—fatty liver, increase in triglycerides and free fatty acids. In pigs, a mild anaemia is observed. Neurological changes have been observed in monkeys after 3–5 years on a vitamin B_{12}-deficient diet, and in fruit bats, after 7 months.

12.8.5 Deficiency: humans

Very strict vegetarian diets containing no fish, poultry, eggs or dairy products, and without vitamin supplements, contain practically no vitamin B_{12}. Such people have low circulating levels of vitamin B_{12}, but clinical symptoms are surprisingly uncommon. Normal body stores of the vitamin are sufficient to last for 3–6 years. Bacteria in the intestine produce some vitamin B_{12} which might perhaps be absorbed from the caecum, but, the bioavailability of such B_{12} is uncertain. Infants breast-fed by strict vegan mothers, are at serious risk of impaired neurological development, anaemia and even severe encephalopathy. Children on macrobiotic diets are at risk of vitamin B_{12} deficiency.

Inadequate dietary intake is not the usual cause of vitamin B_{12} deficiency. Most common is malabsorption due to atrophy of the gastric mucosa so there is inadequate production of IF, or disease of the terminal ileum. The commonest type of vitamin B_{12} deficiency from gastric atrophy is called 'pernicious anaemia' because it used to be untreatable. There are two effects of vitamin B_{12} deficiency: megaloblastic anaemia and/or neurological dysfunction. Anaemia usually precedes neurological symptoms, but not always. Anaemia is megaloblastic, so called because blood cells are characteristically large with reduced nuclear density, and white cells, platelets and epithelial cells are also affected the same way. Vitamin B_{12} deficiency interrupts normal nuclear division by 'trapping' folate, leading to a reduction in the synthesis of DNA (see Section 12.7). The anaemia is morphologically the same in folate and vitamin B_{12} deficiency. Biochemical tests are used to distinguish between them.

The characteristic neuropathy of vitamin B_{12} deficiency has a different biochemical basis, possibly caused by an accumulation of propionate and other odd-chain fatty acids in nerve tissue (lower activity of methylmalonyl-CoA mutase). There is a loss of sensation and motor power in the lower limbs due to degeneration of myelin in the spinal cord.

Spinal cord degeneration is not seen in folate deficiency. The biochemical basis of the pernicious anaemia involves an interaction with folate. The neurological disease does not.

An injection of 100 µg/month will successfully treat pernicious anaemia but high oral doses (working by passive absorption) are also used.

13
VITAMINS C AND E

Murray Skeaff

13.1 VITAMIN C

13.1.1 History

...For some lost all their strength, their legs became swollen, and inflamed, while the sinews contracted and turned as black as coal. In other cases the legs were found blotched with purple-coloured blood. Then the disease would mount to the hips, thighs, shoulders, arms and neck. And all had their mouths so tainted, that the gums rotted away down to the roots of the teeth, which nearly all fell out. The disease spread among the three ships to such an extent, that in the middle of February, of the 110 men forming our company, there were not 10 in good health so that no one could aid the other, which was a grievous sight considering the place where we were.

The above passage describes the condition of Jacques Cartier's expedition in Québec during the winter of 1535–6. It is one of the earliest descriptions of the vitamin C deficiency disease, scurvy, and the first report of a cure. On the advice of the local Indians, Cartier's party made a brew from the bark and leaves of a local tree—probably the white cedar (*Thuja occidentalis*): 'As soon as they had drunk it they felt better which must clearly be ascribed to miraculous causes; for after drinking it two or three times, they recovered health and strength and were cured of all the diseases they had ever had.'

In modern times the needles of the white cedar, like other leaves, have been shown to contain vitamin C. Despite this remarkable cure and Cartier's written record of it, the primitive nature of communication in early medicine meant that French and English voyagers to the same region would suffer the ravages of scurvy for at least another century.

Two centuries later, James Lind, a surgeon in the Royal Navy, after making several voyages during which serious outbreaks of scurvy occurred, undertook to discover the definitive cure for the disease in 1747. In what is now recognized as one of the first controlled dietary trials, Lind not only established 'that oranges and lemons were the most effectual remedies for this distemper at sea' but of equal importance, proved that other curative potions of the time were, with the exception of apple cider, without effect. It was another half century before the British Navy took heed of Lind's research and instituted lemon juice rations for all crews.

The discovery of vitamin C moved a step closer in 1907 when Holst and Frölich, in Oslo, were able to produce scurvy in guinea-pigs. Until that time, experimental scurvy had not been produced in laboratory animals because most of them (e.g. rats, mice, rabbits) are not susceptible to the disease. This breakthrough opened the way for bioassays to be developed to test the relative potencies of antiscorbutic foods and extracts.

Unrelated to the search for the antiscorbutic factor—now named vitamin C—Szent-Györgyi in 1928 isolated a crystalline substance he called 'hexuronic acid' from orange juice, cabbage juice, and adrenal glands. Four years later Szent-Györgyi shared some of these crystals with Svirbely, working in Hungary, who quickly showed it to cure scurvy in guinea-pigs; vitamin C had been discovered.

13.1.2   Terminology and biosynthesis

Vitamin C, formal chemical name L-ascorbic acid, is an odourless, stable, white solid, soluble in water, slightly soluble in ethanol and insoluble in organic solvents. Ascorbic acid can be synthesized from glucose or galactose in a wide variety of plants and in most animal species (Fig. 13.1). The exceptions to this rule are humans and other primates, guinea-pigs, fruit-eating bats, and many fish because they lack the final enzyme, L-gulonolactone oxidase, required to convert L-gulonolactone to L-ascorbic acid. Ascorbic acid is readily oxidized in the body to dehydroascorbic acid which in turn can be reduced back to ascorbic acid. This ability to participate in oxidation–reduction reactions is the basis for most of the known functions of the vitamin.

13.1.3   Functions

Table 13.1 outlines some of the functions of vitamin C, which are discussed in detail below.

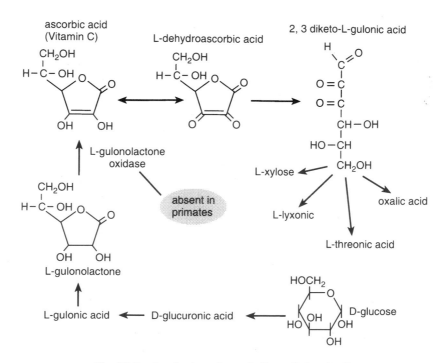

Fig. 13.1   Synthesis and metabolism of vitamin C.

Table 13.1   Metabolic pathways requiring vitamin C

- Hydroxylation of proline and lysine for collagen synthesis
- Synthesis of noradrenaline from dopamine
- Synthesis of carnitine from lysine
- Activation of neuropeptides
- Catabolism of tyrosine
- Synthesis of bile acids

1. The best-defined function of vitamin C is its role in the synthesis of collagen, the principal connective tissue protein found in tendons, arteries, bone, skin and muscle. The protein is first synthesized with an abundance of proline and lysine residues, many of which are then converted by prolyl hydroxylase and lysyl hydroxylase to hydroxy-proline and hydroxylysine, respectively. These hydroxy-amino acids provide the anchor for crosslinking of collagen molecules which increases the strength and elasticity of connective tissue. The enzymes prolyl and lysyl hydroxylase require, along with amino acid substrates, vitamin C, ferrous ions (Fe^{2+}) molecular oxygen (O_2) and α-ketoglutarate to accomplish the hydroxylation reactions. Vitamin C does not participate directly in the hydroxylation reaction; rather, it is required to convert iron on the enzyme from the ferric state (Fe^{3+}) back to the ferrous state (Fe^{2+}). Reduced activity of these two hydroxy-lase enzymes during chronic deficiency of vitamin C leads to the connective tissue defects seen in scurvy. In scurvy, new connective tissue cannot be formed in sufficient amounts to replace ageing or injured connective tissue. Even minor injuries that might normally go unnoticed lead to tissue disruption and extensive bleeding.

2. A second hydroxylation reaction which requires vitamin C is the conversion of dopamine to noradrenaline by dopamine β-monooxygenase. Noradrenaline is an important neurotransmitter produced in neural tissues.

3. Vitamin C is required for conversion of lysine to carnitine (it participates at two steps). Carnitine plays an essential role in the transfer of long-chain fatty acids into the inner mitochondria where they can be converted to energy by way of β-oxidation. In tissues where fat is a significant source of energy, such as in heart and skeletal muscle, low levels of carnitine can impair muscle function. This may explain the fatigue and muscle weakness associated with severe chronic vitamin C deficiency.

4. Activation of various peptide hormones and hormone releasing factors occurs through α-amidation of the hormone by the enzyme, peptidylglycine α-amidating mono-oxygenase. This enzyme requires vitamin C and is involved in the synthesis of calcitonin, melanocyte-stimulating hormone, and releasing factors for corticotropin, thyrotropin and growth hormone.

5. Vitamin C is required for one of the enzymes (4-hydroxyphenylpyruvatehyd-roxylase) involved in the catabolism of tyrosine to carbon dioxide and water.

6. Vitamin C deficiency in animals leads to a reduction in the activity of liver enzymes (i.e. mixed function oxidases) involved in the metabolism of hormones, cholesterol, drugs, and carcinogens.

7. The rate-limiting step of bile acid synthesis in the liver involves the conversion of cholesterol to 7α-hydroxycholesterol by the enzyme 7α-hydroxylase. The activity of this pathway is reduced in vitamin C-deficient animals and is associated with elevated plasma cholesterol concentrations.

8. Considerable attention has recently been focused on the antioxidant function of vitamin C. The water-soluble nature of vitamin C permits it to act as an efficient anti-oxidant against a wide range of intra- and extracellular free radicals. Its role in the regeneration of vitamin E is discussed in Section 13.2.4.

13.1.4   Food Sources

Fruits and vegetables are the major sources of vitamin C in the diet, contributing together up to 90% of the vitamin intake in countries like New Zealand and the United Kingdom (Table 13.2). Fruit juices and drinks fortified with vitamin C are the most significant source in some groups, such as adolescents.

Table 13.2   Vitamin C content of common foods

Food	Vitamin C (mg/100 g)
Blackcurrants	200
Kiwifruit	122
Cauliflower	60
Broccoli	58
Potato crisps	51
Honeydew melon	50
Oranges	50
Strawberries	46
Grapefruit	40
Spinach	34
Pineapple	25
Tomatoes	24
Beef liver	22
Cabbage	21
Beef kidney	13
Potatoes	10
Peaches	10
Apples	9
Pears	3
Chicken liver	3
Milk	1
Wholemeal bread	0

Source: New Zealand food composition database (OCNZ88). Palmerston North: Crop and Food Research Institute.

13.1.5 Digestion, absorption, transport and excretion

Vitamin C is readily absorbed in the small intestine by an energy-dependent mechanism, with 70–90% of average daily vitamin C intake (30–200 mg) being absorbed. The absorption decreases to 20% when a single 5 g dose of the vitamin is ingested and to 16% with a 12 g dose. The bioavailability of vitamin C from foods is similar to that from supplements.

In plasma, vitamin C is transported unbound to protein (i.e. free). Virtually all the extracellular vitamin is present as ascorbic acid (>99.5%) with only trace (<0.5%) amounts as dehydroascorbic acid. An energy-driven uptake mechanism serves to maintain a high concentration of vitamin C in intracellular, as compared to extracellular, fluid. The highest concentration of vitamin C in the body is found in pituitary and adrenal glands, eye lens, leucocytes, lymph glands, brain, and other internal organs. The lowest levels are found in plasma and saliva.

Studies using isotopically labelled ascorbic acid have shown that the amount of vitamin C in the body (i.e. body pool) plateaus at roughly 20 mg/kg body weight or 1500 mg for an average person. This body pool can be maintained with a daily vitamin C intake of 60–100 mg by all but a few in the population. Normal plasma vitamin C concentrations range from 23–87 µmol/l (4–15 mg/l) and it is difficult to raise the upper level even when consuming very large doses. Beyond a daily intake of 200 mg, virtually all the excess vitamin C will be excreted in the urine within 24 hours.

Vitamin C is not stored for long in the body. When a vitamin C free diet is consumed approximately 3% of the total body pool is lost per day, although this proportion decreases considerably with duration of the diet. In the range of usual intake, almost half of the urinary metabolites of vitamin C appear as oxalic acid while ascorbic acid, dehydroascorbic acid, 2,3-diketogulonate, and ascorbate 2-sulphate make up the remainder. When vitamin C intake greatly exceeds physiological requirement, there is some increase in oxalate excretion but most of the vitamin is excreted as unmetabolized vitamin C. Despite the theoretical possibility of increased risk of calcium oxalate stones in the urinary tract of people who take vitamin C supplements, this has not been found in practice.

13.1.6 Factors affecting metabolism

Cigarette smokers have lower concentrations of ascorbic acid in plasma and leukocytes. These lower levels are partly, but not entirely, the result of reduced consumption of vitamin C. Isotopic studies have shown that the metabolic turnover of vitamin C in smokers is twice that in non-smokers. Consequently, smokers require significantly more dietary vitamin C to maintain a body pool of vitamin C equivalent to that of non-smokers. Acute and chronic infections and disease can reduce levels of vitamin C in plasma and leucocytes. However, in chronic disease the poor vitamin C status is often due to poor diet. There is some evidence that excretion of vitamin C increases under acute infections and stressful conditions.

13.1.7 Deficiency

Scurvy is uncommon in populations unless there is a prolonged shortage of fruits and vegetables together with an overall reduced food supply, as in the Irish Potato Famine of the nineteenth century. More recent evidence of outbreaks comes from refugee camps in the Horn of Africa. During the famines of 1985–7 the incidence of scurvy in six refugee camps in Somalia and Sudan ranged from 14–44% of the camp populations. Those who participated in supplementary food programmes did not have a reduced incidence of scurvy. The supplementary foods, cereals, legumes, and oil, were almost completely deficient in vitamin C. Accordingly, the World Health Organization (WHO) now advises that in this area of Africa vitamin C supplements be added to relief food at an early stage of a crisis.

In societies where food supply is plentiful and diverse, scurvy usually occurs only in those consuming extremely poor diets that have a complete lack of fruits and vegetables, for example, in young or elderly men living alone, alcoholics, or illicit drug users. Scurvy can affect infants whose only source of food is cow's milk. There is no known genetic disorder of vitamin C metabolism.

There are several detailed reports of dedicated scientists, prisoners, and paid volunteers in whom scurvy has been produced after adherence to a diet devoid of vitamin C. Symptoms such as weakness, fatigue, inflamed and bleeding gums, impaired wound healing, petechial and other skin haemorrhages, and depression have been observed after 3–6 months on the scorbutic diets. The symptoms usually occur when the plasma concentration of vitamin C falls below 11 µmol/l (2 mg/l) or when the total body pool of the vitamin is less than 300 mg. Full recovery from the clinical manifestations of scurvy requires as little as 10 mg of vitamin C per day.

13.1.8 Nutrient interactions

Vitamin C enhances the absorption of non-haem iron when vitamin C and foods containing non-haem iron are consumed in the same meal (see Chapter 9.4). Vitamin C achieves this effect in the small intestine by helping to convert dietary iron from the ferric state (Fe^{3+}) to the more soluble ferrous state (Fe^{+2}), and by binding to ferric iron (Fe^{+3}) to form soluble complexes. A high enhancing effect can be attained with a vitamin C intake of roughly 100 mg per meal. When body iron stores are low, the enhancing effect of vitamin C on non-haem iron absorption is markedly higher than when iron stores are high. Accordingly, it is common to recommend to vegetarians, many of whom have lower than average iron stores, that foods containing vitamin C be consumed with meals.

In the stomach, vitamin C can inhibit the conversion of nitrates, commonly found in cured and pickled foods, to carcinogenic compounds known as nitrosamines. The incidence of nitrosamine-induced stomach cancer in animals can be reduced by vitamin C. In humans, an epidemiological association has been noted between low intakes of vitamin C, mainly from fruits and vegetables, and high rates of stomach cancer.

13.1.9 Higher dose effects

One of the most commonly ascribed benefits of ingesting large doses of vitamin C (1–10 g/day), in the form of supplements, relates to prevention of the common cold. The most consistent finding from a review of controlled therapeutic supplementation trials is that vitamin C does not reduce the incidence of the common cold; however, some trials have demonstrated a slight decrease in the duration and severity of symptoms.

13.1.10 Toxicity

Toxicity of vitamin C is low, given the widespread chronic and acute use of supplements and the lack of reported harmful effects. There is some concern that vitamin C can increase oxidant stress in those susceptible to iron overload (e.g. with haemochromatosis) by reducing ferritin bound iron from ferric iron (Fe^{3+}) to ferrous iron (Fe^{2+}) thereby promoting its release into the circulation. Discontinuation of high doses of vitamin C does cause a temporary drop in leucocyte ascorbic acid concentrations, below normal dose levels, but there is no evidence in humans that this is harmful or that 'rebound scurvy' occurs.

13.1.11 Biochemical assessment

Measurement of vitamin C in serum and leucocytes is the most common means of assessing vitamin C status (Table 13.3). Both correlate well with dietary intake in populations; in studies where participants follow depletion and repletion diets, serum and leucocyte vitamin C are equally sensitive to changes in dietary vitamin C intake. For practical purposes measurement of vitamin C in serum is preferred over leucocyte measurement.

Urinary excretion of vitamin C falls to undetectable levels during extended deficiency but is otherwise of limited use as a measure of vitamin status because it tends to reflect recent dietary intake. Measurement of urinary vitamin C in patients suspected of scurvy can provide supportive diagnostic information.

There are no reliable functional tests of vitamin C status.

13.1.12 Recommended nutrient intakes

Recommended nutrient intakes vary considerably between countries and depend on the relative importance given to the various criteria for establishing physiological requirement. At one extreme is the amount required to prevent scurvy in adults (approximately 10 mg/day) while the other extreme is the amount of vitamin C above which practically all ingested is excreted (approximately 200 mg/day). Most advisory bodies have chosen

Table 13.3 Assessment of vitamin C status*

Test	Normal	Marginal	Deficient
Biochemical tests			
Serum (μmol/l)	>17	11–17	<11
Leucocytes (nmol/10^8 cells)	>85	45–85	<45
Urine (24 h)			
Saliva			
Body pool size			<300 mg
Functional test			
Capillary fragility test			

* Cut-off values and ranges have only been clearly established for some tests.

a level of intake sufficient to maintain a body pool of vitamin C that will provide a reasonable buffer against the onset of scorbutic symptoms when faced with a vitamin C deficient diet.

The recommended nutrient intake for healthy adults is 40 mg/day in the United Kingdom, Canada, and Australia and 60 mg/day in the United States. Thanks to orange juice, potatoes and the wide availability of green vegetables and fruit, most people in affluent countries consume a good deal more than this.

FURTHER READING

1. Carpenter KJ. *The history of scurvy and vitamin C*. Cambridge: Cambridge University Press, 1986.
2. Davies MB, Austin A, Partridge DA. *Vitamin C: its chemistry and biochemistry*. Cambridge: The Royal Society of Chemistry, 1991.
3. Englard S, Seifter S. The biochemical functions of ascorbic acid. *Ann Rev Nutr* 1986; 6: 365–406.
4. Hemilä H. Vitamin C and the common cold. *Brit J Nutr* 1992; 67: 3–16.
5. Hodges RE, Baker EM, Hood J, Sauberlich HE, March SC. Experimental scurvy in man. *Am J Clin Nutr* 1969; 22: 535–548.
6. Sauberlich HE. Pharmacology of vitamin C. *Ann Rev Nutr* 1994; 14: 371–91.

13.2   VITAMIN E

13.2.1   History

While investigating the relationship between fertility and nutrition, Evans and Bishop discovered in 1922 that female rats fed a diet containing rancid fat and deficient in a lipid-soluble factor were unable to support full-term development of a fetus. The death and ensuing resorption of the fetus could be prevented by adding small amounts of fresh lettuce, wheat germ, or dried alfalfa leaves to the mother's diet. Over the next 10 years, vitamin E-deficient diets were found to produce sterility in male rats and chickens, nutritional muscular dystrophy in rabbits and guinea-pigs, and encephalomalacia (crazy chick disease) in chickens. The unidentified lipid-soluble factor which prevented fetal resorption in rats was named 'vitamin E' and subsequently also became known as tocopherol, (from the Greek 'tokos' for childbirth, 'phereiu' meaning to bring forth, and 'ol' to represent the alcohol in its structure). The vitamin was isolated by Evans in 1936 and the chemical structure identified and synthesized in 1938. The necessity of the vitamin for humans was not clearly established until the 1960s.

13.2.2   Structure and terminology

Vitamin E is unique amongst vitamins because there are eight naturally occurring forms of it found in plants (Fig. 13.2); four tocopherols (alpha, α-; beta, β-; gamma, γ-; and delta, δ-) and four tocotrienols (α-, β-, γ-, and δ-). The structure common to all forms of vitamin E consists of a chromanol ring to which a hydrophobic 16-carbon isoprenoid tail is attached. The α-, β-, γ-, and δ- forms of tocopherol differ in the position and number of methyl groups on the chromanol ring. The only structural difference between the four types of tocotrienols and their respective tocopherols is the presence of three double bonds in the isoprenoid or phytyl tail.

There are three asymmetric centres on the tocopherol or tocotrienol molecule that give rise to stereo isomers; namely, C2 on the chromanol ring, and C4' and C8' on the tail. There are therefore eight theoretical stereoisomers for each of the eight vitamin E compounds. The naturally occurring and most potent form of vitamin E is 2R, 4'R, 8'R-α-tocopherol (formerly termed [d]-α-tocopherol). Chemical synthesis of α-tocopherol results in the production of a mixture of equal amounts of eight stereo-isomers known as all-*rac*-α-tocopherol (formerly termed [dl]-α-tocopherol).

13.2.3 Bioavailability

The abundance and biological activity of each form of naturally occurring vitamin E varies considerably (Table 13.4). The biological activities of the tocopherols and tocotrienols are usually determined by comparing the relative potencies of each form of the vitamin in animal model bioassays (e.g. prevention of rat fetal resorption). Using this

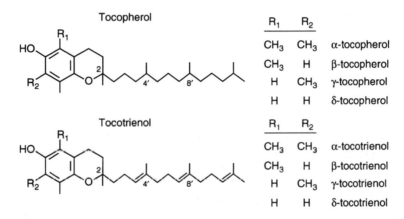

Tocopherol	R_1	R_2	
	CH_3	CH_3	α-tocopherol
	CH_3	H	β-tocopherol
	H	CH_3	γ-tocopherol
	H	H	δ-tocopherol

Tocotrienol	R_1	R_2	
	CH_3	CH_3	α-tocotrienol
	CH_3	H	β-tocotrienol
	H	CH_3	γ-tocotrienol
	H	H	δ-tocotrienol

Fig. 13.2 Structure of tocopherols and tocotrienols.

Table 13.4 Biological activity of vitamin E

Form of vitamin E	Biological activity (IU/mg)	α-Tocopherol equivalents (α-TE/mg)
RRR-α-tocopherol	1.49	1.00
RRR-α-tocopheryl acetate	1.36	0.91
all-*rac*-α-tocopherol	1.10	0.74
all-*rac*-α-tocopheryl acetate	1.00	0.67
all-*rac*-β-tocopheryl acetate	0.45–0.60	0.30–0.40
all-*rac*-γ-tocopheryl acetate	0.11	0.10
all-*rac*-δ-tocopheryl acetate	0.015	0.01
RRR-α-tocotrienol	0.45	0.30

method the synthetic all-*rac*-α-tocopheryl acetate (tocopherol with an acetate molecule attached to the hydroxyl group) has an activity of 1.00 international unit (IU) per mg, while the naturally occurring RRR-α-tocopherol has the highest activity of 1.49 IU/mg; of the tocotrienols only the alpha form shows any significant biological activity (0.45 IU/mg). Although there is a significant amount of γ-tocopherol in the diet, it makes only a minor contribution to overall vitamin E activity because of its low biological activity (0.11 IU/mg). Vitamin E content of the diet is often expressed as α-tocopherol equivalents (α-TE) where 1 α-TE is the activity of 1 mg of RRR-α-tocopherol.

13.2.4 Functions

Vitamin E is a powerful antioxidant which plays an essential role in protecting cell membranes and plasma lipoproteins from free radical damage. Free radicals contain an unpaired electron and react readily with polyunsaturated fatty acids, proteins, carbohydrates, and DNA. Vitamin E is able to 'neutralize' free radicals because the hydroxyl group on the chromanol ring readily gives up an electron or hydride group to the free radical. Through this oxidative reaction, the unpaired electron in the free radical becomes paired (less reactive); however, the hydroxyl group on the vitamin E now has an unpaired electron. This resultant vitamin E radical (Vit E•) can react with another free radical and be permanently inactivated to the stable vitamin E quinone (Vit E=O) or it can be regenerated to active vitamin E (Vit E–OH) by reacting with vitamin C or glutathione.

Fatty acids with two or more double bonds (i.e. polyunsaturated) are abundant in all cell membranes and have an important influence on membrane fluidity and function. However, their double bonds make them susceptible to oxidation by free radicals (Fig. 13.3). Fortunately, most vitamin E in the body is found in cell membranes where it functions to protect polyunsaturated fatty acids from free radical attack. In the event that a fatty acid radical is produced, vitamin E stabilizes the free radical and prevents it from reacting with adjacent polyunsaturated fatty acids and propagating the reaction along the membrane with disastrous consequences.

There is an elaborate interrelationship between vitamin E and other antioxidant nutrient systems in the body. The most direct interaction is with vitamin C which serves to regenerate vitamin E from its radical state. Glutathione can also regenerate vitamin E thus explaining the interaction with sulphur amino acids. Antioxidant systems such superoxide dismutase, catalase, glutathione peroxidase, and vitamin C help to eliminate free radicals, thereby reducing oxidant stress on membranes and preserving vitamin E. However, if membrane vitamin E is deficient, high levels of other antioxidants cannot prevent the peroxidation of membrane polyunsaturated fatty acids, although they may delay the damage.

Plasma lipoproteins, like cell membranes, contain an abundance of lipid including large proportions of polyunsaturated fatty acids. Not unexpectedly, they also contain vitamin E which plays an essential role in protecting the lipoproteins from oxidative damage. This is particularly important in low-density lipoproteins (LDLs) because lipid peroxides can oxidize apolipoprotein B resulting in the formation of oxidatively modified LDL. This oxidized LDL accumulates in the walls of arteries at a greater rate than normal LDL (i.e. non-oxidized) thus accelerating the development of atherosclerotic plaques. (The role of oxidized LDL in the aetiology of cardiovascular disease is discussed in Chapter 18.1.4.)

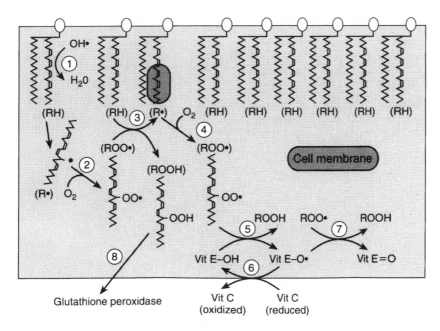

Fig. 13.3 Antioxidant function of vitamin E (1) A free radical (e.g. hydroxyl free radical) abstracts hydrogen from a membrane polyunsaturated fatty acid (RH), converting it into a fatty acid free radical (R•). (2) A shift in the position of the double bond adjacent to the free radical followed by the uptake of oxygen results in the formation of a peroxy-fatty acid radical (ROO•). (3) The peroxy-fatty acid can be stabilized to a hydroperoxy-fatty acid (ROOH) by abstracting a hydrogen from another membrane polyunsaturated fatty acid (RH). The consequence of this is the propagation of the initial free radical damage along the membrane. (4) Isomerization and oxygen uptake occurs. (5) Vitamin E arrests the propagation of the free radical damage by converting the peroxy-fatty acid free radical (ROO•) to a hydroperoxy-fatty acid (ROOH). (6) The resulting vitamin E radical (Vit E•) can be regenerated to vitamin E (Vit E–OH) by oxidation of vitamin C. (7) Alternatively, the vitamin E radical can stabilize another peroxy-fatty acid radical to form the quinone form of vitamin E (Vit E=O). This form of vitamin E cannot be regenerated. (8) Hydroperoxy-fatty acids can be eliminated by glutathione peroxidase.

13.2.5 Digestion, absorption, transport and distribution

Vitamin E is absorbed in a manner similar to most other dietary lipids and requires that fat digestion be functioning normally. The presence of fat in the small intestine enhances vitamin E absorption because the products of triglyceride breakdown in the gut promote the formation of mixed micelles, the vehicle from which vitamin E is absorbed into the mucosal cells lining the small intestine. Absorption is normally quite efficient, ranging from 50 to 70% of usual vitamin E intake but decreases substantially at high doses. Lack of bile acids or fat digestive enzymes, damage to the gastrointestinal lining, or an inability to synthesize chylomicrons will decrease vitamin E absorption. Diseases in which vitamin E absorption is reduced include: pancreatic diseases (e.g. cystic fibrosis), biliary obstruction, coeliac disease, and a rare genetic inability to make chylomicrons (abetalipoproteinaemia).

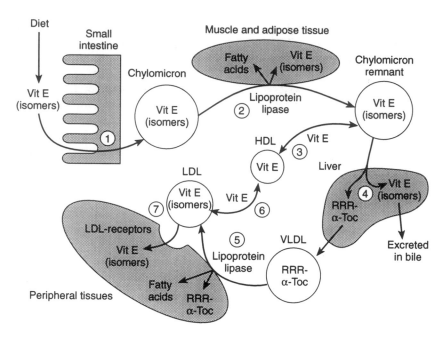

Fig. 13.4 Digestion, absorption, transport, and distribution of vitamin E. (1) Vitamin E isomers of dietary origin are absorbed into the mucosal cell where they are incorporated into chylomicrons which enter the circulation by way of the lymphatic vessels. (2) Vitamin E is transferred from chylomicrons to tissues during the catabolism of triacylglycerols by lipoprotein lipase. (3) Exchange of vitamin E isomers between chylomicron remnants and high-density lipoproteins (HDLs) can occur. (Individuals with familial isolated vitamin E (FIVE) deficiency must rely on this exchange mechanism for dietary α-tocopherol to be distributed to other lipoproteins). (4) The remaining vitamin E isomers of dietary origin are removed from the circulation when chylomicron remnants are taken up by the liver. α-Tocopherol transfer protein preferentially incorporates RRR-α-tocopherol into very low-density lipoproteins (VLDLs) which are secreted from the liver. (5) Metabolism of triacylglycerol in VLDL by lipoprotein lipase leads to the transfer of α-tocopherol to peripheral tissues. (6) Exchange of vitamin E isomers between HDL and low-density lipoprotein (LDL) occurs. (7) Vitamin E is also delivered to the peripheral tissues by way of the receptor-mediated uptake of LDL.

Vitamin E is incorporated into chylomicrons and enters the circulation via the lymphatic system (Fig. 13.4). The profile of vitamin E forms incorporated into chylomicrons reflects that of the diet because there is little discrimination between the different forms of tocopherols and tocotrienols in gut absorption or in incorporation into chylomicrons. During catabolism of chylomicrons to chylomicron remnants by lipoprotein lipase some vitamin E is transferred to muscle and adipose tissue. There is also considerable exchange of vitamin E between chylomicrons and high-density lipoproteins (HDLs). Vitamin E acquired by HDL can be subsequently transferred to VLDLs, (very low-density lipoproteins) and LDL.

Vitamin E is distributed throughout the body mainly associated with cell membranes, plasma lipoproteins, and adipose (i.e. triglyceride) deposits. Higher concentrations of the vitamin tend to be found in organs with a high fatty acid content (e.g. liver, brain, and adipose tissue). The amount of vitamin E in the body reflects dietary intake with excess to requirements deposited in adipose tissue. Adipose tissue vitamin E is not a freely available reserve against deficient intake since only small amounts of the vitamin are mobilized when plasma vitamin E is low. Movement of the excess vitamin E from adipose tissue to plasma can occur, but is the consequence of the breakdown of adipose triglycerides, as would occur during energy restriction, rather than a response to low plasma levels of the vitamin.

13.2.6   Metabolism and excretion

Vitamin E delivered to the liver by chylomicron remnants is incorporated into very low-density lipoprotein (VLDL). However, not all forms of vitamin E (α-, β-, γ-, and δ-) are incorporated equally into VLDL. In the liver, α-tocopherol-transfer-protein preferentially incorporates RRR-α-tocopherol into VLDL as compared to RRR-γ-tocopherol or the other stereoisomers of α-tocopherol (See Fig. 13.4). Consequently, VLDL secreted from the liver is rich in RRR-α-tocopherol while most of the γ-tocopherol and stereoisomers of α-tocopherol are excreted in the bile. This shunting of RRR-α-tocopherol to VLDL helps to explain the fact that RRR-α-tocopherol is the predominant form of vitamin E delivered to the tissues, hence its higher biological activity (i.e. bioavailability).

Metabolism of VLDL to LDL results in the transfer of vitamin E to tissues and HDL in a manner analogous to chylomicron metabolism. Delivery of vitamin E in LDL to the tissues is accomplished by receptor-mediated uptake of the whole LDL particle.

13.2.7   Deficiency

Symptomatic vitamin E deficiency disease has not been produced experimentally in humans; however, a genetically inherited disease called familial isolated vitamin E (FIVE) deficiency provides proof of the essentiality of vitamin E for humans. Individuals with this disease have normal lipid absorption and gastrointestinal function as well as normal incorporation of vitamin E into chylomicrons and subsequent delivery to the liver. Nevertheless, they have low or undetectable levels of plasma vitamin E. They develop reduced tendon reflexes by three to four years of age and more disabling cerebrospinal symptoms such as unsteadiness of gait, loss of touch and pain sense, limb ataxia (lack of co-ordination), ptosis, dysarthria, and impaired eye movements by early adolescence. The genetic defect involves a mutation in the gene for the α-tocopherol-transfer-protein thus blocking the liver's ability to incorporate α-tocopherol into VLDL. The clinical symptoms can be prevented by 1000 mg/day of oral all-*rac*-α-tocopherol. The therapy increases chylomicron vitamin E sufficiently to force enough vitamin E to be redistributed by direct transfer to other circulating lipoproteins from where it can be delivered to the tissues.

In diseases such as cholestatic liver disease, cystic fibrosis, and abetalipoproteinaemia where severe and chronic fat malabsorption is present, neurological symptoms of vitamin E deficiency can develop. Children often develop the clinical symptoms of ataxia, areflexia or hyporeflexia (absent or low/slow reflexes), loss of proprioception (position sense) within two to three years of the onset of fat malabsorption, whereas symptoms in adults may take up to 20 years to manifest. In some cases, there can be yellow/white pigment deposits in the retina. Typical treatment involves oral doses ranging from 5 to 25 IU/kg per day, although intramuscular injection has been used. Once started, the treatment normalizes plasma vitamin E levels rapidly and arrests further deterioration of clinical symptoms; however, full normalization of neurological function can take several years. Individuals with persistent steatorrhea (i.e. fatty stools) should have their plasma vitamin E levels monitored.

13.2.8   Toxicity

Reports of vitamin E toxicity are rare. Intakes of 100–800 mg/day appear to be well tolerated. Thus, vitamin E is one of the exceptions to the earlier belief that high doses of fat-soluble vitamins are toxic while high doses of water soluble vitamins are not.

13.2.9   Food sources

Foods high in fat, particularly polyunsaturated fat, are the best food sources of vitamin E (Table 13.5). Wheat germ oil is the richest source. Tocopherols comprise the bulk of vitamin E in plant foods with the exception of palm oil which contains more tocotrienols. Most vitamin E in animal foods is α-tocopherol (>90%) with small amounts of γ-tocopherol (<10%) and little tocotrienol. The relative amounts of α-, β-, γ-, and δ-tocopherol varies considerably between plant foods, but in a mixed diet α- and γ-tocopherol tend to predominate.

13.2.10   Assessment of vitamin E status

Measurement of plasma vitamin E is the easiest and most common method of assessing vitamin E status (Table 13.6). Normal concentrations ranges from 12 to 30 μmol/l (5–16 mg/l), with more than 90% usually as α-tocopherol. A plasma concentration of vitamin E above 12 μmol/l (5 mg/l) is considered adequate.

When the concentration of plasma lipoproteins is elevated, plasma vitamin E is correspondingly high. To allow for this correlation, plasma vitamin E is frequently expressed per unit of plasma cholesterol. A plasma vitamin E to cholesterol ratio of greater than 2–2.5 μmol/mmol is judged to be normal.

Vitamin E can be measured in platelets, erythrocytes, and adipose tissue although these methods are more time-consuming and reference data are limited.

There are several functional test of vitamin E status involving the measurement of oxidant stress. These test are difficult to standardize and are not entirely specific for vitamin E status because other antioxidant systems can influence the results. The most common test is the erythrocyte fragility test in which erythrocytes are exposed to a standard concentration of hydrogen peroxide (2%) for 3 hours and the amount of haemolysis is measured. Poor vitamin E status is indicated when more than 5% of the

Table 13.5 Vitamin E content of common foods

Food	Vitamin E (mg/100g)
Fats and oils	
wheat germ oil	137.0
palm oil	33.1
soybean oil	16.3
margarine	14.9
Nuts	
almonds (raw)	24.0
peanuts	10.1
Fruits and vegetables	
sweet potato	4.6
spinach	1.7
peaches	1.3
carrots	0.8
tomatoes	0.8
lettuce	0.8
apples	0.4
honeydew melon	0.1
broccoli	0.1
Meat, poultry, fish	
chicken	0.8
cod	0.5
beef	0.3
lamb	0.2
Breads and cereals	
wheat germ	22.6
wholemeal flour	2.0
bran cereal	1.9
rolled oats	1.6
white flour	0.4
brown rice	0.3
wholemeal bread	0.2
Dairy products	
cheddar cheese	0.9
cottage cheese	0.1
Legumes	
mung beans	0.9
lentils	0.4
kidney beans	0.2

Source: New Zealand food composition database (OCNZ97). Palmerston North: Crop and Food Research Institute, 1993.

Table 13.6 Assessment of vitamin E status*

Test	Normal	Marginal-deficient
Biochemical tests		
Plasma (μmol/l)	12–30	< 12
Erythrocytes		
Platelets		
Adipose tissue		
Vitamin E/lipid ratio		
Functional tests		
Erythrocyte haemolysis		
Breath pentane and ethane		
Erythrocyte malondialdehyde		
LDL-oxidation		

* Cut-off values and ranges have only been clearly established for some tests.

erythrocytes haemolyse. The remaining tests involve measurement of metabolites produced during the *in vivo* peroxidation of polyunsaturated fatty acids; these include breath pentane and ethane, urinary malondialdehyde, and lipoprotein diene conjugated fatty acids.

13.2.11 Recommended nutrient intakes

Recommended nutrient intakes for vitamin E are based on the usual intake in apparently healthy populations because clinical deficiency symptoms are rare, and there is no sensitive and specific biochemical measure of vitamin E status. Animal experiments confirm the theoretical prediction that vitamin E requirements (to prevent deficiency effects) are increased if the intake of polyunsaturated fatty acids is high. A ratio of 0.4 mg α-tocopherol per gram of polyunsaturated fat intake is considered sufficient vitamin E to avoid any deficiency. Fortunately, increased intake of vitamin E is not difficult to achieve because of the natural association between vitamin E and polyunsaturated fatty acids in foods. A typical recommended nutrient intake is 10 mg α-tocopherol equivalents per day for healthy men and somewhat less for women.

There is considerable interest in using new criteria to establish nutrient recommendations for vitamin E. Minimizing free radical damage is considered by many the future criterion for establishing recommended vitamin E intakes. The fact that free radicals have both beneficial and pathological effects in the body will make it challenging for nutritionists to decide, within the context of overall oxidant stress and antioxidant status, the level of vitamin E intake that achieves the optimal balance between these opposing effects.

Intakes of 50–200 mg/day appear in prospective epidemiological studies to be associated with a reduced risk of coronary heart disease. But intakes as high as this cannot be achieved by ordinary diets, they require vitamin E supplements. The association between taking vitamin E supplements and reduced risk of coronary disease may be due to other confounding factors (i.e. the lifestyle of people who take vitamin supplements is likely to differ in other ways from people who do not take supplements).

FURTHER READING

1. Kayden HT, Traber MG. Absorption, lipoprotein transport, and regulation of plasma concentrations of vitamin E in humans. *J Lipid Res* 1993; **34**: 343–58.
2. Leth T, Sondergaard H. Biological activity of vitamin E compounds and natural materials by the resorption-gestation test, and chemical determination of the vitamin E activity in foods and feeds. *J Nutr* 1977; **107**: 2236–43.
3. Meydani M. Vitamin E. *Lancet* 1995; **345**: 170–5.
4. Sokol RJ. Vitamin E deficiency and neurological disease. *Ann Rev Nutr* 1988; **8**: 351–373.

VITAMINS D AND K

Stewart Truswell

14.1 VITAMIN D

14.1.1 History

In the first step towards identifying individual vitamins, E.V. McCollum, at the University of Wisconsin postulated (1915) two essential dietary factors as well as macronutrients and minerals—'fat-soluble A' and 'water-soluble B'. Fat-soluble A prevented growth failure and the eye disease, xerophthalmia, in animals fed purified diets. In 1919, Edward Mellanby in London found that some fats would cure experimental dietary rickets in puppies kept indoors but others would not. Cod liver oil was very active against the bone disease rickets and against xerophthalmia (Chapter 11) but when heated, with oxygen bubbled through, its antixerophthalmia activity was lost, not its antirachitic (antirickets) activity, and McCollum realized in 1922 there were two nutritional factors in cod liver oil. He designated the antirachitic factor vitamin D because 'water-soluble C' had been proposed for the antiscorbutic (antiscurvy) factor in 1919. Meanwhile, Harriette Chick, a British scientist, proved that rickets in children in Vienna after World War I could be cured either by cod liver oil or by exposure to an ultraviolet (UV) light lamp. Pure vitamin D_2 was first obtained by irradiating ergosterol with UV light in 1927. Its chemical structure was established by A. Windaus in Germany and F. Askew in England in 1932. In 1936, Windaus published the structure of D_3, the form of the vitamin made by UV light in the skin and present in cod liver oil.

14.1.2 Chemistry and metabolism

Vitamin D_3, cholecalciferol, is derived by the effect of UV irradiation (wavelength 290–315 nm) on 7-dehydrocholesterol (cholesterol with a double bond at carbon 7), a minor companion of cholesterol in the skin. There is a rearrangement of the molecule, with opening of the B ring of the steroid nucleus (Fig. 14.1). Cholecalciferol is the naturally occurring form of the vitamin in man and animals, hence, for example, in cod liver oil, fatty fish, butter and animal liver.

Vitamin D_2 is derived from ergosterol (a fungal sterol) by irradiating it with UV light via the same sequence of chemical changes and is called ergocalciferol. It is used as a pharmaceutical (also called calciferol) and in some of the foods fortified with vitamin D (e.g. milk in North America, margarine). Ergosterol is a phytosterol (plant sterol). It and ergocalciferol differ from 7-dehydrocholesterol and cholecalciferol only in having an extra double bond at carbon-22 and a methyl group at carbon-24 in the side chain

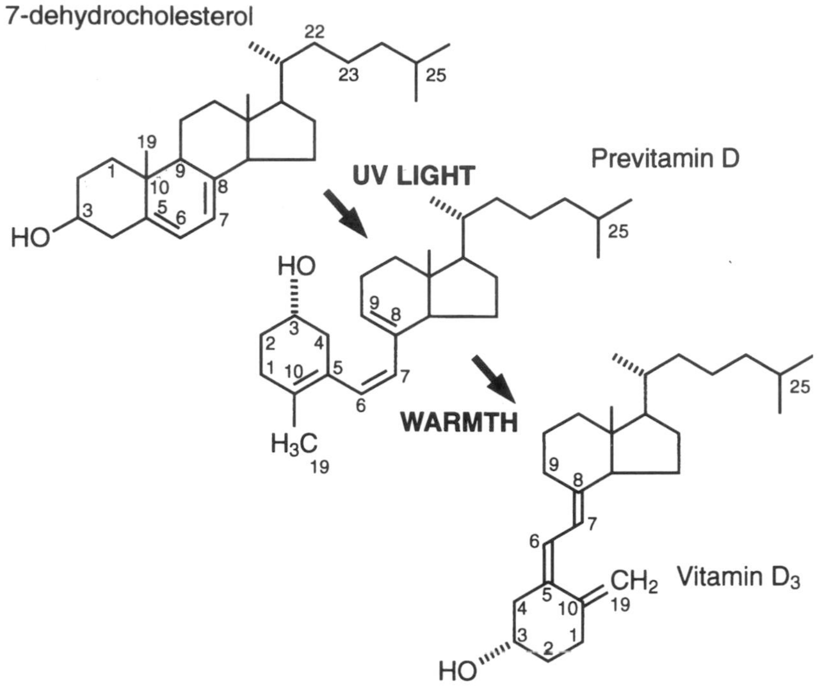

Fig. 14.1 Formation of vitamin D_3 in the skin. 7-dehydrocholesterol is present in the skin as a minor companion of cholesterol. Under the influence of short wavelength UV light (290–315 mm) from sunlight, the B ring of the sterol opens to form a secosterol, previtamin D_3. The first step takes place rapidly. The second stage is a rearrangement of the secosterol to make vitamin D_3 (cholecalciferol). It takes place more slowly, under the influence of warmth.

(Fig. 14.1). The original vitamin D_1 turned out to be an impure mixture of sterols. Other compounds $(D_4–D_7)$ have been made with vitamin D activity by treating several 7-dehydrophytosterols with UV light.

Using the older quantitative unit for vitamin D, one international unit (IU) = 0.025 µg of cholecalciferol (so 1 µg = 40 IU).

In the tropical and subtropical regions of the world, enough vitamin D is made in the skin to meet the body's needs (unless people are housebound or completely covered). Since cholecalciferol is formed in one organ of the body (the skin) and transported by the blood to act on other organs (the bones, gut, kidneys) it can be called a hormone. But when people live in high latitudes, are covered with clothes, spend nearly all their time indoors and the sky is polluted with smoke there is insufficient UV exposure in the winter to make enough vitamin D in the skin. Dietary intake is required, so that the cholecalciferol present in a few foods and the ergocalciferol in fortified foods assume the role of a vitamin.

Inside the body, vitamin D itself is not active until it has been chemically modified (hydroxylated) twice. The first clue to this was the observation of a lag period of eight hours before one could see an effect of administered vitamin D in experimental animals.

Vitamin D, whether of cutaneous origin or absorbed (D_3 or D_2), is carried in the plasma on a specific α_2-globulin, vitamin D-binding protein. In liver microsomes, the end of the side chain is hydroxylated to form 25(OH) vitamin D. This compound has a more stable concentration in the blood than that of vitamin D which rises temporarily as some is absorbed or synthesized in the skin.

25(OH)D is still not the active metabolite. It has to have a third hydroxyl (OH) group put on at carbon-1. This is done by an enzyme, 1α-hydroxylase, in the kidneys (in the mitochondria of the proximal convoluted tubule) to make 1,25-dihydroxy vitamin D (Fig. 14.2). The plasma concentration of $1,25(OH)_2D$ is about one thousand times smaller than that of 25(OH)D. The activity of renal 1α-hydroxylase is tightly controlled so the rate of production of $1,25(OH)_2D$ is increased by any fall in plasma calcium or rise in parathyroid hormone level. $1,25(OH)_2D$ is one of the three hormones that normally act together to maintain the extracellular calcium concentration constant; the other two are parathormone and calcitonin (see Chapter 8). There are about 30 other known metabolites of vitamin D, probably all inactive.

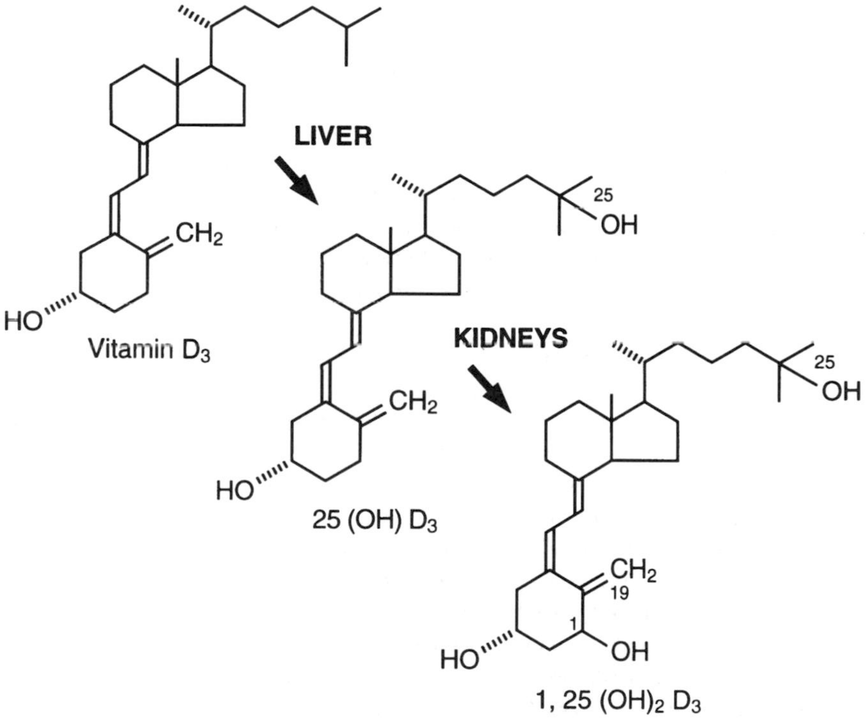

Fig. 14.2 Activation of vitamin D. In the liver parenchymal cells vitamin D_3 (or D_2) is hydroxylated to 25-hydroxy-vitamin D(25(OH)D), which circulates in the blood. A small proportion of the available 25(OH)D is further hydroxylated by a specific 25(OH)D-1α-hydroxylase in the kidneys to the active form, $1,25(OH)_2$ vitamin D. During pregnancy some 1α-hydroxylation also takes place in the placenta.

1,25(OH)$_2$D acts in a similar manner to steroid hormones. There is a specific vitamin D receptor (VDR) protein in the cell nucleus which has great affinity for 1,25(OH)$_2$D. It also has a DNA-binding domain. This receptor, when activated, switches on the gene that induces synthesis of a calcium transport protein (calbindin) in the epithelium of the small intestine. VDR has actually been found in a range of tissues but normally has its main effect in the small intestinal epithelium and the cells in bone osteoblasts (that form new bone) and osteoclasts (that break bone down).

Less vitamin D is made in the skin of dark-skinned people than white-skinned people because the melanin in the former absorbs UV light. Old people also make less vitamin D after exposure to short-wave UV light; their skin contains less of the starting material, 7-dehydrocholesterol. Vitamin D taken by mouth is digested and absorbed then transported from the upper small intestine on chylomicrons, like other lipids. Like other lipids its absorption can be impaired in chronic biliary or intestinal disease with malabsorption. Excretion of vitamin D is in the bile, principally as more polar metabolites.

14.1.3   Deficiency diseases

In rickets, there is reduced calcification of the growing ends (epiphyses) of bones. Thick seams of uncalcified osteoid cartilage are seen histologically. Rickets only occurs in young people whose bones are still growing. Osteomalacia is the corresponding decalcifying bone disease in adults, whose growing ends (epiphyses) have fused so that the bones are no longer growing. Rickets can occur in premature infants and in children in northern Britain (especially of Asian origin). Surprisingly, rickets and osteomalacia can also occur in the tropics in children and women usually staying indoors and fully covered when outdoors. In affluent countries, osteomalacia is possible in elderly people confined indoors. Malabsorption increases the risk. Muscular weakness and susceptibility to infections in rickets or osteomalacia may reflect roles for VDR in the muscles and the immune system. In chronic kidney failure, 1α-hydroxylation is impaired. Renal osteomalacia does not respond to vitamin D (or sunlight), only to 1,25(OH)$_2$D, (pharmaceutical name 'calcitriol') or to 1α(OH)D (pharmaceutical name 'alphacalcidol'). This shows the critical importance of 1α-hydroxylation to normal vitamin D function.

14.1.4   Biochemical tests of vitamin D status

Plasma calcium and phosphate levels fall in severe vitamin D-deficient states. Plasma alkaline phosphatase (the isoenzyme originating in bone) is increased in mild as well as in severe rickets and osteomalacia. It can be elevated in some other bone diseases and does not directly indicate vitamin D status. This is best assessed by assaying plasma 25(OH)D levels and it can be seen how the concentration goes down in population samples at the end of the winter in those temperate countries that have little vitamin D fortification. Plasma 1,25(OH)$_2$D can also be measured but is a specialized investigation.

14.1.5   Food sources

Fish liver oils (e.g. cod and halibut) and some fish and marine animal's livers are rich sources. Moderate sources are fatty fish (sardine, tuna, salmon, etc.), margarines (which in most countries are fortified with vitamin D), infant milk formulas, eggs and beef and lamb liver. Milk is fortified with vitamin D in North America and Scandinavia.

14.1.6   Interactions

Inadequate calcium intake aggravates any insufficiency of vitamin D. Fraser (1995) suggests that low calcium intake increases formation of $1,25(OH)_2D$ and that this acts on the liver to increase destruction or reduce formation of $25(OH)D$. Long-term use of anticonvulsants. (e.g. for epilepsy), by inducing liver microsomes may increase metabolic losses of vitamin D.

14.1.7   Recommended nutrient intake (see Table 32.2)

The United States recommendation is $10\,\mu g/day$ during growth, pregnancy and lactation and $5\,\mu g/day$ in adults. In Canada, the figures are $2.5\,\mu g/day$ for most adults and some children; $5\,\mu g/day$ in toddlers, adolescents and adults over 50 years. In the United Kingdom no vitamin D by mouth is recommended except in infants, adults over 50 years and in pregnant and lactating women (for whom supplements of $10\,\mu g/day$ are suitable).

14.1.8   Toxicity

Exposure of the skin to sunlight if excessive may cause sunburn and brings up the plasma $25(OH)D$ if it was low but does not lead to vitamin D toxicity because with excessive UV light, previtamin D_3 (7-dehydrocholesterol) is photoisomerized to biologically inert products (lumisterol and tachysterol). Vitamin D_3 is also photodegraded if it is not taken inside the body by vitamin D-binding protein. But with oral intake, the margin between the upper limit of the nutritional dose and the lower limit of the toxic dose is quite narrow. Vitamin D is one of the vitamins that should not be sold over the counter. Overdosage causes raised plasma calcium (hypercalcaemia), with thirst, anorexia, raised plasma levels of $25(OH)D$, and risk of calcification of soft tissues and of urinary calcium stones. Infants are most at risk of hypervitaminosis D; some children have developed hypercalcaemia on intakes of only $50\,\mu g/day$ (five times the recommended nutrient intake). More than this should not be taken, except to treat rickets/osteomalacia, for which $25-100\,\mu g$ is the usual therapeutic dose. In some conditions people are unusually sensitive to vitamin D (e.g. in sarcoidosis and a rare condition in infants with elfin facial appearance, Williams syndrome).

FURTHER READING

1. Fraser DR. Vitamin D. *Lancet* 1995; **345**: 104–7.
2. Kodicek E. The story of vitamin D, from vitamin to hormone. *Lancet* 1974; **1**: 325–9.
3. Loomis WF. Skin-pigment regulation of vitamin D biosynthesis in man. *Science* 1967; **157**: 501–6.
4. MacLaughlin J, Holick MF. Aging decreases the capacity of human skin to produce vitamin D_3. *J Clin Invest* 1985; **76**: 1536–8.

5. Reickel H, Koeffler HP, Norman AW. Medical progress: the role of the vitamin D endocrine system in health and disease. *N Engl J Med* 1989; **320**: 980–91.
6. van der Wielen RPJ, Lowik MRH, van der Berg H, de Groot LCPGM, Halter J, Moreiras O, *et al.* Serum vitamin D concentrations among elderly people in Europe. *Lancet* 1995; **346**: 207–10.
7. Webb AR, de Costa BR, Holick MF. Sunlight regulates the cutaneous production of vitamin D_3 by causing its photodegradation. *J Clin Endocrinol Metab* 1989; **68**: 882–7.
8. Webb AR, Kline L, Holick MF. Influence of season and latitude on the cutaneous synthesis of vitamin D_3: exposure to winter sunlight in Boston and Edmonton will not produce vitamin D_3 synthesis in human skin. *J Clin Endocrinol Metab* 1988; **67**: 373–8.

14.2 VITAMIN K

14.2.1 History

The name 'vitamin K' was proposed by Henrik Dam of Denmark in 1935. K was the next letter of the alphabet not already used for a vitamin at that time. It is also the first letter of the German word *Koagulation*, which refers to its best known function. While investigating the essentiality of cholesterol in the diet of chickens (their eggs, of course, are rich in cholesterol) Dam fed them rations from which the lipid had been extracted with organic solvents. They developed haemorrhages and their blood was slow to clot. This bleeding tendency could be corrected with alfalfa or with decayed fishmeal. The alfalfa was soon shown to provide vitamin K_1; bacteria in the fishmeal were responsible for producing vitamin K_2.

14.2.2 Chemistry

H.J. Almquist solved the chemical search in 1939, reporting that a lipid from the sheath of tubercle bacilli, phthiocol, had vitamin K activity (Fig. 14.3A). Vitamin K_1 and the K_2 series are all based on this 2-methyl-3-hydroxyl, 4-naphthoquinone. They have side chains in place of the 3-hydroxyl group. In vitamin K_1 (phylloquinone), the side chain is a 20-carbon terpenoid alcohol (four-fifths of the phytol side chain of chlorophyll) (Fig. 14.3B). It is found in green leaves.

Vitamin K_2 comprises a family of compounds, called menaquinones, whose side chain consists of repeated (5-carbon) isoprene units, from 1 to 14 of them (Fig. 14.3C). Depending on the number of isoprene units they are referred to as MK1–MK14. The menaquinones are synthesized by certain bacteria, some of which occur naturally in the large intestine of animals, including humans.

14.2.3 Functions

In the liver, vitamin K promotes the synthesis of a special amino acid with three carboxylic acid groups, γ-carboxyglutamic acid (Gla) (Fig. 14.4). The enzyme responsible for putting another carboxylic acid on to glutamic acid requires vitamin K as co-factor.

γ-Carboxyglutamic is an essential part of four of the coagulation factors, all proteins: prothrombin (factor II), factors VII, IX and X. Factors II and VII contain 10 Gla residues per molecule; factors IX and X each contain 12. The Gla residues confer on these

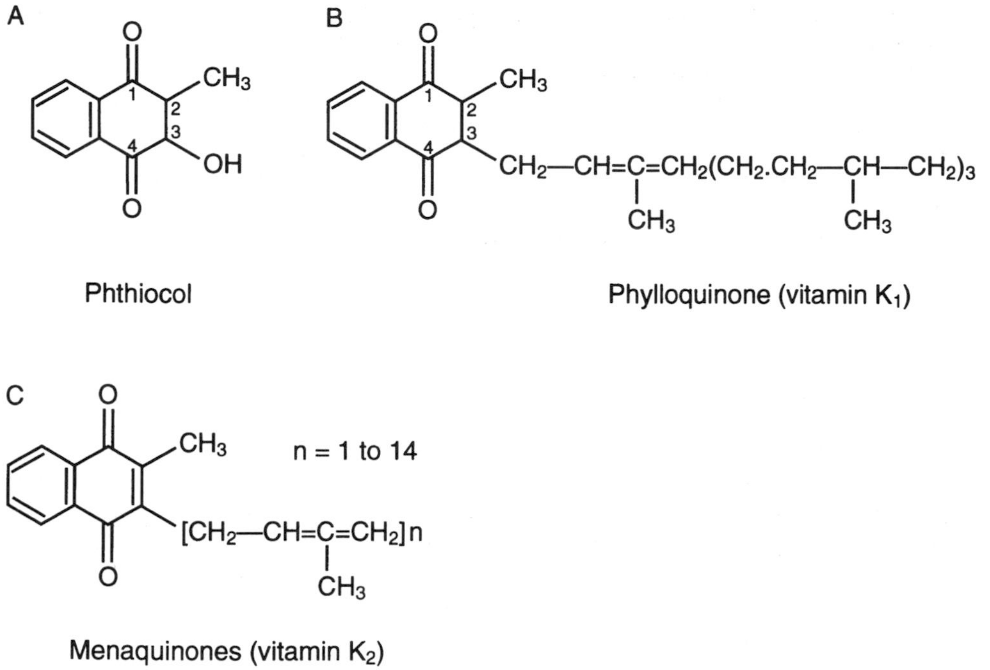

A

Phthiocol

B

Phylloquinone (vitamin K₁)

C

n = 1 to 14

Menaquinones (vitamin K₂)

Fig. 14.3 Structures of (A) phthiocol, (B) phylloquinone (vitamin K₁), (C) menequinones (vitamin K₂).

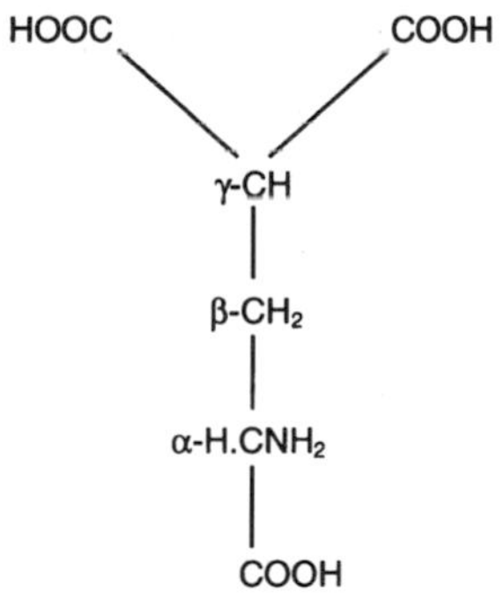

Fig. 14.4 Synthesis of γ-carboxyglutamic acid (Gla) in the liver.

coagulation proteins the capacity to bind to phospholipid surfaces in the presence of calcium ions.

A few other proteins also contain Gla and require the presence of vitamin K for their synthesis. The best known is osteocalcin, a major protein of bone, made by the osteoblasts. It also binds calcium and its plasma concentration indicates osteoblast activity.

Vitamin K, being fat-soluble, requires bile for its absorption. It is transported in the plasma on triglyceride-rich lipoproteins. Analysis of vitamin K in tissues has been difficult because the several compounds are present in very tiny (nanomolar) amounts. In adult liver there is not only vitamin K_1 derived from green leaves in the diet, but also significant amounts of K_2 vitamins, MK7–MK13. As there is little K_2 in wholesome food, these must be synthesized by resident bacteria in the large intestine (bacteriodes and some enterobacteria can synthesize K_2) and absorbed, presumably from the caecum. In plasma, the major form of K vitamin appears to be K_1.

14.2.4 Deficiency disease

In vitamin K deficiency there is a bleeding disorder, characterized by low plasma prothrombin activity (hypoprothrombinaemia). Vitamin K deficiency can occur in obstetric/paediatric practice, in surgical patients and in medical patients.

For most people in developed countries, the first injection of their life is vitamin K_1 given intramuscularly straight after birth to prevent haemorrhagic disease of the newborn. There is a small risk of haemorrhage in the first days after birth because vitamin K, like other fat-soluble vitamins, is poorly transported across the placenta from the mother's blood; the gut of the newborn is sterile (there are no resident bacteria so no vitamin K_2); it is some days before bacteria colonize the large intestine, and human milk usually has a low concentration of vitamin K (K_1).

In surgical practice, vitamin K status is critical in obstructive jaundice in which bile cannot flow into the small intestine so that vitamin K_1 is not absorbed. It is of course very dangerous to operate on someone with a coagulation defect, so before surgery on the bile duct the prothrombin activity must be checked and vitamin K_1 given as a precaution. Vitamin K deficiency also occurs in patients with malabsorption, and following prolonged use of broad-spectrum antibiotics by mouth (which can destroy the colonic bacteria). In serious liver disease the coagulation factors may not be adequately synthesized but this is because of poor liver function, rather than vitamin K deficiency.

In medical practice, the most common cause of vitamin K deficiency is the use of anticoagulant drugs, given to prevent clotting in veins: warfarin and dicoumarol, which owe their therapeutic action to blocking some of the enzymes that recycle vitamin K in the liver.

There are reports of low circulating vitamin K in elderly patients with femoral neck fractures or spinal crush fractures, suggesting that suboptimal vitamin K status may play a role in osteoporosis, presumably because osteocalcin is not made adequately.

It is not possible to measure vitamin K in plasma except as a difficult research procedure because its concentrations are so minute. Plasma prothrombin activity and its response, if it was low, to vitamin K_1 is the usual way of making the diagnosis of deficiency. A more specific method is to measure undercarboxylated prothrombin (i.e. des-γ-carboxyprothrombin or PIVKA, protein induced by vitamin K absence).

14.2.5 Dietary sources

Vitamin K_1 is present in dark-green leaves eaten as foods, some contain more than others. Kale, spinach, brussels sprouts, broccoli, parsley, coriander, endive, mint, mustard greens, cabbage, lettuce are good sources (in descending order). Other good sources are beef liver, some vegetable oils, apples and green tea, and there is some vitamin K_2, in cheese.

The recommended nutrient intake in the United States and in the United Kingdom is based on 1 μg/kg body weight (i.e. around 80 μg/day in men and 65 μg/day in women). Usual adult intakes are variously estimated at 80–300 μg/day.

No application has been devised for supernutritional doses of vitamin K_1 but even milligram doses by mouth have not been found toxic. However, the synthetic water-soluble pharmaceutical with vitamin K activity, menadione, can cause haemolytic anaemia and jaundice in newborn babies. It is now obsolete, superseded by vitamin K_1, since this became available in pharmaceutical form.

FURTHER READING

1. Booth SL, Sadowski JA, Weikrauch JL, Ferland G. Vitamin K (phylloquinone) content of foods: a provisional table. *J Food Comp Anal* 1993; **6**: 109–20.
2. Shearer MJ. Vitamin K. *Lancet* 1995; **345**: 229–34.

OTHER BIOLOGICALLY ACTIVE SUBSTANCES IN FOOD

Mark Wahlqvist and David Briggs

15.1 THE CHEMICAL COMPLEXITY OF FOOD

Food is a complex mixture of a wide variety of chemical components. It is more than just a collection of nutrients. In addition to the nutritionally important components such as protein, fat, carbohydrate, water, vitamins, minerals and dietary fibre, food contains other components which may have biological activity. These include colours, flavours, food additives, natural and artefactual contaminants, and many other products of plant and animal metabolism. This complexity is represented schematically in Table 15.1.

In contrast to nutrients, the other constituents of food are usually more numerous and present in minute amounts. For example, an apple is composed of approximately 98.5% by weight of water and carbohydrate. The remaining 1.5% contains over 100 components, mostly associated with the colour and flavour of the apple (Table 15.2).

We can further systematically consider the major classes of biologically active substances in food which are not regarded as nutrients. Most of these are phytochemicals (plant-derived), but some are uniquely derived from animals. The plant-derived compounds may, however, appear in the animal tissue eaten by humans. They may fall into any one of these categories (Table 15.3): non-provitamin A carotenoids; polyphenols such as flavonoids, isoflavonoids and catechins; indoles, isothiocyanates; sulphoraphane and other organosulphur compounds; monoterpenes; xanthines; non-digestible oligosaccharides and non-digestible protein.

15.2 BIOLOGICALLY ACTIVE COMPONENTS IN FOOD

The biological and health significance of a particular food depends on several factors, including the chemical nature of its components, its physical form, and the amount consumed. Nutrients in food provide energy, regulate body processes and serve as components of body structures. Other food components, which in the conventional sense do not appear to have a nutritive function, can also be important to body functioning and health. Information about the role of diet in health and disease has been obtained from studying human populations and from laboratory investigations. Some of these studies have identified particular foods and food components as important factors in disease prevention and causation. A great deal of scientific research has been directed at evaluating the effect on health of different food components.

Table 15.1 Schematic list showing the chemical complexity of food

Food	Nutrients	Macronutrients	Carbohydrate
			Protein
			Fat
			Dietary fibre
			Water
			Unidentified macronutrients?
		Micronutrients	Vitamins
			Minerals
			Unidentified micronutrients?
	Non-nutrients	Food additives	Synthetic additives
			Nature-identical additives
			Natural additives
		Contaminants	Industrial pollutants
			Production and processing contaminants
			Natural contaminants
			Unknown contaminants
		Processing artefacts	Colours
			Flavours
			Other identified components
			Unidentified artefactual components
		Naturally occurring non-nutrients	Colours
			Flavours
			Other identified components
			Unidentified natural components

It is important to examine the conditions under which biologically active components in food exert their effects. For example, some compounds in food have been shown to exhibit anticarcinogenic behaviour under some conditions yet enhance tumour response when different test carcinogens, animal species, target organs or exposure protocols are used. Careful evaluation is needed to ensure that protective compounds do not compromise normal physiological functions or enhance or promote other risks.

15.3 PROTECTIVE FACTORS IN FOOD

Although nutrients such as dietary fibre, β-carotene and vitamins C and E are considered to be protective against some types of cancer, there is also evidence that other substances in plant foods may provide protective effects. For example, some components found in food which have inhibited the development of cancer in laboratory animals are listed in Table 15.4. Some of these components occur naturally in cruciferous vegetables such as brussels sprouts, cabbage, broccoli and cauliflower (see Table 15.5).

The protective effect against cancer associated with the consumption of cruciferous vegetables is supported by epidemiological studies. This association cannot be entirely

Table 15.2 Components identified in apple aroma

Hydrocarbons	Esters (cont.)	Acids
1-Butoxy-1-ethoxyethane	Ethyl acetate	Acetic
Diethoxyethane	Ethyl butyrate	Benzoic
1-Ethoxy-1-hexoxyethane	Ethyl formate	Butyric
1-Ethoxy-1-methoxyethane	Ethyl hexanoate	Formic
1-Ethoxy-1-(2-methylbutoxy)-	Ethyl 2-methylbutyrate	Hexanoic
ethane	Ethyl 2-methylpropionate	n-Hexenoic
1-Ethoxy-1-propoxyethane	Ethyl octanoate	3-Methylbutyric
1-Methyl-naphthalene	Ethyl pentanoate	4-Methylpentanoic
2-Methyl-naphthalene	Ethyl 2-phenylacetate	2-Methylpropionic
2,4,5-Trimethyl-1,3-dioxolane	Ethyl propionate	Octanoic
	trans-2-Hexen-1-yl-acetate	Pentanoic
	Hexyl acetate	Propionic
Alcohols	Hexyl butyrate	
Butanol	Hexyl propionate	
Ethanol	Methyl acetate	Aldehydes and
Geraniol	2-Methylbutyl acetate	ketones
Hexanol	3-Methylbutyl acetate	Acetaldehyde
n-Hexenol	3-Methylbutyl 3-	Acetone
trans-2-Hexen-1-ol	methylbutyrate	Acetophenone
3-Hexen-1-ol	Methyl butyrate	Butanal
Methanol	Methyl formate	2-Butanone
2-Methylbutan-1-ol	Methyl hexanoate	Diacetyl
3-Methylbutan-1-ol	Methyl 2-methylbutyrate	Formaldehyde
2-Methylpropan-1-ol	Methyl 3-methylbutyrate	Furfural
Pentanol	2-Methylpropyl acetate	Hexanal
Propanol	2-Methylpropyl propionate	2-Hexanone
2-Propanol	Pentyl acetate	2-Hexenal
	Pentyl butyrate	2-Methylbutanal
	Pentyl 2-methylbutyrate	3-Methylbutanal
Esters	2-Phenylethyl acetate	2-Methylpropanal
Benzyl acetate	Propyl acetate	Nonanal
Butyl acetate	2-Propyl acetate	Pentanal
Butyl butyrate	Propyl butyrate	2-Pentanone
Butyl hexanoate	Propyl pentanoate	3-Pentanone
Butyl propionate	Propyl propionate	Propanal

Source: Adapted from Burdock, GA. *Fenarol's Handbook of flavour ingredients*. Vol 2, 3rd ed. Boca Raton: CRC Press, 1995: 816.

explained on the basis of the known nutrients in these vegetables and suggests, that at their level of consumption of these foods, some or all of these substances may effectively inhibit the development of some types of cancer. These foods may also be carriers of other substances whose health significance remains to be identified or recognized.

A more detailed consideration follows for those categories of phytochemicals and other substances under active investigations to evaluate their health properties.

Table 15.3 A general classification of some examples of biologically active components in foods which are not nutrients, additives or contaminants. (This list is by no means exhaustive)

Phytochemicals	Non-provitamin A carotenoids	(e.g. lutein, lycopene)
	Polyphenols	(e.g. flavonoids, isoflavones, lignans, resorcylic acid)
	Organosulphur compounds	(e.g. isothiocyanates, indoles, sulphoraphane, allyl sulphide)
	Monoterpenes	(e.g. limonene)
	Xanthines	(e.g. caffeine)
	Salicylates	(e.g. methyl salicylate)
	Amines	(e.g. L-dopa)
	Non-digestible oligosaccharides	(e.g. fructooligosaccharides)
	Non-digestible protein lignins	(e.g. hydroxyphenylpropane polymers)
Animal-derived compounds	Steroid hormone	
	Morphiceptin (peptide)	
	Immunoreactive thryotrophin releasing hormone (TRH peptide)	
Compounds generated during heat processing	Maillard reaction products	
	Thermally oxidized products (THOPS)	

Table 15.4 Components shown to inhibit the development of some types of cancer in laboratory studies

	Component
Nutrients	Ascorbic acid
	α-Tocopherol
	β-Carotene
	Selenium
Non-nutrients	Phenols
	Flavones
	Indoles
	Isothiocyanates
	Allyl sulphides
	Protease inhibitors

Table 15.5 The known components of Brussel sprouts (*Brassica oleracea* L. var. *Gemmifera* DC)

Allyl-isothiocyanate	Indole-3-acetonitrile	Pantothenic acid
Anteisoheptacosan-1-ol	Indole-3-carbinol	Pentacosan-1-ol
Anteisomontanyl alcohol	Indole-3-carboxaldehyde	Phenylalanine
Antepentacosan-1-ol	Indole-3-carboxylic acid	Phosphorus
Arachidonic acid	Indoyl-3,3'-dimethane-	Phytosterols
Arginine	carboxylic acid	Potassium
Ascorbic acid	Iron	Prop-2-enylglucosinolate
sec-Butyl-isothiocyanate	iso-Hexacosan-1-ol	Protein
Caffeic acid	iso-Leucine	Quercetin
Calcium	iso-Octacosan-1-ol	Quinic acid
Carbohydrates	Triacontan-1-ol	Riboflavin
β-Carotene	Leucine	Rutin
Citric acid	Linoleic acid	Selenium
Copper	α-Linolenic acid	Sinapic acid
p-Coumaric acid	Lysine	1-*O*-*p*-sinapoyl-β-D-
1-*O*-*p*-coumaroyl-β-D-	Magnesium	glucose
glucose	Malic acid	Sodium
Coumestrol	Manganese	Stearic acid
Cystine	Methionine	Succinic acid
Fats	4-Methoxyindol-3-yl-	Tetracosan-1-ol
Ferulic acid	methylglucosinolate	Thiamin
1-*O*-feruloyl-β-D-glucose	Molybdenum	Threonine
Fibre	Montanyl alcohol	α-Tocopherol
Folate(s)	Niacin	Triacontan-1-ol
Fumaric acid	Octacosan-1-ol	Tryptophan
Heptacosan-1-ol	Oleic acid	Valine
Hexacosan-1-ol	Oxalic acid	Vitamin B$_6$
Histidine	Palmitic acid	Water
2-Hydroxybut-3-enyl	Palmitoleic acid	Zinc
glucosinolate		

Source: Adapted from Duke JA. *Handbook of phytochemical constituents of GRAS herbs and other economic plants.* Boca Raton: CRC Press, 1992.

Box 15.1 Tomatoes

Eating foods containing vitamin C has been well correlated with a decreased incidence of gastric cancer. However, this is not the only protective factor. For example, naturally occurring components such as the phenolic antioxidants chlorogenic acid and *p*-coumaric acid found in many plant foods, including tomatoes, have been found to prevent the formation of some carcinogens. Furthermore, tomatoes contain a red pigment, lycopene, a carotenoid which has no provitamin A activity, but which can act as an antioxidant and a trapper of free radicals.

Box 15.2 Cranberry juice

Many bacterial infections are initiated when bacteria become attached to the surfaces of the respiratory, digestive or urinary tracts in the body. Some components of food have been shown to inhibit this attachment and prevent or minimize infection. In studies with animal and human cells, cranberry juice has shown two types of anti-adhesive activity towards pathogens. The activity is believed to be due to fructose and an unidentified high molecular weight constituent in the juice. These studies are supported by recent work in the United States which has shown that cranberry juice is beneficial in the prevention of recurrent urinary tract infections in elderly women.

Box 15.3 Fruits and vegetables

Many fruits and vegetables, as well as tea and wine, contain relatively high levels of naturally occurring phenolic components. Many of these components have antioxidant properties as well as an important influence on the colour and flavour of these foods. Recent population studies have found an association between a lower risk of heart disease in men with increased consumption of phenol-containing foods and beverages.

15.3.1 Carotenoids

Carotenoids possess other biological actions, apart from provitamin A activity, including antioxidant, immuno-enhancement, antimutagenesis and anticarcinogenesis. Owing to the antioxidant property of carotenoids, the possibility exists that these compounds may contribute to protection against coronary heart disease as well as cataract and retinal (macular) degeneration which are linked to oxidative stress, lipid peroxidation and free radical damage. Cells involved in the generation of specific immune responses can also be adversely affected by free radicals and products from lipid peroxidation processes. Incubation with β-carotene has been shown to protect human neutrophils against free radicals. It has also been suggested that antioxidant vitamins may play a role in cancer risk reduction and cancer prevention by reducing premalignant lesions such as cervical dysplasia, leucoplakia and atrophic gastritis. Carotenoids might also enhance an immune response which could lead to reduction of tumour growth.

15.3.2 Flavonoids and isoflavones

Flavonoids are a large group of polyphenolic compounds that occur naturally in vegetables and fruit and in beverages such as tea and wine. The most important groups of flavonoids are anthocyanins, flavonols, flavones and flavonones. Flavonoids have been studied in relation to their improvement of vascular fragility, increase cellular permeability and vitamin C-sparing activities. Some flavonoids such as quercetin, kaempferol and myricetin have antimutagenic and anticarcinogenic effects *in vitro* and *in vivo*. In a large number of epidemiological studies which have investigated relationships between diet and cancer, a protective effect of the consumption of vegetables and fruit on various forms of cancer is found. This protective effect was originally attributed to vitamin C and carotenoids present in these foods. However, the significance of other potentially protective compounds such as flavonoids present in vegetables and fruit has become an important issue. It appears that a number of the biological effects of flavonoids may be explained by their antioxidative activity and ability to scavenge free radicals. Other mechanisms for their reported anticarcinogenic potential include their capacity to inhibit the promotion phase of carcinogenesis; and to modulate the balance between activation and inactivation processes of specific enzymes in the liver.

A small number of isoflavones, such as genistein and daidzein, display oestrogenic activity in animals and humans. This hormonal effect is attributed to the similar spatial arrangement of functional groups on isoflavones and oestrogens, allowing these isoflavones to bind to the oestrogen receptors. Furthermore, genistein is also found to inhibit endothelial cell proliferation and *in vitro* angiogenesis.

Isoflavones occur principally, although not exclusively, in legumes (Leguminosae family). They are at particularly high levels in certain legumes which are regularly consumed by people and animals. Indeed, many traditional human diets which have relatively high legume consumption (soya, lentils, chick pea, etc.) consequently have high isoflavone contents, particularly of those with oestrogenic activity.

15.3.3 Other polyphenols

Several animal models have demonstrated anticarcinogenic effects of polyphenols extracted from green tea in multi-organ carcinogenesis models. A number of investigators have identified epigallocatechin gallate (EGCG) as the principal antimutagenic and anticarcinogenic compound in green tea. The anticarcinogenic activity of EGCG may be related to several factors, such as its effect on the tumour promotion stage of cancer processes; its effect on DNA-adduct formation; on scavenging of free radicals; or the increase of antioxidant activities. There is circumstantial evidence to suggest that simultaneous intake of green tea polyphenols with food products may exert a protective effect. Beneficial effects of drinking tea in relationship to blood pressure, serum cholesterol and other lipids have been reported in human studies.

Several phenolic flavonoids in red wine exert potent antioxidant effects, and as such may act as chemopreventive components. A red wine extract, from which the alcohol has been removed, inhibited the oxidation of low-density lipoproteins. It appears that phenolic components with antioxidant capacity found in red wine may collectively reduce the oxidation of lipoproteins and reduce thrombosis and thereby contribute to the amelioration of atherosclerosis and morbidity and mortality from coronary artery disease.

15.3.4 Isothiocyanates and other organosulphur compounds

Isothiocyanates, indoles and sulforaphane, which are found in cruciferous vegetables such as broccoli, Brussels sprouts and cabbage (see Table 15.5) have been shown to trigger enzyme systems that block or suppress cellular DNA damage, reduce tumour size and decrease the effectiveness of oestrogen-like hormones. Allylic sulphides, found in onions and garlic, enhance immune function, increase the production of enzymes that help to excrete carcinogens, decrease the proliferation of tumour cells, and in large doses may reduce serum cholesterol.

15.3.5 Monoterpenes

Limonene is a monocyclic monoterpene found in the essential oils of citrus fruits, spices and herbs. The presumed potential of limonene as a chemotherapeutic and chemopreventive agent for human breast and possible other cancers is based on results of animal studies showing chemopreventive activity against mammary, skin, liver and lung tumours. Limonene and related monoterpenes may represent a novel class of cytostatic cancer chemotherapeutic agents that induce tumour cell redifferentiation with little toxicity to the host.

15.3.6 Salicylates

Salicylates in food have mainly been of interest to workers investigating food sensitivity. However, health protective effect from food salicylates may, in part, resemble effects of acetyl salicylic acid (aspirin). Aspirin, of course, is of interest in protecting against macrovascular disease, such as coronary heart disease, stroke, and against neoplastic disease of the gut; the same may be true of food salicylates.

15.3.7 L-Dopa

There are anecdotal reports and a paper by Kempster and Wahlqvist (1994) that patients with Parkinson's disease will benefit from meals of broad beans (*Vicia faba*). Broad beans contain rather large amounts of the amino acid dihydroxyphenylalanine (L-dopa) and the response to these beans may even be better than to conventional L-dopa medication in some cases.

15.3.8 Animal-derived compounds

Animal foods may contain certain phytochemicals from the food consumed by the animal. They also may provide peptides following the digestion of animal proteins which have hormone-like action. An example is morphiceptin, which is a peptide with opioid activity, derived from milk proteins. It has been shown to have potent analgesic and cataleptic activities in rats when injected into the cerebral ventricles. Of course, hormones of one animal eaten by another animal may have hormone-like action as the compounds go up the food chain, ultimately in humans. Most cell messenger compounds, commonly known as cytokines—generally labile peptides, are unlikely to survive through the food chain to have biological effects in humans who eat animal-derived foods.

15.3.9 Compounds occurring during food processing

Biologically active compounds are also generated during food preparation. Maillard (carbohydrate-protein derivatives) and THOPS (thermally oxidized products) are produced during food frying. Other biologically active compounds are produced during the preparation of alcoholic beverages such as wine and beer, and in dairy products such as cheese and yoghurt. The biological effect of many of these compounds has been poorly studied.

15.4   FUNCTIONAL FOODS

Functional foods have been defined in the following way (Australian National Food Authority (1994)):

Functional foods are similar in appearance to conventional foods and are intended to be consumed as part of a normal diet, but have been modified to subserve physiological roles beyond the provision of simple nutrient requirements.

What has become clear is that one class of phytochemicals may have several functions (i.e. are multifunctional compounds). A good example is the flavonoids which have been shown to be antimutagenic (and for some, mutagenic), oestrogenic, antioxidant, immuno-modulant and anti-angiogenic. On the other hand, a particular function may be provided by more than one class of phytochemicals. For example, oestrogenic compounds include isoflavones, lignins, and resorcylic acid compounds.

The growing array of phytochemicals (those non-nutrients ultimately derived from plants) which are being shown to have biological effects including those which are health protective, opens up opportunities for development of functional foods to serve particular physiological or pathological needs.

15.5   TOXICANTS IN FOOD

Some biologically active components in food can also contribute to chronic and acute illness. Examples of naturally occurring components in foods and their effects are listed in Table 15.6. Whether consumption of foods containing these toxicants poses a hazard to human health depends on their concentration in the food, the amount consumed and individual susceptibility to the component. Interactions between food components in the same and different foods may also influence their safety. For example, the formation of potentially carcinogenic N-nitrosamines from amines and nitrite can be catalysed by some co-occuring dietary components and inhibited by others. Therefore, under some circumstances, foods containing these substances may be consumed with impunity.

A wide range of extraneous substances are unintentionally or accidentally incorporated into food as a result of agricultural practices, processing, packaging, growth of micro-organisms, storage and industrial pollution (Table 15.7). In addition, these adventitious additives or contaminants can enter the food supply as a result of misuse, unusual growing conditions, accidents or other incidents such as nuclear fallout or illegal waste disposal. These contaminants can affect the quality and safety of food. Whether they constitute a health hazard will depend on a combination of factors that include their concentration in the food, the amount of food consumed, individual susceptibility to the substances, and any interactions that could modify their toxicity. It is often extremely

Table 15.6 Some naturally occurring toxicants that are normal components of plant foods and their effects

Toxicant	Major food source	Effect/action
Caffeine	Coffee, tea, cocoa, cola-type beverages	Diuresis, cardiac stimulant, CNS stimulant, stimulant of gastric acid secretion, smooth muscle relaxant, animal teratogen
Cucurbitacins	Melons, squash, zucchini (bitter varieties)	Cramps, diarrhoea, collapse
Cyanogenic glycosides	Cassava, some varieties of limba bean, apricot kernels, bitter almonds, apple seeds	Cyanide poisoning, tropical ataxic neuropathy?
Cycasin	Cycads (*Cycas circinalis*)	Cancer in animals
Favism-causing compounds	Broad beans (*Vicia faba*)	Acute haemolytic anaemia*
Glycoalkaloids (solanine, chaconine)	Potatoes	Gastrointestinal and neurological symptoms, animal teratogen
Glucosinolates	Brussels sprouts, cabbage, cauliflower, mustard, turnip	Goitrogenic activity
Gliadins	Wheat, rye, barley	Gluten enteropathy (coeliac disease)*
Haemagglutinins	Many species of legume	Agglutination of red blood cells (*in vitro*), growth depression
Hypoglycin	Akee fruit	Acute hypoglycaemia
Lathyrogens	*Lathyrus sativus* (lathyrus pea, chickling vetch)	Paralysis, skeletal abnormalities
Nitrate/nitrite	Cabbage, celery, lettuce, spinach	Methaemoglobinaemia, cancer?
Oxalic acid	Rhubarb, spinach, tea	Gastroenteritis, renal damage, decreased calcium utilization
Oestrogens	Soybeans	Oestrogenic activity in animals
Protease inhibitors	Many species of legume	Decreased growth
Psoralens	Celery, parsnips	Photocarcinogen, mutagen
Pyrrolizidine alkaloids	Comfrey, some herbs	Liver disease, cancer

*Hazardous only for a minority of genetically sensitive individuals. CNS, central nervous system.

Table 15.7 Sources of food contamination

Source	Examples
Agricultural practice	Insecticides, herbicides, rodenticides, fungicides, antibiotics, promoters, coccidiostats, cadmium
Food processing	Cleaning agents, lubricants, pieces of equipment, hair
Food packaging	Inks, plasticizers, monomers, lead, adhesives
Food storage	Insects, insect frass, rodents, rodent excreta
Industrial pollution	Lead, mercury, polychlorinated biphenyls
Microorganisms	Aflatoxins, ergot, *Salmonella*

difficult to assess the effects of long-term exposure to low levels of any food component. Concern about the potential health effects of food contaminants usually follows from their demonstrated effects on occupationally exposed groups (e.g. workers exposed to relatively high concentrations of vinyl chloride in the manufacture of PVC), or those exposed to localized high concentrations resulting from accidental overuse or spillage (e.g. from consumption of fish from the polluted water of Minamata Bay in Japan which contained high levels of mercury). These toxicants are discussed further in Chapter 23.

15.6 CONCLUSIONS

There is emergent need for the following:

1. Food composition tables to reflect phytochemicals and, possibly, substances that are unique to the animal-derived foods, which have health consequence.
2. Nutritional epidemiology which takes into account a possible link between consumption of non-nutrients from food and health outcomes.
3. Clinical nutrition trials which test the potential health protective or therapeutic opportunities that phytochemicals may provide.

A problem in considering the place of phytochemicals in human health is that there are numerous compounds, alongside a few known essential nutrients, and, therefore, that their net interactive effect ultimately requires a study of food itself and food patterns, or that food components intake be subject to sophisticated mathematical modelling. The advance of informatics may help resolve this dilemma.

When particular bodily function or disease processes are considered alongside the phytochemical or other non-nutrient food components which may modulate physiological functions, the potential for making relevant functional foods becomes apparent. For example, products might be designed to prevent or manage obesity through altering appetite, the sensory response to food (taste, smell, look, texture and sound in eating) or energy utilization. Such developments will, however, need to take into account the various caveats outlined above.

FURTHER READING

1. Avorn J, Monane M, Gurwitz JH, Glynn RJ, Choodnovskiy I, Lipsitz LA. Reduction of bacteriuria and pyuria after ingestion of cranberry juice. *JAMA*, 1994; **271**: 751–4.
2. Block G, Patterson B, Subar A. Fruit, vegetables, and cancer prevention: a review of the epidemiological evidence. *Nutr Cancer* 1992; **18**: 1–29.
3. Bronzetti G. Antimutagens in food. *Trends in Food Science and Technology* 1994; **5**: 390–5.
4. Daniel H, Erll G. Opioid peptides derived from dietary proteins: nature and physiological importance. In: Schlierf G (ed.). *Recent advances in clinical nutrition*, Vol 3. London: Smith Gordon, 1993: 55–65.
5. Fotsis T, Pepper M, Adlercreutz H, *et al.* Genistein, a dietary-derived inhibitor of *in vitro* angiogenesis. *Proc Natl Acad Sci* 1993; **90**: 2690–4.
6. Ganly RG. Some unresolved problems of food-medium interactions during deep frying. In: McLean AJ, Wahlqvist ML (eds). *Current problems in nutrition pharmacology and toxicology*. London: John Libbey, 1988.

7. Goldberg I (ed.). *Functional foods: designer foods, pharmafoods, nutraceuticals.* London: Chapman and Hall, 1994.
8. Hertog MG, Hollman PC. Potential health effects of the dietary flavonol quercetin. *Eur J Clin Nutr* 1996; **50**: 63–71.
9. Kempster P, Wahlqvist ML. Dietary factors in the management of Parkinson's Disease. *Nutr Rev* 1994; **52**: 51–58.
10. Mehta RG, Liu J, Constantinou A, *et al.* Cancer chemopreventive activity of brassinin, a phytoalexin from cabbage. *Carcinogenesis* 1995; **16**: 399–404.
11. Morris DL, Kritchevsky SB, Davis CE. Serum carotenoids and coronary heart disease. The Lipid Research Clinics Coronary Primary Prevention Trial and Follow-up Study. *JAMA* 1994; **18**: 1439–41.
12. Parfitt VJ, Rubba P, Bolton C, *et al.* A comparison of antioxidant status and free radical peroxidation of plasma lipoproteins in healthy young persons from Naples and Bristol. *Eur Heart J* 1994; **15**: 871–6.
13. Reilly, C. *Metal contamination of food*, 2nd ed, London: Elsevier Applied Science, 1991.
14. Wilcox G, Wahlqvist ML, Burger HG, Medley G. Oestrogenic effects of plant-derived foods in post menopausal women. *BMJ* 1990; **301**: 905–906.

Part III: Nutrition-related disorders

16

OVERWEIGHT AND OBESITY

Ian Caterson

Overweight and obesity are common conditions. The prevalence of these disorders is increasing in many societies and countries and they are associated with an increased risk of a wide number of diseases and health disorders as well as premature mortality. This chapter will discuss the prevalence, aetiology, consequences and treatment, and possibilities for prevention of excess fat stores (adiposity).

16.1 DEFINITION AND MEASUREMENT

Obesity is a condition in which the fat stores are excessive for an individual's height, weight, gender and race to an extent that produces adverse health outcomes. There are many techniques available for the measurement of total body fat (see Box 16.1, and also Chapter 25). Many of these methods require costly equipment and take time or are uncomfortable for the individual being measured and are generally only used for research. But BIA and DEXA (See Box 16.1) are becoming available and are the most widely used of the more elaborate techniques.

All these measures are too costly, complicated and/or time-consuming for routine clinical use and for much clinical and epidemiological research. Yet, weight alone is not an adequate measure of adiposity so the calculation of the body mass index (BMI), which is weight (in kg) divided by the height (in metres) squared, gives a reasonable approximation of adiposity and this is widely used in both clinical practice and research. It is not as useful in children, the aged or the very fit and muscular. Using the BMI, a simple classification of obesity for adults has been developed and is shown in Box 16.2.

Box 16.1 Techniques for measuring adiposity

- Underwater weighing and densitometry with fat mass calculated from density of individual (based on the principle that fat is lighter than water. More fat the lower a person's body density)
- Bioelectrical impedance (BIA)
- Dual X-ray absorptiometry (DEXA)
- Near infrared spectroscopy (NIR)
- Measurement of naturally occurring isotopes

Box 16.2   Classification of obesity based on BMI for those of European origin

BMI	Grade	
20–24.9	0	Desirable range
25–29.9	I	Overweight
>30	II	Obese
>40	III	Very obese

These cutoff points are based on the extent of risks (discussed below) associated with being overweight or obese. As it was developed for those of European origin, the cutoff points given may not be appropriate for other racial groups. For example, for those of Asian origin the desirable range may be a BMI of 18.5–24.9, whereas for Polynesians the BMI seems to overestimate the degree of adiposity. Some countries use a simple cutoff point, a BMI of 27, with all those greater than this being classified as obese and at risk of the problems produced by excess fatness. The issue remains to be resolved.

Another relatively common indirect measure of adiposity is obtained following the measurement of skinfold thickness at a number of sites (see Chapter 25). This measure requires special calipers and there is a relatively high level of observer error and this reduces the value of this approach. For children a WHO report (1997) suggests that the simplest and best measure would be based on BMI for age charts. A child with a BMI for age above the 97th percentile is obese; above the 85th percentile BMI for age he or she is 'at risk'. These percentile cut-offs correspond to adult BMIs of 30 and 25 kg/m^2 respectively. BMI for age tables for the United Kingdom have been published by Cole et al. (1995).

In addition to the total amount, the site of the increased fat tissue is important. At any weight excess abdominal (visceral) adipose tissue is associated with considerable risk of cardiovascular and metabolic disorders (such as heart attack and diabetes). Therefore it is important to measure abdominal fat. While DEXA and other scans are the most accurate ways to measure abdominal fat, the simplest and most useful way to do this is by measuring the waist circumference. It has been suggested that a measurement >100 cm in men and 95 cm in women indicates increased risk. The waist (W) to hip (H) ratio (W/H ratio) can also be used to indicate abdominal adiposity but it is not as good a measure. (The waist is the narrowest diameter between the ribs and iliac crest, the hips at the maximal protrusion of the buttocks). A ratio of more than 0.8 in women and more than 0.9 in men suggests abdominal obesity. Another indirect measurement of abdominal fat which can be used is the sagittal depth (depth of stomach region while lying flat).

16.2 Prevalence

Obesity and overweight are very common in most affluent and relatively affluent societies and the prevalence has been increasing, despite many public health interventions, over the last 10 years. Obesity increases with age and has a greater prevalence in lower socioeconomic groups in the developed world. In the United States more women and more African-Americans are obese. Overall, the prevalence of obesity in men is about 10% while in women it tends to be higher, ranging from 12% in northern Europe, to 30% in Eastern Europe and to 40% in the former Soviet Republics. Overweight is far more common. In Canada 35% of men and 27% of women have BMIs greater than $27 \, kg/m^2$ while in Australia 38% of the adult population are overweight or obese (BMI $> 25 \, kg/m^2$).

Obesity is not confined to Western societies. Using Western standards, the reported prevalence of obesity ranges from 1.5% in rural China, to 3% in Singaporean men, to 9% in those older than 50 in Bombay, 12% in women of Malay descent in Singapore, to more than 50% in several Pacific Islands and the Pima (American) Indians. In at least some of these countries (e.g. India) obesity is seen primarily among the relatively affluent sections of the population. However, it is important to emphasize that Caucasian standards may well be inappropriate for assessing prevalence in all populations. For example, it has been suggested that among Australian aboriginals the healthy range for BMI appears to be 17–22 with risk increasing rapidly thereafter. Development of appropriate BMI ranges for different populations or finding alternate methods for assessing adiposity are essential aspects of obesity research amongst non-European populations.

16.3 PERCEPTIONS

The perceptions of individuals do have an effect both on obesity and its treatment. In general, those who are obese are perceived poorly by the community and they themselves have low self-esteem. Children see obesity as a worse disability than loss of a limb. Women tend to see themselves as larger than they are and seek to be smaller than is necessary or practically possible. Such unrealistic expectations predispose any overweight or obese woman to failure in a treatment programme. Men are reasonably accurate in the judgement of their size but accept larger sizes, do not see overweight as a problem, and tend not to present for weight control or treatment unless forced by a manifest medical reason or problem. On the other hand, medical practitioners and other health professionals tend to perceive weight problems as the fault of a weak-willed individual and tend not to offer continuing help. This attitude is reinforced by the perceived and real difficulty of treatment and the discouraging long-term success of weight therapy.

16.4 GENETICS OF OBESITY

There are undoubtedly strong genetic influences in weight gain and obesity. The adoption study of Stunkard has shown that the weight of adults adopted as children is related to the weight of their biological parents rather than the weight of their adopting family. In addition Bouchard's overfeeding study with twins demonstrated a strong genetic component in the amount of weight gained with the same amount of overfeeding. It has been estimated that genetic factors contribute 25–40% to the cause of obesity, with a further like amount being contributed by the family and social environment of the individual which cannot usually be separated from the genetic component. Abdominal obesity seems to be more strongly inherited.

There is probably no single gene responsible for the development of obesity, rather it is likely to be a multigene, multifactorial disorder. There is much recent interest in a gene which is responsible for the production of a satiety factor in obese (*ob/ob*) mice. Its protein product, called leptin, given daily will reduce the body weight of obese mice by 30% in three weeks and even lean mice will get a weight reduction when treated with this factor. There are other strains of obese rodents which have abnormalities of the receptor for leptin and are unable to respond. Leptin is produced in adipocytes (fat cells) and the levels in humans and animals are related to the amount of fat tissue in the body. Alterations in nutritional intake and insulin levels alter leptin synthesis. In human obesity, leptin levels are elevated with levels being higher in women than men. These high levels may indicate a receptor defect (and lack of satiety effect) or may demonstrate that we have learned cues about eating that become more important than the normal physiological feedback. It has also been suggested that leptin, rather than simply being a satiety factor, may be a protective factor which, once it has been deposited, keeps fat in its stores so that it becomes available in times of starvation or famine. Obviously, further work needs to be done to understand how the *ob* gene and leptin work, but it seems unlikely that this system will be a key factor as the cause of the major part of human obesity.

16.5 Environmental and Lifestyle Factors

Even though there is a substantial genetic factor underlying obesity, environmental and lifestyle factors are very important in the aetiology. Obesity has increased over the last decades whilst the gene pool has been stable. Overweight and obesity can only occur when there is an imbalance between energy intake as food and the energy expenditure of the body both for essential processes and as exercise or work. The genetic effect may be in part directed at setting either the response to energy input, or the level of energy output at rest, with activity or eating. For example, the resting metabolic rate (RMR) of those who are obese is elevated, not low. It is related to the mass of the body, particularly the lean (non-fat) body mass, so those who are bigger have a greater RMR. But, in the Pima Indians a tribe in Arizona with both the propensity to obesity and the world's highest prevalence, it has been shown that RMRs cluster in families and that those with lower RMRs have a greater risk of gaining 10 kg in the next five years.

16.5.1 Food intake

Obviously the amount of food eaten is important. As societies become more affluent more food is consumed and weight is gained. This has been well demonstrated in the studies in Nauru and Mauritius. Quantity of intake is important, but so is the quality of the food eaten. There is good evidence, accumulated over years, that high fat diets predispose to obesity. Except in exceptional circumstances, such as recovering from periods of starvation or anorexia nervosa, humans do not synthesize fat for storage in the adipose tissue, but any extra fat eaten does tend to go to stores. In addition, Flatt has suggested that those who have a higher resting respiratory quotient (RQ), that is those who oxidize more carbohydrate, tend to store fat whilst good fat oxidizers (low RQ) burn off their fat intake and do not store as much. So what is important is the food quotient (FQ) of food eaten. The FQ is derived like the RQ. It is a measure of oxidation and carbon dioxide production obtained if the food is 'burned'. The lower the FQ the more fat there is in the food. If the FQ of the food eaten is less than the body's RQ, then there will be a tendency to gain weight more easily. This weight gain will be fat gain, and as body fat stores increase so the body's RQ will fall until it reaches the level of the FQ of the food eaten. At this point, a new equilibrium will have been reached between the body's fat stores and the fat eaten, weight (fat) will have been gained without a change in the energy eaten. There is good evidence for this in mice and we have recently demonstrated that weight loss on a very low calorie diet can be predicted by the fasting RQ: those with low RQs lose more. It is possible that the tendency to be a fat or carbohydrate oxidizer (low or high resting RQ) may be inherited. The energy intake and constitution of the diet provided in mental institutions in France for the last 200 years has been calculated. Less energy is consumed now than was eaten in 1900. There has been a slight increase in the protein in the diet but the major change has been a great increase in fat intake, and this change has accompanied the decrease in energy intake and the increase in the prevalence of overweight and obesity. Similarly, there has been a reported decrease in energy intake over the last 20 years in the United Kingdom, but an increase in weight and BMI.

Whilst obese individuals tend to underestimate their intake by as much as 50% (lean individuals may underestimate by 20%) many obese individuals do not overeat all the time. They may eat reasonably normally and healthily but every so often have a 'binge'. This pattern of bingeing, particularly in response to emotional stresses, is particularly common in women but is also found in men.

16.5.2 Exercise

Reduction in voluntary activity is also important in weight gain. This may be as a change in lifestyle (giving up competitive sport, taking on more sedentary job responsibilities, having children), with ageing or with disease (such as arthritis which restricts mobility or with respiratory or cardiovascular disease which reduce capacity). There are also changes in exercise amount and pattern which occur as a consequence of urbanization, affluence and modernization of lifestyle. These changes have meant that overall we are less active. This reduction in activity is probably important in the increase in obesity seen in the last decade. The prevalence of obesity in children has been directly related to hours of television viewed. This may be a result of reduced activity, a result of the advertising viewed or because television viewing reduces the metabolic rate.

16.5.3 Other factors

Other possible factors in the aetiology are cessation of smoking (a 1–4 kg weight gain is usual), pregnancy or initiation of treatment with steroids or hormone replacement therapy or contraceptive therapy (probably through an increase in intake). Hormonal alterations are often blamed as the cause of obesity, but in reality such diseases rarely produce obesity. The weight gain associated with endocrine conditions (see Box 16.3) is not great, usually of the order of 5–10 kg. Non-insulin-dependent diabetes (NIDDM) is often associated with

Box 16.3 Hormonal conditions associated with weight gain

- Hypothyroidism
- Acromegaly
- Cushing's syndrome
- Polycystic ovarian syndrome
- Hyperprolactinaemia
- Insulin resistance

obesity but it is not yet clear whether the two conditions have the same genetic predisposing factors or whether NIDDM is caused by the insulin resistance of obesity.

16.6 CONSEQUENCES OF OBESITY

There is no doubt regarding the adverse health consequences of obesity. Some of these consequences are listed in Box 16.4. Being overweight is associated with a modest increase in the risks discussed below and the risks increase with the degree of obesity so that for those with a BMI greater than 40, total mortality rates are two (for women) to two and a half (for men) to those with BMIs in the desirable range. Again, it needs to be emphasized that the distribution of obesity also plays a role, it is not just mass. The metabolic complications of obesity are associated with visceral fat and with increases in this depot, risk increases even if the BMI is in the desirable range.

The risks to health and life associated with smoking are additive to those of obesity. Although stopping smoking is often associated with some weight gain, it is better for health to stop smoking rather than to keep weight down by continuing to smoke. While weight reduction is associated with a reduction in the various risks discussed below, there is relatively little evidence that life can be prolonged. Stopping smoking, on the other hand, does reduce mortality. The effects of overweight and obesity can be considered under several headings.

16.6.1 Metabolic consequences

Secondary dyslipidaemias (abnormalities in plasma lipids) are common in those who are obese; especially in those with increased abdominal fat (high waist–hip ratio). These dyslipidaemias have raised levels of low-(LDL) and very low-(VLDL) density lipoprotein (the latter shows as raised triglycerides), low levels of high-density lipoprotein (HDL, protective) cholesterol and normal to raised levels of cholesterol. Because of the changes in the LDL particles and other lipids, even a normal level of cholesterol can cause vascular damage and atherosclerosis. Weight loss will improve these detrimental changes. Cellular resistance to insulin action (insulin resistance) occurs in obesity. It is associated with a cluster of abnormalities (raised levels of serum insulin, hypertension, raised triglyceride levels, low HDL cholesterol levels, impaired glucose tolerance or frank diabetes) collectively described as 'syndrome X' or the 'metabolic syndrome'. Whilst for diabetes

Box 16.4   Consequences of obesity

- **Metabolic**
  Impaired glucose tolerance and non insulin-dependent diabetes
  Dyslipidaemia:
  – Increased LDL-cholesterol, triglyceride
  – Reduced HDL cholesterol
  – Impaired apo B lipoprotein (small dense molecules)
  Metabolic Syndrome:
  – Increased insulin, hypertension, raised triglyceride, reduced
    HDL cholesterol
  Fatty liver
  Gallstones
  Infertility in women
- **Cardiovascular**
  Hypertension
  Coronary heart disease
  Varicose veins
  Peripheral oedema
- **Mechanical**
  Osteoarthritis
  Spinal problems
  Obstructive sleep apnoea
- **Social**
  Low self-esteem
  Adverse judgement by society

to occur there must be an abnormality in insulin secretion as well, the insulin resistance produced by abdominal obesity underlies this problem.

There are other metabolic problems seen frequently. These are an elevation in the liver transaminases due to fatty liver and the prevalence of gallstones which increases with increasing age and weight. Infertility is more common in obese women.

16.6.2   Cardiovascular consequences

Obesity is an important risk factor for cardiovascular disease. Some of this may be because of its interactions with blood pressure, diabetes and dyslipidaemia but it does seem that obesity may also increase the risk of coronary heart disease by other mechanisms, particularly in those younger than 50 years of age. Varicose veins and peripheral oedema occur more commonly. Other cardiac abnormalities such as cor pulmonale and lymphoedema may occur with gross obesity.

16.6.3   Mechanical consequences

Osteoarthritis of both weight-bearing and non-weight-bearing joints (e.g. in the hands) is more common in obesity. Sometimes chest pain may be caused by spinal problems in the lower cervical and upper thoracic region. Obstructive sleep apnoea is common in obesity, particularly in men. Snoring, stopping breathing during sleep (apnoeas), morning headache, daytime sleepiness and difficulty in concentration are some of the problems reported. It occurs mainly in males, although women do suffer from this disorder. Sleep apnoea can be treated with weight loss, and/or with continuous positive airways pressure (CPAP) administered by nasal mask whilst sleeping.

16.6.4 Social consequences

Obese people, particularly those who have made many attempts to lose weight, often have lower self-esteem. Obesity and/or its medical consequences may prevent individuals from doing many activities which they enjoy. Children see obesity as a disability. In some societies, there is a poor perception of obesity by the community at large and obese individuals may experience discrimination in various forms, including employment opportunities.

16.7 MANAGEMENT

16.7.1 Whom to treat?

Obesity is common and to treat everybody who is obese individually would require substantial resources. For the healthy overweight and obese and those with no family history of diabetes and heart disease, nutrition advice and encouragement to increase activity may suffice. For those with a BMI more than 28 and abdominal adiposity, with the metabolic syndrome (hypertension, dyslipidaemia, impaired glucose tolerance, and NIDDM or with a strong family history) intensive therapy is probably warranted.

16.7.2 Basic interventions

At the outset, it is important to emphasize that weight loss therapy involves lifestyle changes which need to be maintained long term. There are two phases of therapy, active weight loss and the important maintenance support phase. The basic interventions are eating, exercise and behaviour modification. It is important to set appropriate goals for each individual which should extend beyond the simplistic kilograms to be lost (Table 16.1). Weight loss should be planned in stages. All goals should be recorded, discussed at subsequent visits and the attaining of goals should be noted.

Rather than a diet, an eating plan should be discussed. This plan should be low fat, with high complex carbohydrate, and where appropriate to the culture, it should encourage regular meals. Currently there is a move away from 'calorie-counting' to low fat eating because such eating plans are easier to maintain. A set level of fat intake is decided (e.g. <50 g/day), and within this limit patients may choose foods they wish. If energy reduction is used, it is appropriate to advise a minimal reduction below requirements and not a radical reduction in energy intake. It is clearly necessary to ensure adequate nutrition knowledge but it is interesting to note that many women who are overweight have a 'good' knowledge of nutritional facts and do not need additional education, whereas men often need nutritional education.

Table 16.1 Goals of obesity therapy

- **Weight loss**
  - set realistic losses, in stages
- **Risk factors**
  - weight loss (kg)
  - less abdominal fat
  - lower plasma lipids
  - control of diabetes
  - control of hypertension
- **Mobility**
- **Control of associated disorders**
  - diabetes
  - hypertension
  - sleep apnoea
  - arthritis
- **Reduction in medications**
- **Change in body shape and size**
  - (less abdominal fat)
- **Improved cardiovascular fitness**
- **Psychological and social factors**
- **Individual goals**
  - fitting into clothes
  - need for, or ability to, have surgery
  - reduction in pain

Although it is beyond the scope of this chapter to give an exhaustive descriptions of eating programmes, a few issues deserve special mention. The greater reliance on takeaway or 'fast' food in many societies needs special consideration because such foods tend to be high in fat. These and other convenience foods should not be excluded from an eating plan but they need to be limited and where possible modified. It is necessary to be aware that many obese and overweight people do not have an excessive energy intake all the time but are binge eaters, overeating periodically. Such binges tend to be produced by emotional problems or stress and are often the cause of regaining weight after satisfactory loss. It is important for such people to recognize stress cues and learn alternative ways of dealing with them. Alcohol may be an important source of extra energy intake in some overweight and obese men, and this needs to be taken into account in their eating programme.

Exercise is an important part of any programme. In itself it may not produce major weight losses, but it helps to alter the body composition favourably (reducing fat and increasing muscle). It also improves the metabolic abnormalities of obesity and NIDDM, reduces blood pressure, improves mobility and induces a feeling of well-being. For the obese and overweight, low intensity but prolonged, exercise produces these changes and cardiovascular fitness is not necessary. Behaviour modification is an integral and important part of therapy and it is essential to prevent the regain of weight by aiming to change habits in the long term. The techniques used are the keeping of food and exercise logs, cognitive restructuring (removing the guilt from eating), awareness and changing of habits, improving self-esteem. Such therapy may be given to individuals or in groups.

16.7.3 Additional therapies

After the initiation of the basic interventions, it is proper to consider whether any additional therapies may be necessary. Drug therapy may be of value. Dexfenfluramine is currently the most widely recommended drug and may produce additional weight loss by preventing hunger in those who are big eaters or who eat at night through habit, hunger or boredom. It is also of use when weight loss has stalled on a regular programme. Weight tends to be regained when the drug is ceased. Dexfenfluramine is also of use in those with NIDDM who need to lose weight, as it is a mild hypoglycaemic and improves diabetic control. In those who are depressed, the newer anti-depressant drugs, such as fluoxetine, may assist weight reduction. Other drugs which may be of use in the future are tetrahydrolipstatin (a pancreatic lipase inhibitor which prevents fat absorption) and sibutramine.

Very low calorie diets (VLCDs) which contain between 400 and 800 calories per day are largely protein-based with essential fatty acids, vitamins and minerals and very little carbohydrate. They are extremely effective at producing rapid and early weight loss in the very obese, but the weight loss at longer-term follow-up may not be greater than with a standard programme. They are principally of use when rapid weight reduction is needed for medical reasons. VLCDs should only be used under medical supervision as part of a programme which includes exercise and behaviour modification, regular follow-ups and preparation for the re-introduction of normal eating.

Surgery for the management of obesity is far less commonly performed nowadays. For selected patients gastric banding is sometimes used. A recent development enables the plastic band placed around the stomach to be tightened or loosened from a reservoir placed under the skin. Plastic surgery in the form of breast reductions, local liposuction or lipectomy may be useful in selected patients.

16.7.4 Maintenance therapy

The planned maintenance phase is critical to all weight reduction programmes. These may consist of regular reinforcement visits and regular weigh-ins and the continued application of behaviour modification principles and techniques. Even when weight loss is achieved the predisposing factors remain and so does the propensity for weight regain. It is important for individuals to be aware of regain early and for appropriate therapy to be re-introduced. A weight reduction programme may be undertaken by commercial organizations, but general practitioners working in conjunction with dietitians and other specialists have a particularly important role to play as they know their patients well, and are trusted. Programmes run by dietitians in general practitioners' surgeries can be particularly effective.

A recent suggestion which runs contrary to the traditional approach described here is that it may be better to induce rapid weight loss with drugs, restrictive diets and/or VLCDs and then to have intensive maintenance programmes. This approach has not been tested sufficiently in randomized controlled trials in comparison with the standard approach. Additional information about treatment can be found in published reviews.

16.8   PREVENTION OF OBESITY

The rapidly increasing prevalence of overweight and obesity in many countries and the difficulties involved in achieving and maintaining satisfactory weight loss in those who are already obese mean that preventive approaches should be the solution to reversing the world-wide epidemic of obesity. Many approaches have been tried to date and they have been uniformly unsuccessful in whole population terms. However, the fact that there is less overweight in those of higher socioeconomic status in Western society shows that despite the role of genetic factors, obesity may at least be partially reversible. Targeted preventive programmes need to be developed. For children, the simplest successful way is to ensure that some planned physical activity is done each day at school. Time or cost seem to be the justification for this approach being rejected by schools or education authorities. The development of programmes which aim to prevent excessive weight gain in children and adults and which are appropriate for specific groups must be one of the most important challenges for preventive medicine in both affluent and developing countries.

FURTHER READING

1. Bouchard C, Tremblay A, Despres J-P, *et al.* The response to longterm overfeeding in identical twins. *N Engl J Med* 1990; **322**: 1477–82.
2. Bray GA. The pathophysiology of obesity. *Am J Clin Nutr* 1992; **55**: 448S–94S.
3. Caterson ID. Obesity: effective management in general practice. *Modern Medicine* 1994; **37**: 70–80.
4. Cole TJ, Freeman JV, Preece MA. Body mass index reference curves for the UK, 1990. *Arch Dis Chilh* 1995; **73**: 25–9.
5. Despres J-P. Dyslipidaemia and obesity. *Baillieres Clin Endocrinol Metab* 1994; **8**: 629–60.
6. Dyer RG. Traditional treatment of obesity: does it work? *Baillieres Clin Endocrinol Metab* 1994; **8**: 661–88.
7. Flatt JP. Importance of nutrient balance in body weight regulation. *Diabetes Metab Rev* 1988, **6**: 571–81.
8. Garrow JS. *Obesity and related diseases.* Edinburgh: Churchill Livingstone, 1988.
9. Hodge AM, Zimmet PZ. The epidemiology of obesity. *Baillière's Clin Endocrinol Metab* 1994; **8**: 577–99.
10. Lissner L, Heitmann BL. Dietary fat and obesity: evidence from epidemiology. *Eur J Clin Nutr* 1995; **49**: 79–90.
11. Report of a WHO consultation on obesity. *Obesity: preventing and managing the global epidemic,* Geneva 3–5 June 1997. Geneva: WHO, 1997.
12. Stunkard AJ, Sorensen TIA, Harris C, *et al.* Adoption study of human obesity. *N Engl J Med* 1986; **314**: 193–8.

17
PROTEIN-ENERGY MALNUTRITION (PEM)

Stewart Truswell

People, young or old, who eat less food than they usually eat, and need, lose body weight; the deficit of energy (or calories) in the diet is made up by drawing on the body's energy reserves: first fat, later muscle. The weight loss is carbon dioxide (breathed out) and water (excreted) from oxidation of fat.

$$2(C_{55}H_{106}O_6) + 157O_2 \rightarrow 110CO_2 + 106H_2O + heat$$

(This representative fat molecule is a triglyceride with oleic (18:1), linoleic (18:2) and palmitic (16:0) acids.) This is undernutrition.

Undernutrition can be mild or severe, beneficial (in someone who was obese) or dangerous. The loss of weight is a manifestation of energy depletion. Essential nutrients, protein and micronutrients, are likely to be depleted at the same time but some micronutrients have large stores in the body, and requirements of some others are lower when energy intake is reduced. In children, who have higher protein requirements than adults, important depletion of protein is likely to accompany serious undernutrition.

Protein depletion can affect the body in two different ways:

1. *In somatic protein depletion* the loss of tissue shows as general wasting of muscles, which together contain the largest amount of the body's protein.

2. *In visceral protein depletion* the brunt of the protein loss is borne by the liver, pancreas and gut. This is the less common type of protein malnutrition and nutritional scientists still do not fully agree why it occurs.

Box 17.1   Definitions of malnutrition

- Undernutrition is depletion of energy (calories)
- Malnutrition is serious depletion of any of the essential nutrients (other than energy)
- Fasting is voluntary abstention from food
- Starvation is involuntary lack of food
- Famine is severe food shortage of a whole community
- Wasting is loss of substance, especially muscle (from insufficient food, disuse or disease)

Protein-energy malnutrition (PEM) occurs in three situations:

1. In young children in poor communities, usually in developing countries.
2. In adults, even in affluent countries, due to severe illness (hospital malnutrition).
3. In people of all ages in a famine.

17.1 PROTEIN-ENERGY MALNUTRITION IN YOUNG CHILDREN

There are two forms of severe PEM: marasmus and kwashiorkor.

17.1.1 Nutritional marasmus

Nutritional marasmus is the common form; it is starvation in an infant or young child. (The word is from the Greek, 'marasmos', meaning 'wither'.) The child is very thin and wasted (Fig. 17.1). Weight is less than 60% of the median reference weight-for-age and there is marked wasting (Fig. 17.1). There is no oedema.

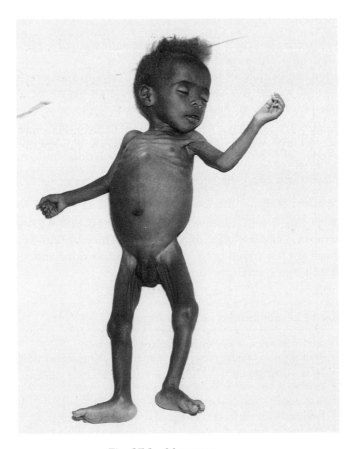

Fig. 17.1 Marasmus.

There is loss of almost all the adipose tissue and (to a smaller extent), wasting of the voluntary muscles. Growth has stopped and it has taken weeks of inadequate feeding for a child to become very wasted like this. The cause is a diet very low in total energy, that is, not enough food, for example, early weaning from the breast on to dilute food, because of poverty or ignorance. Poor food hygiene leads to gastroenteritis, diarrhoea and vomiting. This leads to poor appetite so more dilute feeds are given. Further depletion in turn leads to intestinal atrophy and more susceptibility to diarrhoea.

Not enough food implies not enough protein because most foods contain some protein. It is most unlikely that a child not getting enough food would still be eating a protein-rich food since such foods are expensive. With negative energy balance the major fuel to maintain life is free fatty acids, drawn from the adipose tissue. Blood glucose needed for tissues that can only metabolize glucose (brain, red blood cells) is maintained by gluconeogenesis of glucogenic amino acids (e.g. alanine) drawn from the body's proteins, usually the muscles, sometimes the viscera. Although energy depletion predominates in marasmus, there is inevitably insufficient protein intake and loss of protein inside the body.

Inside the body the heart, brain, liver and kidneys are least wasted but in advanced cases the heart becomes atrophied (wasted) and brain weight is reduced. There is increased mobilization of free fatty acids from adipose tissue, with ketosis (increased concentration of 3(OH) butyrate and acetoacetate). The blood glucose may be subnormal. The basal metabolic rate goes down; an increased proportion of triiodothyronine is in the inactive rT3 form. Plasma insulin is low.

Infections which are only a temporary nuisance in well-nourished children become life-threatening in children with severe PEM. Their bodies are not capable of producing the usual responses to common bacterial infections, of pyrexia and increased white blood cells (leucocytosis). Cell-mediated immunity, the main defence against viruses and tuberculosis, is impaired. Pathogenic bacteria in the intestines can more easily gain access to the blood circulation.

17.1.2 Kwashiorkor

Marasmus has been known for centuries; but the other type of severe PEM, kwashiorkor, was not generally recognized until the 1950s. The classic description was by Cecily

Table 17.1 Classification of protein-energy malnutrition (PEM) in young children

Condition	Body weight as percentage of international standard*	Oedema	Deficit in weight-for-length
Kwashiorkor	80–60	+	+
Marasmic kwashiorkor	< 60	+	+ +
Marasmus	< 60	0	+ +
Nutritional stunting	< 60	0	Minimal
Underweight child	80–60	0	+

* The 50th percentile line of the World Health Organization reference values.

Williams in the *Lancet* in 1935. She wrote from Accra, Ghana and gave the syndrome the name that the mothers used there, in the Ga language.

Typically, a child with kwashiorkor (Fig. 17.2) develops oedema, which is generalized. The child is miserable, withdrawn, obviously ill, and will not eat. Changes can be seen in the skin: there are areas of pigmentation which are symmetrical in distribution, most commonly in the nappy area. The skin later shows cracks and the superficial layer peels off. The hair is thinned and discoloured, blond or red or grey, instead of black. There is diarrhoea. Inside the body the liver is enlarged and its parenchymal cells contain numerous fat droplets. The protein in the liver is reduced and two of the main features of kwashiorkor can be explained by failure of the liver to make two important (export) plasma proteins. Failure to synthesize albumin and the consequent very low plasma albumin may, because of low plasma osmotic pressure, explain the oedema. Failure to synthesize very low-density lipoproteins, and inability to transport fat out of the liver to the periphery explains the accumulation of fat in the liver. There is an abnormal and characteristic pattern of amino acids in plasma (Table 17.2).

Kwashiorkor develops more quickly than marasmus. One day the oedema appears and the mother seeks medical help—though changes in skin and hair must have been developing over a longer period. The child with kwashiorkor is not necessarily underweight. The original meaning of kwashiorkor is 'the deposed child' or 'first second'. Mothers in Accra thought that this was the illness a child can get when a second baby follows and displaces the first one from the breast.

There are two schools of thought on the cause of kwashiorkor. The question is why is there an acute depletion of protein from the liver and other viscera rather than from the muscles in these cases of protein-energy malnutrition.

Table 17.2 Biochemical in kwashiorkor compared to marasmus (on admission to hospital)

	Kwashiorkor	Marasmus
Plasma albumin	Very low	Usually normal
Plasma amino acids	Reduced branch chain and tyrosine	More normal
Serum amylase	Very low	Normal/low normal
Plasma (total) cholesterol	Very low	Normal/low normal
Plasma free fatty acids	Increased	Increased
Plasma growth hormone	Raised	Not as high
Red cell glutathione	Low	Normal
Fasting blood glucose	Low–normal	Low
T lymphocytes	Low	Low
Plasma retinol	Low	Low
Somatomedin-C (IGF-1)	Low	Not as low
Plasma transferrin	Very low	Low normal
Plasma urea	Low	Not as low
Plasma urate	Low	Raised
Plasma zinc	Low	Not as low

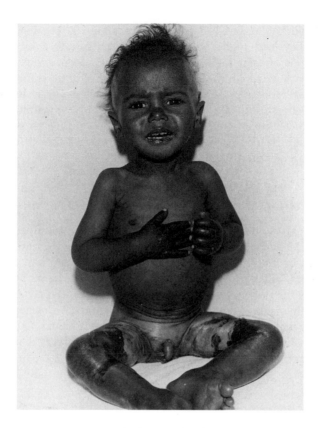

Fig. 17.2 Kwashiorkor.

The original theory is that the child who develops kwashiorkor has been fed on a diet moderately adequate in carbohydrate but very low in protein so that there is a relative deficiency of protein to energy (i.e. protein malnutrition), whereas the diet that leads to marasmus is low in both energy and protein. Researchers who disagree with the classical theory argue that in their experience dietary histories are indistinguishable between children with kwashiorkor and children with marasmus. Something else must explain the visceral protein depletion—'dysadaptation', mycotoxins or free radical damage have been suggested.

Individual dietary histories are not likely to be scientifically reliable from the carer(s) of a child who has become severely malnourished. Kwashiorkor children are not necessarily underweight (= energy-deficient). Their very low blood and urinary urea levels indicate low protein intakes. Cure of kwashiorkor has been initiated with a diet consisting only of 18 pure amino acids plus only 30% energy from glucose. Kwashiorkor occurs in countries where the staple diets for weaned children have very low protein/energy ratios (e.g. cassava, plantains, sweet potato or refined maize). R.G. Whitehead made observations comparing children in The Gambia, where the usual form of severe PEM is marasmus, with children in Uganda, where kwashiorkor occurs. Ugandan children grew more in weight and height and had more subcutaneous fat but lower plasma albumin concentrations. They had higher plasma insulin levels and lower plasma cortisols. Protein/energy ratios of their food were lower. Whitehead suggests that on a very low protein diet, but with adequate carbohydrate, the carbohydrate stimulates insulin which is known to favour deposition of amino acids in muscles. On a very low protein diet amino acids are in short supply, so muscle proteins can only be maintained at the expense of the liver and other viscera, which have a rapid turnover of their proteins. Syndromes resembling kwashiorkor can be produced in monkeys on a diet of cassava with added sugar, and in young rats on a 5% protein ration.

17.1.3 The spectrum of severe protein-energy malnutrition

Kwashiorkor and marasmus are distinct diseases but in communities where both occur cases of severe PEM often have some features of both (e.g. they are very underweight and also have skin or hair changes). This is marasmic kwashiorkor.

PEM does not only affect protein and energy. The Spanish name 'syndrome policarencial infantil' means the polynutritional syndrome of infants. Deficiencies of some micronutrients commonly occur in severe PEM, notably vitamin A deficiency: xerophthalmia (Chapter 11), and potassium depletion from diarrhoea (Chapter 7). There may also be evidence of zinc (Chapter 10), folate and/or niacin (Chapter 12) deficiency.

Children with severe PEM have diarrhoea. An infection may have brought on the severe illness. These children stand infections poorly; measles is especially lethal.

17.1.4 Treatment of severe protein-energy malnutrition

Treatment of severe PEM is in three stages and similar for marasmus and kwashiorkor:

1. *Treatment of acute complications*: correction of dehydration and/or electrolyte disturbance and/or very low blood glucose and/or low body temperature (hypothermia) and start of treatment for infections. Clinical signs of infections are difficult to elicit (e.g. no pyrexia or leucocytosis). Many paediatricians give broad-spectrum antibiotics on the presumption of some infection.

2. *Initiation of cure*: refeeding, gradually working up the energy and protein intake and giving multi-vitamin drops and potassium and magnesium supplements. Children with kwashiorkor have poor appetites. They have to be handfed, with frequent feeds, preferably in the lap of their mother or a nurse they know.

3. *Nutritional rehabilitation*: after about three weeks the child should be obviously better, with oedema cleared, and mentally bright with good appetite but still below the standard for weight-for-height. At this stage, catch-up growth should occur if the child is well looked after and given nutritious combinations of local, familiar foods. If the child has been in hospital they have to go back to their family, unless a nutrition rehabilitation unit is available.

Prognosis   Even in well-equipped hospitals the death rate of children with severe PEM is around 20%. In those who survive are there lasting effects? Follow-up biopsies after kwashiorkor have shown that the liver returns to normal; the fatty change does not progress to cirrhosis (unlike that in alcoholics). In marasmic children, who have become severely wasted in the first two years of life, growth of the skull (easily measured), and the brain inside is retarded and such children may subsequently have impaired intelligence unless they are fortunate thereafter and brought up in an excellent environment.

17.2   Mild to Moderate Protein-Energy Malnutrition

For every florid case of marasmus or kwashiorkor there must be 7–10 children in the community with mild to moderate PEM. Like an iceberg, there is more malnutrition below the surface and not easily recognized. Mothers often do not realize that their child is malnourished because he or she is similar in size and vitality to many of the same age in the neighbourhood. Most children with mild to moderate PEM can be detected, however, by their weight-for-age, which is less than 80% of the international standard (Table 17.1). Such children are either wasted, with subnormal weight-for-height/length or stunted (nutritional dwarfism), with subnormal height-for-age (but not wasted), or both. Wasted children have used up body fat, and some muscle, to maintain their fuel supply. Stunted children have adapted in a different way, by stopping or slowing their growth. Reference tables (or graphs) are available from the World Health Organization (WHO) for weight-for-age, height/length-for-age and weight-for-height for prepubertal children. These are re-calculated from the National Centre for Health Statistics (NCHS) data set (see Chapter 26).

In many developing countries around 2% of preschool children have severe PEM and 20% (in some places more) have mild to moderate PEM. The importance of this mild to moderate PEM is that affected children are growing up smaller than their genetic potential and have increased susceptibility to severe gastroenteritis and respiratory infections. Mild to moderate PEM is probably the main underlying reason why the 1–4 year mortality in developing countries is 30–60 times higher than in Europe or North America (in some places higher).

17.3   Prevention of Protein-Energy Malnutrition

Kwashiorkor most often occurs in the second year of life; marasmus mostly in the first year. Kwashiorkor is more amenable to the medical model of education, for example, education of mothers about the need for protein foods for weaned children and encouraging their provision at the political level. Marasmus is a more intractable problem, bound up with poverty, the status and education of women, lack of contraceptive resources and poor sanitation. UNICEF has achieved reductions in rates of PEM with four simple measures: represented by GOBI (see Box 17.2).

Box 17.2   UNICEFs inexpensive measures to prevent PEM

G *for growth monitoring*   The mother keeps the simple weight-for-age chart in a cellophane envelope and brings the child to a maternal and child health clinic regularly for weighing and advice.

O *for oral rehydration*   The UNICEF formula (NaCl 3.5 g, NaHCO₃ 2.5 g, KCl 1.5 g, glucose 20 g in clear water to 1 litre) is saving many lives from gastroenteritis.

B *for breast-feeding*   This has overwhelming advantages for a baby in a poor community with no facilities for hygiene. It should be continued as long as possible. Additional foods which should be prepared from locally available foods are not usually needed before 6 months of age.

I *for immunization*   For a few dollars a child can be protected against measles, diphtheria, pertussis, tetanus, tuberculosis, poliomyelitis, etc., infections which predispose to and aggravate malnutrition.

The clinical photographs in this chapter were kindly provided by Professor JDL Hansen.

FURTHER READING

Five major books have been written (in English) on PEM of children, the first in 1954. These are the three most recent:

1. Alleyne GAO, Hay RW, Picou DI, Stanfield JP, Whitehead RG. *Protein-energy malnutrition.* London: Edward Arnold, 1977.
2. Suskind RM, Lewinter-Suskind L. *The malnourished child.* New York: Raven Press, 1990.
3. Waterlow JC. *Protein energy malnutrition.* London: Edward Arnold, 1992.

18
CARDIOVASCULAR DISEASES

Jim Mann

18.1 CORONARY HEART DISEASE

Coronary heart disease (CHD) is a common condition in most affluent and some developing societies. In most industrialized countries it is the commonest single cause of death, often accounting for around one-third of all deaths. In addition, each year there are about as many non-fatal cases as there are deaths. A high proportion of the health care budget in these countries is spent treating CHD and its consequences. There is strong evidence that nutritional factors contribute to the aetiology of the condition and that dietary modification is important in the treatment of patients with CHD. Lifestyle modification is undoubtedly the most effective means of reducing CHD risk in high-risk populations and individuals.

18.1.1 Clinical aspects

The basic pathological lesion underlying CHD is the atheromatous plaque which bulges on the inside of one or more of the coronary arteries (Fig. 18.1) that supply blood to the heart muscle (myocardium). In addition, a superimposed thrombus or clot may further occlude the artery. A variety of cells and lipids are involved in the pathogenesis of the atherosclerotic plaque and the arterial thrombus, including lipoproteins, cholesterol, triglycerides, platelets, monocytes, endothelial cells, fibroblasts and smooth muscle cells. Nutrition can influence the development of CHD by modifying one or more of these factors. Two major clinical conditions are associated with these processes:

1. *Angina pectoris* is characterized by pain or discomfort in the chest which is brought on by exertion or stress, and which may radiate down the left arm and to the neck. It results from a reduction or temporary block to the blood flow through the coronary artery to the heart muscle. The pain usually passes with rest and seldom lasts for more than 15 minutes.

2. Coronary thrombosis, or *myocardial infarction*, results from prolonged total occlusion of the artery, which causes infarction or death of some of the heart muscle cells and is associated with prolonged, and usually excruciating, central chest pain. The terms 'coronary thrombosis' and 'myocardial infarction' are used to describe the same clinical condition, although they really describe pathological processes.

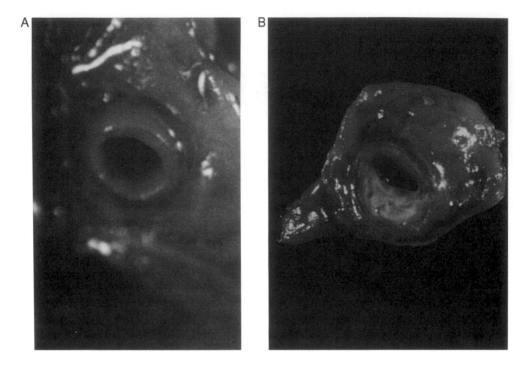

Fig. 18.1   A normal coronary artery is contrasted with an artery showing atheromatous deposits.

18.1.2   Epidemiological aspects

There are marked international differences in rates of CHD (Fig. 18.2). The experience of migrants and changing rates in various countries suggest that environmental and behavioural differences account for much of the variation between countries. Japanese living in the United States have CHD rates approaching those of the host country and Finns living in Sweden have much lower rates than in their country of origin. The rapidly changing rates (increases as well as decreases) shown in Fig. 18.3 are compatible with lifestyle changes which have occurred in these countries, but given the complex interactions between various lifestyle attributes which may influence CHD rates it is very difficult from such data to disentangle individual effects. This may be done using more sophisticated epidemiological and experimental approaches discussed later. In recent years, rates have been decreasing in most Western countries whereas in Eastern Europe rates are increasing. The changes occurring over relatively short time periods encourage the belief that CHD is to some extent preventable if causes can be found and modified. The hope is to reduce morbidity and mortality from CHD in those who are in the prime of life.

18.1.3   Foods and nutrients in the aetiology of CHD

Several approaches have been taken in studies investigating the role of dietary factors in the causation of CHD. The simplest of these involves correlating national dietary intakes

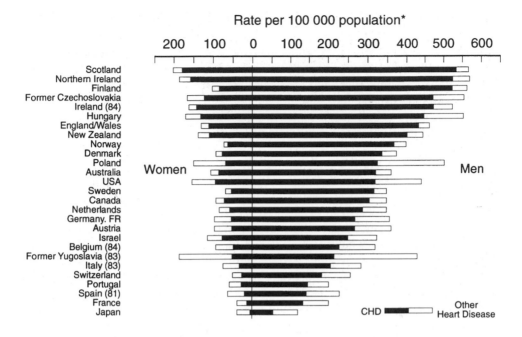

*Rates are age-adjusted and coded to the 9th Revision of the ICD
except in Finland, Norway, Denmark, Sweden, and Switzerland (8th Revision)

Fig. 18.2 International differences in coronary heart disease rates.

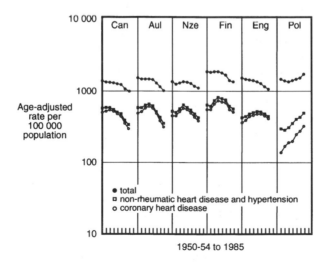

Fig. 18.3 Rates of coronary heart disease over time in men ages 45–64 in Canada, England, New Zealand, Australia, Finland and Poland. *Source*: Thom T. International mortality from heart disease: rates and trends. *Int J Epidemiol* 1989; **18** (suppl.): S20–S8.

281

(based on food balance data) with CHD death rates (mortality) in countries with varying rates or with changes in CHD mortality over time in individual countries. Positive associations between CHD death rate (age-standardized) and saturated fat, sucrose, animal protein and coffee consumption and negative correlations with flour (and other foods rich in complex carbohydrates) and vegetables are some of the most clearly described. However, both food balance data and mortality statistics can be unreliable. Studies that measure food intake of individuals and relate this information about food and nutrients to accurately recorded information regarding CHD events and mortality are much more reliable.

Unfortunately, there are few such studies. In the famous 'Seven Country Study' co-ordinated by Ancel Keys and colleagues, food consumption of people in 16 defined cohorts in seven countries was related to subsequent CHD incidence. The strongest correlation was observed between CHD and percentage of energy derived from saturated fat (Fig. 18.4). Weak inverse associations (suggesting protective effects) were found with percentages of energy from mono- and polyunsaturated fat and CHD. Total fat did not correlate with CHD, and of the other well-known risk factors for CHD (see below) only plasma (total) cholesterol and blood pressure appeared to explain part of the geographical variation in the frequency of this condition. This has led to the suggestion that nutrition-related factors may be particulary important in determining whether countries are likely to have high CHD rates. The Seven Country Study also provided evidence that the degree of risk conferred by other lifestyle factors is strongly influenced by nutrition-related factors: the relationship between cigarette smoking and CHD is much more powerful in those countries where saturated fat intake and mean plasma cholesterol levels are high (e.g. in the United States and Northern European countries) than in Southern Europe and Japan, where saturated fat intake and cholesterol levels are lower.

A more recent study based in a larger number of European countries used a similar approach, and also estimated antioxidant nutrients: CHD rates were inversely related to blood levels of several of these nutrients, in particular vitamin E, carotene and vitamin C

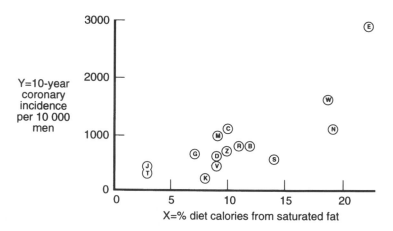

Fig. 18.4 Association between coronary heart disease and percentage energy derived from saturated fatty acids in the Seven Country Study. Keys (1980).

and, to a lesser extent, vitamin A. Coronary heart disease mortality could be predicted by multiple regression analysis with a high degree of certainty from the average intake of vitamin E, carotene and vitamin C. Of the other factors measured, only cholesterol and blood pressure helped to further explain the geographical variation in CHD. This finding may help to explain a phenomenon which has long puzzled epidemiologists, the so-called French paradox. The French have relatively low rates of CHD, but a saturated fat intake and plasma cholesterol levels which do not differ appreciably from countries with much higher rates of CHD. Thus it appears that the geographical variation in CHD is better explained by taking intakes of both saturated fat and dietary antioxidants into account.

Several longitudinal studies have related intakes of foods or nutrients to the subsequent development of CHD. There are particular difficulties associated with establishing nutritional aetiology in this way: no methods for measuring dietary intake are fully reliable and a single assessment does not necessarily provide a truly representative indication of life-long, or even long-term dietary practices. Some more recent studies have used biological markers as surrogate measures of dietary intake (e.g. plasma levels of antioxidants; fatty acid composition of red cells, platelets, or adipose tissue as indicators of the nature of dietary fat). Longitudinal studies have suggested several foods and nutrients which may be protective against CHD: fish, wholemeal bread, walnuts, garlic, red wine, vitamins C and E, flavonoids, non-starch polysaccharides, linoleic acid, and eicosapentaenoic acid, and three which might increase risk: dietary cholesterol, *trans*-unsaturated fatty acids and coffee. Vegetarians appear at lower risk of CHD than meat eaters, but it has not been clearly established which attributes of the vegetarian diet might be protective since there are many aspects other than the absence of meat which characterize these diets.

18.1.4 Cardiovascular risk factors and their nutritional determinants

Attempts to explain the pathological process underlying CHD and to identify individuals at risk suggest that there is no single cause of the disease. An understanding of the characteristics which put individuals at particular risk of developing CHD provides a useful background against which to examine in more detail the role of diet in the aetiology. The term 'risk factor' is used to describe features of lifestyle and behaviour, as well as physical and biochemical attributes which predict an increased likelihood of developing CHD. Potential risk factors are often identified when comparisons are made between people who have developed CHD and healthy controls (case-control studies) and confirmed by cohort (prospective) studies in which these factors are measured in a large group of apparently healthy people who are then followed to see if they develop the disease or not at some future date. The presence, absence, or degree of each factor can then be related to the risk of developing CHD. Table 18.1 lists most of the important risk factors for CHD which have been identified in this way. The irreversible psychosocial and geographical factors, as well as cigarette smoking and physical activity, are reviewed in textbooks of medicine and epidemiology. This chapter concentrates on potentially reversible factors which have been shown to be influenced by diet. Hypertension is considered separately in Section 18.2.

Table 18.1 Risk factors for coronary heart disease

* **Irreversible**
  - masculine gender
  - increasing age
  - genetic traits, including monogenic and polygenic disorders of lipid metabolism
  - body build

* **Potentially reversible**
  - cigarette smoking
  - dyslipidaemia: increased levels of cholesterol, triglyceride, low-density and very low-density lipoprotein and low levels of high-density lipoprotein
  - oxidizability of low-density lipoprotein
  - obesity, especially when associated with high waist/hip ratio
  - hypertension
  - physical inactivity
  - hyperglycaemia and diabetes
  - increased thrombosis: increased haemostatic factors and enhanced platelet aggregation
  - high levels of homocysteine

* **Psychosocial**
  - low socioeconomic class
  - stressful situations
  - coronary-prone behaviour patterns: type A behaviour

* **Geographical**
  - climate and season: cold weather
  - soft drinking water

Dyslipidaemia Altered levels of blood lipids found in lipoproteins (see Chapter 3.3) may place individuals at increased risk of CHD in three ways. First, a relatively small proportion of people have an exceptionally high risk because of a clearly inherited increase of plasma lipids. Second, a large number of people (perhaps as many as half the adult population in high-risk countries) have a slight to moderately increased risk because their blood lipids are higher than desirable as a result of an interaction between polygenic and lifestyle-related factors. They are described as having 'polygenic' or 'common' hyperlipidaemia. Third, some people are also at increased CHD risk because of low levels of high-density lipoprotein (HDL).

Genetically determined disorders of lipid metabolism. The clearly defined genetically determined disorders of lipid metabolism, which are usually characterized by an increase in one or more lipoprotein fractions, are described in Table 18.2. Familial hypercholesterolaemia is the best known. It is characterized by marked elevation of total and low-density lipoprotein (LDL) cholesterol, cholesterol-filled xanthomas (nodules) in tendons, and a very high risk of premature CHD. Untreated, 85% of males with this condition will

Table 18.2 'Genetic-metabolic' classification of hyperlipidaemia. The World Health Organization (WHO) type is also indicated

	Athero-sclerosis risk	Inheritance	Relative prevalence	Lipid abnormalities	WHO type
Familial hypercholest-erolaemia	+++	Autosomal dominant	++	Cholesterol & LDL ↑↑ Triglyceride N or slightly ↑	IIa Occasionally IIb
Familial combined hyperlipidaemia	++	Uncertain	+++	Cholesterol & LDL ↑ Triglyceride & VLDL ↑	IIb Occasionally IIa and IV
Remnant hyperlipo-proteinaemia	++	Apo EIII deficiency and other factors	+	Cholesterol ↑↑ Triglyceride ↑↑ Intermediate-density lipoprotein ↑	III
Familial hypertrigly-ceridaemia.					
Excessive synthesis	Uncertain	Probably autosomal dominant	+	Triglyceride & VLDL ↑↑ Chylomicrons ↑	IV
Lipoprotein lipase/apo CII deficiency	Uncertain	Probably recessive	Rare	Triglyceride ↑↑ Chylomicrons ↑↑ VLDL ↑	IV, V
Common hypercholest-erolaemia	+	Polygenic	++++	Cholesterol & LDL ↑	IIa

↑, raised; ↑↑, markedly raised; N, normal; +, relatively low; ++++, extremely high; LDL, low-density lipoproteins; VLDL, very low-density lipoproteins.
Source: Lewis B. Disorders of lipid transport. In: Weatherall DJ, Ledingham JGG, Warrell DA (eds). *The Oxford textbook of medicine*. 2nd ed. Oxford University Press, 1987.

have had a myocardial infarction before the age of 60 years. The metabolic abnormality and clinical consequences result from impaired removal of LDL from the circulation because of a reduction in LDL receptors on the surface of cells. The other common inherited hyperlipidaemia, familial combined hyperlipidaemia, is characterized by increased LDL and increased very low-density lipoprotein (VLDL) which result from increased production of these lipoproteins. The mode of inheritance is not quite so clearly understood, but the condition is associated with an equally high risk of cardiovascular

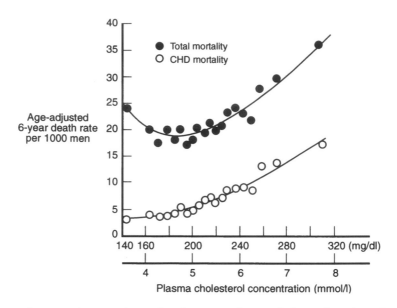

Fig. 18.5 Within population relationship between plasma cholesterol and CHD and total mortality. *Source*: Martin MJ, Hulley SB, Browner WS, *et al. Lancet* 1986; **2**: 933–6.

disease. Remnant hyperlipidaemia and the familial hypertriglyceridaemic states are relatively rare. Diet and other lifestyle factors are relatively unimportant in the aetiology of these conditions, but play a role in their management. By contrast, dietary factors are critically important in polygenic hyperlipidaemia.

Polygenic hypercholesterolaemia. Hypercholesterolaemia, a consequence of elevated LDL or VLDL or both is one of the most clearly described CHD risk factors. In over 40 longitudinal studies in different countries, total cholesterol has been shown to be related to the rate of CHD. The association is independant of other risk factors and characterized by a gradient of risk with increasing plasma cholesterol concentration (Fig. 18.5). Cholesterol is a major constituent of the atheromatous plaque. Average cholesterol levels are similar in adult men and women, but this similarity hides the different age trends observed in cross-sectional studies (Fig. 18.6). Hormonal factors may in part explain the gender differences but the fact that populations and groups with low average cholesterol levels do not show such marked increases with age suggest that lifestyle-related factors may also be involved.

Low-density lipoprotein which transports the bulk of cholesterol in the bloodstream is taken up by macrophages after being oxidized and may then become deposited in the atheromatous plaque. Dietary antioxidants (vitamins E and C and carotenoids, and possibly flavonoids and selenium) may protect LDL against oxidation, help slow the progression of atherosclerosis and thus influence the degree of risk conferred by a particular level of plasma cholesterol.

Levels of total (TC) and LDL cholesterol (LDL-C) are profoundly influenced by the dietary factors described in Chapter 3. It seems very likely that the deleterious effect of

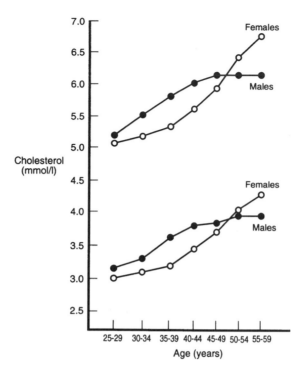

Fig. 18.6 Relationship between total and low-density lipoprotein (LDL) cholesterol, gender and age in the UK. Top: total cholesterol (mmol/l). Bottom: LDL cholesterol (mmol/l). *Source*: Mann JI, Lewis B, Shepherd J, *et al*. *BMJ* 1988; **296**: 1702–6.

saturated fat on CHD in epidemiological studies is explained by the ability of myristic, palmitic, and perhaps also lauric acids to elevate LDL and total cholesterol. Although ω6-polyunsaturated fatty acids help to lower TC and LDL-C, intakes greater than 10% total energy are not advised since the polyunsaturated fatty acids which become incorporated into LDL might increase the oxidizability of LDL. Low ratios of polyunsaturated to saturated fatty acids (around 0.2) are associated with a high average TC level and a high population risk of CHD. Higher ratios (up to 0.8) are found in Mediterranean countries and are associated with lower levels of TC and reduced CHD risk. However, the varying effect of different saturated fatty acids, the need to achieve the right balance of ω6-polyunsaturated fatty acids, the adverse effects of *trans*-unsaturated fatty acids on LDL, HDL and Lp(a) and the potential benefits of *cis*-monounsaturated fatty acids all lead to the conclusion that this ratio, previously used to indicate the effect on cholesterol levels and atherogenic potential of the diet, may be an oversimplified and outmoded concept. For this reason, dietary recommendations (see Section 18.1.6) are based around amounts and proportions of nutrients rather than ratios.

Hypertriglyceridaemia is a less clearly defined risk factor. People who have had myocardial infarctions tend to have higher levels of triglycerides and VLDL than controls and this relation is confirmed by prospective studies. However, it is not clear whether the association between triglycerides and VLDL and CHD is independent of other factors known to be associated with both raised levels of triglycerides and cardiovascular risk (e.g. obesity, hyperglycaemia, hypercholesterolaemia, hypertension). It has been suggested that raised levels of triglycerides may only be important in the presence of reduced HDL-cholesterol. Raised plasma triglycerides appear to be particularly important in determining cardiovascular risk in people with diabetes. Determinants of plasma triglyceride and VLDL levels are discussed in Chapter 3.

Reduced high-density lipoprotein concentrations. There has been considerable interest in HDL as a protective factor. Women have higher levels of HDL and lower risk of CHD. An attempt to aggregate the findings of four large American studies suggests that an increase of 1 mg/100 ml (0.026 mmol/l) HDL-cholesterol is associated with a 2–3% reduction in CHD. HDL levels do not differ markedly with age, are reduced in heavy cigarette smokers, and are increased by physical activity and alcohol intake (Chapter 6). Nutritional determinants are considered in Chapter 3.

Apoproteins and lipoprotein (a). Apoprotein B (apo B) and apoprotein AI (apo AI) are the major apoproteins of LDL and HDL respectively and therefore not surprisingly the former is predictive of CHD and the latter protective against CHD. However, interestingly the effects appear to be independent of total cholesterol, LDL and HDL. The interaction between diet and the apoproteins is complex. Dietary factors which influence LDL and HDL also have an effect on apo B and apo AI, but genetic variation appears to explain some of the variation in LDL and HDL response among individuals to dietary change. Less is known about the effects of dietary factors on other apoproteins. There is interest in lipoprotein (a) as a risk factor. Concentrations of lipoprotein (a), which is assembled from LDL and apolipoprotein (a), may vary from near zero to over 1000 mg/l. Case control studies suggest a strong independent association with CHD, but no data are available from prospective studies. Plasma levels are primarily genetically determined and the only dietary factor which has been shown to appreciably influence levels is intake of *trans*-unsaturated fatty acids, high intakes being associated with increased levels of lipoprotein (a).

Thrombogenesis   Factors that increase the tendency to thrombosis (either as a result of increased platelet aggregation or a high level of coagulability of blood) have received less attention than those influencing lipids and lipoproteins. They are more difficult to study. One clue to the potential for dietary factors to enhance or reduce the tendency for platelets to aggregate stems from observations made on the Eskimo people (Inuits) of Greenland. They have low rates of CHD and reduced platelet aggregation compared with Western nations despite high intakes of total fat. However, this fat comes largely from marine foods rich in ω3-fatty acids (eicosapentaenoate, C20:5, and docosahexaenoate, C22:6) which form the anti-aggregatory prostanoid, PGI_3. Platelet aggregation is largely controlled by a balance between the pro-aggregatory compound thromboxane A_2 (synthesized from arachidonic acid released from the platelet membrane after injury to the blood vessel wall) and the anti-aggregatory substance prostacyclin PGI_2 (also synthesized from arachidonic acid in the endothelial cells of the arterial wall). C20:5 and C22:6 inhibit conversion of arachidonic acid to thromboxane A_2 as well as facilitating the production of the additional anti-aggregatory substance PGI_3 (Fig. 18.7). Polyunsaturated fatty acids of the ω6-series may also reduce platelet aggregation by providing the series

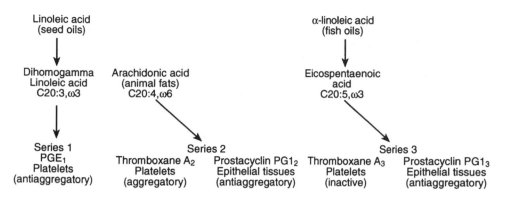

Fig. 18.7   Prostanoids formed from different fatty acids. *Source*: Ulbricht TLV, Southgate DAT. *Lancet* 1991; 338: 985–92.

1 prostanoid PGE_1 which is also anti-aggregatory. Oleic acid may also act as a inhibitor of platelet aggregation, though the effect is less than for polyunsaturated fatty acids.

Although there have been studies of the antithrombogenic effect of polyunsaturated fatty acids in humans, the thrombogenic effect of saturated fatty acids has been more extensively studied in laboratory animals. The findings are consistent: the longer-chain saturated fatty acids ($C14:0$, $C16:0$ and $18:0$) all appear to accelerate thrombosis. One mechanism may be via inhibition of anti-agggregatory prostacyclin. Stearic acid ($C18:0$) which appears not to raise LDL, has thrombogenic properties.

Dietary factors may also influence thrombogenesis via an effect on the coagulation system. The physiological function of coagulation is to secure haemostasis after an injury. Thrombin is produced, which enables the conversion of soluble fibrinogen to insoluble fibrin. Several prospective studies suggest that factors involved in the coagulation system (notably factor VII and fibrinogen) are important predictors of CHD. Too high a level of coagulability might predispose to thrombosis. High levels of fibrinogen are in turn associated with obesity and cigarette smoking. Factor VII is associated to a greater extent with dietary factors: increasing dietary fat can cause elevation of factor VII within 24 hours. Levels of a range of clotting factors, including factor VII, are lower in populations and groups eating a low fat, high polyunsaturated:saturated ratio, high fibre diet, and individuals changing to such a diet show reduction in these factors. While the evidence for an effect of diet on thrombogenesis is strong, there is still insufficient evidence to accurately quantify dietary recommendations concerning the optimal amounts of total fat or the ratio of ω3 to ω6 unsaturated fatty acids.

Diabetes, hyperglycaemia and the metabolic syndrome   Several studies have shown that people with diabetes, impaired glucose tolerance and the metabolic syndrome (hyperglycaemia, hypertension, hypertriglyceridaemia, hyperinsulinaemia associated with insulin resistance, hyperuricaemia) have an increased risk of CHD. Genetic factors play important roles in the aetiology of non-insulin-dependent diabetes and probably also in the metabolic syndrome, but nutrition-related factors are also important. Obesity (body mass index > 30) is associated with a considerable increase in risk of diabetes and there is some evidence that lesser degrees of obesity may also confer some risk. The obesity risk is most marked in those with abdominal obesity. There is less evidence for the role of specific dietary factors. Non-insulin-dependent diabetes is uncommon in populations eating a high fibre, high carbohydrate, low fat diet but there is no definitive evidence that any of these dietary factors are protective, or that fibre depletion or a high intake of fat or sucrose are in themselves predisposing. (These latter factors may influence the risk of diabetes by encouraging increased energy intake.)

Raised plasma homocysteine levels   Patients with inborn errors of homocysteine metabolism have very high levels of plasma homocysteine, homocysteinuria, and a high risk of cardiovascular disease. It has also been found that in the general population there is a gradient of CHD risk associated with increasing levels of plasma homocysteine (i.e. homocysteine is an independent risk factor for CHD). The mechanism by which homo-cysteine influences CHD risk has not been established, but interest in this relatively newly identified risk factor centres around the fact that folic acid can reduce raised homocyst-eine levels. There is as yet no clinical trial to prove that reducing homocysteine levels can reduce clinical CHD.

18.1.5   Clinical trials of dietary modification

There is thus much evidence to suggest that dietary change should reduce coronary disease and no doubt that dietary modification can favourably influence cardiovascular risk factors. However, it is now accepted practice to require proof of benefit of changing epidemiological risk factors from intervention trials which are large enough to examine the effects of dietary change on clinical events. The early trials all attempted to lower cholesterol levels, usually by increasing the polyunsaturated : saturated ratio (i.e. they were single-factor intervention trials). More recent trials have involved multifactorial interventions, including dietary change intended to improve all nutrition-related risk indicators as well as attempts to modify risk factors which are not diet-related (e.g. cigarette smoking). Dietary intervention trials have been undertaken in people with and without evidence of CHD at the time the study was started (i.e. secondary and primary prevention trials). This review describes briefly a few landmark trials (Table 18.3) and presents an overview of all the important investigations of this kind.

Los Angeles Veterans Administration Study   This was the first of the major interven-tion trials, in which 846 male volunteers (aged 55–89 years) were randomly allocated to 'experimental' and 'control' diets taken in different dining rooms. The control diet was intended to be typical North American (40% energy from fat, mostly saturated). The experimental diet contained half as much cholesterol, and predominantly polyun-saturated vegetable oils (ω6-PUFA, polyunsaturated fatty acids) replaced approximately two-thirds of the animal fat, achieving a P : S ratio of two. With skilled food technology, the trial was conducted under double-blind conditions. During the eight years of trial, plasma cholesterol in the experimental group was 13% lower, and coronary events, as well as deaths due to cardiovascular disease, were appreciably reduced, compared with the controls (Table 18.3). The beneficial effect of the cholesterol-lowering diet was most evident in those with high cholesterol levels at the start of the study. Deaths due to other

Table 18.3 Results of selected intervention trials. (Confidence intervals are given in parentheses)

Trial	No. of subjects	% reduction in cholesterol	Odds ratios (Experimental vs. Control)	
			Total mortality	Fatal and non-fatal CHD
Veterans Administration	846	13	0.98 (0.83–1.15)	0.77
Oslo	1232	13	0.64 (0.37–1.12)	0.56
DART				
Fat advice	2033	3.5	0.98 (0.77–1.26)	0.92
Fish advice	2033	Negligible	0.74 (0.57–0.93)	0.85

and uncertain causes occurred more frequently in the experimental group, although no single other cause predominated. This increase in non-cardiovascular mortality in the experimental group raised for the first time the possibility that cholesterol lowering might be harmful in some respects, despite the reduction in CHD. This will be discussed in more detail later in the chapter.

Oslo Trial Middle aged men at high risk of CHD (smokers or those having a cholesterol in the range 7.5–9.8 mmol/l) were divided into two groups; half received intensive dietary education and advice to stop smoking, the other half served as a control group. An impressive reduction in total coronary events was observed (Table 18.3) in association with a 13% fall in serum cholesterol and a 65% reduction in tobacco consumption. There was also an improvement in total mortality and there were no significant differences between the two groups with regard to non-cardiac causes of death. Detailed statistical analysis suggested that approximately 60% of the CHD reduction could be attributed to serum cholesterol change and 25% to smoking reduction. The composition of the experimental diet was quite different from that used in Veterans Administration trial: total and saturated fat were markedly reduced without any appreciable increase in ω6-PUFA, and fibre-rich carbohydrate was increased.

Diet and Reinfarction Trial (Dart) This trial examined the effects of diets high in ω3-PUFA. Burr *et al.* randomized 2033 men who had survived myocardial infarction to receive or not to receive advice on each of three dietary factors: (1) a reduction of fat intake and an increase in the ratio of polyunsaturated to saturated fat; (2) an increase in fatty fish intake; and (3) an increase in cereal fibre. Within the short (two years) follow-up period, the subjects advised to eat fatty fish had a 26% reduction in all causes of mortality compared with those not so advised. The other two diets were not associated with significant differences in mortality, but in view of the fact that fat modification only achieved a 3–4% reduction in serum cholesterol, compliance with the fat-modified and high fibre diets may have been less than that on the fish diet. Furthermore, diets aimed to reduce atherogenicity (ω6-PUFA) are likely to take longer to show a beneficial effect than those aimed to reduce thrombogenicity (ω3-PUFA). These results are the first to find that very simple advice aimed to reduce thrombogenicity (at least two-weekly portions, 200–400 g of fatty fish) appears to reduce mortality appreciably.

Overall perspective of the trials   The dietary trials had sufficient numbers of subjects to see effects on clinical CHD events. None of them had sufficient statistical power to examine the effects of intervention on total mortality, so attempts have been made to aggregate the results of the various trials in order to reduce the margin of error associated with individual trials. This statistical approach, known as a meta-analysis, enables conclusions to be drawn about total mortality and in addition enables a more reliable estimate of the reduction in cardiovascular risk to be made. Meta-analyses are complicated by the facts that different dietary treatments have been used in the various trials, some likely to reduce CHD by cholesterol-lowering, others by reducing tendency to thrombosis, or decreasing oxidative stress. Despite these reservations the meta-analyses enable some firm conclusions to be drawn. For each 1% reduction in serum/plasma cholesterol a 2–3% reduction in coronary events can be expected. When considering all the dietary trials, cardiovascular events appear to be reduced by 13% and total mortality by 6%. However, when considering only those in which appreciable cholesterol lowering was achieved the reductions were 30% and 11%, respectively (Table 18.4). The benefits associated with dietary change are not as great as those achieved by the potent new cholesterol-lowering drugs, simvastatin and pravastatin, which in controlled trials have been shown to nearly halve cardiovascular risk. Nevertheless, dietary change clearly results in appreciable clinical advantage. Increased mortality from non-cardiac causes noted in some early trials of diet or drugs was not confirmed by the more recent trials of statin drugs or the meta-analyses of dietary studies. This suggests that the untoward effects observed in some studies were either chance findings, the results of unusual diets containing exceptionally large amounts of polyunsaturated fatty acids, or a consequence of specific drug regimens.

Table 18.4   Odds ratios for coronary heart disease (CHD) events and all deaths in trials according to various criteria

Trials	Major CHD events	All deaths
All 14 trials	0.87[a]	0.94[a]
Primary prevention trials	0.86	0.96
Secondary prevention trials	0.88	0.87
Seven large trials	0.87	0.95
Trials with largest cholesterol reduction[b]	0.70[a]	0.89[a]

[a] Significantly fewer deaths in the treatment group.
[b] Percentage reduction of cholesterol in intervention group compared with controls multiplied by years in trial greater than 30 (-33 to -180).
Source: Truswell AS. Review of dietary intervention studies: effect on coronary events and on total mortality. *Aust NZ J Med* 1994; 24: 98–106.

A few studies have examined the effects of strict cholesterol-lowering dietary advice or drug treatment on coronary artery narrowing by atheroma as measured by sophisticated angiographic techniques. They show that in comparison with control groups, such interventions can reduce progression of atheroma and possibly induce some regression.

18.1.6 Nutritional strategies for high-risk populations

There is general agreement in most countries with high CHD rates that a population strategy is essential for the overall reduction of the disease. The rationale is well illustrated for cholesterol levels in Fig. 18.8. While risk to the individual increases steadily with increasing levels of cholesterol, only a small number of cases in the community occur in those with very high cholesterol since they represent only a relatively small proportion of the total population. On the other hand, large numbers of people are at modestly increased risk of CHD because of average or slightly above average cholesterol levels. Although the risk to the individuals in this category is not so great, the majority of all CHD cases are drawn from this section of the population. The same principles apply to all risk factors, and the nutritional approach should ideally reduce atherogenic as well as thrombogenic risk by reducing obesity, lowering total- and LDL-cholesterol and triglycerides, increasing HDL-cholesterol, lowering blood pressure, and reducing platelet aggregation and oxidative stress in the population as a whole. The disadvantage of the population approach is that many individuals are being asked to make changes that are likely to produce a relatively small reduction in their personal CHD risk (the 'prevention paradox'). Those at high risk will need to be identified since they are likely to require more radical and individually designed lifestyle changes (or preventive

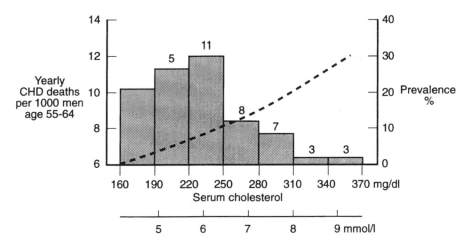

Fig. 18.8 Rationale for population strategy. Prevalence distribution (histogram) of serum cholesterol concentrations related to coronary heart disease mortality (broken line) in men aged 55–64 years. The number above each column represents an estimate of attributable deaths per 1000 population per 10-year period. (Derived from the Framingham Study.) *Source*: WHO Expert Committee (1987).

medical care, including drug therapy). Despite the wide range of risk indicators which may be influenced by lifestyle factors, present knowledge only allows targets to be set for cholesterol. A level of 5.2 mmol/l or lower is regarded as an achievable goal for individual adults in high risk countries, as well as a target population mean for those countries which currently have higher average levels. The justifications for this level are that CHD is relatively infrequent in countries with lower mean levels, and that within individual populations, subgroups with lower levels have the lowest risk of CHD.

Nutritional recommendations for high-risk populations　Broadly similar recommendations are in place in most countries with high CHD rates. The quantitative recommendations are somewhat arbitrary and represent 'best estimates' based upon epidemiological data, studies examining the effects of dietary modification on risk factors, clinical trials and consensus among experts. Table 18.5 shows as an example the dietary reference values for fat and carbohydrate intakes in the United Kingdom. These recommendations emphasize reduction of saturated fatty acids to 10% total energy (an appreciable reduction from present intakes) and acknowledge the particular importance of these nutrients in atherogenesis as well as thrombogenesis. It is impossible in population-based recommendations to distinguish between the different saturated fatty acids even though they do not all have the same effect on lipids and lipoproteins. The suggestion is that *cis*-monounsaturated fatty acids continue to provide on average 12% dietary energy, although the reduction in saturated fatty acids implies that a greater proportion of these fatty acids than at present

Table 18.5　Dietary reference values for fat and carbohydrate for adults

	Individual minimum	Population average	Individual maximum
		(% total energy intake)	
Saturated fatty acids		10 (11)	
Cis-polyunsaturated fatty acids		6 (6.5)	10
	n-3 : 0.2		
	n-6 : 1.0		
Cis-monounsaturated fatty acids		12 (13)	
Trans-fatty acids		2 (2)	
Total fatty acids		30 (32.5)	
Total fat		33 (35)	
Non-milk extrinsic sugars	0	10 (11)	
Intrinsic and milk sugars and starch		37 (39)	
Total carbohydrate		47 (50)	
Non-starch polysaccharide (g/day)	12	18	24

The average percentage contribution to total energy does not total 100% because figures for protein and alcohol are excluded. Protein intakes average 15% of total energy, which is above the RNI. It is recognized that many individuals will derive some energy from alcohol, and this has been assumed to average 5% approximating to current intakes. However, the Panel recognized that some groups chose not to drink alcohol and that for some purposes nutrient intakes as a proportion of food energy without alcohol might be useful. Therefore average figures are given as percentages both of total energy and, in parenthesis, of food energy.
Source: Department of Health. *Dietary reference values for food energy and nutrients for the United Kingdom*. Report on health and social subjects 41, London: HMSO, 1991.

will be derived from vegetable, rather than animal, sources. Recommendations in some other countries suggest that somewhat higher intakes of cis-monounsaturated fatty acids are acceptable. It is suggested that cis-polyunsaturated fatty acids should continue to provide an average of 6% daily energy and that this should be derived from a mixture of $\omega6$ and $\omega3$ polyunsaturated fatty acids. It is not yet possible to recommend optimal proportions of $\omega6$ and $\omega3$ polyunsaturated fatty acids. Polyunsaturated fatty acids should not exceed 10% total energy because of the possibility of HDL lowering and other potential risks associated with the liability to peroxidation of these fatty acids.

Trans-fatty acid intake should not exceed the currrent estimated average of 5 g/day or 2% of dietary energy. Total fatty acid intake should therefore average 30% and total fat (i.e. including glycerol) 33% of total dietary energy (including alcohol), or 35% of energy derived from food. Little emphasis is given to dietary cholesterol, because dietary cholesterol intake in Britain is relatively low and reduction in saturated fat inevitably results in reductions in dietary cholesterol. In countries where there are recommendations about dietary cholesterol, it is usually suggested that intakes should be below 300 mg/day.

Dietary reference values (DRVs) are given for carbohydrates and non-starch polysaccharides. These are not specifically aimed at reducing cardiovascular risk and it is of interest that, whereas an increase of non-starch polysaccharide is recommended, there is no specific advice to increase soluble forms, as has been suggested in other national recommendations. There is also no specific advice regarding antioxidant intake in relation to cardiovascular disease, although a high intake of fruit and vegetables, which is suggested in all dietary guidelines, should ensure adequate intakes.

It is beyond the scope of this chapter to attempt a detailed translation of recommendations and DRVs into guidelines for the population, although a few general comments are offered. A reduction of dairy products and red meat has formed the cornerstone of some guidelines in the past. Dairy products contribute a high proportion of dietary saturated fatty acids in most countries with high CHD rates and reduction of consumption of butter, full-fat milk and cheese, as well as hard margarine, is an important means of reducing intakes of saturated fatty acids. Skimmed or semi-skimmed milk, reduced-fat cheeses, and predominantly unsaturated margarines, particularly those high in oleic acid, are suitable alternatives. However, a change in the composition of many red meats so that lean meat now has less saturated fatty acids and more mono- and polyunsaturated fatty acids than previously has meant that moderate amounts (up to 180 g/day) can be safely incorporated into dietary advice aimed at achieving optimal lipoprotein profiles. The findings of DART also provide reinforcement of the epidemiological findings, which suggest that eating fish (especially oily fish) several times a week may confer additional benefit.

On the basis of Table 3.6 plus an additional effect from other dietary modifications, it might be expected that dietary change along the lines suggested here would reduce cholesterol levels by about 16%. This would mean a reduction in the mean adult population cholesterol levels to the target value of 5.2 mmol/l (or less) in most countries with high CHD rates, and consequently a huge reduction in cardiovascular disease. However, this would involve full compliance with dietary recommendations and in practice much smaller changes are likely to occur.

CHD rates have fallen in some countries (see Fig. 18.3) and this has occurred in parallel with changes in diet and other lifestyle-related factors, most notably a reduction in cigarette smoking. There are a number of reasons why more marked changes have not occured: information and education programmes are sometimes confusing and conflicting; appropriate foods are not always available; food labelling is often unsatisfactory or uninterpretable by the majority of consumers. Maximum compliance with dietary recommendations requires intensive and well-researched educational approaches supported by legislative measures to facilitate change. For example, it is necessary to ensure the widespread availability of healthy foods at relatively low cost and appropriate food labelling. A greater reduction in mean population cholesterol levels will mean that fewer people will remain in the high-risk category, who need to be individually identified in order to receive personal advice to achieve the greater lifestyle change required to reduce their risk of cardiovascular disease.

Dietary advice for high-risk individuals High-risk individuals are those who have markedly elevated levels of a single risk factor (e.g. those with familial hyperlipidaemia), those with multiple risk factors (see Table 18.1)—risk factors for CHD have a synergistic effect—or those who have already developed clinical CHD. They may be identified because of a personal or family history of CHD or in screening programmes. It is clearly important in such individuals to attempt to achieve the lowest possible degree of risk with regard to all identifiable risk factors. From a dietary point of view, the principles are similar to those recommended for the general population, but further changes from the current Western diet are often required (Table 18.6) and regular monitoring is essential. Food lists such as those in Table 18.7 (see Appendix) help make the required changes but individually tailored advice from a dietitian is often necessary. The absence of clinical trial data showing the benefits of dietary change in the elderly does not mean that they should not be given dietary advice. The absolute risk of cardiovascular disease increases steadily with age, although the relative risk associated with individual risk factors might decrease. No doubt there is an age beyond which there are minimal advantages to dietary change, but those who might be expected to otherwise have a reasonable life expectancy should be given advice similar to that given to younger individuals. When giving lipid-lowering advice to older people, it is necessary to ensure an adequate intake of essential nutrients because they usually have a reduced intake of total energy.

18.1.7 Other nutritional issues

The importance of CHD as a major cause of premature morbidity and mortality has led to this disease becoming a highly emotive issue in many high-risk populations. Consequently, the public is bombarded with much nutritional advice, some valid, some with no justification, and some confusingly based on half truths. Fad diets cause particular confusion. An example of the latter was the diet largely based on advice to increase oatbran and niacin. Oatbtan is high in soluble forms of non-starch polysaccharides, which have some cholesterol-lowering properties, and nicotinic acid in megadosage can certainly lower LDL and VLDL. However, the diet as recommended was likely to be far less effective than a simple fat-modified diet in lowering total and LDL-cholesterol and cardiovascular risk.

Similarly, ω3-polyunsaturated fatty acids (sold as concentrates in capsules) are sometimes advertised as a useful means of lowering cholesterol. Although these preparations can have a profound effect on thrombosis and, VLDL, and may indeed reduce the

Table 18.6 Principles of diet modification for individuals with hyperlipidaemia

	Initial advice for hypercholesterolaemia and endogenous hypertriglyceridaemia	Advice for resistant hyper-cholesterolaemia	Advice for chylomicronaemia syndrome
Total fatty acids (% total energy)	< 30	≈ 25	15[b]
saturated fatty acids and trans-unsaturated fatty acids	< 10 (range 6–10)	6–8	
polyunsaturated fatty acids	≈ 8 (range 6–10)	6–8	
monounsaturated fatty acids	up to 18 (range 10–18)	10–15	
Dietary cholesterol (mg/day)	< 300	< 200	< 200
Dietary fibre (g/day)[a]	35	45	35
Protein (% total energy)	12	12	20

[a] Special emphasis given to soluble dietary fibre.
[b] This usually involves reducing total fat to below 25 g/day. Medium-chain triglycerides which are not transported in chyomicrons may be added if liver function is normal. Supplementary fat-soluble vitamins may be required.

risk of CHD, they do not have consistent effects on LDL and total cholesterol, except in high doses. Moderate doses may actually increase LDL-cholesterol. The safety of such preparations in large amounts has not been established, and it is therefore inappropriate to be advising large amounts of these fatty acids in concentrated form until requirements and safety have been established.

Garlic has been used for medicinal purposes since at least 1550 BC. It now seems that garlic can favourably influence several cardiovascular risk factors. Popular interest appears to be greatest in Germany, where garlic preparations have become the largest-selling over the counter 'drugs'. The extent to which garlic as a food or as a diet supplement might reduce cardiovascular disease has not been established.

For a long time, there have been conflicting reports about the association between coffee drinking, cholesterol levels and CHD. Evidence is emerging, however, which suggest that the hypercholesterolaemic effect of coffee may be related to the method of preparation. Boiled coffee, which is most frequently drunk in the Nordic countries, is more hypercholesterolaemic than coffee prepared in other ways. The lipid-containing supernatant of boiled coffee contains the diterpenoid compounds cafestol and kahweol which, fed as extracts, have a powerful effect in elevating total and LDL-cholesterol and triglyceride. The evidence is probably sufficiently strong to inquire about the coffee intake of people with elevated cholesterol levels and where appropriate to recommend a switch in the method of preparation. Instant coffee and filtered coffee do not contain the cholesterol-raising coffee diterpenes.

Another highly controversial issue relates to the effects of alcohol on cardiovascular disease. There is a considerable body of evidence to suggest that a modest intake of alcohol, especially red wine, has a protective effect against CHD, perhaps via a beneficial effect on HDL, fibrinogen and platelet activity, and/or because of the presence of dietary antioxidants. However, the sharp increase in mortality from cerebrovascular disease, cancer, accidents and violence, as well as total mortality associated with more than two drinks per day, suggests that public health recommendations that emphasized the positive health effects of alcohol would be likely to do more harm than good (see Chapter 6).

Given the complexity of the aetiology of CHD, it is quite conceivable that foods and nutrients other than those already extensively investigated will be found to have beneficial or deleterious effects. In view of the potentially powerful effects of advertising by those with vested interests, nutritionists have a critical role to play in the evaluation of, and public commentary on, new findings as well as in the implementation of tried and tested dietary recommendations.

18.2   HYPERTENSION: DIET AND BLOOD PRESSURE

Increasing levels of systolic and diastolic blood pressure are associated with increased rates of coronary heart disease (CHD), strokes (cerebral vascular diseases) and other vascular diseases. A number of dietary factors are associated with hypertension (see Table 18.8); some appear to be sufficiently important determinants of blood pressure that they can influence the increase in blood pressure which typically occurs with ageing in most Western countries. This section deals with the role of dietary factors in the aetiology and management of hypertension.

18.2.1   Salt and sodium

Over 30 years ago, Dahl drew attention to the correlation between salt intake and prevalence of hypertension in populations. This and other similar studies were flawed by methodological difficulties associated with measuring salt intake and blood pressure. Also, the association may not necessarily be causal because increased salt intake is associated with greater acculturation (generally expressed as degree of urbanization). Twenty-four hour urinary sodium excretion provides the best available method of assessing sodium intake. This method and standardized blood pressure measurements were used in the Intersalt study (first results published in 1988) which collected data on 10 000 people aged 20–59 years from 52 centres in 32 countries. Sodium excretion ranged from 0.2 mmol/24 hours among the Yanomamo Indians of Brazil, through around 150 mmol/24 hours in typical Western populations, to 242 mmol/24 hours in north China. The few populations with very low sodium excretion (under 50 mmol/24 h) had low median blood pressures, a low prevalence of hypertension and virtually no increase in blood pressure with age. In the remaining centres, sodium excretion was related to blood pressure levels in individuals, and influenced the extent to which blood pressure increased with age. The overall association between sodium excretion and median blood pressure or prevalence of

Table 18.8 Dietary factors related to blood pressure

Major
- *Salt/Sodium*
- *Body weight*
- *Alcohol*

Less significant/questionable
- Potassium
- Calcium
- Vegetarianism
- Fatty acids
- Caffeine
- Magnesium

hypertension was less striking and was not statistically significant when the four centres with very low sodium intakes were excluded.

There are several possible reasons why the Intersalt study (1988) might have underestimated the relationship between dietary sodium and blood pressure:

- inability of one urinary sodium estimation to measure usual intake;
- narrow range of mean intakes between populations;
- genetic variability;
- existence of a threshold intake (about 60–70 mmol/day) above which amount eaten may not matter;
- long-term rather than current intake may be important; and
- dietary sodium may be an enabling rather than causative factor.

Indeed a re-analysis of the data (published in 1996), taking into account the problem of regression dilution, showed a much more powerful association, so that a difference in sodium intake of 100 mmol/day over a 30-year period would be expected to result in differences of approximately 10 mmHg in systolic blood pressure and 6 mmHg in diastolic blood pressure.

In the light of these observations, the results of recent meta-analyses of observational data among and within populations are of particular interest. Law and colleagues analysed data from published reports of blood pressure and sodium intake for 24 different communities throughout the world, and 14 published studies that correlated blood pressure recordings in individuals against measurements of their 24 hour sodium intake. These analyses confirmed that the initial Intersalt data may have appreciably underestimated the association between blood pressure and sodium intake. For example, at age 60–90 years, the estimated systolic blood pressure reduction in response to a 100 mmol/day reduction in sodium intake was on average 10 mmHg, but varied from 6 mmHg for those on the 5th centile of blood pressure to 15 mmHg for those on the 95th centile.

The results of the intervention trials involving sodium restriction are equally interesting. Examination of the individual studies suggests inconsistent results, but once again Law and collaborators (1991) have aggregated the results of 68 crossover trials and 10 randomized controlled trials of dietary salt reduction. In people aged 50–59 years, a reduction of daily sodium intake of 50 mmol (about 3 g of salt), attainable by moderate dietary salt reduction, would, after a few weeks, lower systolic blood pressure by an average of 5 mmHg and by 7 mmHg in those with high blood pressure; diastolic blood pressure would be lowered by half as much. It is estimated that such a reduction in salt intake by a whole Western population would reduce the incidence of stroke by 26% and of CHD by 15%. Reduction also in the amount of salt added to processed foods would lower blood pressure by twice as much and could prevent as many as 70 000 deaths per year in Britain.

The heterogeneity in the response of individuals to sodium restriction suggests the possible existence of a group of hyper-responders, but there is as yet no clear indication as to how such individuals might be defined.

A fascinating study in a colony of chimpanzees, the species phylogenetically closest to humans, provides strong corroborative evidence concerning the role of sodium in the causation of human hypertension. Half the colony had salt within the typical human range of intakes added to their traditional fruit and vegetable diet (very low in sodium and high in potassium). The addition of salt over 20 months caused a highly significant rise in both systolic and diastolic blood pressure, the change being reversed completely by 6 months after the cessation of salt (Fig. 18.9). The effect of salt differed among individual chimpanzees, some having a large blood pressure rise and others small or no rise.

Several mechanisms have been suggested to explain the association between salt intake and blood pressure, including reduced urinary sodium excretion and fluid retention by some individuals, increased sympathetic nervous system activity and impaired baroreflex function, and alterations of ion transport in vascular smooth muscle.

Despite the overwhelming evidence for the relationship between salt intake and blood pressure, the Salt Institute, the trade organization of salt producers, continues to question the validity of the scientific data. Their arguments have received negligible support among the scientific community which considers that their poorly justified case continues to be made because of commercial considerations.

18.2.2 Body weight

Obese people have higher blood pressures than lean people and if they lose weight their blood pressure falls even if usual salt intake is maintained on the restricted diet. Raised blood pressure is particularly associated with obesity which is centrally rather than peripherally distributed. The Intersalt study showed a highly significant correlation between body mass index as an index of obesity and blood pressure. An Australian trial showed in a clinical trial setting, that dietary weight reduction (mean loss of 7.4 kg) compared favourably with a standard beta blocker drug, metoprolol, in the treatment of mild hypertension and diet was associated with an improvement in the lipid profile which was not seen on the drug.

18.2.3 Alcohol

In epidemiological studies, blood pressure increases progressively when reported alcohol intake increases above three drinks per day. Several intervention studies have shown that reduction of alcohol intake can produce an appreciable reduction in blood pressure amongst hypertensive heavy drinkers. For example, one study showed that replacing

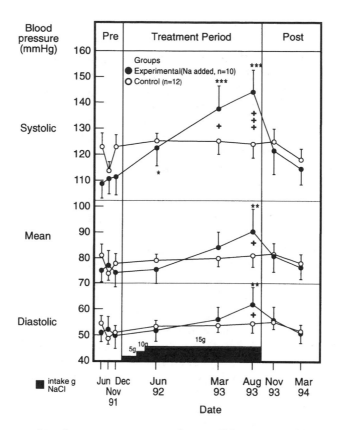

Fig. 18.9 A group of 22 chimpanzees maintained in small long-term stable social groups and fed a vegetable-fruit diet with addition of infant formula as a calorie, protein, calcium and vitamin supplement. Twelve control animals (○) had no change of conditions over 2.4 years and no significant change of systolic, diastolic or mean blood pressure (mean ± s.e.m.). Ten experimental animals (●) had 5 g/day of NaCl added to infant formula for 19 weeks, 10 g/day for 3 weeks, and then 15 g/day for 67 weeks. A 20-week period without salt addition followed. Increase of blood pressure relative to mean of the three baseline determinations (*$P<0.05$, **$P<0.01$, ***$P<0.001$), and experimental group vs. control group (+$P<0.05$, +++$P<0.001$). *Source*: Denton D, *et al*. (1995).

standard beer (5% alcohol) with a reduced alcohol beer (0.9% alcohol) produced a reduction in alcohol intake from 450–64 ml/week and a significant fall in blood pressure.

18.2.4 Potassium

In the Intersalt Study, urinary potassium excretion, an assumed indicator of intake, was negatively related to blood pressure. A pooled analysis of a number of intervention trials suggests that potassium supplementation might reduce blood pressure in both normotensive and hypertensive people by an average 5.9–3.4 mmHg. However, several limitations reduce the applicability of increasing potassium intake as a means of treating hypertension. The effect of potassium appears to be relatively small when sodium intake is reduced. The amount of potassium required to reduce blood pressure is relatively high so that supplements rather than dietary modification would be necessary. No foods contain sufficient to provide the increase in intake achieved in the trials—between 50 and 140 mmol potassium per day.

18.2.5 Calcium

Intracellular calcium is an important determinant of arteriolar tone and some claims have been made that increased calcium intake can reduce blood pressure. However two meta-analyses summarizing the results of more than 20 trials suggest that 1000 mg or more of calcium per day have only a trivial effect on blood pressure levels. Calcium supplements or a high calcium diet might be useful in a very small number of hypertensive patients who have low serum calcium levels or increased plasma parathyroid levels.

18.2.6 Vegetarianism

Vegetarians have lower levels of blood pressure than meat eaters. A series of carefully controlled studies from Perth, Western Australia, have shown that significant reductions in systolic and diastolic pressures occur when healthy subjects are changed from a typical Western diet to a vegetarian diet and salt intake is kept constant (Fig. 18.10). In addition to excluding meat and fish, vegetarian diets provide less saturated fat and cholesterol, and more unsaturated fat, complex carbohydrate and dietary fibre. Also, various differences exist with regard to micronutrients as well as in other biologically active substances in

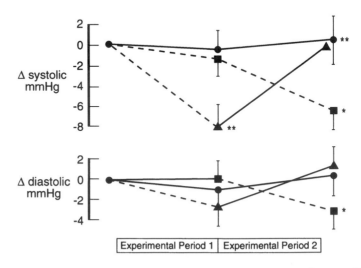

Fig. 18.10 Changes in systolic and diastolic blood pressure in a control group (●) who made no dietary changes throughout the study, and groups randomized to receive either a control (■) or vegetarian (▲) diet and then crossed over to the alternative dietary regime. The broken line represents the period in the vegetarian diet and unbroken line, the control period. *Source*: Beilin, *et al.* (1988).

plant foods (see Chapter 15) when compared with a more usual diet. A recent study has shown the blood pressure lowering potential of increasing fruit and vegetables but more research will be required to disentangle which aspects of the vegetarian diet are particularly relevant in the effect on blood pressure.

18.2.7 Other minor factors

A dietary crossover study in Finland suggested that polyunsaturated fatty acids might reduce blood pressure levels. However, the experimental diet in that study involved several dietary differences when compared with the control diet. Caffeine and magnesium have also been suggested as determinants of blood pressure, but their effect is usually negligible.

18.2.8 Nutritional recommendations aimed at reducing blood pressure levels

Achieving optimal body weight, avoiding excessive intakes of alcohol and taking regular exercise are general health measures likely to reduce blood pressure levels in populations prone to hypertension as well as reducing elevated blood pressure levels in those who already have established disease.

Specific recommendations aimed at hypertension centre chiefly around intake of dietary sodium and salt. Most authorities suggest that the general public should be advised to have intakes below 100 mmol of sodium or 6 g/day sodium chloride. Modest reductions of sodium will not have a major impact on elevated blood pressure levels in individuals but clinically useful reductions are likely to be achieved if intakes are below 50 mmol/day. It is important to appreciate that reducing discretionary salt intake (i.e. salt added at table or in cooking) is insufficient, since in Western countries most of the salt in the diet comes from that added to natural food during processing. For example, most breads have 180 times the salt content of white flour. There is insufficient evidence concerning the other nutritional determinants of blood pressure to offer recommendations for the population at large or for individual patients.

FURTHER READING

1. Ascherio A, Rimm EB, Giovannucci EL, *et al.* Dietary fat and risk of coronary heart disease in men: cohort follow up study in the United States. *BMJ* 1996; **313**: 84–90.
2. Beilin LJ, Rouse IL, Armstrong BK, *et al.* Vegetarian diet and blood pressure levels: incidental or causal association? *Am J Clin Nutr* 1988; **48**: 806–10.
3. Bronte Stewart B, Antonio A, Eales L, Brock JF. Effects of feeding different fats on serum cholesterol level. *Lancet* 1956; **1**: 521–7.
4. de Logeril M, Renaud S, Mamelle N, Salen P, Martin J, Monjaud I, *et al.* Mediterranean alpha-linolenic acid-rich diet in secondary prevention of coronary heart disease. *Lancet* 1994; **343**: 1454–9.
5. Denton D, Weisinger R, Mundy NI, *et al.* The effect of increased salt intake on blood pressure of chimpanzees. *Nature Med* 1995; **1**: 1009–16.

6. Gey KF, Moser UK, Jordan P, *et al.* Increased risk of cardiovascular disease in suboptimal plasma concentrations of essential antioxidants: an epidemiological update with special attention to carotene and vitamin C. *Am J Clin Nutr* 1993; **57** (suppl.): 787S–97S.

7. Hertog MGL, Feskens EJM, Hollman PCH, Katan MB, Kromhout D. Dietary antioxidant flavonoids and risk of coronary heart disease. *Lancet* 1993; **342**: 1007–17.

8. Intersalt Co-operative Research Group. Intersalt: An international study of electrolyte excretion and blood pressure. Results for 24-hour urinary sodium and potassium excretion. *BMJ* 1988; **297**: 319–28.

9. Keys A. *Seven countries: a multivariate analysis of death and coronary heart disease.* Cambridge, MA: Harvard University Press, 1980.

10. Kohlmeier L, Hastings SB. Epidemiological evidence of a role of carotenoids in cardiovascular disease prevention. *Am J Clin Nutr* 1995; **62** (suppl.): 1370S–6S.

11. Law MR, Frost CD, Wald NJ. By how much does dietary salt reduction lower blood pressure? I. Analysis of observational data among populations. *BMJ* 1991; **302**: 811–5.

12. Law MR, Frost CD, Wald NJ. By how much does dietary salt reduction lower blood pressure? III. Analysis of data from trials of salt reduction. *BMJ* 1991; **302**: 819–24.

13. Lewis B, Mann JI, Mancini M. Reducing the risks of coronary heart disease in individuals and in the population. *Lancet* 1986; **i**: 956–9.

14. Mensink RP, Katan MB. Effect of dietary fatty acids on serum lipids and lipoproteins. A meta analysis on 27 trials. *Arterioscler Thromb* 1992; **12**: 911–9.

15. Nestel PJ, Noakes M, Belling GB, McArthur R, Clifton PM, Janus E, *et al.* Plasma lipoprotein lipid and Lp(a) changes with substitution of elaidic acid for oleic acid in the diet. *J Lipid Res* 1992; **33**: 1029–36.

16. Stampfer MJ, Malinov MR. Can lowering homocysteine levels reduce cardiovascular risk. *N Engl J Med* 1995; **332**: 328–9.

17. The WHO MONICA Project. Geographical variation in the major risk factors of coronary heart disease in men and women aged 35–64 years. *Wld Hlth Stat Quart* 1998; **41**: 115–40.

18. Thorogood M, Mann J, Appleby P, McPherson K. Risk of death from cancer and ischaemic heart disease in meat and non-meat eaters. *BMJ* 1994; **308**: 1667–71.

19. Tyroler HA. Review of lipid-lowering clinical trials in relation to observational epidemiological studies. *Circulation* 1987; **76**: 515–22.

20. Truswell AS. Review of dietary intervention studies: effect on coronary events and on total mortality. *Aust NZ J Med* 1994; **24**: 98–106.

21. World Health Organization, Expert Committee. *Prevention of coronary heart disease.* Technical Report Series. Geneva: WHO, 1982.

Appendix

Table 18.7 Guidelines for a lipid-lowering diet

Advisable	May be eaten in moderation	Should be avoided
Fats		
All fats should be limited to a minimum unless otherwise directed.	Equivalent to 5 g fat 1 tsp polyunsaturated margarine, monounsaturated margarine, 1 tsp of the following oils: safflower, soybean, sunflower, corn, wheatgerm, grapeseed, sesame, walnut, olive, rapeseed, peanut. 2 tsp low fat mono- or polyunsaturated spreads.	Butter, dripping, suet, lard, palm oil, coconut oil. Margarines not labelled poly- or monounsaturated. Cooking or vegetable oils of unknown origin. Hydrogenated fats and oils.
Meats		
Average serving 150–200 g Mixed light and dark poultry meat (skinned turkey, veal, chicken, game).	Not more than 100–250 g (cooked weight) 3–5 times a week: lean beef, lamb, pork, steak mince. Average serving liver or kidneys once a fortnight.	Visible fat on meat (including crackling), belly pork, streaky bacon, salami, pate, scotch eggs, duck, goose, pork pies, poultry skin. Sausages and luncheon meat, fried meats, rolled roasts, pressed meats.
Eggs and dairy foods		
Low fat (less than 1% fat) milk, skimmed milk, cottage cheese, low fat quarg, curd, cheese, egg white, low fat yoghurt.	Semi-skimmed 1.5% and 2% fat milk, medium fat cheeses, i.e. those with 24% total fat (45% fat content in dry matter) or less, e.g. Brie, Edam, Camembert, Mozarella. Special processed and Blue (12–13% fat) cheeses 2–4 egg yolks per week including those in cooking and baking.	Full cream milk, evaporated or condensed milk, cream, imitation cream. Full fat cheeses, e.g. Stilton, Cheddar, Cheshire, full fat blue cheeses, cream cheeses, full fat yoghurt.

Table 18.7   (*Continued*)

Advisable	May be eaten in moderation	Should be avoided
Fish		
All white fish, e.g. cod, sole, ling. Oily fish, e.g. herring, mackerel, salmon, sardines. (If possible eat 200–400 g oily fish twice per week.)	Fish fried in suitable oil (oil should not be heated to smoke point or re-used) once per fortnight, avoid using fat in cooking if on a weight-reducing diet. Mussels, oyster, scallops, clams.	Fish roe, shrimps, squid.
Fruit and vegetables		
All fresh and plain frozen vegetables. Peas, beans of all kinds, e.g. haricot, red kidney, butter beans, lentils, chick peas are particularly high in 'soluble fibre' and should be eaten regularly. Jacket or boiled potatoes, eat skins wherever possible. Fresh fruit, dried fruit, unsweetened tinned fruit.	Chips and roast potatoes if cooked in suitable oil. Avocado pears, olives, fruit in syrup, crystallized fruit (restrict the latter two items if triglycerides raised) and avoid all of the above if following a weight-reducing diet.	Chips or roast potatoes cooked in unsuitable fat or oil. Oven chips, potato crisps.
Cereal foods		
Wholemeal flour, wholemeal and especially wholegrain bread, whole grain cereals, oatmeal, cornmeal, porridge oats, sweetcorn, whole grain rice and wholemeal pasta, crispbreads, oatcakes. Low fat crackers.	White flour, white bread, sugary breakfast cereals, commercial muesli, white rice and pasta, plain semi-sweet biscuits, higher fat crackers.	Fancy breads, croissants, brioches, savoury cheese biscuits, bought pastry. Egg noodles, pasta made with eggs.
Madeup dishes		
Low fat puddings, e.g. jelly, sorbet, skimmed milk puddings, low fat yoghurt, low fat sauces.	Cakes, pastry, puddings, biscuits and sauces made with suitable margarine or oil. Low fat or soya-based ice cream. If triglycerides are raised or if following a weight-reducing diet, choose foods mainly from the 'Advisable' column.	Cakes and pastry, puddings and biscuits made with saturated fats. Suet dumplings and puddings, butter and cream sauces. Deep-fried snacks, dairy ice cream.

Table 18.7 (*Continued*)

Advisable	May be eaten in moderation	Should be avoided
Drinks Tea, instant coffee, mineral water, slimline or sugar free soft drinks, unsweetened fruit juice. Clear soups, homemade vegetable soup. Low alcohol beer.	Sweet soft drinks, low fat malted drinks or low fat drinking chocolate and fortified chocolate drinks occasionally. Meat soups, packet soups (avoid if on low salt diet). Alcohol (no more than 1–2 drinks for women, 2–3 drinks for men). Avoid alcohol and sugary drinks if triglycerides raised or if following a weight-reducing diet.	Irish coffee, Irish Cream (a flavouring syrup), full fat malted milk drinks, drinking chocolate, boiled coffee, cream soups.
Sweets, preserves, spreads Unless on a lower salt diet clear pickles, yeast extracts, savoury soup cubes. If on a weight-reduction diet sugar-free sweeteners, e.g. saccharine tablets or liquid, aspartame sweeteners tablets or powder, cyclamate sweeteners-liquid or tablets.	Sweet pickles and chutney, jam, honey, marmalade, syrup, marzipan, lemon curd (made without eggs and butter), boiled sweets, pastilles, sugar, peppermints, wine gums. If triglycerides are raised or if following a weight-reducing diet choose foods mainly from the 'Advisable' column.	Chocolate spreads, mincemeat containing suet. Toffees, fudge, butterscotch, chocolate, coconut bars.
Nuts and seeds	Peanuts, walnuts, almonds, Brazil nuts, hazelnuts, cashews, sunflower seeds, pumpkin seeds, linseed.	Coconut
Miscellaneous Herbs, spices, mustard, pepper, vinegar, Worcester sauce, soy sauce, low fat dressings, e.g. lemon or low fat yoghurt.	Meat and fish pastes. Low calorie salad cream or low calorie mayonnaise bottled sauces. French dressing. If on a weight-reducing diet choose foods mainly from the 'Advisable' column.	Ordinary salad cream, mayonnaise, cream or cream cheese dressings.

Table prepared by Alex Chisholm, Research Dietitian, Department of Human Nutrition, University of Otago, Dunedin, New Zealand.

19
DIET AND CANCER CAUSATION

Sheila Bingham

19.1 GENERAL ASPECTS

19.1.1 Epidemiology

Cancer accounts for about 20% of all deaths in developed countries and is the second most common cause of death after diseases of the circulatory system. The commonest sites of cancer are shown in Table 19.1. Risks of cancer increase with age at virtually all sites, Fig. 19.1 shows rates for bowel, breast, pancreas and prostate cancer at different ages in men and women in England and Wales. There are up to 100-fold variations in the age-standardized incidence rates of some cancers between different geographical areas, e.g. cancer of the skin and of the nasopharynx. Cancer of the colon varies 20-fold (highest United States, lowest India) and of the breast 7-fold (highest United States Hawaiian, lowest Israel non-Jews). Figure 19.2 shows the trends in large bowel cancer incidence in the United Kingdom and in Japan. The rate of bowel cancer is now almost as high in Japan as in the United Kingdom whereas it was virtually unknown in Japan as recently as 30 years ago. The rapidly changing rates over time for some cancers and the fact that migrants acquire the cancer pattern of the host country within a relatively short period of time (e.g. within a single generation for bowel cancer) suggest that much of this variation is due to environmental rather than genetic factors.

Table 19.1 Common sites of cancer (listed in rank order) in developed and developing countries*

Developed countries	Developing countries
Lung	Cervix
Large bowel	Stomach
Breast	Mouth
Stomach	Oesophagus
Prostate	Breast
Bladder	Lung

*Skin cancers are not included because of difficulties involved in estimating incidence. The most serious of these, malignant melanoma, is more common in some countries, especially where fair-skinned people have a high exposure to sunlight (e.g. Australia, New Zealand and South Africa).

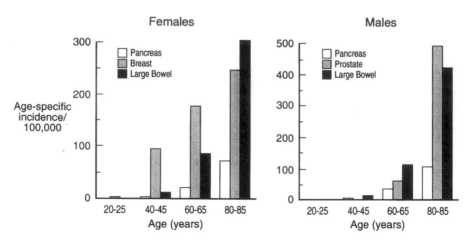

Fig. 19.1 Incidence rates, by age, for different cancers in men and women in England and Wales during the years 1983–87. *Source*: Parkin DM, Muir CS, Whelan SL, Gao YT, Ferlay J, Powell J. *Cancer incidence in five continents*. Vol I–VI. Lyon: IARC, 1992.

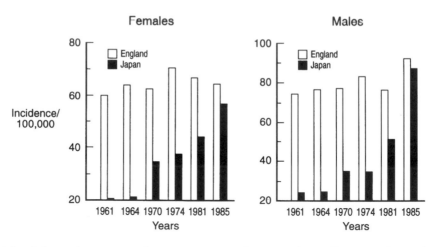

Fig. 19.2 Colorectal cancer incidence in women and men aged 55–60 years in Japan (Miyagi) and England (Birmingham). *Source*: Parkin DM, Muir CS, Whelan SL, Gao YT, Ferlay J, Powell J. *Cancer incidence in five continents*. Vol I–VI. Lyon: IARC, 1992.

19.1.2 Molecular biology of cancer

The development of cancer involves a number of stages, outlined in Fig. 19.3, and generally occurs over a long period of time. The first stage involves damage to the DNA of the healthy cell, either by chance mutation or by some extraneous chemical or radiation. If the DNA is not repaired before the cell divides the mutation is passed on to all subsequent daughter cells, which are said to be initiated. The initiation phase of

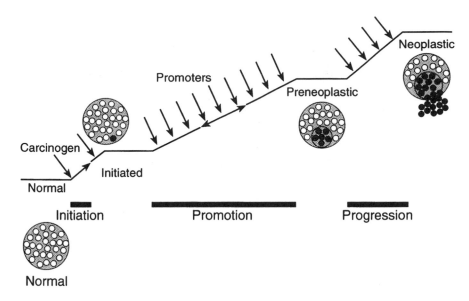

Fig. 19.3   Stages in the development of cancer (see text).

carcinogenesis is short and irreversible. Avoidance of carcinogens, dietary or otherwise, is the best method of prevention at this stage. During the next phase, the promotion phase, initiated cells are exposed to environmental factors (i.e. promoters) that create conditions which can favour initiated cell growth over that of normal cells. Further genetic mutations to genes in the initiated cells that control cell division and differentiation (i.e. oncogenes and tumour suppressor genes) lead to preneoplastic cells that look and function differently from the normal cells that surround them. The promotion phase may be as long as several decades and can be accelerated or slowed down by environmental factors. The role of diet in cancer prevention is most important during this phase of carcinogenesis. The progression phase is characterized by additional mutation in the DNA of preneoplastic cells causing them to be transformed into neoplastic cells that exhibit uninhibited growth. The progression phase may be months to a few years in duration. Diet does not appear to have a great impact during this late phase of carcinogenesis and successful treatment usually requires a combination of surgery, radio- or chemotherapy.

19.1.3   Factors causing cancer

Table 19.2 outlines the many different factors which have been implicated in the development of cancer. The role of diet has been studied in animal models and using the whole range of epidemiological approaches, including ecological and analytical epidemiological studies. Using mainly comparisons between countries, in 1981, Doll and Peto suggested that, on average, 35% of all cancers in the United States are due to diet, but the statistical confidence intervals around this estimate are wide (10–70%). Dietary intervention studies provide the ultimate epidemiological tests of causality, but lengthy, large and immensely costly studies to alter dietary habits would be necessary. As a result,

Table 19.2 Causes of cancer

Genetic
Environmental
• Natural and synthetic chemicals (e.g. workplace, pollution)
• Tobacco smoking, alcohol
• Diet and nutrition
• Infectious agents (e.g. viruses)
• Endogenous and exogenous hormones
• Radiation (UV, nuclear)

no major studies of intervention with diet have been published, although a number of trials with supplements, especially β-carotene and vitamin E, have been conducted. A large-scale initiative of the effect of altering fat intake on breast cancer risk, estimated to cost several hundred million dollars is currently under way in the United States.

This chapter deals principally with the role of diet in the development and prevention of cancer. Dietary treatments intended to suppress the spread of established cancer and influence survival have been widely recommended despite inadequate investigation. They are not discussed here and any benefit of their use is at present uncertain. Cancers at most of the major sites have some link with diet and several dietary factors are associated with cancer at more than one site. Established and possible dietary factors related to cancer at various sites are discussed below, according to their order in the International Statistical Classification of Diseases, Injuries and Causes of Death (ICD). Table 19.3 gives an overview of dietary factors implicated in the cause or prevention of different cancers.

19.2 MOUTH AND PHARYNX

19.2.1 Epidemiology

Mouth and pharyngeal cancers account for about 6% of cancer world-wide and are more common in developing than developed countries. In China and South East Asia the majority of cancers in this group are in the nasopharynx, whereas in India most are in the mouth and tongue. Tobacco and alcohol consumption increase the risk at all sites and there are multiplicative effects for those who drink and smoke. For example, a combination of smoking 16–25 cigarettes and drinking 80–120 g alcohol per day is associated with a 48-fold increase in risk for pharyngeal cancer. Associations between individual foods and cancers at specific sites have also been noted (e.g. salted fish consumption with nasopharyngeal cancer, and betel nut chewing with oral cancer).

There is limited evidence suggesting a protective role for fruit and possibly vegetables in this group of cancers. Intervention trials are in progress with β-carotene, retinol and retinoids in patients with oral leukoplakia, a potential precursor lesion of oral cancer. Some beneficial results have been reported.

Table 19.3 Dietary and nutritional factors that may play a role in human cancers

Factor	Cause + Prevent −	Cancers
Dietary fat	+	Colorectal, breast, prostate, pancreas
ω3-PUFA*	−	Colorectal, breast
ω6-PUFA	+	Prostate, breast, ovary (endocrine-related)
Fish oils	−	Colorectal, breast
Obesity	+	Colorectal, oesophagus, breast, endometrium, gallbladder
Exercise, lack of	+	Colorectal
Meat	+	Colorectal, breast
Protein	+	Colorectal, pancreas, breast, prostate
Soy	−	Breast
Grilled, fried meat	+	Colon
Salt	+	Stomach
Salted foods	+	Stomach, colorectal
Pickled, 'processed' foods	+	Stomach, nasopharyngeal
Mouldy foods (e.g. aflatoxin)	+	Oesophagus, stomach, liver
Sugar	+	Breast, pancreas
Iron	+	Colorectal
Calcium	−	Colorectal
Milk	−	Oesophagus, stomach
Folic acid	−	Cervix, colorectal
Nitrates	+	Stomach
Alcohol	+	Liver, pancreas, oesophagus, colorectal, head and neck, mouth, stomach, breast
Fruits, vegetables	−	Epithelial cancers, especially respiratory and
Antioxidants: selenium vitamins C, E, retinoids (Vitamin A), β-carotene, carotenoids (lycopene, lutein)	−	alimentary tracts: lung, nasopharyngx, oesophagus, stomach, colorectal, mouth, pancreas, breast, bladder, cervix, prostate
Non-nutritive plant chemicals: gluycosinolates, indoles, flavonoids, sulphur-compounds	−/+	Digestive tract
Dietary fibre, non-starch polysaccharides	−	Colorectal
Resistant starch	−	Colorectal
Plant sterols	−	Breast, prostate, hormone-dependent

The evidence for many of the relationships is not yet conclusive; this list is not exhaustive.
* PUFA, polyunsaturated fatty acids.

19.2.2 Mechanisms

The mechanism for the effect of alcohol on cancer is unknown. Alcohol is not a direct carcinogen although alcoholic drinks contain hundreds of different compounds including aldehydes and N-nitroso compounds, some of which are known to be carcinogenic. Acetaldehyde, the main metabolic product, has been shown to be carcinogenic in animal studies, but only when inhaled and administered in high concentrations.

Retinol is well known to control cellular differentiation and proliferation, and some of the beneficial effects in intervention trials may have been due to replenishment or sparing of vitamin A in individuals who were deficient (e.g. in Indian tobacco chewers). In well-nourished populations, postulated effects of β-carotene are attributed to a non-specific antioxidant action. However, there has been little consistent investigation of a direct link between oxidative stress, antioxidant status, and the type of DNA damage in patients with cancer at these sites (Box 19.1).

Box 19.1 Causes of mouth and pharyngeal cancers

Established non-dietary
- Tobacco and betel nut chewing
- Tobacco smoking

Probable non-dietary
- Smoke and fumes (nasopharyngeal)
- Epstein–Barr virus infection (nasopharyngeal)

Established food and drink
- Alcohol

Probable food and drink
- Low fruit
- Low vegetables
- Salted fish (nasopharyngeal)

19.3 OESOPHAGUS

19.3.1 Epidemiology

The aetiology of oesophageal cancer seems to vary according to nutritional status. In well-nourished populations, the most important risk factors are alcohol and smoking. The Calvados region of France has a particularly high age standardized incidence of this cancer. There are three to eightfold increases in risk in individuals who consume 40–100 g alcohol per day and there are multiplicative effects with smoking. These two factors seem to account for the great majority of cases of squamous cell carcinoma, the commonest type of cancer of the oesophagus in Western countries. In developed countries adenocarcinoma is a less common form of cancer of the oesophagus, but its incidence is increasing and the condition appears to be associated with obesity as well as alcohol and smoking. Increasing rates of obesity might explain the increasing rates of this tumour. The effect of obesity may be mediated via increased gastrooesophageal

Box 19.2   Causes of oesophageal cancer

Established non-dietary
- Tobacco smoking

Probable non-dietary
- Opium use
- Very hot drinks

Established food and drink
- Alcohol

Probable food and drink
- Poor nutritional status
- Toxins of *Fusarium moniliforme* (e.g. fumonisins B-1, B-2, fusarin C)
- Obesity
- Low fruit and vegetables

reflux associated with overweight. This is known to be a risk factor for a precursor lesion, Barretts metaplasia. In well-nourished populations, case-control studies suggest that fruit and vegetables may be protective, with low consumers having on average a twofold increase in risk compared with high consumers (Box 19.2).

In less well-nourished countries, a diet restricted in fruit and vegetables seems to be a particularly important risk factor. In the Caspian region of Iran and Linxian county in China, which have very high rates, nutrient deficiencies are common and alcohol and cigarettes are consumed in moderation. A large intervention trial of four combinations of vitamins and minerals in 30 000 adults in Linxian showed no reduction in oesophageal cancer rates, but this could be explained by the general improvement in nutritional status of the non-supplemented group. In a third area where this cancer is very common, the Transkei in South Africa, contamination of poorly-stored maize by toxins from the fungus *Fusarium*, in the presence of deficiencies of B vitamins, may be an important causative factor.

19.4   STOMACH

19.4.1   Epidemiology

Stomach cancer was the most common cancer in the world in 1980, although rates have been steadily decreasing almost everywhere by about 2% every year. There is a 20-fold difference between the highest rates in Japan, and the lowest in The Gambia and Kuwait. Rates in men are about double those in women. High salt consumption bas been proposed as a causative factor but the most consistent link with diet is the protective effect of fruit and vegetables. Case-control studies demonstrate a substantial reduction in risk in individuals who consume higher amounts of fruits and vegetables. There are fewer prospective data, but daily consumption of these foods has been associated with a halving of risk of stomach cancer as compared with infrequent consumption. Smoking, but not alcohol are causally associated with stomach cancer.

315

19.4.2 Mechanisms

Stomach cancer is a progressive disease; initially there is chronic gastritis progressing to atropic gastritis, then metaplasia and carcinoma. Various risk factors have been implicated at one or more of these stages, including high salt intakes and infection with *Helicobactor pylori*, which has been classified as a class I carcinogen by the International Agency for Research on Cancer (IARC). It is suggested that chronic infection with this organism results in a chronic inflammatory response, excessive free radical production and DNA damage leading to carcinoma. As vegetables are sources of the antioxidants vitamin C, carotenoids and vitamin E this may account for their protective effect. An older hypothesis involves the formation of carcinogenic N-nitroso compounds (NOC) in the stomach. These are formed in the presence of nitrite which arises from ingested nitrate, for example in water. More recent evidence suggests that ingested nitrate is unimportant, since people living in areas of high nitrate intake are not at increased risk of stomach cancer and it is now known that substantial amounts of nitrite and nitrate are produced endogenously. Surprisingly, no significant protective effects of vitamin C in stomach cancer were shown in the large Linxian intervention trial referred to above (Section 19.3), but once again it seems likely that vitamin C status was improving even in the non-supplemented group during the course of the study. Combinations of β-carotene, vitamin E and selenium supplements significantly reduced stomach cancer death rates in this study. However, there was no effect of vitamin E and β-carotene in a trial of Finnish smokers (Box 19.3).

Box 19.3   Causes of stomach cancer

Established non-dietary
- *Helicobacter pylori* infection
- Smoking

Probable food and drink
- Low fruit and vegetable consumption
- Salted and preserved foods
- Low vitamin C consumption

19.5   LARGE BOWEL (COLORECTAL)

19.5.1   Epidemiology

Colorectal (large bowel) cancers are the second most common cancer in Western societies, affecting up to 6% of men and women by the age of 75 years. Risks increase markedly with age but there remains at least a 15-fold range in age standardized incidence throughout the world. Countries with the highest rates include the United States, parts of Northern Europe, Australia and New Zealand, and those with the lowest rates include China, India and many African countries. Internationally, there are strong positive associations between fat and meat consumption and large bowel cancer. There are also negative (protective) associations with starch and dietary fibre (non-starch polysaccharide, NSP). Within Western populations, vegetarians are at lower risk than meat eaters

Box 19.4   Causes of large bowel cancer

Established non-dietary
• Genetic mutations
Probable non-dietary
• P450 enzyme genotypic variation
• Lack of exercise
Established food and drink
• Low dietary fibre (non-starch polysaccharide) consumption
• Low vegetable consumption
• Obesity in men
Probable food and drink
• High red and processed meat
• High fat consumption

---

and in the United Kingdom regional differences in colorectal cancer mortality are very strongly related to consumption of vegetables, excluding potatoes (Box 19.4).

About 30 case-control studies in Western countries have generated results which are broadly similar to those of between countries studies: a relatively high intake of meat, protein and fat is associated with an increased risk, whereas those with high intakes of vegetables or dietay fibre-containing foods have approximately half the risk of large bowel cancer compared with those with lower intakes. The IARC estimates of attributable population risk suggest that 25–35% of all colorectal cancers might be attributed to low intakes of vegetables and NSP and 15–25% of these cancers to high fat intakes. Protective effects of vegetables and dietary fibre have been confirmed in cohort studies, as has the risk associated with 'red' or processed meat and total fat intake, although Fig. 19.4 shows that the estimates of relative risk are quite weak. Studies have also shown that a relatively high energy expenditure at work or during leisure time is protective, but this may be because active people eat more food and thus more fibre (NSP). Overweight men are at increased risk of colorectal cancers.

19.5.2   Mechanisms

The molecular biology of colorectal cancer is probably the best worked out of all cancers; Fig. 19.5 shows the current model for the genetic processes involved. Most large bowel cancers are thought to arise from dietary causes which act at various stages in this model. At least 10 different dietary factors have been linked with promoting or preventing colorectal cancers, as outlined in Box 19.5. Several intervention studies have been undertaken to examine whether antioxidant vitamins are responsible for the protective effect of vegetables by treating high-risk individuals (e.g. those with familial adenomatous polyposis) with a range of nutrient supplements. The studies reported to date have shown no benefit, in terms of reducing the risk of polyp recurrence or subsequent large bowel cancer, from taking the antioxidant nutrients, β-carotene, vitamin C or vitamin E as supplements.

However, there are many other constituents of plants which could be of more relevance to colorectal cancer than these vitamins. Flavonoids, other carotenoids, including

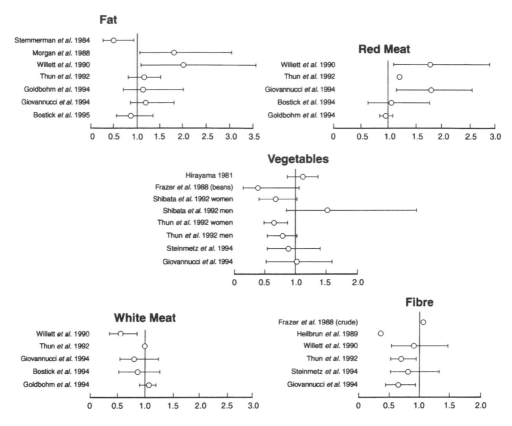

Fig. 19.4 Relative risks for colon cancer and confidence intervals for the highest versus the lowest quartile of fat, meat, fibre and vegetable consumption in prospective studies. Lines show relative risk with mean and 95% confidence interval. *Source*: Bingham S. Epidemiology and mechanisms relating diet to risk of colorectal cancer. *Nutr Res Rev* 1996; 9: 197–239.

lycopene and lutein, and glycosinolates (in brassicas) and other sulphur-containing compounds (in the onion family) are strong candidates. Several of these compounds can stimulate enzymes thought to facilitate the metabolism of potential carcinogens. Vegetables are also a major source of folate, a critical factor in DNA repair.

The high dietary fibre content of many vegetables probably explains much of their protective effect against colon cancer. Fibre (NSP) and other carbohydrate, such as resistant starch, stimulate anaerobic fermentation in the flora when they enter the large bowel. This leads to the production of the short-chain fatty acids (SCFA), acetate, propionate and butyrate, gas, and an increase in microbial cell mass. The stimulation of bacterial growth, together with the binding of water to residual unfermented polysaccharide, leads to an increase in stool weight, dilution of colonic contents and faster transit time through the large gut. This may reduce contact of genotoxins with mucosal cells. Supplements of bran have been found to reduce faecal mutagenicity. Constipation increases risk for colorectal cancer whereas there is a strong inverse association between high stool weight and colorectal cancer incidence. Low stool weight is associated with

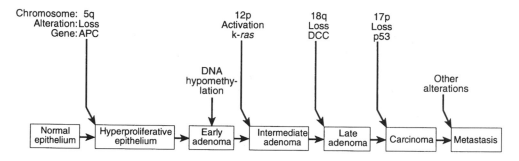

Fig. 19.5 Genetic model for colorectal cancer. The chromosome alterations and the genes involved at each of the stages of progression from normal colonic epithelium through to adenoma, then carcinoma are shown. By the adenoma stage, at least two alterations (loss of the APC gene and activation of the k-*ras* gene) will have occurred and by the carcinoma stage at least five alterations will be present including the loss of tumour suppressing gene p53 in chromosome 17. *Source*: Adapted from Fearon FR, Vogelstein B. A genetic model for colorectal tumorigenesis. *Cell* 1990; **61**: 759–67.

Box 19.5 Diet-related factors in large bowel cancer causation

---

Established
- Low stool weight and constipation from diets containing small amounts of plant polysaccharides

Probable
- Lack of butyrate from diets containing small amounts of plant polysaccharides
- N-nitroso compound formation from high meat diets
- Heterocyclic amines formed in cooked meat
- High colonic levels of ammonia from high meat diets
- High secondary bile acids from high stool pH due to diets low in plant polysaccharides

Possible
- Interference with DNA repair from low folate status
- High iron status initiating free radical reactions
- Low plant constituents such as glucosinolates and flavonoids
- Low intake of ω3-fatty acids

---

bowel disease. The relationship between dietary fibre consumption and stool weight is linear with a 5 g increase for every 1 g of NSP consumed. This is the basis for the United Kingdom and WHO recommendations for population average intake of 18 g NSP per day. This will only be met by an increase of 50% in the fibre intake of the United Kingdom and most Western populations.

Formation of the SCFA may also be important since these are nutrient sources for the colonic mucosa, particularly butyrate. Butyrate is an antiproliferative and differentiation agent, and relatively greater amounts of it are produced from starch than from NSP in fermentation studies. It has been suggested that butyrate induces apoptosis (programmed cell death), which may account for its role in reducing proliferation. The ability of supplements of resistant starch to prevent recurrence of colorectal polyps in familial adenomatous polyposis patients is currently under trial in a European collaborative trial (the CAPP study).

Fermentation and production of SCFA may also interact with high fat diets in protecting against colon cancer, since the fall in pH associated with the production of SCFA inhibits the production of the secondary bile acid, deoxycholic acid, which can promote bowel cancer in rodents by several different mechanisms. It has also been suggested that the damage to the colonic mucosa, caused by bile acids and high levels of free fatty acids associated with a high fat intake, can also be reduced by high intake of calcium which forms insoluble soaps in the colon, thus neutralizing bile acids and fatty acids. Experimental studies suggest that 1.5–2 g of calcium per day may be required for such protection, more than is normally obtained from food. Several intervention trials with these large doses of calcium have been started.

The type of fat may also be important. Supplements of fish oils have been shown to reduce rectal cell proliferation rates when compared with olive oil. This might be the result of the antiinflammatory action of the eicosanoid derivatives of ω3-fatty acids.

Nitrogenous residues from meat enter the colon, and high meat diets induce an increase in colonic ammonia levels. Ammonia enhances cell proliferation and is a promoter of carcinomas in rodents. Amines and amides are also produced by bacterial decarboxylation of amino acids. In the presence of a nitrosating agent, these can be N-nitrosated to a variety of N-nitroso compounds (NOC). In humans, a three- to fourfold increase in protein, as meat, has been shown to increase faecal NOC levels fourfold. NOC are alkylators, and alkylative mutations (e.g. the k-*ras* gene, see Fig. 19.5) are known to be involved in large bowel cancer. However, there are many thousands of NOC, and not all of them are carcinogenic; the compounds formed in faeces are at present under investigation.

There are other possible ways in which high intakes of meat might be carcinogenic. Heterocyclic aromatic amines are formed on the surface of cooked meat especially during grilling and frying. They are known to be colon carcinogens in animal models and are believed to be a cause of a small fraction of all colon cancers. Daily intakes of total heterocyclic amines range from 0.4 to 16 µg per day. This is a minute fraction of the amount found to induce tumours in animals, although high fat diets are known to potentiate the effects of these compounds. A high iron intake is another possible explanation for the association with meat. Free iron is a catalyst in the Fenton reaction which yields hydroxyl radicals. It has been proposed that the oxidative damage which occurs in the colon can be suppressed by phytic acid, a known chelator of iron. Animal studies have shown that very high doses of iron (580 mg/kg diet, 10 times greater than human intakes) induce tumours, and that tumour yield is reduced if phytate is added into the diet. However, no evidence of increased oxidative damage in animals fed iron has been demonstrated.

19.6 LUNG

Lung cancer is the second most common cancer world-wide, and the established cause is cigarette smoking. Peaks and lags in incidence can be related to exposure from smoking

20 years earlier, and the declining rates in younger men in Western countries reflect declining rates of cigarette consumption. Although formerly comparatively rare, there are epidemics of lung cancer in women in line with their increased rates of cigarette smoking. Rates are approaching those for cancer of the large bowel in the United Kingdom. Those smoking a pack of cigarettes per day for 30 years or more have a 20-fold increase in risk of lung cancer compared with non-smokers.

There is a consistent protective effect in both case-control and prospective studies of vegetables and fruit in lung cancer, although the protective effects of these foods are much weaker than the causative effect of smoking. Individuals classified as low vegetable consumers have a 2-fold increase in risk compared with regular consumers of vegetables; cigarette smoking is associated with a 20-fold increase. It is difficult to completely disentangle the separate effects of smoking and fruit and vegetable consumption since smokers generally consume less fruit and vegetables than non-smokers.

The hypothesis that lung cancer risks could be suppressed by β-carotene or vitamin E (which are found in some vegetables and fruits) was tested in a large Finnish trial of over 29 000 smokers given supplements of 50 mg α-tocopherol and/or 20 mg β-carotene or placebos. There was no change in the incidence of lung cancer with vitamin E, and a just significant increase in those given β-carotene (the opposite of what the investigators expected). These effects of β-carotene have been confirmed by another trial so it is unlikely that the carcinogenic effects of prolonged heavy smoking can be ameliorated by vitamin supplements.

19.7 Breast

In developed countries, breast cancer is the commonest cancer in women. Risks increase with age, but there is a slower rate of increase in incidence after the menopause. The incidence of postmenopausal breast cancer is increasing in the United Kingdom, and in countries where this was formerly less common, such as Japan, premenopausal breast cancer is also increasing. Known risk factors are an early menarche, late first pregnancy, late menopause, and, at least for premenopausal breast cancer, possibly not breast-feeding. These factors suggest that hormonal influences, especially oestrogens, are important, but there is no universally accepted mechanism. In postmenopausal women, higher serum levels of oestrogens are associated with increased risk of breast cancer although, of course, levels are generally low in older women. Epidemiological studies have been unable to detect differences in hormone levels between women who develop premenopausal cancer and those who do not, although this would be difficult to establish in large studies because of the large variations from day to day throughout the monthly cycle.

Adipose tissue is able to convert some of the circulating adrenal hormone androsten-dione to oestrogens. After the menopause, adipose tissue is the main source of oestrogens by this route rather than the ovaries, and this may account for the fact that overweight women are at up to a twofold increased risk of postmenopausal breast cancer. Serum oestrogen levels fall in women who lose weight.

The role of diet, particularly fat intake, in breast cancer is a controversial and difficult area, partly due to interlocking effects of fat on obesity, age at menarche, and serum oestrogen levels, which, together with differences in childbearing practices and use of exogenous hormones, such as hormonal replacement therapy, affect lifetime exposure to oestrogens. Animals given chemical carcinogens develop fewer mammary tumours if they are given a low fat diet, although the same effects are achieved by feeding animals a low energy diet. There are strong international correlations between breast cancer incidence and fat intake, and case-control studies in general suggest that in post-menopausal breast cancer, relative risk is increased to 1.4 for a high fat diet (see Fig. 19.6). On this evidence some expert committees have recommended that total fat consumption should be decreased to reduce risk of breast cancer. However, very large prospective studies have failed to show any protective effect of a low fat diet in adult life (see Fig. 19.6). This may be due to limitations of methods used to assess diet in the face of relatively homogeneous fat intakes in single populations. Childhood or teenage exposure to high energy, high fat, low fibre diets, rather than later life exposure, is a determining factor in influencing age at menarche and hence postmenopausal breast cancer. Further, very low fat diets (10–20% total energy) may be required to produce effects. In premenopausal women, such diets have markedly reduced serum oestrogens, particularly when combined with a high fibre intake. A large intervention trial of a very low fat diet in women is now under way in the United States. Alcohol may also be associated with increased risk of breast cancer, although no clear dose response has been shown from existing studies (Box 19.6).

There is evidence from case-control studies that high intakes of plant foods may protect against breast cancer, although few prospective studies have reported vegetable or fibre intakes. Some, although not all, epidemiological studies have found that individuals consuming soya products are protected from breast cancer. Soy, and some other plant foods, contain compounds that are stereochemically similar to mammalian oestrogens. The two main groups of these plant oestrogens (phytoestrogens), the lignans and the iso-flavones, are known to be biologically active in animals when fed in large amounts; they

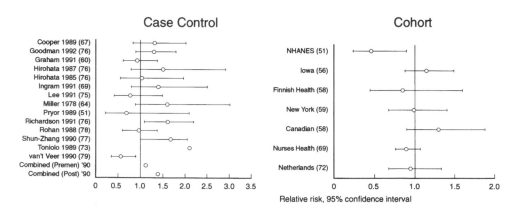

Fig. 19.6 Relative risks for breast cancer and confidence intervals for the highest versus the lowest quartile of fat consumption in (left) case-control studies and (right) prospective studies. *Source*: Margetts B. *Diet and cancer: review of the epidemiological literature.* London: The Nutrition Society, 1993.

Box 19.6   Causative factors in breast cancer

Established risk factors
- Reproductive: early menarche, late first pregnancy, late menopause
- High circulating endogenous oestrogens (postmenopausal)
- Obesity (postmenopausal), small effect

Probable risk factors
- High alcohol consumption
- High fat, and low plant polysaccharide diet causing early menarche

Possible risk factors
- High fat diets in adult life
- Low phytoestrogen intake

have caused fertility problems in sheep. Isoflavones, given as soya foods, have been found to be biologically active in humans, acting as weak oestrogens/antioestrogens in premenopausal women, suppressing output of gonadotrophins and extending the length of the menstrual cycle, especially the follicular phase. This could be important in explaining the relatively low rates of breast cancer in East Asian populations that consume soya foods as part of the staple diet; their menstrual cycles are longer than in Western populations. Longer menstrual cycles would mean fewer over a lifetime and a consequent reduction in exposure to peak oestrogen levels. Lignans have a similar effect on menstrual cycle length, and have been found to have oestrogenic effects in postmenopausal women. Lignans are quite widespread in plant foods such as wholegrain cereals and vegetables; linseed (also called flaxseed) is the richest source. The possible effect of plant oestrogens in protecting against breast cancer is the subject of several research programmes at the present time.

19.8   FEMALE REPRODUCTIVE ORGANS

19.8.1   Cervical cancer

Cancer of the cervix is the most common cancer in many developing countries and the tenth most important in developed countries. It is largely associated with age at first intercourse, numbers of sexual partners, the papilloma virus, parity and cigarette smoking. Risk does seem to be reduced in those individuals who consume greater amounts of vegetables but it is difficult to exclude confounding variables.

19.8.2   Endometrial cancer

Cancer of the endometrium occurs fairly frequently in developed countries, with a similar pattern of hormonal risk factors to breast cancer. However, there is clearer evidence for a role for unopposed oestrogens in increasing risk from studies of different types of the contraceptive pill, and an increased risk from hormonal replacement therapy. After the menopause, the other main source of oestrogens is from endogenous formation in adipose tissue and obesity is a marked risk factor. In the American Cancer Society prospective study of 420 000 women, risks for endometrial cancer increased steadily with increasing body weight, and in those weighing 40% or more than the average, relative risk was 5.4.

19.9 PROSTATE

There is at least a 70-fold variation in incidence of prostate cancer, highest rates occurring in the United States, Europe and Australia. Reported incidence is increasing rapidly, particularly in areas where diagnostic facilities, such as prostate-specific antigen, are now widely available. However, small latent prostatic carcinomas are commonly found at post-mortem examination in older men who have died from other causes, and some of the patterns in incidence may be due to underestimation of prevalence elsewhere. In a cohort study of 47 000 United States health professionals, consumption of tomatoes and tomato products appeared to be protective. In international comparisons of food intake and cancer incidence, high rates of prostate cancer are associated with high fat intake. There are limited detailed dietary studies as yet, and limited evidence that previous high levels of sexual activity is associated with increased risk.

19.10 OTHER SITES: LIVER, PANCREAS, SKIN, BLADDER AND KIDNEY

Alcohol is a cause of liver cancer but other major known risk factors for cancers at these sites are not dietary (e.g. infection with hepatitis B virus in liver cancer, smoking in pancreatic, kidney and bladder cancer, sunlight exposure in skin cancer). However, exposure to aflatoxin is established as a risk factor in liver cancer, and there are a number of ongoing intervention trials of β-carotene and skin cancer. Case-control studies suggest protective effects of fruits and vegetables in cancer of the bladder and of the pancreas.

19.11 DIETARY RECOMMENDATIONS FOR CANCER PREVENTION

It is evident that diet has a role in the prevention of cancer in many sites of the body. However, most of the evidence is based on epidemiological associations with limited information available from intervention studies. As a result, some of the evidence is weak, and relative risks associated with dietary habits are rarely greater than two. In some cases there is only weak mechanistic support for an effect of diet on promotion or initiation of cancer with several hypotheses suggested. Dietary recommendations based on this type of evidence will have to be modified as research advances are made, especially following the outcomes of the new generation of large prospective studies like EPIC (the European [Multicentre] Prospective Investigation into Cancer). However, for the high incidence cancers, even a small alteration in relative risk could represent substantial savings of lives. Current recommendations therefore tend towards the conservative and are made in the expectation that they will not lead to an increase in cancer. They are also compatible with other dietary recommendations for the avoidance of diabetes and cardiovascular disease.

1. Obesity is associated with a somewhat increased risk of breast cancer in women and bowel cancer in men and marked increased risk of endometrial cancer. This is one more reason to avoid overweight.
2. Low fruit and vegetable consumption is associated with increased risk of cancer at virtually all sites. Ideally, consumption probably should double, partly to meet

Box 19.7 Population dietary recommendations for reducing cancer risk in Western countries

- Avoid overweight and obesity
- Increase consumption of fruit and vegetables
- Reduce intake of total fat
- Limit alcohol, salty and pickled foods
- Meat consumption (especially red and processed meat) should not increase
- Avoid mouldy foods

existing recommendations to increase fibre consumption by 50% from 12–18 g NSP per day. (This will increase stool weight by 25% and should reduce population incidence of large bowel cancer by 15%.) Vegetables may have added benefits because they contain antioxidant nutrients and flavonoids, sulphur-containing compounds, and folate, all of which favourably affect factors thought to be important in reducing cancer risk.

3. High fat diets may enhance colon cancer risk. Recommendations to reduce total fat intake to 30% energy and to increase ω3-fatty acid consumption in order to reduce risk of cardiovascular disease may help to reduce bowel cancer rates. There appears to be no effect of fat intake in adult life on breast cancer risk, but low fat diets generally are low in energy content and assist in the avoidance of obesity.

4. Meat consumption, especially of red and processed meats, is linked with higher risk of bowel cancer and possibly breast and prostate cancers. Consumption of these should therefore not increase.

5. Alcohol consumption should be limited to currently recommended 'safe' levels (i.e. no more than 21 units per week).

6. Salty and pickled foods should be reduced (stomach cancer).

7. Foods which have become mouldy should be avoided (aflatoxins and liver cancer).

8. Other specific factors that may protect against cancer are unknown. In humans, the evidence so far relates to food groups, especially vegetables, rather than supplements of vitamins, minerals or purified extracts. Attempts to alter risk with supplements have so far not been successful and are not recommended for the general population.

FURTHER READING

1. Armstrong B, Doll R. Environmental factors and cancer incidence in different countries. *Int J Cancer* 1995; **15**: 617–31.
2. Bingham, S. Epidemiology and mechanisms relating diet to risk of colorectal cancer. *Nutr Res Rev* 1996; **9**: 197–239.
3. Blot WJ, Li JY, Taylor PR, *et al.* Nutrition intervention trials in Linxian China. Supplementation with specific vitamin, mineral combinations, cancer incidence and disease-specific mortality in the general population. *J Nat Cancer Inst* 1993; **85**: 1483–92.

4. Committee on Medical Aspects of Food Policy. *Report on diet and cancer.* London: HMSO (in press, 1997).
5. Doll R, Peto R. The causes of cancer: quantitative estimates of avoidable risks of cancer in the US today. *J Nat Cancer Inst* 1981; **66**: 1191–308.
6. Greenberg RE, Baron JA, Tosteson TD, *et al.* A clinical trial of antioxidant vitamins to prevent colorectal adenoma. *N Engl J Med* 1994; **331**: 141–7.
7. IARC (ed. Tomatis L, *et al.*). *Cancer, causes, occurrence and control.* Chapter 12, 20 IARC Scientific Publication 100. Lyon: IARC, 1990.
8. Layton D, Bogen KT, Knize MG, Hatch F, Johnston VM, Felton JS. Cancer risk of HAA in cooked foods. *Carcinogenesis 2* 1995; **16**: 39–62.
9. Steinmetz K, Potter JD. Vegetables, fruit and cancer prevention: a review. *J Amer Dietetic Assoc* 1996; **96**: 1027–39.
10. The Alpha-Tocopherol, Beta Carotene Cancer Preventioni Study Group. The effect of vitamin E and beta carotene on the incidence of lung cancer and other cancers in male smokers. *N Engl J Med* 1994; **330**: 1029–35.
11. World Health Organization. *Diet, nutrition and chronic disease.* Technical Report Series 797. Geneva: WHO, 1990.

20

DIABETES MELLITUS

Jim Mann

The term 'diabetes mellitus' is used to describe a group of conditions characterized by raised blood glucose levels (hyperglycaemia) and a relative or absolute deficiency of insulin. In non-insulin-dependent diabetes (NIDDM) a key abnormality is resistance to the action of insulin and in the early stages of the disease insulin levels may actually be raised. In some patients with NIDDM the insulin-producing beta cells of the islets in the pancreas may show a degree of failure at some stage during the course of the disease process. Impaired glucose tolerance (IGT) and gestational diabetes (diabetes developing during pregnancy) may represent the earliest stages of NIDDM. Patients with NIDDM are usually treated with 'lifestyle modification' therapy, with or without oral hypo-glycaemic (blood glucose lowering) agents; insulin is not usually required. In insulin-dependent diabetes (IDDM) there is destruction of the pancreatic islet beta cells usually resulting from an autoimmune process and insulin treatment is essential to maintain life.

In both the major types of diabetes a range of metabolic disturbances occurs in addition to the hyperglycaemia and these abnormalities, together with the raised prevalence of hypertension among people with diabetes, help to explain the wide-ranging complications of diabetes. The complications result chiefly from the effects of diabetes on the arterial and nervous systems. They include diabetic retinopathy which may lead to blindness, diabetic nephropathy potentially resulting in kidney failure, and foot ulceration which may lead to gangrene. In addition to these specific diabetes-related complications there is a substantially increased risk of cardiovascular disease in people with diabetes. A full description of the clinical features of diabetes and its complications as well as current theories concerning the causes may be found in textbooks of medicine. The diagnosis of IDDM is usually straightforward because of markedly raised blood glucose levels. For diagnostic features of NIDDM see Table 20.1. This chapter describes the role of nutritional and other lifestyle related factors in the aetiology and management of the two main types of diabetes and their complications.

20.1   Lifestyle Factors in the Aetiology of Non-Insulin-Dependent Diabetes (NIDDM) and its Complications

Diabetes has been recognized as a clinical entity for well over 2000 years. From the earliest times until recently, the sugary urine and raised levels of blood glucose have led to the assumption that an excessive intake of sucrose (table sugar) must be an important cause of the condition. While the causes of NIDDM are still not fully understood it can be said with reasonable certainty that high intakes of dietary sugars *per se* do not play an important

Table 20.1 Criteria for the diagnosis of non-insulin-dependent diabetes (NIDDM) and impaired glucose tolerance (IGT).

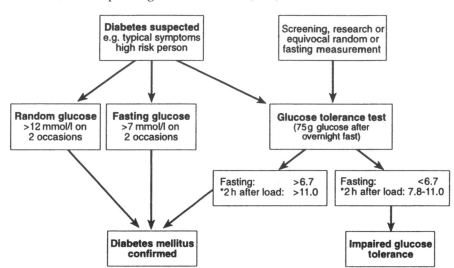

* These figures refer to levels measured on capillary blood. When venous blood is used diagnostic levels are 1 mmol/l lower, i.e. > 10.0 mmol/l confirm diabetes, IGT 6.8–10.0 mmol/l confirm IGT

role. The frequency of NIDDM (as defined in Table 20.1) shows a striking geographical variation (see Fig. 20.1). In some countries the frequency appears to have increased with time. This could be partly due to improved diagnostic facilities but it is generally believed that in most populations of European descent there has been a steady genuine increase in prevalence. In some population groups there have been dramatic increases in prevalence associated either with migration or with a rapid change from a traditional (non-Western) lifestyle to increased consumption of energy-dense foods, high in fats and sugars, and reduced levels of physical activity—characteristics of the way of life in many Western countries. The American Pima Indians, Polynesians and Melanesians in the South Pacific, Australian Aboriginals and Asian Indian migrants to the United Kingdom and other countries are examples of populations in which the process of rapid acculturation has led to diabetes prevalence rates far higher than those observed in European populations. Many epidemiological studies have attempted to disentangle which aspects of the lifestyle changes have been responsible for such emergence of NIDDM.

A totally consistent observation in prospective as well as cross-sectional studies is the striking association between risk of NIDDM and increasing obesity (Fig. 20.2), particularly when the excess body fat is centrally distributed, i.e. in association with a high waist to hip ratio. (The significance of this ratio is discussed in Chapter 16.1.) It is also clear that there is a strong genetic component to this condition. The risk of developing NIDDM is greatly increased when one or more close family members have the condition although the precise mode of inheritance has not yet been resolved. It appears therefore that in predisposed populations or families, genetic and lifestyle factors combine to result in the development of insulin resistance and consequently diabetes. There have been many

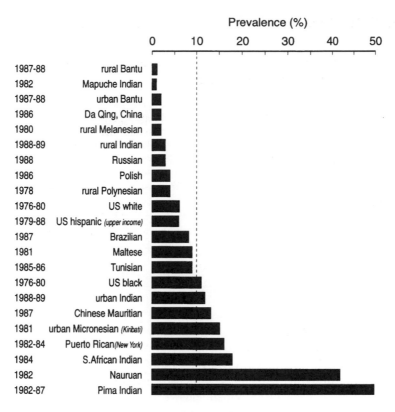

Fig. 20.1 Geographical variation in the prevalence of non-insulin-dependent diabetes (NIDDM) in people aged 30–64 years. *Source*: Survey reported to WHO (1988–91).

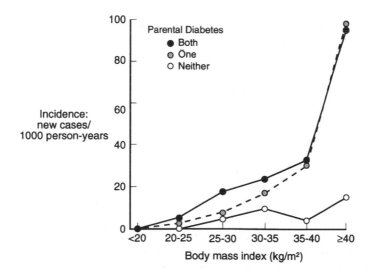

Fig. 20.2 The interaction between obesity and inheritance as risk factors for NIDDM. *Source*: Knowler WC, Pettitt DJ, Savage RJ, Bennett PH. Diabetes incidence in Pima Indians: contributions of obesity and parental diabetes. *Am J Epidemiol* 1981; **113**: 144–56.

Table 20.2 Risk factors for coronary heart disease (CHD) in people with non-insulin-dependent diabetes (NIDDM)

Risk factors which may be of particular relevance in NIDDM	General CHD risk factors which are also relevant in NIDDM
↑ Triglycerides and very low-density lipoproteins	↑ Cholesterol and low-density lipoprotein
↓ High-density lipoproteins	Hypertension
↑ Oxidation of low-density lipoprotein	Cigarette smoking
↑ Platelet aggregation	Obesity, especially when associated with a high waist/hip ratio
↑ Plasminogen activator inhibitor	Physical inactivity
↑ Proinsulin-like molecules	
Microalbuminuria	

attempts to implicate individual nutrients as causal or protective factors in the aetiology of NIDDM, but none of the hypotheses have stood the test of time. It is conceivable that more than one of the attributes that characterise the Western lifestyle (excesive intakes of energy-dense foods, low intakes of vegetables, fruits and lightly processed cereal foods with intact cellular structure, inadequate physical activity) contribute to the aetiology. Thus, while the precise mechanisms remain elusive it is tempting to suggest that altering dietary practices and increasing physical activity might help to prevent, or at least delay, the onset of NIDDM in predisposed individuals. A few encouraging preliminary studies have been published and further large-scale investigations are underway.

Several complications of diabetes (e.g. retinopathy, nephropathy and neuropathy) appear to be a result of hyperglycaemia and other metabolic consequences of diabetes. Diet plays a role in their prevention and treatment by helping to improve blood glucose control (see Section 20.3) but does not appear to be directly involved as a cause. On the other hand, cardiovascular disease which is responsible for the greatest number of deaths and much non-fatal illness in people with NIDDM seems to be more closely linked to dietary factors. There appear to be some risk factors for coronary heart disease (CHD) which are more important in people with diabetes than in the population at large (Table 20.2). They may help to explain the great excess of CHD in this condition. However, other important determinants of atherogenesis and thrombogenesis seem to be similar in those with and without diabetes. Many are diet-related (see Chapter 18). In countries with low CHD rates in the general population, CHD is also relatively infrequent in people with diabetes, so a major focus of dietary recommendations for people with diabetes relates to the need to reduce cardiovascular risk.

20.2 EPIDEMIOLOGY AND AETIOLOGY OF INSULIN-DEPENDENT DIABETES (IDDM)

The prevalence of IDDM also shows marked geographic variation (Fig. 20.3) and in some countries, notably Scotland and Finland, there has been a considerable increase in recent

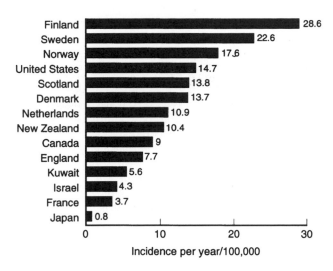

Finland — 28.6
Sweden — 22.6
Norway — 17.6
United States — 14.7
Scotland — 13.8
Denmark — 13.7
Netherlands — 10.9
New Zealand — 10.4
Canada — 9
England — 7.7
Kuwait — 5.6
Israel — 4.3
France — 3.7
Japan — 0.8

Incidence per year/100,000

Fig. 20.3 Geographical variation in insulin-dependent diabetes in selected countries. *Source*: LaPorte RE, Tajima N, Akerblom HR, *et al.* Geographic differences in the risk of insulin-dependent diabetes mellitus: the importance of registries. *Diabetes Care* 1985; 8: 101–7.

years. Note that the prevalence does not exactly parallel that of NIDDM and there is no clear explanation for the variation from one country to another or the change over time. Genetic factors are important in IDDM although only about 10% of people with the condition have a clear family history. It is not clear what triggers the autoimmune process which leads to the destruction of the pancreatic beta islet cells. Various nutritional factors have been suggested but there is reasonable evidence for only one of these. Several epidemiological studies suggest that the early introduction of cow's milk into the diet of infants is associated with an increased risk of developing IDDM later in life, but the extent to which breast milk is protective and cow's milk detrimental remains to be established. The importance of infant nutrition as a risk factor for IDDM and the mechanism by which it might operate are far from clear. It is possible that cow's milk protein might be immunogenic in susceptible individuals. Immunosuppressive drugs have been shown to delay the onset of clinical IDDM when given to children with circulating antibodies to the pancreatic beta islet cell, which are markers of the autoimmune process that precede the early metabolic abnormalities of diabetes. However, these drugs have potentially serious side-effects. A current hope for prevention, centres around the use of large doses of nicotinamide in susceptible individuals before any metabolic abnormalities are detectable. Nicotinamide appears to have an effect on the immune system and has been shown to be both safe and effective in animal experiments and in one uncontrolled study in children in New Zealand. Multicentre controlled clinical trials are now underway. Clinical trials involving various infant dietary regimes have also been suggested.

As with NIDDM, many of the complications of IDDM are associated with unsatisfactory metabolic control, and cardiovascular disease in people with diabetes is associated with risk factors similar to those in the general population. In the aetiology of kidney damage (nephropathy), a high intake of protein, especially animal protein, may be associated, but the evidence is far from conclusive.

331

20.3 LIFESTYLE TREATMENTS FOR DIABETES

Dietary modification is the cornerstone of treatment for people with NIDDM and many of those who manage to comply with dietary advice will show improvement in the metabolic abnormalities associated with this condition to the extent that oral hypoglycaemic drugs and insulin are not required. Even when drug treatment is required attention to diet may further improve blood glucose control and modify blood lipids in a way which might be expected to reduce CHD risk.

In those with IDDM the goals of lifestyle and dietary advice are to minimize short-term fluctuations in blood glucose and especially to reduce the risk of hypoglycaemia by balancing injected insulin with carbohydrate-containing food and physical activity. Dietary modification may also help to reduce the risk of long-term complications by helping to achieve optimal blood glucose control and satisfactory levels of blood lipids.

The principles of dietary advice for people with NIDDM or IDDM are similar to those recommended for entire populations at high risk of CHD and this means that there is no need for people with diabetes to have meals which differ from those of the rest of the family. Dietary recommendations for people with diabetes have been issued in most countries, the most widely quoted are those of the American Diabetes Association (ADA) and the Nutrition Study Group of the European Association for the Study of Diabetes (EASD). The two sets of recommendations are broadly comparable and are summarized in Table 20.3. The most impressive evidence for the value of attempting to achieve blood glucose levels as close as possible to normal comes from the Diabetes Control and Complications Trial (DCCT) which confirmed earlier inconclusive studies. In this trial, people with IDDM were randomized to receive either conventional treatment or intensive lifestyle advice (regarding diet and exercise) plus more intensive insulin regimes than are used in routine practice. The intensively treated group had greatly reduced rates of retinopathy, nephropathy and neuropathy in association with improved blood glucose levels, compared with the control group. Although this study was confined to people with IDDM, it is generally accepted that the results also apply to those with NIDDM.

Recent recommendations have tended to be less rigid than those in the past and acknowledge that quality of life of the individual must be taken into account when defining nutritional objectives. Health care providers are encouraged to achieve a balance between the attempts to achieve optimal control of blood glucose and risk factors and the well-being of the patient. Lifestyle treatments should be adapted to the needs of individuals and may change with time. The recommendations given below are those of the EASD; they are broadly comparable with those of the ADA.

20.3.1 Total energy and body weight

EASD recommendation Detailed recommendations concerning energy intakes are not required for those diabetic subjects with a body mass index (BMI) in the acceptable range (19–25 kg/m^2) for adults. Those who are overweight should be encouraged to reduce their caloric intake and to enhance energy expenditure so that BMI moves toward this range. Advice concerning the reduction of energy-dense foods and, in particular, those high in fat will usually help to achieve weight loss without the need for precise energy prescription. If these measures do not achieve the desired weight reduction, it may be

Table 20.3 Key aspects of the current recommendations for diabetic diet and lifestyle

Dietary energy and body weight	Achieve and/or maintain BMI 19–25 Diet and exercise important
Components of dietary energy	Saturated fatty acids: <10% total energy ω6-polyunsaturated fatty acids: <10% total energy Protein: 10–20% total energy Carbohydrate and cis-monounsaturated fatty acids: make up the remaining 60–70% total energy
Carbohydrate issues	Low glycaemic index foods and those rich in soluble fibre recommended Vegetables, fruits, legumes and cereal-derived foods preferred Sucrose <10% total energy acceptable in certain circumstances Timing of intake essential for those on insulin
Protein and renal disease	Total protein intake at lower end of normal range (0.7–0.9 g/kg per day) for those with incipient or established nephropathy
Vitamins and antioxidant nutrients	Increase foods rich in tocopherols, carotenoids, vitamin C and flavonoids (i.e. a wide range of vegetables and fruits), but supplements not recommended
Minerals	Sodium intake less than 6 g/day Magnesium supplementation may be required in special circumstances
Alcohol	An amount equivalent to 1–2 glasses of wine per day is acceptable for most people with diabetes Special precautions apply to those on insulin or sulphonylureas, those who are overweight and those with hypertriglyceridaemia
Special 'diabetic' or 'dietetic' foods	Non-alcoholic beverages sweetened with non-nutritive sweeteners are useful Other special foods not encouraged No particular merit of fructose and other 'special' nutritive sweeteners over sucrose
Families	Most recommendations suitable for whole family

Source: Derived from the 1995 recommendations of the American Diabetes Association and the Nutrition Study Group of the European Association for the Study of Diabetes.

necessary to offer more precise advice concerning the dietary modifications needed to produce a sustained energy deficit of at least 500 kcal/day. It should be noted that energy restriction even in the absence of weight loss improves the metabolic abnormalities. The amount of physical activity needs to be taken into account when considering total energy requirements.

Comment The energy requirements for an individual to maintain weight and ensure adequate intakes for growth, pregnancy and lactation are usually met by physiological appetite control. Prescriptive advice concerning energy intake is only necessary for those who are clearly overweight or steadily gaining weight over the years. A wide range of clinical and metabolic disturbances associated with centrally distributed obesity (hypertension, hyperglycaemia, raised levels of LDL and VLDL, reduced HDL and insulin resistance) improve with even modest weight loss. The use of very low calorie diets should be confined to special cases (BMI $\geqslant$ 35) and to experienced medical centres. Regular physical activity may help to improve glucose tolerance, influence the lipid profile favourably, facilitate weight control and maintain muscle mass.

20.3.2 Components of dietary energy

EASD recommendation Saturated fatty acids should provide under 10% total energy. A lower intake may be beneficial if LDL cholesterol is elevated. Polyunsaturated fatty acids are recommended up to 10% of dietary energy. Protein intake should range between 10% and 20% total energy. The rest of dietary energy (more than 50%) should come from a combination of carbohydrates and monounsaturated fatty acids with *cis*-configuration. Carbohydrate-containing foods that are rich in soluble fibre or have a low glycaemic index are especially recommended.

Comment The high rates of CHD in people with diabetes and the strong evidence for benefit of reducing total and LDL-cholesterol provide the justification for the strong recommendation concerning the reduction of saturated fats. A large Scandinavian trial of the cholesterol-lowering drug, simvastatin, showed that people with diabetes had a significant reduction in cardiovascular and total mortality in association with reduction in cholesterol similar to that observed in non-diabetics. Although dietary modification alone cannot achieve cholesterol lowering to the extent that can be achieved by this powerful drug, diet can produce the degree of cholesterol-lowering which might be expected to reduce CHD by about 30% (see Chapter 18.1). People with diabetes in most Western countries appear to have an intake of saturated fatty acids much the same as that of the population at large and exceeding current recommendations (Fig. 20.4). In general, recommendations concerning saturated and polyunsaturated fatty acids apply equally to those with and without diabetes (Chapter 18.1).

There has been controversy concerning the respective merits of carbohydrates and *cis*-monounsaturated fatty acids as sources of replacement energy for saturated fatty acids. It has been suggested that *cis*-monounsaturated fatty acids might be associated with more favourable levels of blood glucose, lower levels of triglyceride and VLDL, higher levels of HDL and reduced oxidation of LDL. However, these differences seem not to be apparent when the carbohydrate foods are rich in soluble fibre or have a low glycaemic

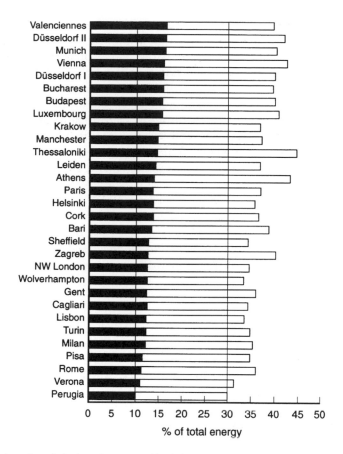

Fig. 20.4 Intake of total (□) and saturated (■) fatty acids as proportion of total dietary intake, calculated from 4-day diet records. Data from European centres participating in the EURODIAB study. *Source*: From Toeller M, Klischan A, Heitkamp G, *et al. Diabetologia* 1996; **39**: 929–39.

index. There are no grounds for recommending exceptionally high intakes of either carbohydrates or *cis*-monounsaturated fatty acids. The percentage of energy contributed by each may vary according to local or individual preferences or clinical circumstances. For example, fibre-rich carbohydrate may be especially useful in those attempting to lose weight, and *cis*-monounsaturated fatty acids for those who have particularly low levels of HDL. Fruit, vegetables, legumes and lightly processed cereals are the preferred sources of carbohydrate since they are often rich in soluble fibre as well as vitamins and other potentially beneficial substances. Intact foods and those with a low glycaemic index (e.g. legumes, oats, pasta, parboiled rice, certain raw fruits) may help to improve blood glucose control and lipid levels (see Chapter 2.6.3).

For insulin-treated patients, it is important that the timing and dose of insulin match with the amount and time of carbohyrate-containing food intake to avoid both hypoglycaemia and excessive postprandial hyperglycaemia. An adequate amount of carbohydrate food, preferably rich in soluble fibre, before going to bed is often important in reducing the risk of low blood glucose during the night in insulin-treated patients. Self-monitoring of blood glucose is helpful for patients with IDDM and NIDDM in determining the most appropriate timing of food intake as well as optimal food choices.

Moderate intakes of total sucrose (table sugar), < 10% total energy, are acceptable, if desired, in both types of diabetes. A sucrose intake above this may result in an increase in triglyceride levels in some people because of its fructose content. Sucrose should preferably be included within meals and considered within the overall diet prescriptions. Drinks high in sucrose and/or glucose should only be used to treat hypoglycaemia. In overweight and obese patients sucrose needs to be reduced as far as possible because of its high energy density.

20.3.4 Protein and renal disease

EASD recommendation Protein intake should be between 10% and 20% total energy except in those with incipient (abnormal microalbuminuria) or established nephropathy when intake should be at the lower end of the normal range (0.7–0.9 g/kg body weight per day).

Comment In most Western countries, adult protein intake (approximately 0.8 g/kg per day or 10% total energy) exceeds recommended daily intake. There is at present insufficient evidence to justify a general reduction in diabetics, although protein intakes greater than 20% total energy may increase the risk of renal disease. However, among those with evidence of (early or established) renal impairment, protein restriction has been shown to delay the progression of nephropathy. An intake below 0.6 g/kg per day is not recommended. There is limited information to suggest that protein from vegetable sources may have a less deleterious effect than animal protein in those with nephropathy.

20.3.5 Vitamins and antioxidant nutrients

EASD recommendation Foods naturally rich in dietary antioxidants (tocopherols, carotenoids, vitamin C and possibly flavonoids) should be encouraged.

Comment The disturbed equilibrium between pro- and antioxidants in people with diabetes and the evidence that increased oxidative stress increases cardiovascular risk provide the justification for this recommendation. Pharmacological doses of vitamin E have been shown to reduce oxidation of LDL, but present evidence does not justify the routine use of vitamin E or other micronutrients taken in pharmacological quantities as supplements.

20.3.6 Inorganic nutrients

EASD recommendation Particular advice for people with diabetes is only given for sodium. As in the general population, people with diabetes should be advised to restrict salt intake to under 6 g sodium chloride/day. More marked reductions should be considered in those whose blood pressure levels show any degree of persistant elevation.

Comment   For most inorganic nutrients there are no grounds for recommendations which differ from those for the general population but the importance of hypertension in diabetes justifies special mention of sodium. However, some insulin-dependent diabetic patients with poor metabolic control or during pregnancy can develop a magnesium depletion. An increased intake of magnesium-rich foods (Chapter 8.2.3) is the preferred treatment. Supplements are very rarely required.

20.3.7   Alcohol

EASD recommendation   Precautions regarding alcohol intake that apply to the general public also apply to people with diabetes. For those who choose to drink alcohol, an amount equivalent to two glasses of wine per day is acceptable for most of them. When alcohol is taken by those on insulin or sulphonylurea drugs it should be consumed with carbohydrate-containing foods because of the risk of severe hypoglycaemia.

Comment   General recommendations regarding alcohol for people with diabetes are complicated by the fact that alcohol may have both untoward and beneficial effects. Alcohol may be an important energy source in overweight people. As well as its association with accidents, it can also be associated with raised levels of blood pressure, increased triglycerides, an increased risk of hypoglycaemia and it favours body fat deposition. On the other hand, moderate intakes (equivalent to approximately one or two glasses of wine per day) may confer benefit in middle aged patients by elevating levels of high-density lipoproteins, reducing coagulability and decreasing lipid oxidation through the antioxidant nutrients present in wine. Recommendations must therefore depend on the characteristics of individual patients.

20.3.8   Diabetic foods

EASD recommendation   Non-alcoholic beverages sweetened by non-nutritive sweeteners may be used for people with diabetes. For other foods, there are no known grounds for encouraging specially formulated 'diabetic' or 'dietetic' foods.

Comment   Non-nutritive sweeteners (e.g. aspartame) may be helpful when used in drinks. Fructose and other nutritive sweeteners do not have substantial advantages over sucrose for people with diabetes (other than decreased cariogenicity) and should not be encouraged. Many foods currently marketed as suitable for people with diabetes are high in fat and energy and are often more expensive than regular products. Their continued promotion may detract from, rather than facilitate, compliance with the nutritional recommendations.

20.3.9   Translating nutritional principles into practice

Many medical practitioners do not have the training or the time to help people with diabetes translate the nutrition principles described here into practice. Dietitians or appropriately trained nutritionists play a key role in translating these general principles into specific advice for individuals. The importance of increased physical activity as well as dietary advice for those who are overweight cannot be overemphasized. Behaviour modification techniques and various special lifestyle programmes can be of considerable value. Ongoing encouragement and reinforcement of lifestyle changes are essential, one-off advice is rarely adequate.

20.4   FAMILIES AND COMMUNITIES

Individual compliance with dietary advice is improved if the general aspects of advice are understood by the family and are of potential benefit to them. In view of the strong genetic component to NIDDM, the possibility that lifestyle changes might reduce the risk of developing the condition and that the dietary principles are similar to those which reduce CHD risk, it seems perfectly reasonable to suggest that foods and meals which are suitable for people with diabetes are appropriate for their families. In countries with high rates of NIDDM, community programmes are needed but, as with CHD prevention, appropriate food labelling and availability of appropriate foods at reasonable cost are essential components of such initiatives. There is at present insufficient evidence to justify programmes aimed at identifying people at risk of IDDM. However, if high dose nicotinamide or other safe methods of preventing IDDM prove to be of value in the clinical trials which are presently underway, screening high-risk families or even populations may be feasible in the future.

FURTHER READING

1. American Diabetes Association. Nutrition recommendations and principles for people with diabetes mellitus. *Diabetes Care* 1994; **17**: 519–22.
2. Brand Miller J. Importance of glycemic index in diabetes. *Am J Clin Nutr* 1994; **59** (suppl.): 747S–52S.
3. Diabetes and Nutrition Study Group of the European Association for the Study of Diabetes. Recommendations for the nutritional management of patients with diabetes mellitus. *Diabetes Nutr Metab* 1995; **8**: 1–4.
4. Diabetes Control and Complications Trial Research Group. The effect of intensive treatment of diabetes on the development and progression of long term complications in insulin-dependent diabetes mellitus. *New Engl J Med* 1993; **329**: 977–86.
5. Garg A. High monounsaturated fat diet for diabetic patients. *Diabetes Care* 1994; **17**: 242–46.

21
EATING DISORDERS: ANOREXIA NERVOSA AND BULIMIA NERVOSA

Christopher G. Fairburn

The term 'eating disorders' refers to anorexia nervosa and bulimia nervosa, and their variants. Together, the two disorders are a major source of morbidity among young women in Western societies. Anorexia nervosa has long been recognized, with particularly good descriptions being published in France and Britain in the last century. In contrast, the first series of patients with bulimia nervosa was described as recently as 1979.

21.1 DEFINITIONS

21.1.1 Anorexia nervosa

Three features are required to make a diagnosis of anorexia nervosa (see Table 21.1). The first is the presence of a characteristic set of attitudes and values concerning shape and weight. Various expressions have been used to describe them, including the 'relentless pursuit of thinness' and a 'morbid fear of fatness'. The essential feature is that these individuals judge their self-worth almost exclusively in terms of their body shape and weight. Their level of concern about shape and weight is far more intense than the dissatisfaction with appearance experienced by many women today. The second diagnostic feature is the active maintenance of an unduly low weight. The definition of what constitutes 'low' varies: a widely used threshold is having a body mass index (BMI) below 17.5. The low weight is achieved by a variety of means, including strict dieting or fasting, excessive exercising and, in some, self-induced vomiting. Laxatives and diuretics may also be taken for this purpose. The third diagnostic feature is amenorrhoea (in post-menarchal females who are not taking an oral contraceptive).

21.1.2 Bulimia nervosa

Three features are also required to make a diagnosis of bulimia nervosa (see Table 21.1). The first is the presence of attitudes to shape and weight similar to those found in anorexia nervosa. The second is frequent episodes of bulimia (binge eating). By definition, these 'binges' involve the consumption of unusually large amounts of food, given the circumstances, and loss of control at the time of eating. The third feature is the practice

Table 21.1   Diagnostic criteria for anorexia nervosa and bulimia nervosa

Anorexia nervosa
1. Characteristic extreme concerns about shape and weight
2. Active maintenance of a very low weight (BMI < 17.5)
3. Amenorrhoea

Bulimia nervosa
1. Characteristic extreme concern about shape and weight
2. Binge eating
3. Extreme weight-control behaviour (e.g. strict dieting, self-induced vomiting, misuse of laxatives)

of extreme weight-control behaviour such as strict dieting, self-induced vomiting and the misuse of laxatives or diuretics.

The great majority of people who meet the three diagnostic criteria for bulimia nervosa have weights that are in the normal range. However, there are some who are significantly underweight and also meet diagnostic criteria for anorexia nervosa. In practice, both diagnoses are not given: instead, the diagnosis of anorexia nervosa takes precedence over that of bulimia nervosa.

21.2   Epidemiology

Anorexia nervosa is largely confined to women aged between 10 and 30 years and to Western countries in which thinness for women is considered attractive. Estimates of the incidence of the disorder range from 0.24 to 14.6 per 100 000 female population per annum, and it seems that the incidence may have increased in recent decades. Estimates of the prevalence of the disorder amongst adolescent girls (11–18 years), the group most at risk, range from 0.2% to 1.1%. Anorexia nervosa is rarely encountered among men (less than 10% of cases are male) and is uncommon among non-whites. The social class distribution appears to be uneven with cases from upper socioeconomic groups being over-represented.

Bulimia nervosa is more common than anorexia nervosa. Among young women (aged 16–35 years) in Western countries the prevalence rate is between 1% and 2%. Most of these cases are not in treatment. Whilst there are no satisfactory data on the incidence of bulimia nervosa, it seems that the disorder has become much more common over the past 25 years. People with bulimia nervosa are on average somewhat older than those with anorexia nervosa, most being in their twenties, and they have a broader social class distribution. The disorder is rarely seen in men.

21.3   Anorexia Nervosa

21.3.1   Development of the disorder

The onset of anorexia nervosa is usually in adolescence, although prepubertal cases are encountered. Occasionally the disorder does not begin until adulthood. Usually it starts as normal adolescent dieting which then gets out of control. As the dieting intensifies, weight falls and the physiological and psychological effects of starvation develop. Additional methods of controlling shape and weight may be adopted at any stage. The characteristic overconcern with shape and weight may not be present at the outset.

21.3.2   Clinical features

The weight loss is mainly achieved through a marked reduction in food intake. The amount consumed may be very small and some patients fast at times. Typically, the range of foods eaten is restricted with those foods viewed as fattening being avoided. Vegetarianism is common. The average energy intake is in the region of 2.5–3.7 MJ/day (600–900 kcal/day) with the proportion of energy derived from fat being particularly low. Mineral intake is also low, although frank mineral deficiencies are rarely seen. It is possible that zinc deficiency may contribute to the maintenance of the disorder through an effect on appetite and taste. Except in longstanding cases, appetite persists and for this reason the term 'anorexia' is not appropriate. Frequent intense exercising is common and adds to the weight loss. A minority of patients lose control over their eating at times and some induce vomiting and misuse laxatives or diuretics.

Accompanying the disturbed eating is a disturbance of body image. This has various components. It may include a perceptual element such that all, or parts, of the body are seen as larger than their true size, and there is an attitudinal element characterized by an intense dislike of the body or parts of it. Neither feature improves as weight is lost: indeed, both tend to get worse.

Feelings of depression, anxiety and irritability are common in anorexia nervosa. In more chronic cases there may be hopelessness and thoughts of suicide. Outside interests decline as weight is lost and there may be marked social withdrawal. Obsessional features are frequently present and often these affect eating. There is also preoccupation with thoughts about food, eating, shape and weight, and concentration may be impaired.

21.3.3   Physical health

Anorexia nervosa is associated with many physiological abnormalities. These are now thought to be secondary to the disturbed pattern of eating and low weight. While many patients have no physical complaints, systematic enquiry often reveals heightened sensitivity to cold and a variety of gastrointestinal symptoms including constipation, fullness after eating, bloatedness and vague abdominal pains. Other symptoms include restlessness, lack of energy, low sexual appetite and early morning wakening. In post-menarchal females who are not taking an oral contraceptive, amenorrhoea is by definition present and some patients present complaining of infertility. On examination, the patients are found to be emaciated and underweight. Those with a prepubertal onset may be short in stature and show a failure of breast development. Often there is fine downy hair (lanugo) on the back, arms and side of the face. The skin tends to be dry and the hands and feet cold. Blood pressure and pulse are low and there may be dependent oedema. The findings on investigation are listed in Table 21.2.

Table 21.2   Anorexia nervosa: common abnormalities on investigation

Endocrine
- Low levels of female sex hormones (luteinizing hormone, follicle-stimulating hormone and oestradiol)
- Low levels of thyroid hormones (T_3 and T_4)
- Raised growth hormone and cortisol levels

Haematological
- Slightly lowered white cell count
- Anaemia (normocytic, normochromic)
- Low erthyrocyte sedimentation rate (ESR)

Other metabolic abnormalities
- Raised blood cholesterol
- Increased serum β-carotene
- Low blood sugar
- Dehydration
- Electrolyte disturbance (in those who vomit frequently or misuse large quantities of laxatives or diuretics)

Other findings
- Skeletal abnormalities (osteopenia and osteoporotic fractures)
- Delayed gastric emptying and prolonged gastrointestinal transit time

21.3.4   Aetiology

Predisposing factors   There is no single cause of anorexia nervosa. Dieting appears to be a general vulnerability factor. It is a common precursor of anorexia nervosa and bulimia nervosa, and the two disorders seem to be largely confined to countries in which young women diet. However, whilst dieting is common, few people develop an eating disorder. Therefore, other aetiological factors must operate, some of which may interact with dieting.

A variety of risk factors have been implicated. These include premorbid obesity and longstanding low self-esteem and perfectionism. The parents often report that as children these patients were exceptionally compliant and well behaved. There is an increased rate of eating disorders and clinical depression in these patients' families. Communication between family members is often disturbed, but this is difficult to interpret since it is not clear whether this disturbance is a cause or consequence of the eating disorder.

Maintaining factors   As food intake decreases and weight is lost, secondary effects develop, some of which perpetuate the disorder. For example, delayed gastric emptying results in fullness even after eating small amounts of food, and social withdrawal isolates the person from his or her peers. Those who have been overweight in the past are often understandably pleased with the weight loss and may be complimented on it. Refusing to eat gives a sense of self-control and may enhance self-esteem. It may also have gratifying effects within the family.

21.3.5 Assessment

Few patients with anorexia nervosa refer themselves for treatment. Usually, they are persuaded to seek help by concerned relatives or friends and as a consequence they often attend somewhat reluctantly.

Careful history-taking from both the patient and, if at all possible, an informant will make the diagnosis clear. It will be evident that the low weight is self-induced and is associated with the characteristic attitudes to shape and weight. No physical tests are required to make the diagnosis, and unless there are positive reasons to suspect the presence of another physical condition, no tests are required to exclude other medical disorders.

Some patients present complaining of features associated with anorexia nervosa rather than the disorder itself. For example, they may present with gastrointestinal symptoms, amenorrhoea or infertility, or with depressive or obsessional features. However, once the weight loss has been identified, and it has been recognized to be self-induced, the diagnosis should be clear.

Whilst physical tests are not required to make the diagnosis, all patients with anorexia nervosa should have a thorough physical examination and whatever investigations are indicated on the basis of the findings. Those who vomit frequently or misuse significant quantities of laxatives or diuretics should have their electrolytes checked.

21.3.6 Management

Patients with anorexia nervosa vary; some present with short histories and are willing and able to change, while others have an entrenched disorder and resist attempts to help them.

In principle, there are two aspects to treatment. One is establishing healthy eating habits and a normal weight, and the second is the removal of those factors which have been maintaining the disorder. Except in mild cases of short duration, both are essential. The normalization of eating habits and weight is mainly achieved though a combination of common sense advice and support in conjunction with nutritional counselling. Refeeding should start slowly and it may be achieved on an outpatient, daypatient or inpatient basis. Addressing the factors that have been maintaining the disorder generally involves the use of more specialized treatments such as family therapy and cognitive behaviour therapy. Drugs have almost no role, although dietary supplements may be used during weight restoration.

21.3.7 Course and outcome

For some, anorexia nervosa is a relatively benign self-limiting disorder; for others, it becomes a long-term problem. Few consistent predictors of outcome have been identified, the exceptions being a long history and late onset both of which are associated with a poor prognosis. A very low weight and a history of premorbid psychosocial problems also tend to be associated with a poor outcome.

Whilst at least half the patients recover in terms of their weight and menstrual function, the disturbed attitudes to shape and weight often persist and eating habits may remain disturbed. Up to a quarter develop bulimia nervosa. Standardized mortality ratios range between 1.36 and 6.01, the deaths being either a direct result of medical complications or due to suicide. The more recent follow-up studies have obtained lower figures suggesting that the mortality rate is falling. The outcome in males appears to be essentially the same as that in females.

21.4 Bulimia Nervosa

21.4.1 Clinical features

Anorexia nervosa and bulimia nervosa have similar clinical features. There are the same extreme concerns about shape and weight and the same methods of weight control. However, there are two features which distinguish people with bulimia nervosa from those with anorexia nervosa: first, their weight is generally within the normal range; and second, there are frequent bulimic episodes. These 'binges' generally take place in secret and are often followed by compensatory behaviour such as self-induced vomiting and the misuse of laxatives or diuretics. The binges vary greatly in size, many involving the consumption of 2000 kcal (8.3 MJ) or more, and most consist of foods the person is otherwise attempting to avoid eating. The term 'carbohydrate craving' is sometimes used to describe the urge to binge but it is misleading since binges do not generally contain a disproportionate amount of carbohydrate. Between binges, people with bulimia nervosa severely restrict their food intake much as in anorexia nervosa, a behaviour that perpetuates the problem. Figure 21.1 shows a monitoring record illustrating the eating habits of a typical patient.

Depressive and anxiety symptoms are common in bulimia nervosa, more so than in anorexia nervosa. A significant minority also have problems with alcohol or drugs. Interpersonal functioning is often impaired.

The majority of patients with bulimia nervosa have few physical complaints. Those most commonly encountered are irregular or absent menstruation, weakness and lethargy, vague abdominal pains and toothache. On examination, appearance is usually unremarkable. Parotid gland enlargement may be present and there may be significant erosion of the dental enamel particularly on the lingual surface of the upper front teeth. The most important abnormality on investigation is the electrolyte disturbance which is encountered in those who vomit frequently or take large quantities of laxatives or diuretics. Clinically serious electrolyte disturbance is not often found and rarely does it merit direct treatment: instead, it is better to focus on the treatment of the eating disorder. Other abnormalities are occasionally found and these resemble those present in anorexia nervosa, but are not as severe.

21.4.2 Aetiology

Many patients with bulimia nervosa give a history of disturbed eating stretching back into adolescence, and about a third have previously fulfilled diagnostic criteria for anorexia nervosa. Most of the remainder started with an anorexia nervosa-like picture although the weight loss was not severe. Given this sequence of events, and the fact that the two conditions are so similar, it may be assumed that most factors of relevance to

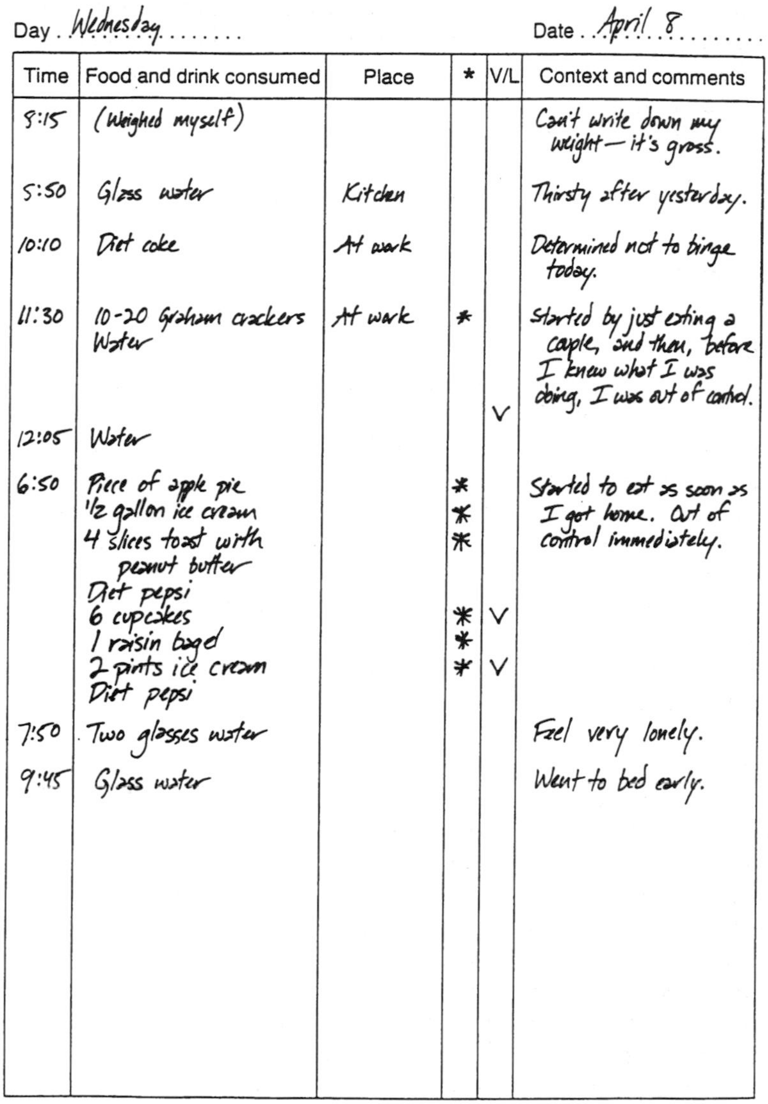

Day . *Wednesday* . . . .   Date . *April 8* . . . .

Time	Food and drink consumed	Place	*	V/L	Context and comments
8:15	(Weighed myself)				Can't write down my weight — it's gross.
5:50	Glass water	Kitchen			Thirsty after yesterday.
10:10	Diet coke	At work			Determined not to binge today.
11:30	10-20 Graham crackers Water	At work	*		Started by just eating a couple, and then, before I knew what I was doing, I was out of control.
				V	
12:05	Water				
6:50	Piece of apple pie ½ gallon ice cream 4 slices toast with peanut butter Diet pepsi 6 cupcakes 1 raisin bagel 2 pints ice cream Diet pepsi		* * * * * *	V V	Started to eat as soon as I got home. Out of control immediately.
7:50	Two glasses water				Feel very lonely.
9:45	Glass water				Went to bed early.

Fig. 21.1 A monitoring record showing the eating habits of a typical patient with bulimia nervosa. V, vomiting, L, laxative mususe, *eating viewed by the patient as excessive. *Source:* Reprinted with permission from Fairburn CG. *Overcoming binge eating.* New York: Guilford Press, 1995.

the aetiology of anorexia nervosa are also relevant to the aetiology of bulimia nervosa. Nevertheless, it seems that some factors preferentially increase the risk of developing bulimia nervosa. These include vulnerability to obesity, affective disorder and substance abuse, the rates of all three disorders being raised in the relatives of these patients. Sexual abuse predating the onset of the eating disorder is reported by about a quarter of the patients. This rate is higher than that among matched subjects in the general population but is no higher than that among young women with other psychiatric disorders.

21.4.3 Assessment

Most patients with bulimia nervosa are ashamed of their eating habits and have kept them secret for many years. Like those with anorexia nervosa, they may present complaining of features associated with the disorder rather than the disorder itself. For example, they may present with depression or substance abuse, or with gastrointestinal or gynaecological symptoms. Under these circumstances making the correct diagnosis can be difficult since there may be no pointers to the eating disorder.

Those who present with bulimia nervosa itself complain of the loss of control over eating. Assessment is relatively straightforward and the diagnosis can be made with little difficulty. As with anorexia nervosa, no physical tests are needed to establish the diagnosis. However, the electrolytes should be checked of all those who vomit frequently or misuse large quantities of laxatives or diuretics.

21.4.4 Management

The great majority of patients with bulimia nervosa may be managed on an outpatient basis, the most effective treatment being a specific form of cognitive behaviour therapy. This is a specialized psychological treatment which is designed to modify not only the disturbed eating habits but also the extreme concerns about shape and weight. It usually involves about 20 sessions over five months and results in substantial improvement in all aspects of the psychopathology. Some patients respond to less intensive interventions and self-help manuals based on cognitive behavioural principles have a role. Antidepressant drugs are the only drug treatment to have shown promise. They result in a decline in the frequency of binge eating and an improvement in mood, but the effect is not as great as that seen with cognitive behaviour therapy and, more importantly, it is usually short-lived.

21.4.5 Course and outcome

Little is known about the long-term course and outcome of bulimia nervosa. Many of the cases identified in community surveys appear to be relatively benign in that they are transitory. In contrast, patients who present for treatment usually have an enduring disorder, the mean length of history being five years. About two-thirds respond well to cognitive behaviour therapy with the changes being well maintained.

21.5 ATYPICAL EATING DISORDERS

In addition to anorexia nervosa and bulimia nervosa, various 'atypical eating disorders' are encountered. These have not been well characterized. Most common are disorders resembling anorexia nervosa or bulimia nervosa but not quite meeting their diagnostic criteria. For example, about a quarter of those who present for the treatment of obesity have recurrent binges similar to those seen in bulimia nervosa. However, the binges do not occur against the background of extreme dietary restraint nor are they accompanied by self-induced vomiting or the misuse of laxatives or diuretics. Patients with this eating pattern are sometimes said to have 'binge eating disorder'. The evidence to date suggests that it responds well to a modified version of the cognitive behavioural treatment for bulimia nervosa.

Further Reading

1. American Dietetic Association. Nutrition intervention in the treatment of anorexia nervosa, bulimia nervosa, and binge eating. *J Am Dietet Assoc* 1994; **94**: 902–7.
2. Brownell KD, Fairburn CG (eds). *Eating disorders and obesity: a comprehensive handbook.* New York: Guilford Press, 1995.
3. Rock CL, Yager J. Nutrition and eating disorders: a primer for clinicians. *Int J Eating Disorders* 1987; **6**: 267–80.

Part IV: Foods

22

FOOD GROUPS

Margaret Allman-Farinelli

with coauthors named at the head of each section

22.1 BREADS AND CEREALS

with Trish Griffiths

Cereals, the 'seeds of civilization', have constituted much of the food eaten by humans for thousands of years. It was not until the nomadic hunter–gatherers learned to farm crops that permanent settlements arose. Cultivation of wheat can be traced back to about 7000 BC in the Euphrates valley while cultivation of rice, dates back to around 3000 BC in China and shortly after in India. Maize was first cultivated about 5000 BC in Mexico. Food patterns were, and still are, most often built around a cereal. Wheat and barley were the staple foods of ancient Egypt, Greece and Rome; maize, the staple of the early Americans; oats and rye staples in the colder regions of Europe and millets (including sorghum) were important in Africa and parts of Asia. Early breads were made from crude flours produced by pounding grains with a stone. Water was then added and the dough baked to a flat bread. Leavened bread dates back to Egypt in about 2000 BC.

Wheat, rice and maize (corn) are currently the predominant cereals in terms of the land devoted to them and their consumption. Wheat covers more of the earth's surface than any other crop having largely replaced rye, barley and oats in Northern Europe, and increasingly replacing sorghum and millet in Africa. About 50% of the food protein available on the globe is derived from cereals, with consumption greatest in the developing countries (providing two-thirds of energy and protein). With increasing income, cereal consumption tends to decrease, while the intake of animal products and refined carbohydrates increases.

The nutritional values of all cereal grains are essentially similar, with some variation due to genetic factors and environmental conditions such as soil type and temperature (Table 22.1). Cereals are an important source of energy, providing between 1400 and 1600 kilojoules per 100 grams of whole cereal. Cereals provide starch and dietary fibre (soluble and insoluble) which together comprise 70–77% of the grain. Grains are usually processed and cooked so that the starch is digestible. Protein accounts for 6–15% and the limiting amino acid is lysine, with maize additionally low in tryptophan. Gluten is the major protein in wheat and rye and oryzenin the major protein in rice. All cereals are low in fat, oats have slightly more; most of the fat is polyunsaturated. Whole grains are a good source of thiamin, their germ is rich in vitamin E and they contain significant amounts of minerals especially potassium, phosphorus, magnesium, iron and zinc.

Table 22.1 Nutrient content of grains

Nutrient	Nutrients per 100 g (raw grains)				
	Wheat[a]	Brown rice[b]	Maize[b]	Millet[b]	Oats[b]
Water (g)	11.0	12.0	13.8	11.8	8.3
Protein (g)	12.6	7.5	9.0	10.0	15.0
Fat (g)	2.7	1.9	3.9	2.9	7.0
Carbohydrate (g)	72.4	77.4	72.2	72.9	69
Thiamin (mg)	0.5	0.34	0.37	0.73	0.6
Niacin (mg)	6.1	4.7	2.2	2.3	1.0
Calcium (mg)	35.0	32.0	22.0	20.0	53.0
Iron (mg)	3.7	1.6	2.1	6.8	4.5

Based on [a] Bread Research Institute of Australia Inc.
[b] Lorenz KJ and Kulp K (eds). *Handbook of cereal science and technology*. New York: Marcel Dekker, 1991.

However, the contribution of cereals to mineral intake may be less than anticipated because phytate in the outer bran layers binds some minerals and inhibits their absorption. Bioavailability of minerals is better from refined products but because the mineral content is less, overall more minerals will be provided by whole grains. During fermentation, as in bread making, phytase is produced which breaks down phytate.

22.1.1   Processing of cereal grains for human consumption

Wheat   requires some processing to increase its digestibility. This is achieved by milling which involves a series of grinding and sifting steps to produce flour. The nutritional value of flour varies with the extraction rate (the number of parts by weight of flour produced after milling 100 parts of grain). Typically fibre, vitamins and minerals are concentrated in the outer bran and aleurone layers of grains and the extent to which these layers are removed determines the nutrient content. White flour will have a lower micronutrient content compared to wholemeal but the amounts still make a significant contribution to the diet. In some countries, cereal products are fortified with added vitamins or minerals (e.g. thiamin, niacin, calcium, iron). Starch and protein concentrated in the endosperm of the grain are less affected by processing. The protein content and 'hardness' of flour determines its application, for example, hard high protein wheat is most suitable for bread, soft low protein wheats are most suitable for biscuits and hard durum wheat is used exclusively for the production of pasta. In addition to flour, milling produces bran, germ and semolina. Bread, breakfast cereals, gluten (used predominantly by the baking industry) and wheat starch are also products of wheat processing. Bread, one of the most widely eaten foods in the world, is the major product made from wheat flour. White, wholemeal and mixed grain breads are popular in Western countries; white flatbreads and Chinese steamed breads are common in the Middle East and China.

Rice   is the staple food of over half of the world's population. After harvesting, paddy rice is cleaned and dehulled but the bran layer retained to produce brown rice.

Alternatively, the brown rice can be further milled and polished to give white rice. Brown rice has a higher protein, mineral and vitamin content than milled rice but also has a higher content of phytate and fibre. The practice of extensive abrasive polishing of rice is of concern in many Asian nations because the majority of food eaten is rice. Because of this any loss of nutrients like protein, thiamin and iron becomes critical. The practice of parboiling rice before milling is encouraged as this results in an inward migration of water-soluble vitamins to the endosperm. The process of rice enrichment may also improve nutrient intake. This involves mixing the ordinary white rice in a fixed proportion with rice that has been treated with a vitamin mixture. In developed countries people have been enticed to eat more rice by a range of novel products such as rice cakes, rice bran, rice noodles and rice crackers.

Maize (corn) may be either dry-milled (the protein and starch fractions are not separated) or wet-milled (the protein and starch is separated). Dry milling produces grits, meals, flour and hominy feed, while wet milling yields starch, dextrose, corn syrup solids and glucose. Immature maize is often eaten fresh as a vegetable—sweet corn. Maize kernels can also be frozen or canned. Maize is used in the production of corn meals, corn flour, corn chips, tacos and tortillas, the consumption of which is no longer confined to Mexico. In African countries maize is widely consumed as a porridge, either a stiff porridge (ugali) or thin gruel (uji) which can be used as the basis for alcoholic or non-alcoholic beverages. Maize is also processed to make flaked breakfast cereals.

While maize contains little niacin or its amino acid precursor, tryptophan, the traditional alkali cooking method (using a lime cooking step) for tortillas increases the availability of niacin and may have prevented widespread pellagra in populations relying on maize tortillas as a staple food.

Oats are processed by steaming or kiln drying before de-hulling. The resultant 'groats' can be cut to produce a coarse meal which is steamed, then rolled to make oat flakes, or granulated to produce a fine oat meal. Oats are generally eaten as a breakfast cereal. Consumption of oat bran became popular because of the cholesterol-lowering properties of its soluble fibre. However, the amounts usually consumed will have only a minor effect.

Barley is used in the form of pearled grains for soups, flour for flatbreads and ground grain for porridge. Barley flour is generally milled by conventional roller milling as used for wheat. Malted barley is important in the brewing and baking industries and is also used in the making of vinegar and for flavouring breakfast cereal.

Rye is milled in a similar fashion to wheat. Cracked rye is used for porridge and other breakfast cereals and rye flour can be baked into bread, pumpernickel and crispbreads. The distillation of gin, whiskey and beer may include rye in the process.

Millet is a name given to a group of cereals that includes sorghum. It is consumed in Africa, parts of India, Pakistan and China. The grains are pounded into flour and mixed with water to make porridge. In parts of Africa, finely ground millet grains are left to ferment slightly before being baked into flatbreads called injera.

FURTHER READING

1. Bourne GH (ed.). *Nutritional value of cereal products, beans and starches.* Vol 60. World Review of Nutrition and Dietetics. Basel: Karger, 1989.
2. Juliano B. *Rice in human nutrition.* FAO Food and Nutrition Series. No 26. Rome: IRRI and FAO, 1993.
3. Munck L. Barley for food, feed and industry. In: Pomeranz Y, Munck L (eds). *Cereals: a renewable resource, theory and practice.* St Paul, MN: AACC, 1981: 427–59.
4. Rooney LW, Serna-Saldivar SO. Food uses of whole corn and dry milled fractions. In: Watson SA, Ramstad PE. *Corn, chemistry and technology,* St Paul, MN: AACC, 1987: 399–429.

22.2 LEGUMES

with Sue Munro

Legumes are the edible seed from the Leguminosae family (*Fabaceae*) and include dried peas, beans, lentils and dhal. Peanuts are also legumes. Cultivated since earliest civilizations, legumes have assumed a major secondary nutritional role for humanity. Legumes were often considered an inferior food eaten by peasants, described as being 'poor man's meat'. They never assumed the importance of a staple food as did the cereal crops of wheat, rice, maize or barley. Yet, they played an important synergistic role with staple foods both in meeting nutritional requirements and fertilizing the soil.

The cereal-and-bean combination is a feature of many cuisines. Mexicans eat kidney beans and tortillas, Indians top their rice with dhal, the Chinese enjoy soy products with rice, those in the Middle East combine lentils with rice, while the English put baked beans on toast. The ratio of quantities of cereal and beans consumed is similar with cereal foods assuming the role of staple, the main source of energy, and the legumes used as accompaniments.

Of all foods, legumes most adequately meet the recommended dietary guidelines for healthful eating. They are high in carbohydrate and dietary fibre, mostly low in fat, supply adequate protein while being a good source of vitamins and minerals. Cooked legumes contain about 6–9% protein, about twice as much protein as in cereal foods. The exceptions are soybeans and peanuts, which contain 14% and 24%, respectively, when cooked. The limiting amino acids of legumes are the sulphur-containing methionine and cysteine but, being rich in lysine, legume proteins are well complemented by cereals. Recent reports suggest that the amount of indispensable amino acids in soy protein products is sufficient to meet protein requirements for normal human growth and development.

Legumes provide 10–13 g of carbohydrate and 6–9 g of fibre per 100 grams of cooked beans. Some of the fibre is soluble fibre which might lower blood cholesterol. Legumes also contain oligosaccharides which escape digestion in the gut to be fermented by bacteria in the large bowel. This is responsible for the abdominal discomfort and flatulence and is perhaps the factor limiting consumption. Legumes are low in fat (∼2.5%) but soybeans and peanuts contain 8% fat and 47%, respectively. This fat is mostly monounsaturated or polyunsaturated.

Table 22.2   Nutrient content of legumes

Nutrient	Nutrients per 100 g cooked beans			
Protein (g)	6.2	(cannelini)	to 24.7	(peanuts)
Fat (g)	0.4	(lentils)	to 7.7	(soybeans)
Carbohydrate (g)	1.4	(soybeans)	to 12.6	(haricot beans)
Dietary fibre (g)	3.7	(lentils)	to 8.8	(haricot beans)
Thiamin (mg)	0.6	(lima beans)	to 0.79	(peanuts)
Riboflavin (mg)	trace	(kidney beans)	to 0.7	(soybeans)
Niacin equivalents (mg)	1.6	(lima beans)	to 19.8	(peanuts)
Calcium (mg)	13.0	(split peas)	to 76.0	(soybeans)
Iron (mg)	1.0	(split peas)	to 2.2	(soybeans)
Zinc (mg)	0.6	(split peas)	to 1.6	(soybeans)

Source: English R, Lewis J. *The composition of foods Australia*. Canberra: Australian Government Publishing Service, 1990.

Legumes supply vitamins and minerals including thiamin, niacin, iron, zinc, calcium and magnesium (Table 22.2). Soybeans contain isoflavones and lignans which are phytoestrogenic compounds possessing anti-cancer and antioxidant properties. There are, however, several substances in uncooked legumes that inhibit their nutritional quality. Most of these toxic substances are destroyed or inactivated by normal cooking or processing. Trypsin inhibitors, may reduce the effectiveness of the digestive process; haemagglutinins appear to reduce the efficiency of absorption of digestive products; phytate binds metals, like zinc and iron, decreasing their absorption; goitrogens interrupt the absorption of iodine. Apart from antinutrient toxins other substances in beans can cause specific diseases. Lathyrus sativus is drought-resistant but can precipitate lathyrism (a neurological disorder) when consumed in large amounts, and broad beans may result in favism, a haemolytic anaemia, in individuals of Mediterranean descent who are genetically susceptible to this disease. Some legumes contain toxic cyanide and alkaloids. Peanuts are common food allergens especially for children. Peanuts are susceptible to *Aspergillus* mould which produces aflatoxin which is a potent liver carcinogen. Careful storage and monitoring are essential to avoid contamination.

22.2.1   Products from the basic food

Uncooked dried legumes are virtually indigestible, tasteless and too hard to eat anyway. Processing is essential to make beans edible and to improve the nutritional quality and digestibility of the bean. Cooking and processing inactivates most antinutrients and toxins. Germination and fermentation improve the nutritional quality of the bean resulting in increases in vitamin C, niacin, riboflavin and thiamin and vitamin E content of beans.

There are distinct differences in preparation between the East and West. In India and some parts of Africa, raw legumes are milled to remove fibrous seed coats. Cotyledons are split along natural cleavage lines to form two split peas or dhal. The peas or beans are then boiled, roasted, fermented, germinated or ground into flour or paste, as required. In Western countries and South America and much of Africa, the seeds are soaked and cooked for long periods of time to inactivate toxic substances and improve digestibility.

The beans are either eaten whole, pureed and fried or made into cakes. In Asia, various methods of processing the soybean evolved, along with its cultivation. Immature beans are eaten whole in salads, vegetable dishes or soups, but mature soybeans are not usually eaten as whole beans but rather processed into curd, cheese, sauces, pastes or sprouted as a vegetable.

Today, peanuts and soybeans account for most of the legume products. Soybeans are made into a range of products, including, soy protein concentrates or isolates, extrusion-textured products, soyflour, soymilk and tofu. Many soy products are used in manufactured food products, including bread and baked goods, processed meat products, soy ice cream, sauces and low fat spreads. Peanuts are made into butters and used in confectionery and baked goods.

FURTHER READING

1. Food and Agriculture Organization. *Legumes in human nutrition.* Nutritional Studies No. 19. Rome: FAO, 1964.
2. Food and Agriculture Organization. *Utilization of tropical foods: tropical beans.* Food and Nutrition Paper 47/4. Rome: FAO, 1989.
3. Golbitz P. Traditional soyfoods: processing and products. *J Nutr* 1995; **125**: 570S–2S.
4. Lusas EW, Mian NR. Soy protein products: processing and use. *J Nutr* 1995; **125**: 573S–80S.
5. Young VR. Soy protein in relation to human protein and amino acid nutrition. *J Am Dietet Ass* 1991; **91**: 828–35.

22.3 NUTS AND SEEDS

with Sue Munro

Nuts and seeds have been valued for their oils as much as a food and were an important source of nutrients and energy since the earliest civilizations. Traditional cuisines have

Table 22.3 Nutrient content of raw nuts and seeds

Nutrient	Nutrients per 100 g raw nuts (kernel only)			
Protein (g)	2.0	(chestnuts)	to 24.4	(pumpkin seeds)
Fat (g)	2.7	(chestnuts)	to 77.6	(macadamias)
Carbohydrate (g)	3.1	(Brazil nuts)	to 36.6	(chestnuts)
Dietary fibre* (g)	1.9	(pine nuts)	to 7.9	(sesame seeds)
Thiamin (mg)	0.11	(Barcelona nuts)	to 0.93	(sesame seeds)
Riboflavin (mg)	0.06	(macadamias)	to 0.75	(almonds)
Niacin equivalents (mg)	0.9	(chestnuts)	to 9.1	(sunflower seeds)
Calcium (mg)	11.0	(pine nuts)	to 670.0	(sesame seeds)
Iron (mg)	1.6	(macadamias)	to 10.4	(sesame seeds)
Zinc (mg)	0.5	(chestnuts)	to 6.6	(pumpkin seeds)

* Englyst method (see Chapter 24.2.4).
Source: Holland B, Unwin ID, Buss DH. Fruit and nuts. First supplement to *McCance and Widdowson's, The composition of foods.* 5th ed. London: Royal Society of Chemistry, MAFF, 1992.

utilized the locally grown nuts and seeds for both savoury and dessert dishes. Today, nuts and seeds are processed for their oil, ground into pastes, used as ingredients in baked goods or eaten raw or roasted as snack foods.

Common types of nuts include almonds, walnuts, pecans, cashew, Brazil nuts, macadamias and hazelnuts. Sunflower, sesame and pumpkin are the most common seeds eaten as foods. Caraway and poppy seeds are usually used as seasonings.

Nuts and seeds have similar nutritional qualities; their high content of energy, protein, vitamins and minerals makes them a very nutritious food (Table 22.3). The energy content of nuts is mostly due to their high fat content. The fat in nuts varies in both quantity and type. Chestnuts are low in fat, but other nuts contain from 45–75% fat. The majority of nuts contain unsaturated fatty acids either polyunsaturated (walnut) or monounsaturated (macadamia). The protein content of nuts ranges from 2–25%; lysine is the limiting amino acid. They are good sources of dietary fibre, B vitamins, (thiamin, riboflavin and niacin), vitamin E, and iron, zinc, magnesium, potassium and calcium.

Nuts are known to be both detrimental and beneficial to health. For some people, walnuts can trigger an allergic reaction, whereas for others they help lower plasma cholesterol.

22.4 FRUIT

with Stewart Truswell

In its strict botanical sense a 'fruit' is the fleshy or dry ripened ovary of a plant enclosing the seed and so includes corn grains, bean pods, tomatoes, olives, cucumbers, and almonds and pecans (in their shells). We usually restrict the term 'fruit' to mean the ripened ovaries that are sweet and either succulent or pulpy and usually eaten as an appetizer or a dessert. Fresh fruits were formerly only available seasonally but with technology and imports, many are available most of the year. Most of us eat more species in the fruit food group than in any other food group, for example, 30 or more species: some daily (e.g. apples, oranges, bananas) and others rarely (e.g. goldenberries, elder-berries, mulberries, loganberries, passion fruit).

Our ancestors originally ate fruits for their sweetness. They learned that fruits that were not bitter were unlikely to be toxic. The sugar provides energy and may be as fructose and/or glucose and/or sucrose and others (such as sorbitol) (Table 22.4). Fruits generally provide useful amounts of potassium, β-carotene, vitamin C and folate. Avocados are unusual because they have a high content of fat (mostly monounsaturated) and contain a 7-carbon sugar.

Fruits are preserved in jams by boiling with sugar; the pectin (soluble dietary fibre) they contain makes a gel. Some fruits are dried: especially grapes, plums, dates, bananas, apricots (dried fruits do not contain vitamin C).

Quite large amounts of some fruits, especially citrus and apples are consumed in the form of fruit juices, which contain most of the nutrients but less of the fibre, and give less satiety.

Grapes are high in sugar (glucose), which makes crushed grapes a good substrate for fermentation into wine; apples are fermented to make cider.

Table 22.4   Nutrient content of raw fruits

Nutrient	Nutrients in fruits per 100 g raw edible portion			
Protein (g)	0.3	(apples)	to 2.6	(passionfruit)
Fat (g)	trace	(most)	to 19.3	(avocado)
Sugars (g)	trace	(olive)	to 20.9	(bananas)
Dietary fibre (g)	0.1	(watermelon)	to 3.8	(kumquat)
β-Carotene (mg)	5.0	(lemon)	to 1800	(mango)
Vitamin C (mg)	3.0	(durian)	to 230	(guava)
Folate (mg)	3.0	(grapes)	to 34	(blackberries)
Vitamin B$_6$ (mg)	0.02	(gooseberries)	to 0.29	(banana)
Vitamin E (mg)	0.2	(strawberries)	to 2.4	(blackberries)
Potassium (mg)	88.0	(watermelon)	to 400	(banana)

Source: Holland B, Unwin ID, Buss DH. Fruit and nuts. First Supplement to *McCance and Widdowson's, The composition of foods*. 5th ed. London: Royal Society of Chemistry, MAFF, 1992.

Most fruits taste somewhat sour, because they contain organic acids such as citric, malic, tartaric and in some cases, benzoic or sorbic acids. Only citric and malic acid provide small amounts of energy in the mammalian body. Because of the sourness, sugar is added to some fruits to make them palatable.

Fruits contain other substances, not nutrients, which can be biologically active (e g salicylates, flavonoids, limonoids). Tiny amounts of many different natural esters, aldehydes and ketones contribute the distinctive volatile flavours of fruits (e.g. in an apple, 103 flavour compounds have been identified, see Table 15.2).

People cannot live for long on fruits alone. They are inadequate in protein, sodium, calcium, iron and zinc. Nutritionists, however, look very favourably on fruit as part of a mixed diet and urge people to eat plenty of fruits each day. This is because they are low in energy, fat and sodium and make valuable contributions to the intakes of vitamin C, β-carotene, folate and dietary fibre. Numerous epidemiological studies have shown that people who eat above average amounts of fruit and vegetables (intakes of these two food groups are often recorded together) have below average rates of major degenerative diseases. This may be partly because more fruit is eaten in more privileged sections of society, partly because of good things in fruits, such as antioxidant nutrients (vitamin C and β-carotene) or other substances yet to be fully elucidated.

There is little to be said about fruits on the negative side, except that in the orchard they are often sprayed with pesticide. These pesticides should have decomposed before sale but it is safer to wash fruits before eating. The seeds or stones of some fruits contain cyanogenic glycosides which are potentially toxic.

22.5   VEGETABLES

Vegetables comprise any plant part, other than fruit which is used as food. They include roots and tubers such as potatoes, taro, turnips, parsnips, carrots and yams; bulbs such as onions, stems like celery, leaves such as lettuce, cabbage and flowers such as broccoli and cauliflower. Some fungi (e.g. mushrooms) are also consumed as vegetables. Marrows, although strictly fruits, are usually considered as vegetables by the consumer (e.g. zucchini and squash). Peas and beans are legumes but when immature and green are treated as vegetables. The nutritional composition and the usage pattern of the roots and tubers is somewhat different to that of the stems, leaves and flowers.

Potatoes had their origin in the New World, being staples of the Incas; other tubers such as yams and taro have been staple foods in the Pacific Islands for many years. Leafy vegetables were grown in monastery gardens during the Middle Ages. Today, most nations have cereal staples like rice or wheat but some countries have vegetable staples. Cassava is a staple energy source for about 200 million people in tropical countries. Potatoes whether as potato chips, boiled or baked, or French fries remain a much consumed commodity in developed nations like the United States. While leafy vegetables are commonly eaten in developed countries they are less popular in developing nations. It is estimated that in India there were 40 species of leaves grown 70 years ago and the number has now diminished to about four.

Potatoes, yams and taro will supply moderate amounts of protein in people's diets. The biological value is good with the limiting amino acid being methionine. The stem, bulb, leaf and flower vegetables usually provide smaller amounts of protein to the diet although their content may be similar. All vegetables contain negligible fat. Starch predominates in tubers, mainly amylopectin; the other vegetables contain sugars. Vegetables are a good source of dietary fibre. The fibre includes the soluble-type (e.g. pectin) but also includes insoluble fibre, like cellulose.

Green leafy vegetables have a very high water content and are exceptionally low in energy while relatively high in micronutrients so in a weight-conscious community they are a good food choice. Some vegetables are rich in micronutrients: potatoes are a major source of vitamin C, carrots are exceptionally high in β-carotene and spinach is rich in folic acid. Broccoli is relatively rich in calcium and spinach in iron, although neither is necessarily consumed in sufficient quantities to make a large contribution to the mineral intake. The other factor to consider is the bioavailability. Some studies suggest that β-carotene from vegetables may be more poorly absorbed than the pharmaceutical preparation; others refute this finding. This is unfortunate because leaves are very rich in β-carotene and blindness from vitamin A deficiency remains a major public health risk in many developing countries. It is well recognized that the absorption of non-haem iron from vegetables is not as good as the haem form found in meat but the presence of vitamin C will enhance non-haem iron absorption (Table 22.5).

Apart from the well-recognized nutrients, vegetables contain a variety of substances that may be beneficial for health. Epidemiological studies indicate that vegetable consumption is associated with a lower prevalence of certain types of cancer like bowel, lung and stomach. Initially this was attributed to their high content of antioxidant vitamins but other constituents may be more important. Flavonoids like quercetin and kaempferol found in onions and broccoli and glucosinolates found in cruciferous vegetables like brussels sprouts and cabbage may protect against cancer. The flavonoids may also be cardioprotective because they function as antioxidants and decrease the aggregation of blood platelets which leads to thrombus formation.

While eating vegetables is desirable there are a few potential toxic effects. Potatoes, especially green ones, contain solanine which is a neurotoxin and this is harmful if excessive amounts are eaten. Sweet potatoes if infected with a certain fungus may contain

Table 22.5 Nutrient content of vegetables

Nutrient	Nutrients per 100 g raw edible portion			
Energy (kJ)	27.0	(lettuce)	to 441.0	(taro)
Protein (g)	0.6	(celery)	to 4.7	(broccoli)
Fat (g)	0.0	(chinese cabbage)	to 0.6	(pumpkin)
Carbohydrate (g)	0.4	(lettuce)	to 30.4	(cassava)
Fibre (g)	0.8	(globe artichoke)	to 4.0	(broccoli)
β-Carotene (mg)	0.0	(potato)	to 10.35	(carrots)
Vitamin C (mg)	4.0	(lettuce)	to 110.0	(brussels sprouts)
Calcium (mg)	4.0	(potato)	to 82.0	(okra)
Iron (mg)	0.2	(pumpkin)	to 3.2	(English spinach)
Flavonoids* (mg)	0.0	(spinach)	to 35.3	(onion)

* Hertog MGL, Hollman PCH, Katan MB. Intake of potentially anticarcinogenic flavonoids and their determinants in adults in the Netherlands. *J Agric Fd Chem* 1992; **41**: 1242–6.
Source: English R, Lewis J. *The composition of foods Australia.* Canberra: Australian Government Publishing Service, 1990.

furanoterpenes that cause lung disorders. Cassava contains cyanogenic glycosides which liberate cyanide but this is largely removed by peeling and cooking.

Vegetables are an enjoyable, nutritious food commodity. A number of major epidemiological studies have lead to the advice to consume five servings of vegetables and fruit per day. Whether the planet can provide this for all people is another problem that will need to be addressed.

FURTHER READING

1. Block G, Patterson B, Subar A. Fruit, vegetables, and cancer prevention a review of the epidemiological evidence. *Nutr Cancer* 1992; **18**: 1–30.
2. Hertog MGL, Hollman PCH, Katan MB, Kromhout D. Intake of potentially anticarcinogenic flavonoids and their determinants in adults in the Netherlands. *Nutr Cancer* 1993; **20**: 21–9.
3. Johns L, Stevenson V. *The complete book of fruit.* Sydney: Angus and Robertson, 1979.
4. Martin FW. *Handbook of tropical food crops.* Boca Raton, FL: CRC Press, 1984.
5. Wolfe J. *The potato in the human diet.* Cambridge University Press, 1987.

22.6 MILK AND MILK PRODUCTS

with Soumela Amanatidis

All mammals produce milk and man consumes a variety of milks from cows, sheep, goats, horses, reindeer, yaks, water buffalos and camels. It is impossible to identify when the use of animals' milk as a food source began, but it is reasonable to assume it coincided with the domestication of animals around ten thousand years ago. Sheep and goats were domesticated first, probably about 8000–9000 BC. Cave paintings show that dairy animals were domesticated by 4000 BC, and traces of cheeses have been found in Egyptian tombs dating back to 2000 BC. Hippocrates recommended milk as a health food and medicine about 400 BC.

Milk and milk products, yoghurt, cheese and cream are widely used throughout Europe but are not to any extent in Asia or the smaller Pacific islands. With a few exceptions, milk is the most commonly used milk product in Northern Europe and cheese is the dominant milk product in Southern Europe. In North America, Australia and New Zealand, dairy industries are well established and milk and milk products are widely consumed.

Milk   Cow's milk is about 88% water and 3% protein. The two main proteins are casein and whey proteins which include lactalbumin and lactoglobulin. Casein comprises about 82% of the total protein. It is of high nutritional value and contains all the essential amino acids with relatively high amounts of the amino acid, lysine. Goat's milk has a similar protein content and casein to whey ratio.

The fat content of cow's milk varies from 3.2–4.5%, depending on the breed of cow. Milk fat or butter fat is over 60% saturated, 33% monounsaturated, and less than 5% polyunsaturated. Milk contains a significant proportion of volatile short-chain fatty acids which are easily digested by humans and other mammals. Goat's milk has a fat content of about 4.5%.

Milk is an excellent source of readily absorbable calcium and phosphorus and milk and milk products provide over 75% of the calcium in the human diet in Western countries. Milk also contains moderate amounts of potassium, sodium, magnesium and zinc but is low in iron. Milk can be an important source of iodine because the sterilizing solutions used in some dairies contain iodine and traces get into the milk.

Milk carries B group vitamins, particularly riboflavin and vitamin B_{12}, and the fat-soluble vitamins A and D. Goat's milk has less folic acid and vitamin B_6 than cow's milk. Milk in glass bottles exposed to direct sunlight may lose up to 50% of the riboflavin in two hours. Paperboard cartons reduce the penetration of sunlight but do not block it completely.

Lactose is the principal sugar in milk and milk is the only source of lactose in nature. The lactose enhances the absorption of calcium and phosphorus from the intestine. Around two-thirds of the world's population have difficulty digesting lactose because the lactase enzyme that breaks down lactose in the gut is lost after weaning. The undigested lactose ferments and causes abdominal pain and diarrhoea. Lactase deficiency is common among Southern Europeans, Asians, Australian Aborigines, Black Africans, and those from Middle Eastern countries but they can usually include small amounts of milk in their diet.

Milk is pasteurized to destroy any disease-causing bacteria, particularly tuberculosis and brucellosis bacteria. During pasteurization, milk is heated to 72 °C for 15 seconds then cooled immediately. This causes small losses of nutrients but these are not significant nutritionally. Milk can be kept for about one week in the refrigerator.

Long life or ultra heat treatment (UHT) milk is heated to 142 °C for two seconds. This process destroys more bacteria than pasteurization. Long life products unopened have a shelf life of several months without refrigeration. Once opened, they should be refrigerated and treated in the same way as the pasteurized products.

Milk is available in different forms. Skim milks have all the fat taken out and do not contain the fat-soluble vitamins A and D; reduced fat milks generally have 50–60% of the fat removed. Fortified milks are also becoming popular. These consist of either skim milk or a mixture of skim milk and whole milk, with some concentrated skim milk added. Evaporated milk has half its water removed while condensed milk undergoes a similar process but has about 40% added sugar. Powdered milk has most of its moisture removed and keeps indefinitely in a cool dry place. Buttermilk is a soured milk made by adding a bacterial culture to skim or part-skim milk.

Less than 5% of infants appear to be allergic to cow's milk protein. About 80% of infants who are allergic to cow's milk protein are also allergic to goat's milk protein. Most children grow out of their allergy to milk as their digestive system matures.

Yoghurt   One of the most popular fermented foods is yoghurt. It originated in Asia and was introduced to Europe in the eighteenth century from the Balkans. Yoghurt is made by warming milk of various fat levels and introducing a special culture of bacteria: *Lactobacillus acidophilus* or *L. bulgaricus*. Milk sugars are broken down, releasing lactic acid which acts to coagulate the milk into a curd consistency. Yoghurt offers all the nutrients in milk, except for less lactose. Full cream yoghurt made from whole milk contains around 4% fat; reduced fat yoghurt has 1–2% fat; and low fat yoghurt has less than 0.2% fat.

Cheese   has been made for centuries and is one of the most effective ways of preserving milk. There are over 400 different cheeses, which vary because of differences in treatment of the starting material (bacteria or rennet) and the way the curd is subsequently treated and matured. Basically, cheese is made by using specific bacteria or renin to coagulate the casein of milk so that it separates into a thick curd and watery whey. The whey is removed and the curd undergoes further processing to produce the different cheeses.

Nutritionally, 30 g of cheese is similar to 250 ml of milk except that a large amount of salt is added and some of the B group vitamins are removed during the process of making hard cheese. The fat content of cheese varies from almost none in skim milk cheeses to around 35% in hard cheeses (i.e. 74% of energy, calories). The calcium content is high and there is no lactose except for those cheeses made from whey such as ricotta and cottage cheese which contain a small amount. Many cheeses contain tyramine, a protein-related substance formed when bacteria digest the protein of milk. In some sensitive people it can cause headaches. Tyramine can also raise blood pressure and has

Table 22.6   Nutrient content of milk and dairy products

Nutrient	Nutrients per 100 g				
	Milk (pasteurized whole)	Skim milk	Trim milk*	Cheese (Colby, Cheddar)	Yoghurt (fruit-flavoured, fat reduced, sweetened)
Protein (g)	3.3	3.5	4.3	22.9	4.5
Fat (g)	4.0	0.2	0.4	34.1	1.8
Carbohydrate (g)	4.4	4.6	5.2	0.1	14.8
Vitamin A (µg) (RE)	28.0	5.0	3.0	194	56.0
Riboflavin (mg)	0.2	0.2	0.3	0.4	0.2
Calcium (mg)	114	122	145	650	112

*Trim milk is fat-reduced (0.4%) with added skim milk solids. RE, Retinol equivalents.
Source: N.Z. Food Composition Database. New Zealand Institute for Crop and Food Research, 1997.

to be avoided by people taking monoamine oxidase-inhibiting drugs for depression. One positive effect of cheese is that it helps to protect teeth from dental caries.

Cream   is made from the fat portion of milk and comes in different thicknesses. In Australia, cream has 35% fat, except reduced fat or light cream which has half this level. In the United Kingdom, single cream has 21% fat, whipping cream has 35% fat and double cream has 48% fat. Sour cream is made by adding a bacterial culture to cream. Creams contain large amounts of vitamin A, a riboflavin content similar to milk, but less than half the calcium of milk (Table 22.6).

FURTHER READING

1. Campbell JR, Marshall RT. *The science of providing milk for man.* New York: McGraw-Hill Publications, 1975.
2. Renner E. *Milk and dairy products in human nutrition*, 4th ed. Munich: Volkswirtschaftlicher Verlag, 1983.
3. Rosenthal I. *Milk and dairy products: properties and processing.* New York: VCH, 1991.

22.7   MEAT AND POULTRY

There is evidence of primitive man hunting for animals from around 500 000 BC but it was not until the end of the last Ice Age (10 000–12 000 years ago) that humans began to domesticate animals along with the development of agriculture. The term 'meat' encompasses not only the muscle tissues but also organs like liver, kidneys and pancreas (termed offal). The major animals produced for human consumption are pigs, cattle, and sheep and birds like chicken and turkey. More unusual meats which are consumed include seals by the Eskimos, kangaroo in Australia, deer in Europe (venison), antelope in Africa, and guinea-pigs in South America.

Muscle meat is generally a good source of protein and minerals while offal meats may also offer a rich source of vitamins. Muscle is rich in essential amino acids, particularly sulphur amino acids. The greater the proportion of muscle to connective tissue the greater the digestibility of the protein and its biological value. The mineral content is high with potassium and phosphorus accounting for the largest proportion. Meat is a major source of readily available iron and zinc, and a good source of magnesium. Liver and kidney are richer in iron and zinc than muscle, and pig liver contains more than that from sheep or beef. The bioavailability of minerals from meat is superior to that from cereal and other plant foods. Meat provides a valuable source of thiamin, niacin and riboflavin, with pork higher in thiamin than the other meats. Organ meats contain more vitamin A and vitamin B_{12}, especially liver because this is where these vitamins are stored (Table 22.7). Liver is so rich in vitamin A that in Britain it is no longer advised for pregnant women because too much vitamin A is teratogenic.

In a number of countries, such as Australia, there has been a decline in the consumption of meat especially red meat. One of the reasons is the perceived threat to good health. In the past meats have had a higher fat content. The fat was largely saturated and it is now well known that saturated fat will raise plasma cholesterol. However, there is some

Table 22.7 Nutrient content of meats

Nutrient	Nutrients per 100 g cooked meats			
	Beef (grilled steak)	Lamb (grilled chop)	Pork (grilled chop)	Chicken (roast, no skin)
Protein (g)	28.6	27.8	32.3	24.8
Fat (g)	6.0	12.3	10.7	5.4
• saturated fatty acids	2.5	5.9	3.8	1.6
• monounsaturated fatty acids	2.8	4.6	4.1	2.5
• polyunsaturated fatty acids	0.2	0.6	1.5	1.0
Carbohydrate (g)	0.0	0.0	0.0	0.0
Vit B_{12} (mg)	0.002	0.002	0.002	trace
Iron (mg)	3.5	2.1	1.2	0.8
Zinc (mg)	5.3	4.1	3.5	1.5

Source: Holland B, Welch AA, Unwin ID, Buss DH, Paul AA, Southgate DAT. *McCance and Widdowson's, The composition of foods*. 5th ed. London: Royal Society of Chemistry, MAFF, 1991.

question as to whether the major fatty acid constituents of meat, palmitic and stearic acid, will raise cholesterol. Animal producers have made a large effort over the past couple of decades to breed leaner animals and butchers have been altering the type of cuts and trimming meats. This means that the fat content of lean meat is less than many consumers perceive. Meat also contains unsaturated fat including the very long-chain fatty acid, arachidonic acid, which is a predominant polyunsaturated fatty acid in cell membranes. Humans can produce this from polyunsaturated fat in vegetable oils but an intake of preformed arachidonic acid may be important in pregnant and lactating women and the infant for optimal development of the infant brain and retina.

Meat is made into a range of products by curing (e.g. ham and bacon) and by the addition of cereals (e.g. sausages). There is some concern about the nitrate used to cure meat because the nitrites formed have been linked with nitrosamine and cancer in animals. However, the amount permitted to be used has been lowered to the minimum which prevents bacterial growth and we actually obtain more nitrites via conversion of nitrates from plant foods.

Meat has a short shelf-life and must be kept at low temperatures and be adequately cooked to prevent microbial growth. The mode of cooking may be important. Frying or grilling on a hot plate may lead to the development of heterocyclic amines shown to be mutagenic. However, it cannot necessarily be extrapolated that these cause cancer in humans. The most recent concern for meat eaters was the development of 'mad cow disease' (bovine spongiform encephalopathy) in British beef. The link between eating affected meat and neurological disease in man (Creutzfeldt–Jakob) is questionable but as a precaution thousands of cattle have been destroyed.

Chicken and turkey meats are consumed in growing amounts in countries like the United States and Australia. Much of this is because people are selecting 'white' meat over red meat for health reasons. More exotic birds consumed include pigeon, pheasant and partridge. It is not only the muscle which is consumed but also parts like the feet (in China), the liver (goose paté), and even the head. Poultry is a good source of protein, with the fat content dependent on the individual bird, for example, turkey is leaner than chicken, which is leaner than goose or duck. Much of the fat is located just under the skin and can be easily removed.

Like red meat, poultry is a good source of protein and minerals including iron and zinc. Processed turkey meats such as a ham substitute and turkey bologna and sausages are increasing their share of the market because of the growing demand for lower fat meats.

FURTHER READING

1. Lawrie RA. *Meat science*. 4th ed. Oxford: Pergamon Press, 1985.
2. Lawrie R (ed.). *Developments in meat science*. Vol. 5. New York: Elsevier Applied Science, 1991.
3. Sinclair AJ, O'Dea K. The lipid levels and fatty acid compositions of the lean portions of Australian beef and lamb. *Food Tech Aust* 1987; 39: 229–31.

22.8 FISH

with Samir Samman

Most fish are caught in the oceans, rivers and lakes but some are produced under intensive farm conditions. Usually, the main edible parts are the flesh but other components such as roe are also eaten. Fish, like meat, contains protein of high biological value. The nutritional interest in fish, however, is the fat content which ranges from 0.5% to 15%. It varies according to season and environmental factors such as water temperature. In canned fish, more of the fat is often the oil used in packaging or cooking. Fish oils contain long-chain $\omega3$-polyunsaturated fatty acids, mainly eicosapentaenoic acid and docosahexaenoic acid. There is very little carbohydrate in fish and a moderate amount of cholesterol but more in fish roe. Fish decomposes rapidly. It is not usually a good source of fat-soluble vitamins, particularly those with antioxidant activity but whole body fish like sardines provide vitamin D. It is, however, a source of vitamin B_6, B_{12}, riboflavin, folate and most inorganic nutrients including iodine and fluoride. Calcium, although not found in high amounts in the fish flesh, can be eaten as part of the edible soft bones (as in sardines). Sodium content is usually low but as for fat, it can be introduced as part of the processing (e.g. fish canned in brine) (Table 22.8).

Table 22.8 Nutrient content of fish

Nutrient	Nutrients per 100 g raw edible portion			
Protein (g)	11.2	(oreo dory)	to 20.6	(John Dory)
Fat (g)	0.6	(red cod)	to 12.6	(silver warehou)
Calcium (mg)	5.44	(rig)	to 42.9	(NZ sole)
Iron (mg)	0.39	(hake)	to 1.66	(kahawai)
Zinc (mg)	0.26	(oreo dory)	to 1.0	(lemon sole)

Source: *Food Data*. Palmerston North, NZ: Biotechnology Division, DSIR, 1988.
N.Z. Food Composition Database. New Zealand Institute for Crop and Food Research, 1997.

The flavour of fish is generally favourable, with fish obtained from cold, clear, deep water generally more flavoursome than those obtained from warm, muddy, shallow water. The cooking methods are determined by the fish's fat content: fatty fish, for example, salmon or mullet, is usually grilled or baked, whereas lean fish, for example, whiting or cod, is fried. Sauces and garnishes are often used to enhance the flavour of fish. Undercooked fish can present some problems such as: tapeworms which deplete vitamin B_{12} and thiaminase which destroys thiamin. Other potential hazards associated with the consumption of fish are: toxic metal contamination (e.g. mercury, also known as Minimata disease), tetradoxin poisoning (mainly associated with puffer fish), poisoning by dinoflagellates (*Ciguatera*), and bacterial spoilage, particularly in tuna.

The health effects of fish consumption are considerable. Long-term fish consumption may reduce death from heart disease as shown in the Zutphen study. These effects may be attributable to the ω3-fatty acids in the fish flesh which may reduce thrombotic tendency by an array of mechanisms.

FURTHER READING

1. Ruiter A (ed.). *Fish and fishery products. Composition, nutritive properties and stability.* Wallingford: CAB International, 1995.

22.9 EGGS

Since prehistoric times humans have raided nests, seeking eggs. Eggs are a central ingredient in many cuisines but they have received adverse publicity in recent years, mainly centred around the high cholesterol content of the yolk. However, it is frequently forgotten that hen's eggs have the highest quality dietary protein for nutrition and a relatively inexpensive one. Eggs also contribute calcium, B vitamins and vitamins A and B_{12} (Table 22.9). The fat, cholesterol and micronutrients are confined to the yolk while the white contains mainly protein. Those people on cholesterol-lowering diets can limit the amount of yolk consumed but many studies show no effect of daily egg consumption

Table 22.9 Nutrient content of eggs

Nutrients per 100 g raw egg (shell excluded)	
Protein (g)	12.7
Fat (g)	10.1
• saturated (g)	3.6
• monounsaturated (g)	5.3
• polyunsaturated (g)	1.2
Cholesterol (mg)	375
Carbohydrate (g)	0.3
Calcium (mg)	39.0
Iron (mg)	1.6

Source: English R, Lewis J. *The composition of foods Australia.* Canberra: Australian Government Publishing Service, 1990.

on cholesterol concentrations in healthy normocholesterolaemic people. Food scientists have assisted the farmers to produce eggs with lower cholesterol content over the years. A recent innovation has been the development of eggs enriched with ω3-fatty acids by feeding hens meals rich in α-linolenic acid. Consumption of these fatty acids is believed to be cardioprotective although the contribution the eggs make to ω3 intake is small compared to fish and oils.

FURTHER READING

1. Marshall AC, Kubena KS, Hinton KR, Hargis PS, Van Elswyk ME. *n*-3 fatty acid enriched table eggs: a survey of consumer acceptability. *Poult Sci* 1994; 73: 1334–40.
2. Stadelman WJ, Cotterill OJ. *Egg science and technology*. 2nd ed. Wesport: Avi Publishing Co, 1977.

22.10 FATS AND OILS

with Louise Macan

The type and amount of fats consumed today is very different from the days of the hunter–gatherer when lean animals were eaten and fat came from some seeds and nuts. It is necessary for the diet to provide the essential fatty acids but in most developed countries obtaining sufficient amounts of fat is rarely a problem. Overconsumption of fats and oils, particularly saturated fat, is of far greater concern. The main sources of dietary fat are meats, dairy products and vegetable oils and spreads and their associated products. During the past 20 years the type of fat consumed has changed from predominantly animal sources like butter and lard towards vegetable-derived fats and oils. The knowledge that saturated fat is associated with raising blood cholesterol and risk of coronary heart disease has resulted in the emphasis on the consumption of more unsaturated fats. Consumer demand has seen the development and production of new oils and margarines. However, the diet remains high in saturated fats because of lifestyle changes. These have resulted in greater use of pre-prepared foods inside the home and more food outside the home which are manufactured with saturated fats and oils (Table 22.10).

The bulk of edible fats and oils is made up of triglycerides (i.e. three fatty acids on a glycerol backbone). The predominant fatty acid present in the oil or fat will determine whether it is classified as a saturated, monounsaturated, or polyunsaturated fat (see Table 22.11). Hence, canola which has oleic acid as its major fatty acid, is called a monounsaturate, safflower with linoleic acid as the predominant fatty acid is a polyunsaturate and butter is a saturate. Fats and oils also contribute fat-soluble vitamins to the diet especially vitamin E. Table 22.11 lists the minor constituents of fats and oils.

Animal fats are usually obtained by a process called rendering. This involves heating or steaming to remove the adipose tissue from the animal carcass. These fats are most commonly obtained from pigs (lard) and cattle (tallow). After rendering they may contain residual amounts of free fatty acids, water and protein, all of which must be removed for

Table 22.10 Composition of common animal and vegetable fats and oils

Fat/oil	Saturates (%)	Monounsaturates (%)	Polyunsaturates (%)
Butter fat	64	33*	3
Canola	7	63	30
Coconut	91	7	2
Cottonseed	26	22	51
Olive	14	76	10
Palm	51	39	10
Peanut	19	45	36
Safflower	9	14	77
Soybean oil	15	23	62
Sunflower (high oleic)	10	85	5
Sunflower	11	23	66
Tallow	50	47*	3

* Tallow and butter fat contain about 5% *trans*-fatty acids and appear as monounsaturates in this table.

Table 22.11 Minor constituents of fats and oils

Monoglycerides and diglycerides	one or two fatty acids esterified to glycerol
Free fatty acids	not combined with any other molecule
Phospholipids	also known as phosphatides
Sterols	phytosterols (in plant oils), cholesterol (in animal fats)
Tocopherols	vitamin E (antioxidant) compounds
Carotenoids	yellow red colours
Chlorophyll	green pigment
Vitamins	vitamin E and perhaps A and D

a high quality product. Fats and oils derived from animal sources contain cholesterol and are usually high in saturated fat.

Vegetable oils and fats are obtained from a wide variety of plants. They can be obtained from seeds (canola [rapeseed], sunflower, cottonseed, safflower and palm), legumes (soybean and peanuts), fruits (olive) and nuts (almond and walnut). Vegetable oils are pressed from plants and then the unwanted components, such as colour pigments, phosphatides and free fatty acids are usually removed. Solvent extraction may also be used to remove residual fat from the meal. Further processing or refining is usually required when specific sensory properties or functions are required. This produces a clear high quality oil that is suitable for use as an ingredient, for frying, salad dressings, mayonnaise and the production of margarine and shortenings. Most crushing of seeds, nuts, and fruits requires a cooking stage prior to pressing to increase oil yields. A cold pressed oil has this step omitted and the temperature during pressing is controlled. Cold pressed oils tend to have stronger flavours and odours which may be desirable in certain foods but there is little nutritional difference between the two types. Close attention is paid to minimize the loss of vitamin E during the extraction process.

Margarine is a water-in-oil emulsion produced from vegetable oils (liquid at ambient temperature) and fat (solid or semi-solid 'hard' fraction). The hard fraction is essential to give solidity to the margarine and is produced by either hydrogenation (produces some *trans*-fatty acids) or interesterification (avoids *trans*) with the latter giving a less solid margarine. By blending hydrogenated fats with liquid oils in varying proportions the functional and nutritional properties can be altered. Water, skim milk powder, salt, lecithin emulsifiers, colours, flavours and vitamins are added to the blend. Low-fat margarine spreads contain about half the fat and have a gel with gelatin and maltodextrin providing the texture of the spread.

Other commodities based around fats and oils include animal and vegetable shortenings (with no water, salt or milk) used by the baking industry and frying oils (stable to heat and moisture) for domestic, small-scale food outlets and large-scale food production. Salad dressings and mayonnaises are oil-in-water emulsions. Mayonnaise is about 80% oil which is 'winterized' to prevent crystal formation upon refrigeration that would break the emulsion. For baking and frying, saturated fats such as palm oil and coconut oil and tallow and lard are still commonly used because they provide the sensory and functional properties that are required as well as being stable. The way a biscuit melts in the mouth is important and also a more saturated oil avoids the problem of oxidation producing off-flavours. Newer products such as high oleic sunflower oil and blends of vegetable and hydrogenated vegetable fat are now finding their way into the baking and frying sector of the food industry.

FURTHER READING

1. Cambie RC. *Fats for the future*. Chichester: Ellis Horwood Ltd, 1989.
2. Rossell JB, Pritchard JLR. *Analysis of oilseeds, fats and fatty foods*. London: Elsevier Applied Science, 1991.

22.11 FAT REPLACERS

The push to produce low fat and fat-free products becomes stronger as the consumers in developed nations battle obesity and heart disease. Fat replacers are ingredients which recreate the attributes of fat without providing the energy. The success of fat replacement in foods is dependent on the ability to recreate the texture, mouthfeel, appearance and flavour of the original food. Fat mimetics replace the mouthfeel and texture of fats but do not possess all of the physical and chemical properties. Fat substitutes, however, resemble the triglyceride structure and can be used to replace fat on a gram-for-gram basis (Table 22.12).

Fat mimetics may be based on starch, cellulose or protein or be hydrophilic colloids. Starch may be modified by acid or enzymic hydrolysis to yield smaller polymers like maltodextrin or β-glucan, or glucose may be polymerized to give polydextrose. Cellulose may be modified to microcrystalline aggregates. Protein-based products include those made from skim milk and egg whites which are microparticulated. Hydrocolloids and gums will provide mouthfeel, juiciness, and thickening. All the mimetics are soluble or dispersible in the water phase and will retain moisture. They cannot be used to replace

Table 22.12   Examples of fat replacers

Mimetics	Name
Starch-based	Starch hydrolysis product (SHP)
	N-Oil™ (National Starch and Chemical Corp. Bridgewater, NJ)
	Maltrin M040 Maltodextrin™ (Grain Processing Corp. Muscatine, IA)
Gums	Carrageenan (Carrageenan Marketing Corp. Santa Ana, CA)
	Gum arabic
	Alginates
Polysaccharide-based	Cellulose (microcrystalline, modified)
	Fibercel™ (Alpha-Beta Technologies, Cambridge, MA)
	Oatrim™ (Rhône Poulenc, Cranbury, NJ)
Protein-based	Simplesse™ (NutraSweet Co. Skokie, IL)
	Dairylite (John Labatt Ltd., Ault Foods London, Canada)
Synthetic 'triglyceride-like' substitutes	Caprenin™ (Procter & Gamble, Cincinnati, OH, Grinsted Products, Kansas City, MO)
	Dialkyldihexadecylmalonate (DDM) (Frito-Lay Inc. Dallas, TX)
	Olestra (Procter & Gamble, Cincinnati, OH)

oil for frying because they may denature and burn or will not melt. Applications of mimetics include their use in ice cream, frozen desserts, confectionery, salad dressings, cheese spreads, dairy-type foods, and baked goods.

Fat substitutes will have the same functionality as fat. Synthetic substitutes are either resistant or partially resistant to the action of lipase in the gut and hence contribute none or a lower energy content. The best known is sucrose polyester which consists of a sugar backbone with fatty acids esterified to the sugar. They have the possibility to replace fat in a wide variety of foods including fried foods like potato chips and snack food. Some caution needs to be exercised because diarrhoea or malabsorption of fat-soluble vitamins may occur with excessive consumption. Other fat substitutes on the horizon include esterified propoxylated glycerol (EPG), malonate esters (DDM), and trialkoxytricarbyllate (TATCA) which all exhibit triglyceride-like properties.

It is apparent that fat replacement is a growing market for the food industry. As biotechnology develops it should be possible to provide all the attributes of fat without the energy value.

FURTHER READING

1. Akoh CC, Swanson BG (eds). *Carbohydrate polyesters as fat substitutes*. New York: Marcel Dekker Inc, 1994.

22.12 HERBS AND SPICES

with Sue Munro

Herbs and spices are derived from various parts of plants. Spices can be divided into four types: pungent spices, aromatic fruits and seeds, aromatic barks and coloured spices. Herbs are the green or dried leaves of plants. It is the essential or volatile oils that give each herb or spice its characteristic aroma and flavour. For as long as recorded time, herbs and spices have assumed a significant role in society. They have been the panacea of all ills, a status symbol and a means to economic success.

Originating in the Asias and South America, spices were introduced into Western cuisine by the Crusaders and Marco Polo. They brought welcome culinary relief, by adding colour and flavour to the plain fare of Europe. Spices are known to stimulate the appetite and thus increase total consumption. Herbs and spices have been just as important to medicine. Chinese medicine is characterized by its use of herbs. Many modern drugs were discovered in plants (e.g. digitalis).

The demand for spices initiated world trade. That trade still continues. India is the world's biggest producer; Sri Lanka, Indonesia, Jamaica and Brazil also produce significant amounts of spice for export.

Different combinations of herbs and spices are the distinguishing features of many cuisines around the world, providing distinctive flavours, colour and aroma. What the curry paste is to Indian cuisine, the chilli powder is to South Americans and the fine herbs are to French cooking. Little is known about the actual quantities of herbs and spices consumed.

Herbs and spices contain all the macronutrients but because they are used in small quantities their contribution to nutrient intake is assumed to be minimal. Surveys in India have found that regular use of spices can make a small but significant contribution to the total intakes of essential amino acids, calcium and iron. Spices and herbs are rich in minerals like calcium, iron, phosphorus, manganese and zinc. Fresh herbs contain significant amounts of β-carotene and vitamin C although the drying and grinding of herbs and spices will reduce these. The dietary fibre content of herbs and spices ranges from 14–53%. Garlic is a source of soluble fibre. Antinutrients in spices include tannins, and phytic acid.

Herbs and spices are claimed to cause a variety of physiological effects. These include carcinogenic effects (capsicin found in chillies) and anticarcinogenic effects (garlic, mace, rosemary, saffron and tumeric); thermogenic effects (capsicin); antioxidant, lipid-lowering and anticoagulant effects and antibacterial or antifungal effects. Seasonings contain high levels of salicylates. In cases of food intolerance or an allergic reaction, herbs and spices may need to be avoided. Garlic is reported to have a range of beneficial physiological effects: antibacterial activity, lipid-lowering effects, antiplatelet activity, detoxification activity and anticarcinogenic properties, especially stomach cancer.

Toxins in seasonings may be naturally occurring or due to contamination. Spices and herbs are usually irradiated to reduce microbial contamination. Naturally occurring toxins do not usually pose a threat since the amounts used in cooking are very small. Nutmeg contains hallucinagenic compounds, comfrey is poisonous and piperine, the pungent ingredient in pepper, reacts with nitrites found in cured foods to produce carcinogenic compounds. A common fungal contaminant is aflatoxin, a known liver carcinogen.

FURTHER READING

1. Greenberg S, Ortiz EL. *The spice of life*. London: Mermaid Books, in association with Channel 4 TV, 1983.

22.13   SWEETENERS: NUTRITIVE AND NON-NUTRITIVE

with Janette Brand-Miller

All through human history, we have sought concentrated forms of sweetness. Honey, honey ants, maple syrup, dates and other dried fruit came well before sucrose was refined from sugar cane and sugar beet. Today, the choice is even wider, with the advent of industrially produced sugar alcohols (sorbitol, lactitol) and high intensity sweeteners (e.g. saccharin, aspartame). The new sweeteners can be classified into those that provide energy and those that do not, nutritive and non-nutritive sweeteners, respectively. Some people prefer to use the names 'carbohydrate sweeteners' and 'intense sweeteners' instead.

Nutritive sweeteners   Some of the new carbohydrate sweeteners provide energy but not as much as the equivalent amount of sucrose. These include isomalt (trade name Palatinit™) which is a disaccharide alcohol made from sucrose. It has half the energy value of sucrose and is non-cariogenic. In Europe, a lot of 'tooth-friendly' confectionery is being manufactured from this new sweetener.

Oligofructose (trade names Raftilose™, Actilight™) is made from the breakdown of the polysaccharide inulin, a polymer of fructose that occurs naturally in many plants (e.g. onions and leeks). Oligofructose tastes sweet, resists digestion in the small intestine and has only one-third of the energy of sucrose. It can also stimulate the growth of friendly *Bifidobacteria* in the large intestine. Its physical properties mean it can replace both sugar and fat in foods.

Sorbitol is the alcohol derivative of glucose. It is absorbed slowly and does not raise plasma insulin or cause dental caries and has found its way into many 'sugar-free' and diabetic products. The energy value of sorbitol ($16\,kJ/g$) is the same as that of glucose unless so much is eaten ($>15\,g$ at a time) that its slow rate of absorption results in malabsorption and diarrhoea. There are no real advantages to the use of sorbitol in diabetic diets.

Non-nutritive sweeteners   Cyclamate and saccharin were the first non-nutritive sweeteners, both discovered by accident when scientists happened to lick their fingers during the course of experiments. Cyclamate is 30 times sweeter than sucrose and saccharin >250 times sweeter. Both can be used in tiny amounts to sweeten beverages such as tea, coffee and soft drinks. Their taste profile is better when used together than alone. Cyclamate was banned in the United States in 1969 after animal experiments involving huge doses showed it caused bladder cancer. More than 30 other countries around the world (e.g. Australia), considered it was safe in the amounts generally used. There was no evidence of increased cancer rate in individuals with diabetes who used greater amounts of saccharin and cyclamate than the general population. In 1971, it was saccharin's turn to be accused but this time the American public demanded it remain on the shelves because the perceived benefits to health outweighed the risks.

Several more intense sweeteners have been discovered, rigorously tested for safety and then marketed. Aspartame (trade name Nutrasweet™) is a dipeptide of aspartic acid and phenylalanine, 200 times sweeter than sucrose and has a better taste profile than saccharin and cyclamate, leaving no bitter aftertaste. Concerns that it might cause hyperactivity in children or headaches in adults have been disproven. It should not be used by people with phenylketonuria. Acesulphame K is also 200 times sweeter than sucrose without aftertaste and can be used in cooking and baking. It is excreted through the human digestive system unchanged.

Newer intense sweeteners include sucralose (trade name Splenda™) and alitame (trade name Aclame™). Both offer advantages over the older generation of intense sweeteners in flavour profile, heat and storage stability, thereby widening the types of food product that can be developed. Sucralose is 400–800 times sweeter than sucrose, made by substituting chlorine atoms for three hydroxyl groups on the sucrose molecule. It is not absorbed and survives heat treatment so it can be used in baking.

Alitame is a dipeptide of aspartic acid and alanine and is 2000 times sweeter than sucrose. Thaumatin has recently been introduced into products. It is a protein of 207 amino acids isolated from a West African berry and is heat-stable.

The increase in the number of intense sweeteners has been fuelled by public concerns about weight gain as well as sugar *per se*. Although it is safer to have a wide range of intense sweeteners on the market (the safety-in-numbers concept), there is little evidence that people who use them are slimmer or have fewer dental caries. Similarly, there is little evidence that they improve glycaemic control in individuals with diabetes. In fact, the recognition of the sugar–fat 'seesaw' may mean that people who avoid sugar and increase their use of non-nutritive sweeteners may eat a diet that is higher in fat. Millions of dollars have been poured into the development of sugar substitutes and low joule products, money which might have been better spent on research into the pathogenesis of diabetes and obesity. Nonetheless, low joule soft drinks now occupy 20% of the total market in carbonated beverages and intense sweeteners are probably here to stay.

FURTHER READING

1. Editorial. Saccharin and bladder cancer. *Lancet* 1980; i: 855–6.
2. Horwitz DL, Bauer-Nehrling JK. Can aspartame meet our expectations. *J Am Diet Ass* 1983; **83**: 142–6.

22.14 FOOD PROCESSING

with Stewart Truswell

All the foods we eat are living matter made of cells containing enzymes, and many foods, especially those of animal origin, are inhabited by microorganisms. Hence, food processing is necessary to prevent food decaying and to keep it safe for consumption. Food processing destroys the growth of microorganisms including pathogens (e.g. *Salmonella* and *Listeria*) and will inactivate some natural toxins (e.g. trypsin inhibitors). The storage life of the food is increased which means that it can be grown some distance from the point of consumption. This enables us to benefit from economies of scale by growing large quantities of food on the most suitable land. Not all processing involves food preservation, some also improve the appearance and flavour of foods and convenience. One of the major considerations of modern consumers is the ease and speed with which a meal can be prepared and more meals are now consumed away from the home. Food processing is essential to meet these consumer needs.

22.14.1   Methods of food processing

Many methods involve reduction of water content so that microorganisms cannot grow and autolytic enzymes are inhibited. One of the earliest methods of food preservation used was drying. The Ancient Greeks sun-dried grapes to produce raisins, which lasted longer than the fresh fruits because of their low water content. In addition to sun drying and smoking of foods, modern technology includes tunnel drying, spray drying and freeze drying of food to make milk powders, egg powders, and coffee powders. Freezing while not removing the water changes it into a form that is unavailable for normal enzyme functions and the low temperature decreases both bacterial growth and enzyme activity. The addition of salt such as salting of fish or inclusion of sugar as in jams, also prevents bacterial growth by their osmotic effects.

Heat is used in several ways to prevent food spoilage and microbial growth. Pasteurization of milk by heating to 72 °C for 15 seconds destroys pathogenic organisms. Blanching of food (100 °C for 1–8 minutes) before freezing and canning inactivates autolytic enzymes. Canned and sealed foods are sterilized by the application of heat. Food irradiation is a newer technique which can be applied to foods, the flavour of which would be altered by heating (e.g. spices and strawberries). However, the employment of irradiation is an emotive issue and the practice is restricted by legislation in many countries at present.

Many fruits and vegetables are foods with particularly short shelf-lives. If people are to meet the recommendations made by various health authorities to increase fruit and vegetable consumption some processing is essential. Fresh fruits need to be harvested and stored using modern technology to increase year-round availability and distribution around the globe. Bananas are picked before they are ripe and shipped and stored at a controlled temperature until they are ripened by exposure to ethylene gas (which is naturally given off during ripening of bananas). Californian oranges may be consumed in New Zealand and New Zealand kiwi fruit in California when local production ceases seasonally.

Other food processing methods include milling and pressing. Most cereal products such as wheat, maize and rice are subjected to varying amounts of crushing with metal rollers and sieving to separate course and fine components which eventually produces the different flours and brans. Pressing is used to crush the juice from fruits like grapes and to press edible oils from oilseeds like canola, and sunflower seeds.

Packaging and refrigeration also assist in preventing spoilage of food. Sealing sterilized foods in vacuum packs prevents microbial growth because oxygen is unavailable. Refrigeration retards the multiplication of microorganisms although some will still reproduce at 4 °C.

Food irradiation can be used to inhibit sprouting of vegetables, delay the ripening of fruits, and kill insect pests in fruit, grains or spices, reduce or eliminate food spoilage organisms and reduce microorganisms on meats and seafoods.

22.14.2   Food additives

Chemical preservatives may be added to specific foods to prevent bacterial growth. Examples include benzoic acid, propionic acid, sorbic acid, and sodium metabisulphite. Antioxidants may be added to slow the oxidation of oils and fats, preventing rancidity. Fermentation of products will produce acid or alcohol, both of which inhibit autolytic enzymes and bacterial growth (Table 22.13).

Other food processing includes the addition of chemicals to provide a variety of functions. Additives such as emulsifiers keep the oil and aqueous phases together in mayonnaises and sauces. Humectants prevent food from drying out (e.g. glycerol in cake frostings). Thickeners may be added to sauces or jams to improve texture. Anticaking agents may be added to ensure that powdered foods do not become lumpy (e.g. flavoured coffee mixes). Food acids may be used for flavour or to adjust the pH for preservation reasons. Some foods have their organoleptic properties enhanced by the addition of colours and flavours. About half of the colours used are from natural sources (e.g. β-carotene). Flavours are usually a 'trade secret' so that the names of individual flavours are not declared on the label but in most developed nations food legislation only permits those that have been shown to be safe. In the United States they are known as GRAS, 'generally regarded as safe'.

Other types of food additive are vitamins or minerals (see Table 22.13). Some foods may be restored with micronutrients (e.g. the thiamin removed during milling of flour is replaced), while other food may be fortified, for example, there are requests to fortify foods with folic acid because of the difficulty for women of childbearing age to obtain adequate amounts in the diet. Vitamins may be added to a food which becomes a replacement for a food in which the vitamin naturally occurs: such an example is margarine to which vitamin A and D are added, both occurring in butter.

22.14.3   Safety aspects of food additives

There are a series of strict tests which must be conducted before a food additive is permitted. The Food and Agriculture Organization/World Health Organization (FAO/ WHO) has a joint expert committee on food and most countries have an expert body that prepares food legislation (e.g. the United States Food and Drug Administration, the European Scientific Committee for Food, and the National Food Authority in Australia). The acute toxicity of the additive must be tested in both male and female animals in a minimum of three species and the distribution of the compound in the body is assayed. Short-term feeding trials are conducted in at least two species of animal (only one can be rodent) and reproduction is studied over two generations. After this, both mutagenicity

Table 22.13 Some common food additives, the number used in the European Union and one of the foods to which it is added

Food additive	Code No.	Foods
Preservatives		
benzoic acid	210	Fruit juices
lactic acid	270	White bread
fumaric acid	297	Confectionary
propionic acid	280	Bread
sodium metabisulphite	223	Wine
sorbic acid	200	Cheesecake
Antioxidants		
ascorbic acid	300	Stock cubes
butylated hydroxyanisole	320	Ice cream
propyl gallate	310	Gelatin desserts
α-tocopherols	307	Oils
Emulsifiers		
lecithins	322	Chocolate
mono- and diglycerides of fatty acids	471	Potato crisps
Humectants		
glycerol	422	Pastilles
sorbitol	420	Chewing gum
Thickeners		
alginic acid	400	Ice cream
guar gum	412	Salad dressings
methyl cellulose	461	Jelly
pectin	440	Jams
xanthan gum	415	Bottled sauces
Anticaking agents		
magnesium carbonate	504	Icing sugar
Food acids		
acetic acid	260	Tomato ketchup
citric acid	330	Marmalades
malic acid	296	Canned tomatoes
Colours		
β-carotene	160a	Margarines
canthaxanthin	161g	Biscuits
curcumin	100	Curry powder
erythrosine	127	Glacé cherries

and carcinogenicity are tested for in bacteria and tissue culture. Effects of food additives in humans are continually reviewed. It is not realized that the most likely toxic substances in our foods are naturally occurring ones rather than food additives. Additives are the most thoroughly monitored and tested of all chemicals in the food supply chain.

Table 22.14 The effect of freezing on vitamin C content of selected vegetables

Food	Vitamin C mg/100 g
Cauliflower (boiled)[a]	56
Cauliflower (frozen, boiled)[a]	14
Peas (boiled)[b]	16
Peas (frozen, boiled)[b]	12
Spinach (boiled)[c]	26
Spinach (frozen, boiled)[c]	26

Source:
[a] English R, Lewis J. *The composition of foods Australia*. Canberra: Australian Government Publishing Service, 1990.
[b] Holland B, Welch AA, Unwin ID, Buss DH, Paul AA, Southgate DAT. *McCance and Widdowson's, The composition of foods*. 5th ed. London: Royal Society of Chemistry, MAFF, 1991.
[c] United States Department of Agriculture. Human Nutrition Information Service. *Composition of Foods. 1976–1986*. Agriculture Handbook 8. Washington: US Government Printing Office, 1989.

22.14.4 Effects of food processing on nutrient content

Some nutrient losses will occur during processing but domestic cooking also results in appreciable losses of vitamins and leaching of minerals. Most labile of the vitamins are C and folate which are unstable, although low pH will protect vitamin C (Table 22.14). The losses during processing by the food industry are standardized and easily quantified unlike those in domestic kitchens. In some cases the nutrient content may be greater when using a processed food than preparing it from the raw product in a domestic kitchen.

22.14.5 Conclusion

Food processing allows an abundant year round pathogen-free food supply. No pregnant woman would debate the importance of pasteurization of milk to remove bacteria which would cause miscarriage. Some nutrient losses are inevitable upon processing but they are not usually sizeable. The impact of nutrient loss will be dependent on the overall composition of the diet (e.g. milling and polishing of rice would only precipitate thiamin deficiency in those people who eat nothing else). If it were not for processing, the food would be unavailable for consumption throughout the year and the nutrient may be missed altogether.

FURTHER READING

1. Branen AL, Davidson PM, Salminen S. *Food additives*. New York: Marcel Dekker, 1990.
2. Karmas E, Harris RS. *Nutrition evaluation of food processing*. 3rd ed. New York: Van Nostrand Reinhold, 1988.
3. MacCarthy D (ed.). *Concentration and drying of foods*. London: Elsevier Applied Science, 1986.
4. Thorne S (ed.). *Food irradiation*. London: Elsevier, Applied Science, 1991.

23
FOOD TOXICITY AND SAFETY

Peter Williams

All chemicals, including all those naturally found in foods, are toxic at some dose. Laboratory animals can be killed by feeding them glucose or salt at very high doses, and some micronutrients such as vitamin A and selenium can be hazardous at doses only a few times greater than normal human requirements. Even very common foods, such as pepper, have demonstrated carcinogenic activity. Toxicity testing of a food or ingredient can tell us what the likely adverse effects are and at what level of consumption they may occur, but by itself this does not tell us whether it is safe to eat in normally consumed amounts.

'Hazard' is the probability that a substance will produce injury under defined conditions of exposure. The concept of hazard takes into account the dose and length of exposure as well as the toxicity of a particular chemical, and is a better guide to the safety of a food. Thus, although it is well known that potatoes contain solanine, a poisonous alkaloid, eating potatoes as they are normally prepared is not a risk to health at normal levels of consumption; in other words, the solanine in potatoes is toxic but not usually hazardous.

Consequently, any attempt to examine the safety of the food supply should not be based on the question 'Is this food or ingredient toxic?' (the answer is always 'Yes'), but rather by finding out if eating this substance in normal amounts is likely to increase the risk of illness significantly (i.e. 'Is it safe?').

23.1 HAZARDOUS SUBSTANCES IN FOOD

Three general classes of hazardous substances are found in foods: (1) microbial or environmental contaminants, (2) naturally occurring toxic constituents, and (3) intentional food additives. The most dangerous contaminants of foods are those produced by infestations of bacteria or moulds, which can produce toxins that remain in the food even after the biological source has been destroyed. Other contaminants, such as pesticide residues or heavy metals, are usually well controlled in modern food supplies but can be significant hazards in particular localities. Naturally occurring toxic constituents can be considered normal and unavoidable. They are usually present in amounts that are too small to produce harmful effects when foods are eaten normally, except in the cases of atypical consumers who may be allergic to individual ingredients. Food additives are generally the least dangerous hazards because their toxicology is well studied and the levels of use are tightly controlled. Table 23.1 summarizes the types of hazardous substances that may be present in food.

Table 23.1 Potential hazards in foods

Hazards	Examples
Microbial contamination	
Pathogenic bacteria	Toxins from *Clostridium botulinum*
Mycotoxins	Aflatoxin from mould on peanuts
Environmental contamination	
Heavy metals and minerals	Arsenic and mercury in fish
Criminal adulteration	Aniline in olive oil
Packaging migration	PVC from plastics
Industrial pollution	PCB, radioactive fallout
Changes during cooking or processing	Carcinogens produced in burnt meat
Natural toxins	
Inherent toxins	Cyanide is cassava
Produced by abnormal conditions	Ciguatera poisoning from fish
Enzyme inhibitors	Protease inhibitors in legumes
Antivitamins	Avidin in raw egg white
Mineral-binding agents	Goitrogens in brassica vegetables
Agricultural residues	
Pesticides	DDT
Hormones	Bovine somatotrophin
Intentional food additives	
Artificial sweeteners	Cyclamate
Preservatives	Sodium nitrite

The United States Food and Drug Administration (FDA) has ranked the relative importance of health hazards associated with food in the following descending order of seriousness:

1. Microbiological contamination.
2. Inappropriate eating habits.
3. Environmental contamination.
4. Natural toxic constituents.
5. Pesticide residues.
6. Food additives.

This list is very different from that found in public opinion polls, which show that most people rate food additives as one of their major concerns about the safety of the food supply.

23.2 MICROBIAL CONTAMINATION

23.2.1 Pathogenic bacteria

Outbreaks of acute gastroenteritis caused by microbial pathogens are usually called food poisoning. They can be caused by foodborne intoxication—where microbes in food produce a toxin that produces the symptom, or foodborne infection—where the symptoms are caused by the activity of live bacterial cells multiplying in the gastrointestinal system. Table 23.2 lists the most common bacterial causes of food poisoning, in order of the rapidity of onset of symptoms. In general the intoxications have a more rapid onset.

The most important pathogens are *Clostridium botulinum*, *Staphylococcus aureus*, *Salmonella* species and *Clostridium perfringens*. The last three organisms account for about 70–80% of all reported outbreaks of foodborne illness, but there are also many others as well as some viral and protozoan agents. The four most frequently identified factors contributing to food poisoning incidents are improper cooling of food (44%), lapses of

Table 23.2 Common bacterial food poisoning organisms

Organism	Symptoms	Time after food	Typical food sources
Toxins			
Staphylococcus aureus	Vomiting, diarrhoea, abdominal pain	1–6 h (mean 2–3 h)	Custard and cream-filled baked goods, cold meats
Clostridium perfringens	Diarrhoea and severe pain, nausea	8–24 h (mean 8–15 h)	Meat products incompletely cooked or reheated
Bacillus cereus	(a) nausea, vomiting; (b) abdominal pain, watery diarrhoea	(a) 1–5 h (b) 6–16 h (mean 10–12 h)	Rice dishes, vegetables, sauces, puddings
Clostridium botulinum	Dry mouth, difficulty swallowing and speaking, double vision, difficulty breathing. Often fatal	2 h–8 days (mean 12–36 h)	Home-canned foods (usually meat and vegetables), and inadequately processed smoked meats
Infection			
Vibrio parahaemolyticus	Diarrhoea, abdominal cramp, nausea, headache, vomiting	4–96 h (mean 12 h)	Fish, crustaceans
Salmonella spp.	Diarrhoea, fever, nausea, vomiting	8–72 h (mean 12–36 h)	Undercooked poultry, reheated food, cream-filled pastries
Yersinia enterocolitica	Fever, abdominal pain, diarrhoea	24–36 h	Raw and cooked pork and beef
Escherichia coli	Fever, cramps, nausea, diarrhoea	8–44 h (mean 26 h)	Faecal contamination of food or water
Shigella spp.	Diarrhoea, bloody stools with mucus, fever	1–7 days (mean 1–3 days)	Faecal contamination of food
Campylobacter jejuni	Fever, abdominal pain, diarrhoea	1–10 days (mean 2–5 days)	Raw milk, poultry, eggs, meat
Listeria monocytogenes	Septic abortion, septicaemia, meningitis, encephalitis. Often fatal	1–7 wks	Milk and dairy products, raw meat, poultry and eggs, vegetables and salads, seafood

12 hours or more between preparing and eating (23%), contamination by food handlers (18%) and contaminated raw foods or ingredients (16%).

The reported incidence and cost of foodborne illness in most countries is increasing, although it is difficult to determine the exact extent of the problem. Collection of data on foodborne illness is notoriously unreliable, relying on medical practitioners to report cases to a central authority. In 1993, the World Health Organization (WHO) estimated that 'in industrialised countries, reported cases of foodborne illness could be under-estimated by a factor of 10'. What is clear is that in recent years a number of new pathogens have emerged.

Control of food poisoning   The trend in all countries today is to require more formal training of all food handlers and the development of food safety plans wherever food is prepared and served to the public, based on the principles of Hazard Analysis of Critical Control Points (HACCP). HACCP is a preventive approach to quality control, identifying potential dangers for corrective action. The principles include:

- assessing potential hazards at each step in the food chain;
- identifying those points in the operation where the hazards may occur;
- deciding which points are critical for consumer safety and food quality;
- setting up control procedures and standards for each critical control point;

    The following are examples of control procedures:
    – washing hands
    – sanitizing food preparation surfaces and tools
    – cooking food to specific temperatures
    – rapid chilling of food
    – storage of food at correct temperatures

- planning the corrective actions to be taken if a deviation occurs;
- establishing a system to document performance of the process;
- verifying that the HACCP process is working.

Table 23.3 outlines an example of some parts of a HACCP plan for a commercial food product sold as ready-to-eat.

23.2.2   Mycotoxins

Moulds, or fungi, are capable of producing a wide variety of chemicals that are biologically active. Humans have used some of these as effective antibiotics, but there are also a number of diseases resulting from accidental exposure to fungal products that contaminate food. Some examples are as follows.

Aflatoxins   These are a group of closely related compounds from the common *Aspergillus* fungus species that have been shown to be highly toxic and carcinogenic mycotoxins, causing liver damage. They are stable to heat and survive most forms of food processing. Aflatoxin contamination can occur whenever environmental conditions are suitable for mould growth, but the problem is more common in tropical and semitropical regions. Aflatoxins were first recognized in the 1960s in peanuts and contamination of peanut

Table 23.3 An example of six steps from a HACCP Plan for chilled chicken salad

Step	1. Growing and harvesting	2. Raw material processing	3. Supply storage temperatures
Hazard	Chemicals, antibiotics	Chemical, microbiological	Microbiological
Control	Raw material specifications	Certified supplier	Raw material specifications
Limit	Regulatory approved residues	Free of pathogens and foreign material	Chicken $< -12\,°C$ Vegetables $< 4\,°C$
Monitoring	Certificate of compliance	Monitor supplier HACCP programme	Check coolroom records daily
Action if limit exceeded	Reject lot	Reject as supplier	Investigate time/ temp. abuse
Responsibility	Receiving operator	Purchaser	Store person

Step	4. Ingredient assembly	5. Bagging	6. Labelling
Hazard	Microbiological	Microbiological	Incorrect dates, traceability
Control	Temperature control specs	Correct seal settings	Legible, correct dates and codes
Limit	Food $< 4\,°C$	Upper tolerance limit on sealer	Use proper labels
Monitoring	Check temp. once per shift	Check setting every 15 min.	Each batch at changeover
Action if limit exceeded	Report to supervisor	Examine all packages	Destroy incorrect labels
Responsibility	Cook	Seal inspector	Packer

Source: Adapted from Microbiological and Food Safety Committee, National Food Processors Association. *HACCP implementation: a generic model for chilled foods. J Food Prot* 1993; **56**: 1077.

butters remains a problem. On a world-wide basis, maize is the most important food contaminated with aflatoxin.

Patulin is an antibiotic that is produced by the mould *Penicillium caviforme*. It has been implicated as a possible carcinogen from one study in rats although other studies have not confirmed this. Patulin in primarily associated with the apple rotting fungus and so apple juices and some baked goods with fruit can contain patulin.

Fusarium toxins The *Fusarium* family of moulds produce several potent toxins that cause disease in farm animals and also in humans. During World War II in Russia, famine forced people to eat bread made from mouldy, overwintered cereals. They suffered from alimentary toxic aleukia, with suppression of white cells in the blood, gastrointestinal disorders and haemorrhages. The toxin, 'T2 toxin', a tricothecene, was produced by *Fusarium* moulds on the wheat. It has also been suggested that a similar toxin on maize may have been involved in some of the historical outbreaks of pellagra (see Chapter 12.3.5).

Another species, *Fusarium moniliforme* produces the fumonisin group of toxins. In the Transkei of South Africa there is a very high incidence of cancer of the oesophagus. It was found that mouldy maize was used for making native beer, causing it to be contaminated with *F. moniliforme* and fumonisins. The carcinogenic potential of fumonisin has been shown in laboratory rats.

23.2.3 New foodborne diseases

Over the past two decades a number of new foodborne pathogens have emerged as important causes of illness. The reason for this is still uncertain, but centralized production of food products and the widespread use of refrigeration to hold food for long periods may have contributed to the emergence of bacteria able to grow at low temperatures, including *Yersinia, Listeria,* and some strains of *Escherichia coli.* The presence and relative importance of these newer diseases varies from region to region. Some of the more important new organisms are:

Campylobacter jejuni which was a well-known bacterium in veterinary medicine before it was considered a human pathogen. It is now recognized as one of the most common causes of gastroenteritis in humans, of greater importance than *Salmonella.* It is present in the flesh of cattle, sheep, pigs and poultry and can be introduced wherever raw meat is handled.

Escherichia coli 0157:H7 is a bacterium that can damage the cells of the colon, leading to bloody diarrhoea and abdominal cramps. Raw or undercooked hamburger meat was a major vehicle of transmission in a number of well-publicized outbreaks in the United States in 1993.

Norwalk virus This virus is found in the faeces of humans and illness is caused by poor personal hygiene among infected food handlers. Symptoms include nausea, vomiting, diarrhoea, abdominal pain and fever. Because it is a virus, it does not reproduce in food, but remains active until the food is eaten.

Listeria monocytogenes is widely distributed in nature but is unusual in that it grows at refrigeration temperatures (down to 0 °C). Listeriosis can cause death in the elderly and those with compromised immune systems, such as people with AIDS, as well as abortions. Listeria has been linked to the consumption of contaminated pâtés, milk, soft cheese and undercooked chicken, and is often found in preprepared chilled foods.

'Mad cow disease' (bovine spongiform encephalopathy) is a major concern in Europe. Over half of the dairy herd in Britain has suffered this prion-type disease, which is believed to have been caused when feeds contaminated with the remains of dead sheep, with a similar brain disease called scrapie, were fed to cattle. There has been widespread public concern that eating contaminated meat may be linked to a rare human disorder called Creutzfeldt–Jakob disease, although there is little scientific evidence to support this.

23.3 ENVIRONMENTAL CONTAMINATION

23.3.1 Heavy metals and minerals

Selenium is one of the most toxic essential trace elements. The level of selenium in foods usually reflects the levels in the soil and in a few high-selenium areas, such as North Dakota and parts of China, excessive selenium intake has been associated with gastrointestinal disturbances and skin discoloration. In China in the early 1960s, selenium intoxication affected up to 50% of the population in certain villages; brittle hair, skin lesions and neurological disturbances were the main symptoms in affected individuals.

Mercury Fish can contain 10–1500 mg/kg of organic mercury, and even higher levels when mercury wastes are released into lake waters. Serious poisonings from mercury in fish have occurred in Japan, the most famous being that in Minamata Bay (from 1953 to 1960). Another example of widespread mercury intoxication occurred in Iraq in 1971–2 as a result of bread made from seed wheat treated with mercury-based pesticides. Most countries have now established maximum permitted levels for mercury in fish in the range of 0.4–1.0 mg/kg.

Cadmium is a toxic element that accumulates mainly in bone and kidneys. Chronic exposure at excessive levels can lead to irreversible kidney failure. Plants readily take up cadmium from the soil, and there has been a slow increase in the cadmium levels in soils due to the use of phosphate fertilizers and the effect of air and water pollution. The average cadmium intake from food is now approximately 10–50 μg/day, which is approaching the provisional tolerable weekly intake of 7 μg/kg body weight per week. Measures to control cadmium contamination include controls on waste disposal, and development of new crops that accumulate less cadmium.

23.3.2 Criminal adulteration

Modern food regulations began in the nineteenth century when adulteration of food was often widespread to increase profits. Milk was diluted with water, cocoa with sawdust; some operators preserved milk with formaldehyde and butter with borax. Today, regulations and the standards of the food industry are much higher and risks from illegal adulteration are rare. However, there have been some notorious instances. For example, in Spain in 1981 there was an outbreak of an apparently new disease characterized by fever, rashes and respiratory problems. Many thousands were hospitalized and over 100 people died. The agent responsible was identified as cooking oil that had been fraudulently sold as pure olive oil but in fact was mostly rapeseed oil which was intended for industrial uses and contaminated with aniline.

23.3.3 Packaging migration

The materials used to package food can sometimes result in contamination of the food itself. At one time the lead used in the solder of metal cans was a significant source of contamination of infant formulae, but this problem has been eliminated by the introduction of non-soldered cans. Polyvinyl chloride (PVC), the parent compound for many polymers used in food packaging materials, has been detected in a variety of products stored in PVC containers. Although there is some evidence that PVC is carcinogenic in humans, the level of exposure from this route is very low and not regarded as a significant risk to health.

23.3.4 Industrial pollution

Throughout the industrial era, many potentially hazardous substances have been released into the environment and are now widely distributed in the food chain. Among the most important are the polychlorinated biphenyls (PCBs). PCB is a generic term for a wide range of highly stable derivatives of biphenyl that have been used in a vast number of products, including plastics, paints, and lubricants. Although manufacture has now ceased, their stability and solubility in lipids has meant that they accumulate in fatty tissue and they have become widespread, particularly in seafood. They can be found at low levels now even in human milk. The health effects of PCBs are not well established, although they are thought to be mild carcinogens. In one incident in Japan in 1978, when rice oil was contaminated with 2000–3000 ppm PCB, growth retardation occurred in young children and the fetuses of exposed mothers.

23.3.5 Radioactive fallout

The most important dangerous radioisotopes in fall-out are strontium-90 and caesium-137, with half-lives of 28 and 30 years. Strontium is absorbed and metabolized like calcium and stored in bones. Because it is concentrated in milk it is particularly dangerous for infants and children. Since the Nuclear Test Ban Treaty of 1963, the level of radioactive contamination from atmospheric dust is negligible, but accidental exposure can still occur, such as that after the Chernobyl disaster, and lead to dangerous food contamination over widespread areas.

23.3.6 Changes during cooking or processing

Food is frequently exposed to high temperatures during cooking. In roasting and frying, localized areas of food may be subjected to temperatures that lead to carbonization and under these circumstances any organic substance is likely to give rise to carcinogens. The major compounds are polycyclic aromatic hydrocarbons (PAH), produced mainly by burning of fats, and heterocyclic amines (HCA) produced from amino acids. Char-broiling or barbecuing is particularly likely to lead to carcinogen formation.

23.3.7 Irradiation

Irradiation can be used to sterilize foods, control microbial spoilage, eradicate insect infestations and inhibit undesired sprouting. Despite the great potential of the technology, there has been substantial opposition from consumer groups concerned about the process producing toxic chemicals in foods. Extensive studies have shown the products formed are no different from those produced in normal cooking and over 250 toxicological studies have consistently found no adverse effects from feeding irradiated food to animals or humans. Food irradiation is approved by the WHO and currently more than 30 countries have approved some form of use.

23.4 Natural Toxins

Many plant species contain hazardous levels of toxic constituents. Intoxications from poisonous plants usually result from the misidentification of plants by individuals harvesting their own foods, but many ordinary foods also contain potential toxicants at less harmful levels. Toxins occurring naturally in foods are not subject to regulatory control and many would not receive approval if they were proposed as new food additives.

23.4.1 Inherent natural toxins

There are many examples of potentially dangerous toxins in natural food products: cyanogenic glycosides in plants such as cassava and sorghum, alkaloids in herbal teas and comfrey, lathyrus toxin in chickpeas. However, natural toxicants are a generally accepted hazard because the foods that contain them have been eaten in traditional diets for many generations. We are protected from their harmful effects in three ways: avoidance, removal and detoxification. First, traditional knowledge has been passed down to us about which foods are safe and which are not. Thus, we know it is safe to eat certain mushrooms and not others. Second, traditional food preparation methods have evolved to reduce the harmful effects of natural toxins. People in South America and Africa use complex chopping and washing procedures in their preparation of cassava that removes much of the cyanide naturally found in the raw product. Third, the body has numerous detoxification systems, mainly enzymes in the liver, to deal with the toxins that we do ingest. So we can still happily eat very small amounts of nutmeg and sassafras, even though they both contain the naturally occurring carcinogen, safrole.

23.4.2 Abnormal conditions of the animal or plant used for food

Some foods only become hazardous during particular conditions of growth or storage. Ciguatera poisoning is a serious human intoxication, caused by eating contaminated fish, that causes gastrointestinal disorders, neurological problems and, in severe cases, death. There are over 400 species of fish that may become ciguatoxic, but almost all of the two dozen or so fatal cases annually are attributable to barracuda. The poisoning is particularly insidious because it can occur in fish that are normally safe to eat. The precise nature of the intoxication is not yet known but most likely occurs when certain tropical and subtropical fish have been feeding on dinoflagellates that produce toxins which accumulate in the flesh of the fish.

Paralytic shellfish poisoning (PSP) It has been known for many centuries that shellfish can occasionally become toxic. Symptoms of PSP include numbness of the lips and fingertips and ascending paralysis, which can lead to death within 24 hours. PSP, which primarily affects mussels and clams, is also associated with the growth of dinoflagellates in the water. When the dinoflagellates are undergoing periods of rapid growth ('blooms', or 'red tides') in areas where the shellfish are growing, the toxin, saxitoxin, accumulates to hazardous levels in the hepatopancreas of the shellfish.

Glycoalkaloids in potatoes Solanine is one of a range of glycoalkaloid compounds found in the green parts of the potato plant that are toxic above concentrations of 20 mg/100 g. In normal peeled potatoes there are about 7 mg solanine/100 g. Solanine synthesis can be induced by exposing the tubers to light so that they go green and also by simple mechanical injury. In very green potatoes, the levels can reach up to 30 mg/100 g. These glycoalkaloids possess anticholinesterase activity which can produce gastrointestinal and neurological disorders, and deaths have occasionally been reported from consumption of excessive amounts of green potatoes.

23.4.3   Enzyme inhibitors

Protease inhibitors Substances that inhibit digestive enzymes are widespread in many legume species and trypsin inhibitors are found in oats and maize as well as brussels sprouts, onions and beetroot. These inhibitors are proteins and therefore are denatured and inactivated by cooking. Thus, for humans these substances are not a problem, although feeding raw legumes to animals can result in pancreatic enlargement.

23.4.4   Antivitamins

One of the best known antivitamins is the biotin-binding protein, avidin, in raw egg white. Biotin deficiency induced by eating raw egg white is rare because biotin is adequately provided in most human diets. The few cases that have been reported involved abnormally large amounts of raw egg white, so the occasional raw egg is perfectly safe. Avidin is inactivated when heated.

Other antivitamins, such as the pyridoxine antagonist amino-D-proline in flax seeds, the antithiamin compound caffeic acid found in bracken fern, and a tocopherol oxidase in raw soy beans, are only of importance in animal feeding.

23.4.5   Mineral-binding agents

Goitrogens There are a number of glucosinolate and thiocyanate compounds found in foods that interfere with normal utilization of iodine by the thyroid gland and can result in goitres. Goitrogens are widely distributed in cruciferous vegetables such as cabbage, brussels sprouts and broccoli. The average intake of glucosinolates from vegetables in Great Britain is 76 mg/day and clinical studies have found that intakes of 100–400 mg/day may reduce the uptake of iodine by the thyroid. There is no evidence that normal consumption of these foods by humans is in any way harmful, but it is possible that eating large amounts of brassica plants might contribute to a higher incidence of goitre in areas of the world where dietary iodine intakes are low (see Chapter 10.3.4).

Phytate in wholemeal cereals can bind minerals and make them less available for absorption. In leavened bread, phytases in the yeast break down the phytate, but in some parts of the Middle East, where unleavened bread is a dietary staple, phytate has been reported to be the cause of zinc deficiency (see Chapter 10.1.6). It may also affect calcium (Chapter 8.1), and iron (Chapter 9) nutrition.

Oxalate Certain plants, including rhubarb, spinach, beetroot and tea, contain relatively high levels of oxalate. Oxalate can combine with calcium to form an insoluble complex in the gut that is poorly absorbed and high intakes can lower plasma calcium levels. Kidney damage and convulsions can accompany oxalate poisoning. However, the average diet supplies only 70–150 mg oxalate/day which could theoretically bind 30–70 mg calcium. Since calcium intakes are usually 10 times this amount there is no good evidence that food oxalates have any detrimental effect on mineral balance under normal conditions.

Tannins (polyphenols) These are present in tea, coffee and cocoa as well as broad beans. Tannins inhibit the absorption of iron and regular consumption of stewed beans has been associated with anaemia in Egyptian children with low iron intakes. High levels of tea consumption may contribute to low iron status in people with marginal iron intakes.

23.5 AGRICULTURAL RESIDUES

23.5.1 Pesticides

The most common agricultural chemicals found in foods are pesticides, albeit at very low levels. The chlorinated organic pesticides (such as DDT and chlordane) were among the first modern pesticides to be used. In general, they have low toxicity to mammals and are highly toxic to insects. However, they are very stable compounds and persist in soils. Due to their fat solubility, they are stored in the fat tissue of animals. Because of concern about their effect on the reproduction of certain birds and possible carcinogenic activity, the use of these compounds has been restricted. Surveys show that the levels of organochlorine compounds in food have been in decline over the last decade. The alternative insecticides now in use, such as the organophosphates, do not accumulate in the environment. No food poisonings have ever been attributed to the proper use of insecticides on foods.

23.5.2 Fungicides and herbicides

Most fungicides and herbicides show very selective toxicity to their target plants and therefore present very little hazard to humans. In addition, most do not accumulate in the environment.

23.5.3 Hormones

The use of hormones such as bovine somatotrophin (bST) to improve yields of meat and milk, and to reduce the percentage of carcass fat, has been a subject of controversy in many countries. Although low levels of bST can be detected in the milk of treated cows, the hormones are inactive in humans even when injected and, because they are proteins, are digested and inactivated in the stomach when consumed in food. The United States FDA approved the commercial use of bST in 1993 and it likely that a number of other biotechnology hormones will be approved for animal husbandry in the future.

23.6   INTENTIONAL FOOD ADDITIVES

23.6.1   Approval process for food additives

Each country has its own legislation to control the approval of additives in foods, but most follow the same general principles that are used by the two main international bodies of experts organized by WHO and FAO: the Joint Expert Committee on Food Additives (JECFA) and the Codex Alimentarius Committee on Food Additives and Contaminants. The aim of the evaluation of a food additive is to establish an acceptable daily intake (ADI). The ADI is usually expressed in mg/kg of body weight and is defined as the amount of a chemical that might be ingested daily, even over a lifetime, without appreciable risk to the consumer. The evaluation process consists of a number of steps, as follows:

1. Toxicity testing is carried out in experimental animals, usually mice and rats, but other species may also be employed. Three types of testing are performed: (i) acute toxicity studies at high doses to determine the range of possible toxic effects of the chemical; (ii) short-term feeding trials at various doses; and (iii) long-term studies of two years or more to examine the effect of lifetime exposures over several generations.

2. From the feeding trials, the level of additive at which observed health effects do not appear in the animals is determined. This is called the 'no observed effect level' (NOEL).

3. The lowest NOEL is divided by a safety factor to derive a level of exposure that is regarded as acceptable for human exposure, the ADI. Most commonly, a safety factor of 100 is used, but for some substances factors of up to 1000 have been used. This safety factor allows for possible differences in susceptibility to the additive between experimental animals and humans and also the differences in sensitivity of individual people.

Not all additives have been evaluated for safety using modern testing procedures. Some additives have been used for many years without apparent harm and in the United States, 675 ingredients not evaluated by prescribed testing procedures have been classified as generally recognized as safe (GRAS). This list includes commonly used ingredients such as salt and sugar, seasonings and many food flavourings.

While the 100-fold safety factor is accepted for most additives, in the United States, the Delaney Clause prohibits the use in any amount of substances known to cause cancer in animals or humans. When the Bill was introduced in 1958, chemicals could be detected down to 100 parts per billion; anything less was considered zero. Improved analytical techniques can now detect substances at parts per trillion and it has been argued that the trivial risk from such minute quantities should be put into perspective against the benefits of additives in improving the quality, quantity and convenience of the modern food supply. The United States FDA has now changed the interpretation of the Delaney Clause so that if a food additive increases the chance of developing cancer over a lifetime by less than one case per million, the threat is considered too small to be of concern.

Ames has recently ranked the level of carcinogenic risk associated with a variety of chemicals we may be commonly exposed to. The human exposure/rodent potency index (HERP) expresses the typical human intakes as a percentage of the dose required to produce tumours in 50% of rodents. The values in Table 23.4 show that the HERP (i.e. the risk) for the alcohol in a glass of wine is almost 100 times higher than that from the aflatoxins in a peanut butter sandwich or the saccharin in a can of diet cola, and more than 10 000 times the hazard from the residues of the pesticide EDB. That the risks from wine appear more acceptable to most consumers seems to relate to the fact that benefit is easily perceived, that wine is seen as 'natural', and because the risk is voluntary. Although the risks from other additives and contaminants may be far smaller, they arouse suspicion because they are risks that people generally cannot control.

23.6.2 Artificial sweeteners

Saccharin is one of the oldest artificial sweeteners, having been used in foods since the last century. Studies in rats have linked high doses (7.5% of the diet by weight) of saccharin with bladder cancer and because of this there have been attempts to ban its use in human foods. However, at lower doses, such as 1%, no adverse effects are found

Table 23.4 Rankings of possible carcinogenic hazards

Daily human exposure	Carcinogen and dose per 70 kg person	Index of possible hazard*(HERP, %)
Natural dietary toxins		
Wine (250 ml)	Ethyl alcohol, 30 ml	4.7
Basil (1 g of dried leaf)	Estragole, 3.8 mg	0.1
Peanut butter (32 g, 1 sandwich)	Aflatoxin, 64 ng	0.03
Cooked bacon (100 g)	Dimethylnitrosamine, 0.3 µg	0.003
Food additives		
Diet cola (1 can)	Saccharin, 95 mg	0.06
Pesticides		
DDE/DDT (daily diet intake)	DDE, 659 ng	0.00008
EDB (daily diet intake)	EDB, 420 ng, from grain	0.0004

Reprinted with permission from Ames BN, Maga WR, and Gold LS. Ranking of possible carcinogenic hazards. *Science*, **236**: 271–80. Copyright 1987 American Association for the Advancement of Science.

and large epidemiological studies of diabetics who have had lifetime exposures to saccharin have found no increased incidence of cancer in humans.

Cyclamate Dietary cyclamate appears to promote bladder cancer and induce testicular atrophy in rats although carcinogenicity testing in mice, dogs and primates have all been negative. The United States FDA banned the food use of cyclamate in 1969, but in many other countries it is still a permitted sweetener, and there is no good evidence from mutagenicity testing or epidemiological studies that it is a health risk to humans.

Aspartame is a dipeptide of two amino acids, phenylalanine and aspartic acid. Aspartame is metabolized to phenylalanine and therefore carries a risk for people with phenylketonuria, but for the normal population it is an extremely safe sweetener that is digested like any other protein.

23.6.3 Preservatives

Preservatives are used in foods as antioxidants and to prevent the growth of bacteria and fungi. Most pose no toxicological problems, but a few have generated some concerns.

Sodium nitrite is used as an antimicrobial preservative that is very effective in preventing the growth of *Clostridium botulinum*, as well as acting as a colour-fixing agent (to preserve the red colour) in cured meat products such as bacon and ham. Nitrite reacts with primary amides in foods to produce N-nitroso derivatives, many of which are carcinogenic. There has been some concern over exposure of infants to nitrites in infant foods but the risk to human health from dietary nitrite is difficult to assess. While food additive nitrites are significant, a substantial amount is also produced by bacterial reduction of naturally occurring nitrate in vegetables. In recent years, manufacturers have worked to reduce the levels of nitrite used in cured meats, and have added agents such as ascorbic acid which help to prevent the formation of nitrosamines in the stomach.

Sulphur dioxide and its salts (sulphites) are commonly used as inhibitors of enzymic browning, dough conditioners, antimicrobials and antioxidants. Although sulphites have been used for many centuries, with no adverse effect for most consumers, 1–2% of asthmatics are sensitive to sulphites, and in those individuals the reaction can be fatal.

23.7 SUMMARY

Despite the many potential health risks associated with foods, in practice the degree of risk associated with the modern food supply is extremely low. The life span of humans in Western countries is steadily increasing and age-specific death rates for most cancers that might be associated with food ingredients are either decreasing or stable. By far the most important hazards of significance are those from biological agents: pathogenic bacteria, viruses, fungi and a few toxic seafoods. All of these hazards are avoidable by following established food handling practices. The other categories of hazard (contaminants and additives) are closely monitored and regulated and represent only a theoretical risk to most consumers.

FURTHER READING

1. Bryan FL. *Hazard analysis critical control point evaluations. A guide to identifying hazards and assessing risks associated with food preparation and storage.* Geneva: WHO, 1992.
2. Cliver DO (ed.). *Foodborne diseases.* San Diego: Academic Press, 1990.
3. Institute of Food Technologists Expert Panel on Food Safety and Nutrition. The risk/benefit concept as applied to food. *Food Technol* 1988; **42**: 119–26.
4. Riley RT, Norred WP, Bacon CW. Fungal toxins in foods: recent concerns. *Ann Rev Nutr* 1993; **13**: 167–89.
5. Shibamoto T, Bjeldanes LF. *Introduction to food toxicology.* San Diego: Academic Press, 1993.
6. World Health Organization. *Principles for the safety and assessment of food additives and contaminants in food.* IPCS Environmental Health Criteria No. 70. Geneva: WHO, 1987.
7. World Health Organization. *Safety and nutritional adequacy of irradiated food.* Geneva: WHO, 1994.

Part V: Nutritional assessment

24

FOOD ANALYSIS AND FOOD COMPOSITION TABLES

Philippa Lyons Wall

Food composition tables or nutrient databases are designed to describe the composition of the foods in the country of origin. They contain data on foods eaten on a regular basis by the population and generally include some less widely consumed foods that are unique to the culture or eaten on special occasions. The values for nutrients and antinutrients are based on chemical analyses, sometimes performed by the compiler of the tables (or databases) or in an associated laboratory. Some food composition values may be 'borrowed' from a major overseas food table, or represent estimated averages from reports in the literature. The United Kingdom food composition tables (*McCance and Widdowson's, The composition of foods*) and the United States data (USDA Handbook, no. 8) are widely used reference sources. Alternatively, they may be imputed from analytical values existing for a similar food or derived from the ingredients of a mixed food. The origins of the nutrient composition values should be specified, although in practice this is not always done.

When compiling food composition data there are two important considerations. First, food items must be relevant; sampling of an individual food should be representative of the types commonly consumed by the population on a year-round, nation-wide basis, and pertinent to the current food supply. Second, the food composition data must be of high quality; analyses of the foods should be conducted in a rigorous, scientific environment so that values are precise and accurate. Well-established food composition tables have evolved over many years and often combine old and new analytical methods from a variety of different sources. Clear and detailed documentation of sampling and analytical procedures at all stages is as critical as the choice of the analytical procedure itself, so that compilers of tables faced with the challenge of inevitable changes in the food supply can continue to evaluate the relevance of the item and quality of the data.

24.1 SAMPLING

How does one sample foods that are truly representative of a particular food item? Does the analyst just go out to the corner shop nearest the laboratory and buy some food or try to include the varieties of that food across the nation? Foods are ultimately based on parts of plants or animals that vary naturally according to many factors. For example, varieties of sweet potato differ widely in β-carotene content according to whether the flesh is orange, yellow or white in colour. Seasonal variation can markedly influence water and vitamin content, and fruits and vegetables tend to increase their concentration of sugars as they ripen, a process that is highly temperature-dependent. Fat depots in animal foods are also extremely variable according to degree of exercise, type of feed, and age of the animal. Guidelines for sampling protocols that take these variations into account are detailed by Greenfield and Southgate (1992). In general, the greater the natural variation in a particular food the larger the number of samples required. National food production figures may also indicate the types of foods most widely consumed and therefore most representative of the population.

When the food arrives in the laboratory for analysis, it must first be unambiguously identified with both scientific and local names. Full descriptions are required for the part of the animal or plant used, its stage of maturity, size, shape and form. Any cooking or processing methods used in preparing the item must be documented and the edible portion must be carefully separated from inedible refuse. Analyses may then proceed in one of two directions. Individual samples of the same food from different locations can be analysed separately in order to provide information on the variation between samples as well as their average nutrient content. This approach, however, may be a luxury that many laboratories cannot afford. Alternatively, a composite sample can be prepared by pooling several individual subsamples of a food from many locations to give a single sample for analyses. Often, a weighting scheme is used to ensure that those varieties and/or locations where the food item is consumed more frequently are proportionately represented in the final composite. Whether derived from an individual or composite sample, the edible portion must be homogenized or ground thoroughly to ensure that the aliquot taken for analyses is representative of the original sample. For trace minerals, it is also important that the sample is not exposed to adventitious sources of contamination during the collection, homogenization, sample preparation, and analytical stages. Similarly, care must be taken that vitamins and other susceptible organic components are not degraded by air or light, for example.

24.2 ANALYSIS

The ultimate aim of food tables or databases is to provide nutrient information on food components that are of nutritional importance to the health of the population, over their lifetime and in different disease states (Table 24.1). Some of the more common methods used to analyse food components are described below. It is important to document the accuracy and precision of all analytical methods and to use reference materials of a similar matrix to the food sample and certified for the nutrient of interest. Reference materials can be obtained from the United States National Institute for Standards and Technology, Washington, DC and the International Atomic Energy Agency, Vienna.

24.2.1 Moisture

Moisture (water) is the first component to be analysed in a food and it is probably the single most important piece of food composition data. Underestimation of water content will lead to an overestimation of other components which are subsequently determined in the dried food. Water can be gained or lost during the cooking process, with changes in

Table 24.1   Food components of nutritional importance

Basic components[a]
- Moisture
- Energy
- Protein, fat, and carbohydrate
- Up to 13 vitamins, and 10 or more minerals or trace elements

More detailed profiles[b]
- Fatty acid profile (up to 20 fatty acids)
- Amino acid profile (around 18 amino acids)
- Carbohydrate components (sugars, starches)
- Dietary fibre and components (soluble, insoluble)
- Alcohol

Optional components[c]
- Cholesterol
- Vitamin A-inactive carotenoids (lycopene, lutein, zeaxanthin and others)
- Organic acids (malic, citric, lactic, formic, oxalic, salicylic acids)
- Physiologically active components (e.g. flavonoids)

[a] Essential for growth and maintenance of body tissues and always listed in food tables.
[b] Useful for research into diet and disease risk and usually included in well-established tables.
[c] Not essential nutrients but may influence nutritional status indirectly by exerting physiological effects within the body; not routinely listed in food tables but may be cited in appendix sections.

the apparent content of an array of nutrients, as well as energy. Water content is an important preliminary consideration when comparing the nutrient content of similar items in tables from different countries, as may happen if a specific food is not available in the local database. Furthermore, a high moisture content, typical of many fresh fruits and vegetables, indicates a low energy value while the reverse is true for items of low moisture content.

The moisture content in foods is determined by simply evaporating off the water and calculating the difference in weight at the beginning and end. Different methods are used. Water may be driven off in an oven at temperatures around its boiling point, provided the sample itself does not decompose or oxidize or contain other volatiles that would contribute to the weight loss. Alternatively, evaporation can be achieved at lower temperatures by vacuum drying under reduced pressure, or by freeze-drying. In practice, a wide range of methods varying in temperature, time interval, and sample preparation have evolved to optimize this apparently simple process.

24.2.2   Protein and amino acids

Protein in foods is determined indirectly by measuring the content of amino-nitrogen, a major constituent of the amino acid units which combine to form proteins. For the amino-nitrogen assay, the food sample is digested in hot concentrated sulphuric acid to convert the nitrogen into ammonium ion, which is then quantified by either distillation and titration in the classic *Kjeldahl method* or by *spectrophotometric analysis*. The protein content in the original food is then estimated by multiplying the total nitrogen value by specific conversion factors for different foods as shown in Table 24.2. Alternatively, the

Table 24.2 Sample calculations of protein content from nitrogen

Item (100 g)	Total nitrogen (g)		Conversion factor*		Protein (g)
Rump steak	3.02	×	6.25	=	18.9
White rice	1.23	×	5.95	=	7.3

* Conversion factors for converting nitrogen in foods to protein: milk and milk products, 6.38; eggs, meat, fish, 6.25; rice, 5.95; barley, oats, rye, whole wheat, 5.83; soybeans, 5.71; peanuts, brazils, 5.46; almonds, 5.18.

conversion factor of 6.25 is used because nitrogen is assumed to represent about 16% of the protein content.

From a nutritional viewpoint, the importance of a particular dietary protein lies in its ability to sustain growth or replenish tissues, functions that depend more on the quality of the protein (or pattern of content of indispensable amino acids) than the total amount (see Chapter 4). Gelatin, for example, is a food that comprises over 80% protein, one of the highest values listed in the food composition tables, yet as the sole protein source it cannot sustain life no matter how much is eaten because it is deficient in the indispensable amino acid, tryptophan. *Amino acids* are measured by hydrolyzing the protein with strong acid or alkali to break down the peptide bonds, followed by separation and measurement of the free amino acids using ion-exchange chromatography. Food tables may list the amino acid composition of major foods in addition to the total amount of protein, either in the main tables or in an appendix. The profile of indispensable amino acids can then be compared with that of a reference protein, such as hen's egg (a protein known to be utilized very efficiently) for adults, or human milk for babies, to develop a measure of the protein quality, referred to as the amino acid score or chemical score. Table 24.3 shows the indispensable amino acids in two common food proteins compared with those in hen's egg.

Table 24.3 Content of indispensable amino acids in food proteins (mg amino acid per g of protein)

	Hen's egg	Cheese	Wheat flour
Isoleucine	54	67	42
Leucine	86	98	71
Lysine	70	74	20*
Methionine + cystine	57	32	31
Phenylalanine + tyrosine	93	102	79
Threonine	47	37	28
Tryptophan	17	14	11
Valine	66	72	42

The nutritive value of a dietary protein can be estimated by comparing its pattern of indispensable amino acids with those in a reference protein such as hen's egg. The amino acid score is the content of the most limiting (inadequate) amino acid, as a percentage of the reference value for this amino acid. For wheat flour (*), the most limiting amino acid is lysine and the amino acid score is 20/70 or 28%. In real life, however, wheat flour (as bread) is frequently eaten with another protein (e.g. cheese), which has even more lysine than egg, so the amino acid score of whole meals is usually much higher than for individual foods. The limiting amino acid in an equal mixture of wheat and cheese protein is methionine + cystine and amino acid score is 55%.

24.2.3 Fat

A characteristic property of fats is their solubility in organic solvents such as *n*-hexane, petroleum ether or chloroform. Estimation of fat in foods involves extraction with one of these solvents followed by evaporation of the solvent and weighing of the final fat residue. The accuracy of this estimation depends on the type of fat as well as the mix of other components in the food. The traditional *Soxhlet method* tended to underestimate fat that was bound to other food components such as protein. To overcome this problem the sample is now predigested in concentrated acid or alcoholic ammonia to release the bound portion before extraction. The fat residue may be further analysed in various ways. Thin layer chromatography can separate the fat into lipid classes including triglycerides, phospholipids and sterols. If lipids are hydrolyzed to liberate their fatty acids, these can be separated by gas–liquid chromatography. Fatty acid profiles of major foods are provided in several comprehensive food tables such as USDA Handbook, no. 8 and the New Zealand Food Composition Tables. Total saturated fatty acids (including branched-chain acids), monounsaturated (*cis* and *trans* together) and polyunsaturated fatty acids are given in a supplement to the United Kingdom's *McCance and Widdowson's, The composition of foods*.

The presentation of the fat content of foods differs among food tables. In addition to providing the total fat content, compilers may sum the individual fatty acids into groups: polyunsaturated, monounsaturated, and saturated, and list each class separately, or they may present these as a ratio of polyunsaturated and monounsaturated fatty acids to that of saturated fatty acids, termed the P:M:S ratio. Alternatively they may list each fatty acid according to its chain length and degree of saturation. The P:M:S ratio provides a crude estimate of overall atherogenic risk; the higher the proportion of unsaturates the more favourable the ratio. For research purposes, however, the content of individual fatty acids is more useful because each may exert independent effects. (Chapters 3 and 18.1.4 discuss further the role of individual fatty acids in health and disease.)

24.2.4 Carbohydrates

Food composition tables vary widely in the methods used to measure carbohydrate. Probably the commonest approach is 'by difference' which defines carbohydrate as the difference between 100 and the sum of the percentages for protein, fat, water, and ash. However, inaccuracies arise using this approach because of the summation of the errors in estimating these four constituents. In addition, such values are of limited use because they do not distinguish between different carbohydrates, especially those that are available to the body (i.e. digested, absorbed and utilized) and those that are unavailable. More accurate methods quantify the available and unavailable carbohydrate by direct measurements.

Available carbohydrate includes sugars (monosaccharides and disaccharides), and starches and dextrins (polysaccharides). Individual sugars can be extracted with aqueous alcohol and measured by high performance liquid chromatography or using specific enzymatic colorimetric tests. Starches and dextrins, which are glucose polymers, are measured in the same way after an initial hydrolysis step to liberate free glucose. Food tables that report carbohydrate by direct analysis may list the monosaccharide equivalents because this is the form in which the carbohydrate is estimated. To obtain the actual values for disaccharides and starch (polysaccharide) in the food, these values should be divided by 1.05 and 1.10, respectively.

Unavailable carbohydrate or dietary fibre is the mixture of plant components that are resistant to digestive enzymes in the small bowel of the human intestinal tract. The chemical diversity of fibre makes it a very challenging and elusive component to analyse in the laboratory. Accordingly, a number of methods have evolved. All begin with the defatted, dried food sample but each measures a different chemical fraction. *The Englyst method* is the most sensitive and perhaps the most useful from a nutritional perspective because it can distinguish between soluble and insoluble fibres, both of which have physiologically distinct effects in the body in relation to chronic diseases such as diabetes, heart disease, and cancer. In the Englyst method starch is initially removed by digestion with strong amylases and then the constituent sugars of dietary fibre are measured directly after acid hydrolysis to produce the free sugars. This yields estimates of both soluble (pectin, gums, mucilages and hemicelluloses) and insoluble (cellulose and other hemicelluloses) fibre components, collectively called non-starch polysaccharides (NSP). Lignin escapes detection because it is not a carbohydrate but a polymeric phenolic compound. The older *Southgate method* gives a higher value for dietary fibre content as it measures lignin, as well as NSP.

Other methods are less precise because they measure fibre 'by difference' but they involve less analytical work and so are more economical. In the widely used *Association of Official Analytical Chemists* (AOAC) *procedure* developed by Prosky and Asp, starch is first removed by enzymatic hydrolysis and the undigested residue is weighed, analysed for nitrogen, and then ashed. Protein and ash contents are then subtracted from the residue weight. *Van Soest's neutral detergent fibre* (NDF) *method* measures only the insoluble cellulose and lignin, and not the soluble fibre. Hence, this method underestimates total dietary fibre. The 'crude fibre' method is the least accurate, involving rigorous treatment with boiling acid and alkali which removes much of the dietary fibre itself.

A further complication in the analysis of dietary fibre is the recognition that a variable but small proportion of the dietary starch found in beans, whole grains, potatoes (especially if eaten cold), or unripe bananas, is not completely digested and is unavailable to the body for absorption. This starch, termed 'resistant starch', escapes digestion because it is physically inaccessible to the enzymes, and instead, it is probably fermented in the colon, thus behaving like soluble dietary fibre. Current values for dietary fibre in food tables do not include separate values for resistant starch, although the AOAC and Southgate methods include some of the resistant starch in the fibre value.

Different analytical methods can result in several fold variations in the estimate of fibre for the same item, as shown in Table 24.4. Most food tables, however, are internally consistent in their choice of analytical method(s) and these should be stated clearly in the introductory section or in the main tables alongside the nutrient values. Special care should be taken when comparing carbohydrate values from different food composition tables. For reasons outlined above, values from those tables in which total carbohydrate is analysed by difference (i.e. including dietary fibre) are not compatible with others in which carbohydrate constituents are analysed directly.

Table 24.4 Dietary fibre content of dried red kidney beans estimated by five different methods

Method	Fibre content (g/100 g)	Fibre components
Englyst[a]	15.7	Soluble + insoluble fibre (not lignin or resistant starch)
Southgate[a]	23.4	Soluble + insoluble fibre, lignin
AOAC (Prosky and Asp)[b]	21.5	Soluble + insoluble fibre, lignin
Neutral detergent fibre (Van Soest)[c]	10.4	Insoluble fibre only
Crude fibre[c]	6.2	Part of the insoluble fibre

Note: Red kidney beans contain both soluble and insoluble dietary fibre. AOAC, Southgate, and Englyst methods measure total dietary fibre, but Englyst fibre is lower because it does not measure lignin or resistant starch. Neutral detergent fibre is lower because it does not measure soluble fibre.
Sources:
[a] Holland B, Welch AA, Unwin ID, Buss DH, Paul AA, Southgate DAT. *McCance and Widdowson's, The composition of foods.* 5th ed. Cambridge: Royal Society of Chemistry, 1991.
[b] English R, Lewis J. *Nutritional values of Australian foods.* Canberra: Australian Government Publishing Service, 1991.
[c] USDA. *Composition of foods: legumes and legume products.* Handbook no. 8–16. Washington, DC: US Department of Agriculture, 1986.

24.2.5 Energy

The total energy of a food is measured by *bomb calorimetry* in which a sample of the food is burned with oxygen in a sealed chamber until completely oxidized. The heat released corresponds to the chemical or gross energy of the food. Food energy is reported in kilojoules (kJ) or kilocalories (kcal), where $1 kJ = 0.24 kcal$. When a food is eaten, however, the energy yielding components, protein, fat, carbohydrate and (where present) alcohol, are oxidized by enzymatic processes within the body to provide energy, but not with 100% efficiency. Some energy is lost into the faeces as not all food components are fully absorbed from the digestive tract. Further energy is lost into urine since dietary protein, unlike carbohydrate and fat, is not completely oxidized by the body and its excretory product, urea, still retains some of the chemical energy from the original protein. The eminent American physiologist, Atwater, measured the energy losses into faeces and urine by a series of meticulous experiments in humans fed a mixture of foods. In his experiments 92% of protein, 95% of fat, and 97% of carbohydrate were absorbed by the body, but for every gram of protein ingested about one-quarter of its gross energy was lost into the urine.

Atwater's experiments, conducted at the turn of the nineteenth century, represent landmark studies from which the energy content of foods in today's food composition tables are derived. Atwater developed a system of four conversion factors which represent the energy available in: (1) protein (17 kJ/g, 4 kcal/g), (2) fat (37 kJ/g, 9 kcal/g), (3) carbohydrate (16 kJ/g, 4 kcal/g) and (4) alcohol (29 kJ/g, 7 kcal/g), taking into account the estimated energy losses into faeces and urine. The value is slightly higher for starch (due to lower hydration) than that given for all carbohydrates and slightly lower for sugars. These factors provide values for food energy as it is utilized by the body (i.e. metabolizable energy). The energy content of each food is calculated by first multiplying the weight of each component by its Atwater conversion factor, and second, summing

Table 24.5 Calculation of metabolizable energy content in raw soybean using Atwater conversion factors

Component	Weight (g/100 g)		Atwater factor (kJ(kcal)/g)		Energy content (kJ(kcal)/100 g)
Water	8		–	=	– –
Protein	31	×	17 (4)	=	527 (124)
Fat	20	×	37 (9)	=	740 (180)
Available carbohydrate	7	×	16 (4)	=	112 (28)
Dietary fibre	20		not included	=	– –

Note: The energy content of individual components is then summed to give a grand total of 1379 kJ/100 g or 332 kcal/100 g.

the energy from each component to give a grand total for the food, as shown in Table 24.5. Note that the total weight of each nutrient is obtained by direct analysis of the food, as described previously. The biggest variable is the carbohydrate value and whether this includes fibre, because Atwater factors are applied to the total carbohydrate content irrespective of whether this is analysed directly or by difference. In practice, the value for energy is somewhere between the two extremes of 16 kcal/g for available carbohydrate and 0 kJ/g for unavailable carbohydrate. This is because a proportion of dietary fibre is fermented in the colon to short-chain fatty acids which can be absorbed from the large bowel and oxidized for energy. Livesey (1991) has estimated that about half the dietary fibre can be utilized by the body in this way and proposes an average energy conversion factor of 8 kJ/g (2 kcal/g) for unavailable carbohydrates, about half the value for available carbohydrate. Current values in food tables do not incorporate estimates of the energy from fibre.

The energy conversion factors used today vary somewhat from Atwater's original factors. The German, British, Australian and New Zealand food composition tables, for example, apply the same four factors to all foods, whereas the United States and East Asian tables use a range of slightly differing conversion factors, rather lower for components in plant foods than in animal foods, reflecting Atwater's initial observation that the energy from plants was less available. The conversion factors selected to calculate energy should be specified in the introduction or appendix section of all food composition tables and the reader is referred to these for more in-depth information.

24.2.6 Inorganic nutrients and vitamins

The range of inorganic nutrients in foods including calcium, iron, magnesium, zinc, copper, manganese, potassium and sodium can be determined by *flame atomic absorption spectrophotometry (AAS)*, a method whereby a solution of the ashed or acid-digested food sample is sprayed into the flame of an atomic absorption spectrophotometer and quantified by the degree of absorption at a specified wavelength. For selenium, direct AAS with a Zeeman background correction is required. Graphite furnace AAS is used for analysing the ultratrace elements such as chromium, nickel and manganese. Alternatively, all the minerals can be measured in the one sample using inductively coupled plasma spectrophotometry or X-ray fluorescence. Minerals are a very stable component of foods and these procedures can be highly accurate provided any interfering substances such as plant pigments or organic constituents have first been removed. This is achieved by reducing the food sample to a dry ash by thorough heating in a muffle furnace, or by breaking down and oxidizing the organic components by wet ashing with boiling concentrated acids. For trace element analysis, precautions must be used to avoid adventitious contamination by the use of ultrapure acids, acid-washed glassware, plastic materials for sample preparation and analysis, and high grade deionized water.

In contrast to the minerals, many of the vitamins in foods are not very stable. Riboflavin and vitamin A are sensitive to light; thiamin, folate and vitamin C are sensitive to heat, and vitamin E to oxidation. Vitamins are either analysed by the traditional but more time-consuming microbiological methods or by newer, faster chemical techniques. *Microbiological assays* are conducted with a culture of organisms that have a specific growth requirement for the particular vitamin. The assumption is made, however, that the microorganism reacts in the same way as the human organism. Such methods are available for a wide range of B vitamins including thiamin, niacin, riboflavin, vitamins B_6 and B_{12}, folate, biotin and pantothenate, and have the advantage of estimating the total biological potential of the vitamin. Alternative chemical methods, such as *high performance liquid chromatography*, can be used for vitamins A, C and E. They require an initial extraction step to remove other components in the food, but are useful for separating and quantifying different chemical forms of the vitamin. It should be borne in mind that many of the existing values for vitamins, as well as minerals, in food tables were obtained with older, less specific colorimetric methods that are now obsolete.

Values in food composition tables represent the total content of each mineral or vitamin in the food and do not address the complex problem of bioavailability, defined as the proportion of a nutrient that is actually absorbed from the food and utilized. When a vitamin exists in two or more forms which are utilized differently in the body, some food composition tables tabulate each form separately. Vitamin A, for example, has two major components obtained from quite different food sources, preformed vitamin A (or retinol), which is found in many animal products, and the pro-vitamin A carotenoids derived from plants. The compiler may further attempt to calculate the overall potency of the vitamin in the body by summing the different forms, taking into account their relative biological activities. Some of the assumptions and calculations made in food tables regarding the different forms of niacin, and vitamins A, C and E are shown in Table 24.6.

24.3 COMPILATION OF FOOD COMPOSITION DATA

Compilation of food composition data either in the form of tables or computerized databases is a very large task. It requires painstaking inspection of a wide range of sources that use a variety of sampling and analytical procedures. Data analysed outside the compiler's laboratory must frequently be traced back to its source and any items without clear documentation discarded because there is no way to evaluate their quality. Values from different sources must be compared and statistical calculations made to provide a meaningful average for the nutrient content of a food. As food patterns within a population are constantly changing and evolving, data must also be scrutinized to determine its relevance in the current food supply.

Not only should data be accurate and relevant, but the format must be clear so that the user may easily understand the data. Food items are listed alphabetically and usually

Table 24.6 Presentation of different vitamin forms in food composition tables

Vitamin	Main forms	Unit of total vitamin activity
Niacin[a]	1. Preformed in foods (nicotinic acid + nicotamide) 2. Derived from tryptophan	Niacin equivalents (NE)
Vitamin A[b]	1. Retinol 2. Provitamin A carotenoids	Retinol equivalents (RE)
Vitamin E[c]	1. Tocopherols $(\alpha, \beta, \gamma, \delta)$ 2. Tocotrienols (α, β, γ)	α-Tocopherol equivalents
Vitamin C[d]	1. Ascorbic acid 2. Dehydroascorbic acid	Vitamin C

[a] Because approximately 1% of protein is tryptophan and $\frac{1}{60}$ th tryptophan is converted to niacin in the body:

$$NE \ (mg) = preformed\ niacin\ (mg) + dietary\ protein\ (g) \times 0.16.$$

[b] Because β-carotene has $\frac{1}{6}$ th activity of retinol and twice the activity of other carotenoids:

$$RE \ (\mu g) = retinol \ (\mu g) + \frac{\beta\text{-carotene} \ (\mu g)}{6} + \frac{\alpha\text{-carotene} + cryptoxanthin \ (\mu g)}{12}.$$

[c] α-Tocopherol is the most abundant form with over twice the activity of other tocopherols and tocotrienols. Activities of individual vitamin forms are cited in *McCance and Widdowson's, The composition of foods*. 5th ed. Cambridge: Royal Society of Chemistry, 1991.

[d] Both forms have equal activity and are summed to give total vitamin C.

grouped according to food sources with similar nutritional properties (e.g. vegetables, fruits, grains, meats, dairy products); or by product use (e.g. snacks, desserts, breakfast cereals). In cases where foods are collected or prepared with inedible matter, the percentage edible portion, sometimes expressed indirectly as percentage refuse, is also given. However, irrespective of the proportion of edible matter or the accustomed serving size, nutrient values for items are always presented in terms of 100 g edible portions. Consequently, this does not include the core or stone in fruit, or the bones in meat and chicken, but it does include optional material like certain vegetable skins and trimmable meat fat, unless specified otherwise. Most food tables cite both scientific and local names for each item, and some specify the number of food items analysed, and whether a single or composite sample was used for analysis. Rarely do tables include the natural variation around the mean value but rather provide a single mean representative value. The German (Souci *et al.* 1994) and the United States (USDA Handbook, no. 8) tables are exceptions, citing the range (i.e. highest and lowest values known) or the standard error of the mean, respectively, in addition to the mean value.

Ideally, food composition tables or databases should include analyses for all food components of nutritional relevance to the potential user, whether this be a dietitian prescribing advice to a client, a research worker investigating certain nutrients in relation to disease risk, or a food manufacturer seeking accurate nutrient information on their products for the purposes of marketing and food legislation. In practice, however, inclusion is determined more by the analytical resources and public health priorities of the country concerned. Nevertheless, a wealth of analytical and descriptive information on food habits and customs already exist within different cultures. Yet many of these

Table 24.7 INFOODS guidelines for describing foods

Name and identification	Name of food in national language of the country
	Name in local language or dialect
	Nearest equivalent name in English, French or Spanish
	Country or area in which sample of food was obtained
	Food group and code in database used in the country
	Food group and code for food in regional nutrient database
	Codex Alimentarius or INFOODS food indexing group
Description	Food source (common and scientific name)
	Variety, breed, strain
	Part of plant or animal
	Manufacturer's name and address
	Other ingredients (including additives)
	Food processing and/or preparation
	Preservation method
	Degree of cooking
	Agricultural production conditions
	Maturity or ripeness
	Storage conditions
	Grade
	Container and food contact surface
	Physical state, shape, or form
	Colour

Source: Truswell AS, Bateson DJ, Madafiglio KC, Pennington JAT, Rand WM, Klensin JC. INFOODS guidelines for describing foods: a systematic approach to describing foods to facilitate international exchange of food composition data. *J Food Comp Anal* 1991; 4: 18–38.

data are not widely accessible outside the country, often because local names are idiosyncratic or culture-specific making it difficult to identify the food. In this regard the INFOODS guidelines (Table 24.7) were established to ensure foods are named and described in a standardized manner with a view to facilitating interchange of food composition data at the international level.

FURTHER READING

1. Greenfield H, Southgate DAT. *Food composition data. Production, management and use.* London: Elsevier Applied Science, 1992.
2. Holland B, Welch AA, Unwin ID, Buss DH, Paul AA, Southgate DAT. *McCance and Widdowson's, The composition of foods.* 5th ed. Cambridge: Royal Society of Chemistry, 1991.
3. Leung W-TW, Bukum RR, Chang FH, Rao MN, Polacchi W. *Food composition tables for use in East Asia.* Rome: FAO, 1972.
4. Livesey G. Calculating the energy values of foods: towards new empirical formulae based on diets with varied intakes of unavailable complex carbohydrates. *Eur J Clin Nutr* 1991; 45: 1–12.
5. Souci SW, Fachmann W, Kraut H. *Food composition and nutrition tables.* Stuttgart: Medpharm Scientific Publishers, 1994.
6. Burlingame BA, Milligan GC, Spriggs TW, Athar N. *The concise New Zealand food composition tables.* 3rd ed. Palmerston North, NZ: New Zealand Institute for Crop and Food Research, 1997.

25

DIETARY ASSESSMENT

Rosalind Gibson

There is increasing interest in the relationships between diet and health and disease. As a result, research has centred on improving the quality of dietary intake data collected by existing dietary assessment methods. This chapter describes the three stages in a dietary assessment protocol with emphasis on food consumption methods suitable for individuals. The three stages include: (1) measurement of food intakes; (2) calculation of nutrient intakes; and (3) evaluation of nutrient intakes in relation to recommendations. The nature, magnitude, and impact of measurement errors on dietary assessment methods are also discussed together with ways of minimizing these errors.

25.1 MEASURING FOOD CONSUMPTION OF INDIVIDUALS

Methods for measuring food consumption of individuals can be classified into two major groups—quantitative and qualitative—the choice depending primarily on the objectives of the study. Quantitative methods consist of recalls or records designed to measure the quantity of food consumed over a one-day period. By increasing the number of measurement days, quantitative estimates of recent food intake, or—for longer time periods—habitual food intake of individuals can be obtained.

Qualitative dietary assessment methods are used most frequently to assess habitual intake of foods or specific classes of foods rather than intakes of nutrients. With some modification, however, they can provide data on habitual nutrient intakes. Two qualitative dietary assessment methods exist: (1) the dietary history; and (2) the food frequency questionnaire. Both obtain retrospective information on the patterns of food use during a longer, less precisely defined time period than that associated with the quantitative assessment methods. Table 25.1 compares the procedures, uses, and limitations of both quantitative and qualitative methods of assessing food consumption of individuals.

25.1.1 Twenty-four hour recall

The purpose of the 24-hour recall method is to provide information on the respondent's exact food intake during the previous 24-hour period or preceding day. Such information can be used to characterize the mean intake of a group, provided the sample is truly representative and that all the days of the week are adequately represented. If habitual intakes of individuals are required, multiple replicate 24-hour recalls must be used.

The recall interviews are conducted in four stages on the subjects, their parents, or caretakers using a standardized protocol. In *stage one*, a complete list of all foods and

Table 25.1 Uses and limitations of commonly used methods to assess the food consumption of individuals

Methods and procedures	Uses and limitations
Twenty-four hour recall Subject or caretaker recalls food intake of previous 24 hours in an interview. Quantities estimated in household measures using food models as memory aids and/or to assist in quantifying portion sizes. Nutrient intakes calculated using food composition data.	Useful for assessing average usual intakes of a large population, provided that the sample is truly representative and that the days of the week are adequately represented. Used for international comparisons of relationship of nutrient intakes to health and susceptibility to chronic disease. Inexpensive, easy, quick, with low respondent burden so that compliance is high. Large coverage possible; can be used with illiterate individuals. Element of surprise so less likely to modify eating pattern. *Limitations.* Relies on memory and hence unsatisfactory for the elderly and young children. Single 24-hour recalls likely to omit foods consumed infrequently. Multiple replicate 24-hour recalls used to estimate usual intakes of individuals.
Estimated food record Record of all food and beverages as eaten (including snacks), over periods from one to seven days. Quantities estimated in household measures. Nutrient intakes calculated using food composition data.	Used to assess actual or usual intakes of individuals, depending on number of measurement days. Data on usual intakes used for diet counselling and statistical analysis involving correlation and regression. *Limitations.* Accuracy depends on conscientiousness of subject and ability to estimate quantities. Longer time frames result in a higher respondent burden and a lower co-operation. Subjects must be literate.
Weighed food record All food consumed over defined period is weighed by the subject, caretaker, or assistant. Food samples may be saved individually, or as a composite, for nutrient analysis. Alternatively, nutrient intakes calculated from food composition data.	Used to assess actual or usual intakes of individuals, depending on the number of measurement days. Accurate but time-consuming. *Limitations.* Condition must allow weighing. Subjects may change their usual eating pattern to simplify weighing or to impress investigator. Requires literate, motivated, and willing participants. Expensive.
Dietary history Interview method consisting of a 24-hour recall of actual intake, plus information on overall usual eating pattern, followed by a food frequency questionnaire to verify and clarify initial data. Usual portion sizes recorded in household measures. Nutrient intakes calculated using food composition data.	Used to describe usual food and/or nutrient intakes over a relatively long time period which can be used to estimate prevalence of inadequate intakes. Such information used for national food policy development, food fortification planning, and to identify food patterns associated with inadequate intakes. *Limitations.* Labour-intensive, time-consuming and results depend on skill of interviewer.

Table 25.1 (*Continued*)

Methods and procedures	Uses and limitations
Food frequency questionnaire Uses comprehensive list or list of specific food items to record intakes over a given period (day, week, month, year). Record is obtained by interview, or self-administered questionnaire. Questionnaire can be semi-quantitative when subjects asked to quantify usual portion sizes of food items, with or without the use of food models.	Designed to obtain qualitative, descriptive data on usual intakes of foods or classes of foods over a long time period. Useful in epidemiological studies for ranking subjects into broad categories of low, medium, and high intakes of specific foods, food components or nutrients, for comparison with the prevalence and/or mortality statistics of a specific disease. Can also identify food patterns associated with inadequate intakes of specific nutrients. *Limitations.* Method is rapid with low respondent burden and high response rate but accuracy is lower than other methods.

beverages consumed over the previous 24-hour period is obtained. In *stage two*, detailed descriptions of all the foods and beverages consumed, including cooking methods and brand names (if possible) are recorded, and the time and place of consumption. In the *third stage*, estimates of the amounts of all foods and beverages consumed are obtained, usually in household measures. Finally, in the *fourth stage*, the recall is reviewed to ensure that all items have been recorded correctly on the 24-hour recall form (Table 25.2). At this time, interviewers should also ensure that vitamin and mineral supplement usage has also been recorded and that the day of the recall represented a 'normal' day.

To reduce errors associated with memory lapses and/or portion size estimates, coloured photographs or food models are often used. Graduated food models such as those developed by Nutrition Canada (Fig. 25.1) are preferred. Simulated plastic food models representing 'average' portion sizes should not be used because they tend to direct responses. If the interviews are conducted in the respondent's home, household cups, glasses, bowls and spoons can also be used to estimate amounts, provided they are calibrated prior to use. Respondents can also be trained to estimate food portion sizes using food models or household measures to improve the accuracy of recalled portion size estimates.

When conducting the interview, both interpersonal and technical skills are important: for example, the interview must always be conducted with an open and pleasant manner, with the aim of being friendly, diplomatic, empathetic, and determined, as appropriate. Leading questions, judgemental comments, and questions about specific meals (e.g. breakfast, lunch, supper) or about snacks should be avoided. Respondents should not be told in advance when a 24-hour recall will be conducted to avoid any changes in the food intake of the subject.

The advantages of the 24-hour recall method include a low respondent burden, high compliance, low cost, ease and speed of use, use of a standardized interview, element of surprise (so that the respondent is less likely to modify his or her eating habits), and its suitability for illiterate respondents. Disadvantages include its reliance on memory, making it an unsatisfactory method for the elderly and young children, and the errors

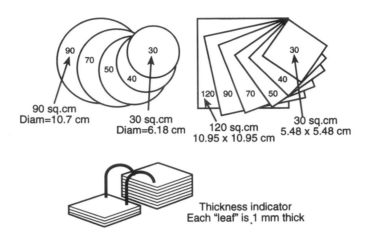

Fig. 25.1 Models for use in the estimation of portion size developed by Health and Welfare Canada (1973).

that may occur in the estimation of portion sizes of foods. The 'flat slope syndrome' may be a problem in the 24-hour recall method: in this syndrome, individuals appear to overestimate low intakes and underestimate high intakes—sometimes referred to as 'talking a good diet'. Subjects completing single 24-hour recalls also tend to omit foods that are infrequently consumed. Some of these advantages and disadvantages are summarized in Table 25.1.

The success of the 24-hour recall depends on the subject's memory, the ability of the respondent to convey accurate estimates of portion sizes consumed, the degree of motivation of the respondent, and the skill and persistence of the interviewer.

25.1.2 Food records

For the food record, subjects, parents, caretakers, or local field investigators are instructed to record all foods and beverages consumed by the subjects during a specified time period. Details of methods of food preparation and cooking, description of foods, and brand names (if known) should also be documented, as shown in Table 25.2. For composite dishes such as spaghetti bolognese, the amount of each raw ingredient used in the recipe, the final weight of the composite dish, and the amount consumed by the subject, should be recorded. Both weekdays and weekend days should be proportionately represented to account for potential day-of-the-week effects on food and nutrient intakes.

For estimated food records, the amounts of all food and beverages in the form they are consumed is estimated using household measures. For example, standard measuring cups can be used for soups, casseroles, and drinks whereas measuring spoons can be used for small quantity food items (e.g. for butter, sugar, coffee, jam). Portion sizes for meat, fish, and cakes can be estimated by measuring with a ruler; counts can be used for eggs and bread slices as shown in Table 25.3. The practice of describing quantities of foods consumed in terms of standard servings should be avoided.

Table 25.2 Form used to record detailed food intakes

Date		Day of the week		
Subject ID		Name of subject		
Place Eaten	Time	Description of Food/Drink	Brand	Amount

Table 25.3 The correct and incorrect methods for describing and quantifying foods when using household measures

Group	Incorrect		Correct	
	Description	Amount	Description	Amount
Meat and fish	Hamburger	medium patty	Beef hamburger	75 g (3 oz)
	Lamb	medium chop	Lamp chop, lean and fat	2 × 4 × 1″
	Fish	small portion	Cod fried in batter	2 × 3 × 1″
Fruits and vegetables	Apple	medium dish	Stewed apple	1 cup
	Tomato	small amount	Fried tomato	2 tbs
Prepared foods	Bread	a few slices	Wholemeal bread	2 slices
	Muffin	small portion	Bran muffin	1 × 2″
	Spaghetti	large serving	Campbell's spaghetti and tomato sauce	$\frac{3}{4}$ cup
Others	Small candies	handful	Smarties	6

For weighed food records, the edible portion sizes consumed are weighed using dietary scales. Hence, accuracy and precision are greater for the weighed compared to the estimated food record. Nevertheless, misreading the weighing scale and errors in recording may still occur. For occasional meals eaten away from home, respondents are generally requested to record descriptions of the amounts of food eaten. The nutritionist can then buy and weigh a duplicate portion of each reported food item, where possible, to assess the probable weight consumed.

Generally, respondents must be numerate and literate when a food record is used, unless the recording is undertaken by a field investigator, as may occur in a developing country. They must also be highly motivated because the method is more time-consuming than a 24-hour recall, and the respondent burden is higher. In addition, respondents may change their usual eating pattern to simplify the measuring or weighing process, or, alternatively to impress the investigator (Table 25.1). Nevertheless, because food intake is recorded at the time of consumption, errors from memory lapses are less likely in a food record compared to 24-hour recall.

25.1.3 Dietary history

The purpose of the dietary history is to obtain retrospective information on the usual food intake and meal patterns of individuals over varying periods of time. The time periods covered often include the previous month, six months, or (sometimes) the previous year. The maximum time period that can be used has not been established, although measurements of food intake over a one-year period are probably unrealistic if seasonal variations in food intake occur. A dietary history is usually conducted by a nutritionist during a personal interview which may be 1.5–2.0 hours in length.

The dietary history technique was developed by Burke in 1947 as an interview method consisting initially of three components:

(1) a 24-hour recall of actual food intake, as well as the collection of general information on the overall eating pattern at mealtimes and between meals;

(2) a questionnaire on the frequency of consumption of specific food items, which was used to verify and clarify the information on the kinds and amounts of foods given as the usual intake in the first component; and

(3) a three-day estimated food record which was used as a cross-check. The latter was found to be least helpful and consequently is often omitted.

Advantages of the dietary history include its ability to provide information on habitual dietary intake and its relatively low respondent burden compared to that of a food record. A major disadvantage, however, is its reliance on the respondent's memory and ability to estimate portion sizes correctly, making it unsuitable for children less than 14 years of age and for the elderly. The method is also unsuitable for those with erratic meal patterns: it tends to underestimate any irregularities in food intake and meal patterns because of its emphasis on regular eating patterns. The maximum time period over which a dietary history method can be used has not been firmly established. When shorter time frames (i.e. one month) are used, precision and validity are apparently higher than for longer periods.

25.1.4   Food frequency questionnaire

A food frequency questionnaire is designed to obtain qualitative or semi-quantitative descriptive information about usual food consumption patterns. This is accomplished by assessing the frequency with which certain food items (e.g. milk and cheese) or food groups (e.g. fruits and vegetables) are consumed during a specified time period (e.g. daily, weekly, monthly or yearly) during a standardized interview. Alternatively, a self-administered questionnaire can be completed by the respondent.

The food frequency questionnaire has two main components: (1) a list of foods; and (2) a set of frequency-of-use response categories (Table 25.4). The list of foods may focus on specific foods or groups of foods, or foods consumed periodically in association with special events or seasons. Alternatively, the food list may be extensive, to enable estimates of total food intake—and hence dietary diversity—to be made. If the questionnaire is modified to quantify the usual portion sizes consumed for each food item, then semi-quantitative food frequency data can be obtained. Usual portion sizes can be estimated by means of photographs or pictures of average portion sizes, or by using food models. Data for the average portion sizes for males and females by age should be derived from national nutrition survey data. In some food frequency questionnaires, small and large portion sizes, based on the 25th and 75th percentiles for food portions from national survey data are also included and the respondent is requested to indicate the usual portion size consumed for each food item as small, medium, or large, as shown in Table 25.4.

The advantages of a food frequency questionnaire include a high response rate and a low respondent burden (Table 25.1). The method is also speedy, relatively inexpensive, and can be designed to measure usual food intake. The questionnaire can be administered

415

Table 25.4 An example of part of the self-administered semi-quantitative food frequency questionnaire

Food	Medium Serving	Serving			How often				
		S	M	L	D	W	M	Y	N
Apples, apple sauce, pears	(1) or $\frac{1}{2}$ cup								
Bananas	1 medium								
Peaches, apricots (canned)	(1) or $\frac{1}{2}$ cup								
peaches, apricots (fresh)	1 medium								
Cantaloupe melon	$\frac{1}{4}$ medium								
Watermelon	1 slice								
Strawberries	$\frac{1}{2}$ cup								
Oranges	1 medium								
Orange Juice	150 ml (6 oz glass)								
Grapefruit or grapefruit juice, etc.	$\frac{1}{2}$ or 6 oz glass								

S, M, L, small, medium, and large relative to the medium serving; D, W, M, Y, N, daily, weekly, monthly, yearly, and never.
Source: Modified from Block G, Hartman AM, Dresser CM, Carroll MD, Gannon J, Gardner L. A data-based approach to diet questionnaire design and testing. *Am J Epidemiol* 1986; **124**: 453–69.

by non-professional interviewers in the home or via telephone; alternatively, it can be self-administered.

Data from a food frequency questionnaire can be used to rank respondents into broad categories of low, medium, and high intakes of certain foods, based on tertiles, for example. In epidemiological studies, such rankings are often compared with the prevalence and/or mortality statistics for a specific disease within the population studied. The example given in Fig. 25.2 demonstrates an association between death rate for cancer of the prostate and the frequency of consumption of green/yellow vegetables. Such data are very preliminary and only provide a guide for more extensive investigations. For example, several dietary components may be associated with the relationship presented in Fig. 25.2, including dietary fibre, β-carotene, or vitamin C.

Alternatively, food scores can be calculated based on the frequency of consumption of certain food groups, and compared with the optimum number of servings of the major food groups per person per day, derived from an accepted standard such as Canada's Food Guide.

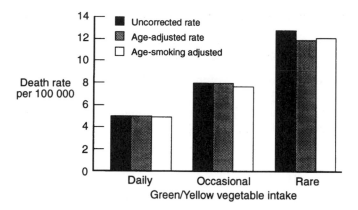

Fig. 25.2 Death rate for cancer of the prostate by frequency of green/yellow vegetable intake. *Source*: Redrawn from Hirayama (1981) by permission of Lawrence Erlbaum Associates Inc.

If a semi-quantitative food frequency questionnaire is used, the frequency-of-use categories should first be converted to a daily basis with, for example, once per day equal to one, and assuming 30 days per month. For example: tomato juice consumed four times per month is equivalent to 4/30 per day, ∼ 0.13 per day. For seasonal fruits and vegetables, the yearly category is used so that peaches consumed 15 times over the summer will be equivalent to 15/365 per day, ∼ 0.04 per day. Then the frequency per day is multiplied by the usual portion size (in grams) to provide the weight of each food item consumed in grams per day. The nutrient content of the latter is then obtained from appropriate food composition data. Sometimes, semi-quantitative food frequency questionnaires are designed to obtain information on intakes of single nutrients (e.g. fat, vitamin A, or calcium). Using these nutrient intake data, subjects are often classified into the lowest or highest quintiles or tertiles within the distribution.

25.1.5 New developments for measuring food consumption in individuals

New developments for measuring food intakes of individuals include telephone-assisted approaches, use of photographs to record both food items consumed and leftovers, electronic devices for recording food intakes directly, use of list-based tools designed to minimize compliance bias, and computer-assisted interviewing techniques, such as the fully automated dietary history program developed in Germany. All these developments aim to reduce respondent burden and hence increase compliance and thus reduce compliance bias, reduce errors resulting from memory lapses and under-reporting, and in the case of electronic devices, eliminate the tedious process of coding the food records.

25.2 SELECTION OF THE METHOD TO MEASURE FOOD CONSUMPTION

The number of measurement days, their selection, and spacing, and the method chosen for measuring food consumption of individuals depends on a variety of factors which are outlined below.

25.2.1 Study objectives

The selection of the method for measuring food intakes depends primarily on the study objectives. Four levels of objectives are possible:

1. The mean intake of a group is required. This objective can be met by measuring the food intake of each subject by a recall or record over a one-day period, provided all the days of the week are proportionately represented in the final sample, and the subjects are representative of the study population.
2. An estimate of the proportion of the population 'at risk' of inadequate nutrient intakes is required. This is achieved by measuring the food consumed by each subject over more than one day. Hence, repeated 24-hour recalls, or replicate weighed or estimated one-day food records are the methods of choice.
3. Nutrient intakes of individuals are ranked within the distribution. This necessitates measuring multiple replicates of an individuals daily food intake.
4. When usual nutrient intakes of individuals are required for individual counselling or for correlation and regression analysis, an even larger number of measurement days for each individual are required. Sometimes, dietary histories or semi-quantitative food frequency questionnaires are used to obtain this level 4 data on usual nutrient intakes.

The number of replicate 24-hour recalls, or weighed or estimated one-day food records required to obtain level two, three or four data depends upon the nutrient of interest, the population group, and the degree of precision required. Generally, for nutrients found in high concentrations in only a few foods, such as vitamins A and D and cholesterol, the number of replicates required is greater than for those found in a wide range of food items (e.g. protein).

25.2.2 Validity

Validity describes the degree to which a dietary assessment method measures what it purports to measure. Absolute validity can only be determined for those dietary methods covering a short time frame and which are conducted in institutional settings. Methods used include surreptitious observation, or weighing duplicate portions of the actual intake of foods recalled by the same subjects over the same 24-hour period. In general, the 24-hour recall tends to underestimate mean dietary intakes in the elderly and children but produces valid mean intakes for other population groups. For dietary methods undertaken in non-institutional settings and designed to characterize usual intakes, and hence covering a longer time period, absolute validity cannot be measured because the truth is never known with absolute certainty. Subjects may eat atypically during a dietary period, even though every effort is made to discourage this. Therefore, relative validity rather than absolute validity can only be measured. In this approach, the performance of the 'test' dietary method is evaluated against another 'reference' method. Choice of the reference method must take into account:

(1) accuracy and precision which must be high in the reference method;
(2) ability of reference method to measure food intake over the same time frame as the test method;

(3) spacing of the test and reference methods so that completion of the test method does not influence responses to the reference method; and

(4) errors in the two methods should be independent. Effects of season, day of the week, and training should also be taken into account during both the test and the reference method.

The appropriate method for validating the dietary history is a weighed food record, provided it is completed over the same time frame. Studies have shown that a dietary history over a relatively long time period (six months to one year) tends to produce higher estimates of group mean intakes than the weighed food record. In cases where a shorter time frame for the dietary history has been used, smaller differences in mean intakes have been reported. Food records themselves have been validated by collecting intermittent duplicate diets. However, duplicate diets are not an ideal method for validating food record methods because food intake changes during a duplicate diet collection period—sometimes resulting in a decrease in energy intake of as much as 20%. For semi-quantitative food frequency questionnaires, dietary histories or weighed food records can be used, provided they cover the same time frame. Studies using this combination have shown relatively good agreement for food intakes determined for a group but not for individuals.

It is important to note that for any combination of dietary methods used to determine relative validity, good agreement between the two methods does not necessarily indicate validity: agreement may merely indicate similar errors in both methods. Recognition of this problem has prompted the development of more objective measures, independent of the measurement of food intake, to validate dietary intake data. In this approach, external variables such as biochemical indices or markers are used to validate dietary assessment methods. These include:

- the doubly labelled water method to estimate energy expenditure,
- 24-hour urinary nitrogen excretion as a measure of protein intake,
- urinary excretion of sodium and potassium as measures of sodium and potassium intakes, and
- the fatty acid composition of subcutaneous adipose tissue as a measure of fatty acid composition of the diet.

A detailed discussion of biochemical markers of dietary intake can be found in Hunter (1990).

25.2.3 Precision

A dietary assessment method is considered precise (reliable/reproducible) if it gives very similar results when used repeatedly in the same situation. The precision of a dietary assessment method depends on:

(1) time frame of the method;

(2) population group under study;

(3) nutrient of interest;

(4) technique used to measure the foods and quantities consumed; and

(5) variation in dietary intakes among individuals (inter-subject variation) and within one individual (intra-subject variation).

True precision cannot be measured in dietary assessment because nutrient intakes vary daily. Instead, it is conventionally estimated using a test–retest design, in which the same dietary method is repeated on the same subjects after a preselected time interval, followed by an assessment of the extent of the agreement between the nutrient intakes obtained on the two separate occasions, either on a group or individual basis. The selection of the time interval in the test–retest design depends on the time frame of the dietary method selected. Care must be taken to avoid the second measurement being influenced by the earlier one, as a result of recollection of the first interview. The effects of season or changes in food intake over time must also be minimised.

Results of tests of precision suggest that the 24-hour recall and dietary histories over a short time frame provide a relatively precise estimate of the average usual intake for most nutrients for a large group, but not for individuals. Weighed dietary records, especially those completed for seven days, yield more precise nutrient intakes on an individual basis, with the notable exception of vitamins A and C, and polyunsaturated fat.

25.2.4 Measurement errors

Both systematic and random errors occur during the measurement of food consumption; the major sources of error are summarized in Table 25.5. The direction and extent of these errors vary with the method used as well as the population and nutrients studied. Random errors affect the precision of the methods; such errors can be reduced by increasing the number of measurement days but cannot be entirely eliminated. In contrast, systematic measurement errors cannot be minimized by extending the number of measurement days. Systematic measurement errors are important as they can introduce a significant bias into the results which cannot be removed by subsequent statistical analysis.

Both types of measurement errors can be minimized by incorporating appropriate quality control procedures during each stage of the measurement process. For example, respondent and interviewer bias can be minimized by training the interviewers, and by developing standardized interviewing techniques and questionnaires. Errors arising from respondent memory lapses can be reduced by probing questions and/or by using visual aids such as food models or photographs. To improve the accuracy of estimating food portion sizes for recall methods, graduated food models can be used.

25.2.5 Additional factors

Additional factors which should be considered when selecting a method for measuring food intake include: (1) characteristics of the subjects within the study population; (2) respondent burden of the method; and (3) available resources. For instance, certain methods (e.g. 24-hour recalls) are unsuitable for elderly subjects with poor memories, for busy mothers with young children, or for illiterate subjects. Generally, the more accurate methods are associated with higher costs, greater respondent burden, and lower response rates.

Table 25.5 Major sources of error in the collection and recording of food composition data

Respondent biases may lead respondents to overestimate facts such as income and age. Consumption of 'good' foods such as fruits and vegetables may also be over-reported, whereas the consumption of 'bad' foods, such as snack or 'fast' foods, and the use of alcohol and tobacco, may be under-reported. Overweight respondents tend to under-report food intakes whereas underweight persons may over-report food intakes.

Interviewer biases may occur if different interviewers probe for information to varying degrees, intentionally omit certain questions and/or record responses incorrectly.

Respondent memory lapses may result in the unintentional omission or addition of foods in recall methods.

Incorrect estimation of portion size occurs when respondents fail to quantify accurately the amount of food consumed. Alternatively, the respondent's concept of an average 'serving' size may deviate from the standard, or an interviewer may assume an answer such as an average serving size.

Supplement usage may be omitted from the dietary record or recall, causing significant errors in the calculated nutrient intakes.

The 'flat slope syndrome' is a bias that may be introduced by a tendency to overestimate low intakes and underestimate high intakes in recall methods. The observed relationship, however, may be an artefact of the statistical analysis and the result of regression towards the mean.

Coding and computation errors arise when portion size estimates are converted from household measures into grams, or when food items are incorrectly coded (e.g. 2% milk is coded as whole milk). When computerized nutrient databases are used, the computer program and the associated database may be major sources of error.

25.3 CALCULATION OF NUTRIENT INTAKES

Nutrient intakes can be calculated from food consumption data provided quantitative or semi-quantitative methods for measuring food intake have been used. Food composition values, representative of the average composition of a particular foodstuff on a year-round nation-wide basis, are most frequently used to calculate nutrient intakes. These values generally indicate the total amount of the constituent in the food, rather than the amount actually absorbed. Hence, intakes of most nutrients calculated from food intake data, represent the maximum available to the body. Therefore, when nutrient intakes are evaluated in relation to nutrient requirements (Section 25.4), the potential bioavailability of the nutrients from the diets must also be considered.

Food composition values are available in food composition tables or in nutrient databases stored on a computer, and appropriate for the country of interest. A detailed discussion of food composition tables is given in Chapter 24. Nutrient intakes can be calculated using a computer program and a nutrient database. Before selecting a computer program, both the source of the accompanying nutrient database, its completeness—both in terms of the range of foods listed and in the availability of the nutrient values for individual foods—must be assessed, as well as the validity of the computer program for calculating the nutrient intakes. Both of these features can be checked using the diagnostic tool developed by Hoover and Perloff (1981).

There are two stages in the computer calculation of nutrient intakes: (1) coding the food intake data into a defined machine readable form; and (2) using a software package to calculate energy and nutrient intakes from the food intake data. Generally, coding is done manually and usually involves assigning a numerical code to the subject, day, meal, food, and amount. The food identification code can define the food group, major and minor subgroup, and finally the individual food. The code may also provide information on preserving or processing techniques, storage conditions, etc.

Duplicate coding of recalls or records by independent coders should be used as a quality control for coding. Gross errors in coding can be reduced if 'coding rules' are established to deal with incomplete or ambiguous descriptors of the foods. Check digits can be included in the food code so that incorrect codes can be rapidly identified by the computer program. Systematic detection of wrongly coded weights of foods is more difficult but can be facilitated by including a routine in the computer program which flags subjects with the 10 highest and 10 lowest daily intakes of energy and selected nutrients. Checks can then be made for weight errors in the coded data for the reported subjects. Finally, spot checks should be undertaken on subsamples of the stored data against the original data forms.

It is recommended that the software package selected to calculate energy and nutrient intakes should generate output as:

(1) total nutrients per meal and per day;

(2) average nutrient intake per day and per food group;

(3) average daily intake (in grams) of major food groups; and

(4) the average frequency of consumption of food groups.

25.4 Evaluation of Nutrient Intakes

Most of the methods for evaluating nutrient intakes involve comparison with tables of recommended nutrient intakes. Recommended nutrient intakes are set for a particular group of healthy individuals with specified characteristics, consuming a typical dietary pattern of the country and are discussed in detail in Chapter 33. They refer to the average recommended intake for a nutrient consumed over a reasonable period of time. Values for the recommended nutrient intakes for the same nutrient vary among countries because of differences in the sources and interpretation of the nutrient requirement data, incomplete or non-existent data for some nutrients and/or specific age groups, discrepancies in age, sex, physiological subgroupings, criteria used to define nutrient adequacy, judgement by the committees, and in the habitual dietary patterns among countries. When tables of recommended intakes for a particular country are not available, the FAO and/or WHO (Food and Agriculture Organization/World Health Organization) requirements are often used.

All the methods used to evaluate nutrient intakes provide an estimate of the risk for nutrient inadequacy of a population and/or individual. The reliability of this risk estimate depends on the method of evaluation used; none of the methods identify actual individuals in the population who have a specific nutrient deficiency. This can only be achieved if biochemical and/or clinical assessments are also carried out with the dietary investigation. To evaluate nutrient intakes of individuals, food intakes must be determined over more than one day for each individual. The percentage of individuals with intakes below the recommended nutrient intake, or an arbitrary proportion of the recommended nutrient intake, is then calculated. Because recommended intakes for nutrients are generally set at the average requirement (for a particular age and sex category) plus two standard deviations, the recommended nutrient intakes exceed the needs of all but 2–3% of individuals in the population. Therefore, individuals should not be classified as 'deficient' or 'inadequate' in any nutrient just because their short-term nutrient intake appears to fall below the recommended intake. Indeed, when the recommended nutrient intake is used as a cut-off value, the prevalence of individuals with intakes below their own requirements will always be overestimated. Nevertheless, the more the habitual intake of an individual falls below the recommended intake and the longer the duration of the low intake, the greater the risk of nutrient deficiency for that individual.

This conservative approach has been adopted because most of the health risks are associated with inadequate rather than excess intakes of nutrients. In contrast, recommended intakes for energy are based on estimates of the average energy requirements, and not on the average requirement plus two standard deviations, because excessive energy intake is injurious to health (Fig. 25.3).

More recently, a probability approach has been used to assess more reliably the prevalence of inadequate intakes of a group. The method predicts the number of individuals within the group with nutrient intakes below their own requirements. It is essential to note that this procedure does not identify with certainty which individuals are 'at risk' because of the absence of information about the actual requirements of each individual. Table 25.6 illustrates the use of the probability approach for assigning 'risk' to six classes of observed intakes expressed as proportions of the Canadian Recommended Nutrient Intake.

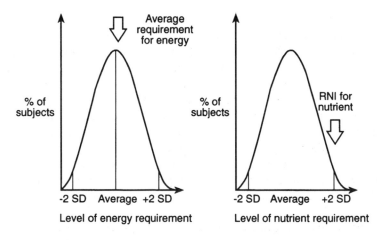

Fig. 25.3 Comparison of the average requirement for energy and the recommended intake of a nutrient. It is assumed that in both cases individual requirements are normally distributed about the mean. *Source*: From Health and Welfare Canada (1990). Reproduced with permission.

Table 25.6 Assignment of 'risk' or probability statements to six classes of observed intakes expressed as proportions of the Canadian Recommended Nutrient Intake (RNI)

	Class 1	Class 2	Class 3	Class 4	Class 5	Class 6
A	< -2 SD of RNI	-2 SD to -1 SD	-1 SD to mean	mean to $+1$ SD	$+1$ SD to $+2$ SD	$> +2$ SD of RNI
B	$<54\%$	54% to 65.5%	65.5% to 77%	77% to 88.5%	88.5% to 100%	$>100\%$
C	1.0	0.93	0.69	0.31	0.07	0.0

Note: Assumptions in this model are: requirements are normally distributed with the coefficient of variation = 15%; the recommended intake is set at the average requirement +2 SD. Row A shows the individual's intake in terms of the distribution of requirements; B gives the intake in terms of the percentage of the RNI; C indicates the probability that the individual's intake does not meet the requirement.
Source: Modified after Beaton GH. Uses and limits of the use of the recommended allowances for evaluating dietary intake data. *Am J Clin Nutr* 1985; **41**: 155–64. © *Am J Clin Nutr* American Society for Clinical Nutrition.

The absence of reliable estimates of the mean nutrient requirements and their variability for many nutrients, and the limitations of food composition data for certain nutrients, limit the general applicability of the probability approach to estimate the prevalence of inadequacy for every nutrient at the present time. Nevertheless, it has been recommended by the United States Subcommittee on Dietary Evaluation (NRC, 1986) for most nutrients in future national nutrition surveys, with the exception of vitamin C, vitamin A, folate, and energy.

FURTHER READING

1. Anderson SA. *Guidelines for use of dietary intake data*. Life Sciences Research Office, Bethesda, Maryland: Federation of American Societies for Experimental Biology, 1986.
2. Black AE, Bingham SA, Johansson G, Coward WA. Validation of dietary intakes of protein and energy against 24 hour urinary N and DLW. *Euro J Clin Nutr* 1997; **51**: 405–13.
3. Buzzard IM, Willett WC. *Dietary assessment methods. Am J Clin Nutr* 1994; **59** (suppl.): 143S–306S.
4. Cameron ME, Staveren WA van. *Manual on methodology of food composition studies*. Oxford University Press, 1988.
5. Consumer and Food Economic Institute. *Composition of foods—raw, processed, and prepared*. Agriculture Handbook 8, Nos. 1–21, Washington, DC: US Government Printing Office, 1976–1992.
6. FAO/WHO/UNU (Food and Agriculture Organization/World Health/United Nations University). *Energy and protein requirements*. WHO Technical Report Series No. 724. Geneva: WHO, 1985.
7. Gibson RS. *Principles of nutritional assessment*. New York: Oxford Unviersity Press, 1990.
8. Gibson RS. *Nutritional assessment: A laboratory manual*. New York: Oxford University Press, 1993.

9. Hoover LW, Perloff BP. *Model for review of nutrient data base system capabilities.* University of Missouri, Columbia, Missouri, 1981.

10. Hunter D. *Biochemical indicators of dietary intake.* In: Willett WC. Nutritional epidemiology. New York: Oxford University Press, 1990.

11. NRC (National Research Council). *Nutrient adequacy. Assessment using food consumption surveys.* Subcommittee on Criteria for Dietary Evaluation, Co-ordinating Committee on Evaluation of Food Consumption Surveys. Food and Nutrition Board, Commission on Life Sciences. Washington, DC: National Academy Press, 1986.

12. Thompson FE, Byers T, Kohlmeier L (eds). Dietary assessment resource manual. *J Nutr* 1994; **124** (suppl.): 2245S–317S.

26

Determining Nutritional Status

Rosalind Gibson

Nutritional status is defined as the health status of individuals or population groups as influenced by their intake and utilization of nutrients. A variety of methods are used to determine nutritional status; they can be used either alone, or more effectively, in combination. The methods are based on a series of dietary, laboratory, anthropometric, and clinical measurements designed to characterize each stage in the development of a nutritional deficiency state. Dietary assessment is described in Chapter 25. This chapter describes anthropometric, laboratory, and clinical methods used to assess nutritional status with emphasis on their biological basis, scientific principles, and advantages and limitations, together with some discussion on the effect of confounding factors on the interpretation of the results.

26.1 Anthropometric Assessment

Anthropometric assessment comprises measurements of the variations of the physical dimensions and the gross composition of the body. It provides information on past nutritional history, which cannot be obtained with equal confidence using the other assessment methods.

Anthropometric measurements are of two types: growth and body composition. The latter can be further subdivided into measurements of fat-free mass and body fat, the two major compartments of total body mass; the advantages of anthropometric measurements are summarized below:

- The procedures use simple, safe, non-invasive techniques which can be used at the bedside and are applicable to large sample sizes.
- Equipment required is inexpensive, portable, and durable and can be made or purchased locally.
- Relatively unskilled personnel can perform measurement procedures.
- The methods are precise and accurate, provided that standardized techniques are used.
- Information is generated on past long-term nutritional history, which cannot be obtained with equal confidence using other techniques.
- The procedures can assist in the identification of mild to moderate malnutrition, as well as severe states of malnutrition.

- The methods may be used to evaluate changes in nutritional status over time and from one generation to the next, a phenomenon known as the secular trend.
- Screening tests, to identify individuals at high risk to malnutrition, can be devised.

Errors may occur in nutritional anthropometry which affect the precision, accuracy, and validity of the measurements/indices. The errors can be attributed to three major effects:

1. *Measurement errors.* These may be random or systematic and may include examiner error resulting from inadequate training, instrument error, and measurement difficulties. Some of these measurement errors can be minimized by training personnel to use instruments that are precise and correctly calibrated, and standardized, validated measurement techniques.
2. *Alterations* in the composition and physical properties of certain tissues. These may occur in both healthy and diseased subjects, resulting in inaccuracies in certain anthropometric measurements/indices. Even in healthy individuals, body weight may be affected by variations in tissue hydration with the menstrual cycle, whereas skinfolds may be influenced by alterations in compressibility with age and site of the measurements. Generally, anthropometric measurements are not corrected to account for these effects.
3. *Use of prediction equations* developed on healthy lean subjects for patients with certain diseases in whom increases in total body water and alterations in the distribution of body fat may occur.

26.1.1 Growth measurements

The most widely used anthropometric measurements of growth are those of stature (height or length) and body weight. These measurements can be made quickly and easily, and with care and training, accurately. Head circumference measurements are often taken in association with stature. Details of the standardized procedures for these growth measurements are given in Gibson (1993).

Head circumference   Chronic malnutrition during the first few months of life, or intra-uterine growth retardation, may decrease the number of brain cells and result in an abnormally low head circumference. Consequently, measurement of head circumference is important because it is closely related to brain size and can be used as an index of chronic protein-energy nutritional status during the first two years of life. Beyond two years, growth in head circumference is so slow that its measurement is no longer useful. Head circumference is often used with other measurements to detect pathological conditions associated with an unusually large (hydrocephalic) or small (microcephalic) head. Certain non-nutritional factors, including disease and pathological conditions, genetic variation, and cultural practices (such as binding of the head during infancy) may also influence head circumference.

Head circumference is measured with a narrow, flexible non-stretch tape made of fibreglass or steel about 0.6 cm wide; alternatively a fibre glass insertion tape can be used.

Body weight   Body weight represents the sum of protein, fat, water, and bone mineral mass. Hence, changes in body weight may reflect a change in one or more of these

Box 26.1   Calculation of percentage weight loss and rate of change

---
Percentage usual weight = (actual weight)/(usual weight) × 100%
Percentage weight loss = ((usual weight) − (actual weight))/(usual weight) × 100%
Rate of change (kg/day) = $(BW_p - BW_i)/(Day_p - Day_i)$
BW_p and BW_i indicate present and initial body weights on the respective days.

---

chemical compartments. In healthy persons, daily variations in body weight are generally small (i.e. less than ± 0.5 kg). In conditions of acute or chronic illness, however, negative energy-nitrogen balance may occur resulting in a decline in body weight. In conditions of total starvation, the maximal weight loss is approximately 30% of the initial body weight, at which point death occurs. In chronic semi-starvation, body weight may decrease to approximately 50–60% of ideal weight. When persistent positive energy balance occurs, there is an accumulation of adipose tissue, and body weight increases.

To measure body weight in infants and children, a paediatric scale is recommended, although in the field, a suspended spring balance and a weighing sling may be used. For older children and adults a beam balance with non-detachable weights is recommended. All equipment should be calibrated regularly and whenever it is moved to another location. To assess weight changes, the actual and usual weight of the patient must be known from which the percentage of usual weight, percentage weight loss, and rate of change can be calculated as shown in Box 26.1.

Recumbent length and stature   The distribution of length and height measurements at a given age within most populations is usually narrow, so that accurate measuring techniques are essential. As a deficit in recumbent length or height takes some time to develop, assessment of nutritional status based on recumbent length- or height-for-age alone may result in an underestimation of malnutrition in infants. The influence of possible genetic and ethnic differences must also be considered when evaluating recumbent length and stature for age.

Recumbent length should be measured for infants and children less than two years of age using a measuring board, or infantometer, made of perspex or wood. For field use, a portable infant-length measuring scale or a plastic measuring mat can be used. Children over two years of age and adults are generally measured in the standing position using a stadiometer or portable anthropometre. In the field, vertical surfaces are not always available. In such circumstances, modified tape measures such as the Microtoise, which measure up to two metres, can be used.

Knee height   This may be used to estimate height in persons with severe spinal curvature or who are unable to stand. It is highly correlated with stature. Knee height is measured on the left leg with a caliper consisting of an adjustable measuring stick with a blade attached to each end at a 90 degree angle. A nomogram or formula (below) can be used to estimate stature from knee height (Chumlea *et al.*, 1984).

Male stature (cm) = (2.02 × knee height [cm]) − (0.04 × age [yr]) + 64.19

Female stature (cm) = (1.83 × knee height [cm]) − (0.24 × age [yr]) + 84.88

26.1.2 Growth indices

To assist in the interpretation of anthropometric measurements, indices based on two or more raw measurements (e.g. weight-for-age and weight-for-height) are derived.

Indices constructed from the measurement of body weight and/or stature include:

• *Weight-for-age*. This index is frequently used as an index of acute malnutrition for children from 6 months to 7 years provided the exact age of the child is known. In some countries, local calendars of special events can be constructed to assist in identifying the birth date of a child. Weight-for-age, however, overestimates the prevalence of malnutrition in small children because it does not take into account height differences. Children who are genetically short, or 'stunted' will have a low weight-for-age but will not necessarily be wasted; their weight may be appropriate for their short stature.

• *Weight-for-height*. This index has been recommended by the World Health Organization (WHO) instead of weight-for-age because it differentiates between nutritional stunting, when weight may be appropriate for height, and wasting, when weight is very low for height as a result of deficits in both tissue and fat mass. For children weight-for-height is relatively independent of age between 1 and 10 years and ethnic group for those aged 1 to 5 years. Unfortunately, oedema and obesity may complicate the interpretation of weight-for-height measurements. A further disadvantage is that it classifies children with poor linear growth as 'normal'. Weight-for-height is more sensitive to changes in current nutritional status than height-for-age.

• *Length- or height-for-age*. This index has been recommended for use by WHO to detect 'stunted' children in combination with weight-for-height. Stunting is a slowing of skeletal growth and of stature, defined as 'the end result of a reduced rate of linear growth'. The condition results from extended periods of inadequate food intake and increased morbidity and hence is an index of chronic nutritional status. The highest prevalence of stunting is between 2 to 3 years of age, whereas it is during the post-weaning period (i.e. from 12 to 3 months) for wasting.

• *Quetelet's index* (weight/height^2). This is considered to be the best body mass index (BMI) for most adult populations, as it is the least biased by height and easily calculated. In adults, Quetelet's index correlates with many health-related indices such as mortality risk. Nevertheless, Quetelet's index does not distinguish between excessive weight

Box 26.2 Classifications for body mass index (BMI)

Body mass index		Evaluation
Canada	New Zealand	
Under 20	Under 20	May be associated with health problems for some individuals.
20–25	20–25	'Ideal' index range associated with the lowest risk of illness for most people.
25–27	25–30	May be associated with health problems for some people.
Over 27	Over 30	Associated with increased risk of health problems such as heart disease, high blood pressure, and diabetes.

Table 26.1 Simple classification of adult chronic energy deficiency using BMI

BMI	<16.0	16.0–16.9	17.0–18.4	>18.5
CED grade	III	II	I	Normal

Source: From Ferro-Luzzi A, Sette S, Franklin M, James WPT. A simplified approach to assessing adult chronic energy deficiency. *Eur J Clin Nutr* 1992; 46: 173–86.

produced by adiposity, muscularity, or oedema. The range of acceptable values for Quetelet's index varies among countries. The classifications (in metres and kilograms) used in Canada and New Zealand are shown in Box 26.2. These classifications are not valid for those under 20 or over 65 years of age, or for those women who are pregnant or lactating.

• *Chronic energy deficiency* (CED) in adults in less industrialized countries is also classified by Quetelet's index (Table 26.1). In this classification, three grades of CED have been set, the upper limit being less than 18.5 for both men and women. Studies in less industrialized countries have shown that low BMIs in a community are consistently associated with a decline in work output, productivity, and income-generating ability, and a population whose ability to respond to stressful conditions is compromised.

26.1.3 Body composition measurements

Most anthropometric methods used to assess body composition are based on a model in which the body consists of two chemically distinct compartments: fat-free mass and fat. Anthropometric techniques can indirectly assess these two body compartments, and variations in their amount and proportion can be used as indices of nutritional status.

Fat-free mass consists of skeletal muscle, nonskeletal muscle and soft lean tissues, and the skeleton. Body muscle is composed largely of protein. Hence, assessment of body muscle can provide an index of the protein reserves of the body; these reserves become depleted during chronic undernutrition, resulting in muscle wasting.

The body fat content is the most variable component of the body, differing among individuals of the same sex, height, and weight. On average, the fat content of women is higher than that of men, representing 27% of their total body weight compared to 15% for men. Fat is the main storage form of energy in the body and is sensitive to acute malnutrition. Alterations in body fat content provide indirect estimates of changes in energy balance. A large and rapid loss of body fat is indicative of severe negative energy balance. Small changes in body fat (i.e. <0.5 kg) cannot be measured accurately using anthropometry. Body fat can be measured either in absolute terms (the weight of total body fat, expressed in kilograms) or as a percentage of the total body weight.

Mid upper-arm circumference The arm contains subcutaneous fat and muscle; a decrease in mid upper-arm circumference may therefore reflect either a reduction in muscle mass, a reduction in subcutaneous tissue, or both. In developing countries, where the amount of subcutaneous fat is frequently small, changes in mid upper-arm circumference tend to parallel changes in muscle mass and hence are particularly useful in the diagnosis of protein-energy malnutrition or starvation. Between the ages of six months and five years, mid upper-arm circumference varies little, and as a result mid upper-arm circumference measurements are frequently used in areas where the ages of the children are uncertain.

Mid upper-arm circumference measurements should be taken with a flexible, non-stretch tape made of fibreglass or steel; alternatively, a fibreglass insertion tape can be used. The measurement is taken to the nearest millimetre at the midpoint of the upper left arm, between the acromion process and the tip of the olecranon.

Skinfold thicknesses   One-third of the total body fat in reference man and woman is estimated to be subcutaneous fat. Skinfold thickness measurements are said to provide an estimate of the size of the subcutaneous fat depot, which in turn is said to provide an estimate of the total body fat. Such estimates are based on two assumptions: (1) the thickness of the subcutaneous adipose tissue reflects a constant proportion of the total body fat, and (2) the skinfold sites selected for measurement, either singly or in combination, represent the average thickness of the entire subcutaneous adipose tissue. Neither of these assumptions is true. Variations in the distribution of subcutaneous fat do occur with sex, race, age, disease states, body weight, and malnutrition. Hence, the most representative skinfold site is not the same for both sexes, nor is it the same for all age and ethnic groups.

Skinfold measurements are best made using precision skinfold thickness calipers: they measure the compressed double fold of the fat plus skin. Three types of precision calipers can be used: Harpenden, Lange, and Holtain. Low-cost plastic McGaw calipers are also available. The following skinfold sites are commonly used:

1. *Triceps skinfold* measured at the midpoint of the back of the upper left arm, between the acromion process and the tip of the olecranon, as noted for mid upper-arm circumference (Fig. 26.1).
2. *Biceps skinfold* measured as the thickness of a vertical fold on the front of the upper left arm above the centre of the cubital fossa, at the same level as the triceps skinfold.
3. *Subscapular skinfold* measured just below and laterally to the inferior angle of the left scapula, with the shoulder and arm relaxed (Fig. 26.2).
4. *Suprailiac skinfold* measured in the midaxillary line immediately superior to the iliac crest. The skinfold is grasped obliquely just posterior to the midaxillary line and parallel to the cleavage lines of the skin (Fig. 26.2).

Of these four skinfold sites, the triceps is most frequently selected because it is assumed to be most representative of the whole of the subcutaneous fat layer. However, because subcutaneous fat is not uniformly distributed about the body, a body skinfold site such as the subscapular skinfold, as well as a limb skinfold, are often used with the triceps skinfold to improve the estimate of total body fat and provide information on the distribution of body fat. The optimum combination of skinfold measurements sites varies with age, race, sex, and with the presence of particular disease states.

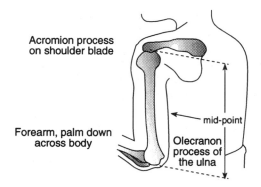

Fig. 26.1 Location of the midpoint of the upper arm. Source: Robbins GE and Trowbridge FL. In: Nutritional assessment (eds Ms Simko *et al.*), 1987.

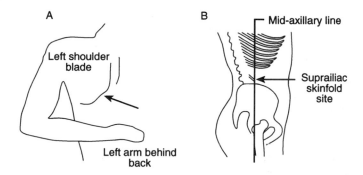

Fig. 26.2 Location of the subscapular and suprailiac skinfold sites.

26.1.4 Body composition indices

Several indices of fat-free mass and body fat are calculated from the mid upper-arm circumference and/or skinfold thickness measurements. Some of these are discussed below:

• *Mid upper-arm muscle circumference* represents the circumference of the inner circle of muscle mass surrounding a small central core of bone; it is calculated using the following equation:

$$\text{mid upper-arm muscle circ.} = \text{mid upper-arm circ.} - (\pi \times \text{TSK})$$

where TSK = triceps skinfold thickness. Note that this equations is only valid when all the measurements are made in the same units (preferably millimetres). Alternatively, a nomogram can be used. The equation for calculating mid upper-arm muscle circumference assumes that the limb is cylindrical, with fat evenly distributed about its circumference, and also makes no allowance for variable skinfold compressibility. Mid upper-arm

433

muscle circumference can be used to assess body muscle mass, and is frequently used for this purpose in field surveys.

• *Mid upper-arm muscle area* provides a more valid index of body muscle mass and hence protein nutritional status than mid upper-arm muscle circumference because it reflects more adequately the true magnitude of muscle tissue changes. The following equation may be used to estimate mid upper-arm muscle area:

$$\text{mid upper-arm muscle area} = \frac{(C - (\pi \times TSK))^2}{4\pi}$$

where C = mid upper-arm circumference and TSK = triceps skinfold thickness. Again, all the measurements should be made in the same units (preferably millimetres). This equation overestimates mid upper-arm muscle area by 20–25%, and, as a result, may underestimate the severity of muscle atrophy.

• *Corrected mid upper-arm muscle area* calculates absolute bone-free arm muscle area using the following equation:

$$\text{corrected mid upper-arm muscle area} = \frac{(C - (\pi \times TSK))^2}{4\pi} - 6.5 \text{ (for women)}$$

$$\text{corrected mid upper-arm muscle area} = \frac{(C - (\pi \times TSK))^2}{4\pi} - 10 \text{ (for men)}$$

The revised equations have not been validated for use with elderly persons and are not appropriate for obese patients. They take into account errors resulting from the non-circular nature of the muscle compartment and the inclusion of non-skeletal muscle tissue (e.g. neurovascular tissue and bone), reducing the average error for a given subject to 7–8%.

• *Mid upper-arm fat area*, the cross-sectional area of the fat of the upper-arm, is also calculated from the mid upper-arm circumference and triceps skinfold thickness. It provides a better estimate of total body fat (i.e. fat weight) than a single skinfold thickness at the same site, because it is more highly correlated with total body fatness. It is also independent of age for children between one and seven years of age. The equation for calculating arm fat area (A) is:

$$A = \frac{TSK \times C}{2} - \frac{\pi \times (TSK)^2}{4}$$

where TSK = triceps skinfold thickness (mm) and C = mid upper-arm circumference (mm). Alternatively, a nomogram can be used in the field.

• *Sum of skinfolds* is sometimes used to assess total body fat and to provide information on the distribution of subcutaneous fat. The optimum combination of skinfold measurements has not been established; the triceps and subscapular are often used.

• *Waist–hip circumference ratio* is used to describe the distribution of both subcutaneous and intra-abdominal adipose tissue. It can be measured more precisely than skinfolds. Waist–hip ratios greater than 1.0 for men and 0.8 for women are said to be indicative of increased risk of cardiovascular complications and related deaths. Changes of waist–hip circumference ratio with age and excessive weight are not yet established.

26.1.5 Body fat from skinfold measurements via body density

Skinfold thickness measurements, preferably from multiple anatomical sites, can also be used to predict body density from which the percentage of body fat can be calculated using the following procedures:

• *Determination of appropriate skinfolds* and other anthropometric measurements for the prediction of body density, the selection of the sites depending on the age, sex, and population group under study.

• *Calculation of body density* using an appropriate regression equation. A variety of population-specific and generalized regression equations are available. More research is needed to identify empirical equations for specific population groups such as under-nourished persons. An example of a generalized regression equation and based on sum of four skinfolds (biceps, triceps, subscapular, suprailiac) for male subjects aged 20–29 years is given below:

$$D(kg/m^3) = 1.1631 - (0.0632 \times \log_{10}(SK4[mm]))$$

where D = body density and SK = skinfold thickness.

• *Calculation of percentage body fat* from body density using empirical equations which relate fat content to body density (D); examples of three equations are given below:

$$\text{Siri: } \%F = \left\{ \frac{4.95}{D} - 4.50 \right\} \times 100\%$$

$$\text{Brozek et al.: } \%F = \left\{ \frac{4.57}{D} - 4.142 \right\} \times 100\%$$

$$\text{Rathburn and Pace: } \%F = \left\{ \frac{5.548}{D} - 5.044 \right\} \times 100\%$$

• *Calculation of total body fat* content and/or the fat-free mass.

$$\text{total body fat (kg)} = \frac{\text{body weight (kg)} \times \% \text{ body fat}}{100}$$

$$\text{fat-free mass (kg)} = \text{body weight (kg)} - \text{body fat (kg)}$$

26.1.6 Evaluation of anthropometric indices

Anthropometric indices can be used to identify malnourished individuals and/or to assess the nutritional status of population groups. Such procedures require the selection of appropriate anthropometric reference data for comparison. Both local and international reference data may be used. The World Health Organization (WHO) have recommended the use of the United States National Centre for Health Statistics (NCHS) reference growth data as an international standard for comparisons of health and nutritional status of children among countries (see Fig. 29.1). Use of an international reference data set for body composition measurements is not appropriate because they are more influenced by ethnic and genetic differences than growth measurements.

To identify individuals 'at risk' of malnutrition classification schemes comprised of at least one anthropometric index and one or more cutoff points are used. The simplest use a single cutoff point drawn from a percentile or standard deviation score of the reference data; older classification schemes use percentage of the reference median for the cutoff point.

• *Percentiles* refer to the position of the measurement values in relation to all (100%) of the measurements for the reference population, ranked in order of magnitude. The percentiles often used as cutoff points to classify individuals as 'at risk' to malnutrition are either below the 3rd or 5th percentiles or above the 95th or 97th percentiles depending on the reference data. The percentile for a subject of known age and sex can be calculated exactly, provided the numerical percentile values are available for the reference data. Alternatively, the percentile range within which the measurement of an individual falls can be read from graphs of the reference data.

• *Standard deviation (SD) score* is a measure of an individual's value with respect to the distribution of the reference population. It is recommended for evaluating anthropometric data from developing countries because SD scores can be defined beyond the percentile limits of the original reference data. Cutoff points used with SD scores vary; often scores of below -2.0 are designated as indicating risk of severe protein-energy malnutrition whereas scores above $+2.0$ are taken to indicate risk of obesity. An important advantage of cutoff points based on SD scores is that the same SD score values (e.g. -2.0 SD) represent the same degree of malnutrition, irrespective of the anthropometric index used (e.g. weight-for-age or weight-for-height) or the age of the child. Standard deviation scores can be calculated for individuals using selected reference standard deviation values and the equation shown below:

$$\frac{\text{weight of subject}-\text{median reference value of weight-for-height}}{\text{median reference value}-1 \text{ SD below median reference value}}$$

• *Percentage of the reference median* is used as a cutoff point by many of the older classification schemes. For example, a scheme such as the Gomez classification utilizes weight-for-age for the anthropometric index and cutoff points corresponding to $<60\%$, 61–75%, and 76–90% of the Harvard weight-for-age reference median to indicate severe, moderate and mild malnutrition. There is an important distinction between the use of cutoff points based on SD scores and percentage of the reference median. Unlike SD scores, a constant percentage of the reference median (e.g. 60%) cannot be used as the cutoff point across all growth indices and across all ages because it does not represent the same severity of malnutrition. The percentage of the reference median is calculated as:

$$\% \text{ median} = \frac{100 \times \text{observed weight}}{\text{median weight-for-age and sex}}$$

For population studies the distribution of the anthropometric indices can be compared using percentiles and/or standard deviation scores derived from appropriate reference data. As well, the number and proportion of individuals with indices below predetermined cutoff points can also be tabulated or presented as a histogram. Percentiles are recommended in Western countries. Standard deviation scores are preferred in developing countries because the study population often have growth indices below the extreme percentiles of the international reference data population.

26.2 LABORATORY ASSESSMENT

Laboratory assessment is used primarily to detect subclinical deficiency states or to confirm a clinical diagnosis. It provides an objective means of assessing nutritional status, independent of emotional and other subjective factors. Both static and functional tests can be used. However, they are often affected by biological and technical factors other than depleted body stores of the nutrient, which may confound the interpretation of the result. These factors are listed in Box 26.3. Their impact (if any) on each test should be determined before carrying out the tests because often these confounding effects can be minimized or eliminated by standardizing the sampling and collection procedures, and by an appropriate experimental design.

Generally, a combination of laboratory tests should be used rather than a single test for each nutrient; several concordant abnormal values are more reliable than a single aberrant value in diagnosing a deficiency state. All techniques may be subject to random and systematic measurement errors and hence personnel should be trained to use standardized and validated techniques which are continuously monitored by appropriate quality control procedures. A summary of recommended biochemical laboratory tests is shown in Table 26.2.

26.2.1 Static biochemical tests

Static biochemical tests measure either a nutrient in biological fluids or tissues or the urinary excretion rate of the nutrient or its metabolite. Tables A26.1–A26.4 in the Appendix summarize the most commonly used static biochemical tests for assessing minerals, trace minerals, fat-soluble and water-soluble vitamins, respectively.

Whole blood or some fraction of blood (e.g. serum, erythrocytes, leucocytes) is the most frequently used biopsy material for measuring a nutrient in a biological fluid or tissue. For example (see Table 26.2), selenium levels can be measured in whole blood, folate in red blood cells, and magnesium and vitamin C in leucocytes. A wide range of nutrients or their

Box 26.3 Factors that may confound the interpretation of static biochemical tests

• Homeostatic regulation	• Recent dietary intake
• Diurnal variation	• Haemolysis: for serum/plasma
• Sample contamination	• Drugs
• Physiological state	• Disease states
• Infections	• Nutrient interactions
• Hormonal status	• Inflammatory stress
• Physical exercise	• Weight loss
• Age, sex, ethnic group	• Sampling and collection procedures
• Accuracy and precision of the analytical method	• Sensitivity and specificity of the analytical method

Table 26.2 Recommended biochemical laboratory tests

Test	Analytical method
Minerals	
Calcium	
Serium ionized calcium	Ion-specific electrodes
Phosphorus	
Serum phosphorus	Colorimetry using molybdenum blue
Magnesium	
Leucocyte magnesium	Separation of leukocytes with Ficoll-Hypaque gradient followed by analysis via atomic absorption spectrophotometry (AAS)
Trace minerals	
Copper	
Erythrocyte superoxide dismutase	Involves inhibition of oxidation-reduction reactions catalysed by the superoxide anion
Iodine	
Thyroid-stimulating hormone in whole blood or serum	ELISA with dried whole blood spots on filter paper or in serum
Iron	
Serum ferritin (in absence of infection) in conjunction with haemoglobin	Radioimmunoassay (RIA) or ELISA
Haemoglobin	Via cyanmethaemoglobin method
Serum transferrin receptor	ELISA
Selenium	
Whole blood selenium	AAS with a Zeeman background correction or instrumental neutron activation analysis or fluorometric method
Glutathione peroxidase in whole blood or erythrocytes in countries where Se intakes are habitually low	Glutathione peroxidase activity measured by oxidation of NADPH with cumen peroxidase via glutathione reductase
Zinc	
Hair zinc in children in presence of low height per-centile and/or hypogeusia	AAS or instrumental neutron activation analysis
Serum/plasma zinc (in absence of infection)	AAS
Fat-soluble vitamins	
Vitamin A	
Liver retinol stores	High performance liquid chromatography (HPLC)
Modified relative dose response	Serum retinol and dehydroretinol assayed via HPLC 4–6 hours after an oral dose of 3, 4-didehydroretinylacetate (100 µg/kg)
Vitamin D	
Serum 25-hydroxy vitamin D	Separation of serum 25(OH)-D by HPLC followed by assay by a competitive binding assay
Vitamin E	
Ratio serum tocopherol: serum lipids	Reverse-phase HPLC with a high sensitivity fluorescence detector

Table 26.2 *(Continued)*

Test	Analytical method
Water-soluble Vitamins	
Thiamin	
Erythrocyte activity of transketolase enzyme with and without added thiamin pyrophosphate	Semi-automated spectrophotometry using glyceraldehyde as internal standard
Riboflavin	
Erythrocyte activity of glutathione reductase with and without the added prosthetic group flavin adenine dinucleotide	Enzyme-coupled kinetic assay whereby glutathione reductase activity measured spectrophotometrically via oxidation of NADPH to $NADP^+$
Niacin	
Ratio of erythrocyte nicotinamide adenine dinucleotide (NAD) and NADP nucleotide	Uses cycling mixture of thiazoylblue and phenazine methosulphate
Pyridoxine	
Plasma pyridoxal-5'-phosphate	Cation-exchange HPLC followed by fluorometric assay
Vitamin C	
Leucocyte ascorbic acid	HPLC
Folic acid	
Erythrocyte folate in combination with serum folate	Microbiological assay using *Lactobacillus casei*
	Serum folate via RIA
Vitamin B$_{12}$	
Serum vitamin B$_{12}$	RIA
Protein	
Serum transthyretin	Radial-immunodiffusion or ELISA

metabolites can be measured in serum; certain minerals (e.g. phosphorus and magnesium), trace minerals (chromium, copper, selenium, zinc), fat-soluble (A, D, E) and water-soluble vitamins (folate, vitamin B$_{12}$, ascorbic acid and pyridoxine (as pyridoxal 5'-phosphate). Other body fluids and tissues less widely used include hair for certain trace minerals (e.g. chromium, selenium, zinc) and finger- or toenails for selenium (see Tables A26.1–A26.4 in the Appendix).

Appropriate precautions must be undertaken to avoid adventitious contamination during the collection, transfer, storage, handling, and/or analyses of these biopsy materials for trace element analyses. Standardized washing procedures employing non-ionic or ionic detergents or organic solvents have been recommended for hair samples; aqueous detergents are preferred for washing fingernails and toenails. As well, when collecting blood samples, care must be taken to avoid haemolysis and the use of inappropriate anticoagulants.

Box 26.4   Types of urine specimens

- 24-hour urine samples
- First voided fasting urine samples
- Non-fasting casual urine samples

Some of these static biochemical tests monitor short-term or acute changes in nutritional status; others provide a long-term or chronic index of nutrient status. For example, nutrient levels in serum almost always reflect acute nutritional status, whereas those of erythrocytes reflect chronic status because the erythrocyte half-life is quite long (i.e. 120 days). Similarly, trace element concentrations in hair, fingernails and toenails provide a chronic and retrospective index during the period of hair or nail growth.

Static tests which measure the *urinary excretion rate* of a nutrient or its metabolite also monitor short-term or acute changes, provided renal function is normal. They include tests for certain minerals (calcium, magnesium, phosphorus), trace minerals (zinc, selenium, chromium), water soluble B-complex vitamins (e.g. thiamin, riboflavin) or their metabolites (e.g. 4-pyridoxic acid for pyridoxine), and vitamin C. The methods depend on the existence of a renal conservation mechanism that reduces the urinary excretion of the nutrient and/or metabolite when body stores are depleted. Urine cannot be used to assess the fat-soluble vitamins A, D, E, and K, as metabolites are not excreted in proportion to the amount of these vitamins consumed, absorbed, and metabolized. The types of urine specimens which can be collected are shown in Box 26.4.

Twenty-four-hour urine samples are preferred for measuring urinary excretion of thiamin, riboflavin, ascorbic acid and 4-pyridoxic acid. To monitor their completeness, urinary creatinine excretion is often measured. This approach, however, will only detect gross errors in 24-hour urine collections. As a result, another marker, *para*-aminobenzoic acid (PABA) has been used to assess completeness of urine collection. This substance is taken with meals, is harmless, easy to measure, and is rapidly and completely excreted in urine.

Twenty-four-hour urine samples are difficult to collect in non-institutionalized population groups. Instead, first-voided fasting urine specimens may be collected as they are not affected by recent dietary intake, although sometimes it is only feasible to collect non-fasting casual urine samples. When first-voided or casual urine specimens are collected, urinary excretion is expressed as a ratio of the nutrient to urinary creatinine (e.g. mg nutrient per g creatinine) to correct for both diurnal variation and fluctuations in urine volume.

26.2.2   Functional biochemical tests

Functional biochemical tests measure the extent of the functional consequences of a specific nutrient deficiency, and hence have greater biological significance than the static laboratory tests. Some examples of functional biochemical tests are given in Tables A26.5–A26.7 in the Appendix. They include measurement of:

- *Abnormal metabolic products in blood or urine* arising from reduced activity of a nutrient-dependent enzyme (Table A26.7). They include measuring urinary excretion of xanthurenic acid, formiminoglutamic acid (FIGLU), and methylmalonic acid as a test of vitamin B_6, folate, and vitamin B_{12} deficiency, respectively.

• *Reduction in activity of enzymes* which require a nutrient as a coenzyme or prosthetic group (Table A26.5). The activity of the enzyme is sometimes measured with and without the addition of saturating amounts of the coenzyme added *in vitro*. For example, thiamin is a component of the coenzyme thiamin pyrophosphate (TPP) required for the action of transketolase in the pentose phosphate pathway. For the test, erythrocyte activity of the transketolase enzyme, with (i.e. stimulated activity) and without (i.e. basal activity) added TPP is measured, and then expressed as a ratio, termed the 'activity coefficient' (AC) or percentage stimulation. Similar enzyme tests are carried out for riboflavin and pyridoxine, employing the activities of erythrocyte glutathione reductase, and erythrocyte aminotransferases, respectively. The basal and stimulated activities can be expressed per gram of haemoglobin, per number of erythrocytes, or in terms of the volume of erythrocytes (in ml). In general, the higher the value of the AC or 'percentage stimulation', the greater the degree of vitamin deficiency.

• *Changes in blood components* related to intake of a nutrient (Table A26.6). A well-known example is the measurement of haemoglobin concentration in whole blood for iron deficiency anaemia; iron is an essential component of the haemoglobin molecule. Other examples include measurement of the transport proteins transferrin, thyroxine binding pre-albumin (transthyretin) and retinol-binding protein as indices of iron, iodine and vitamin A status, respectively.

• *Load tests* conducted on the subject *in vivo* are used to assess deficiencies of water-soluble vitamins (e.g. tryptophan load tests for pyridoxine, histidine load test for folic acid, vitamin C load test) and certain minerals (e.g. magnesium, zinc, and selenium) (Table A26.7). For the load test, basal urinary excretion of the nutrient must first be determined on a timed preload urine collection. Then a loading dose of the nutrient or associated compound is administered orally, intramuscularly, or intravenously. After the load, a timed sample of the urine is collected and the excretion level of the nutrient or a metabolite determined. The net retention of the nutrient is calculated by comparing the basal excretion data with net excretion after the load. In a deficiency state, when tissues are not saturated with the nutrient, excretion of the nutrient or a metabolite will be low because net retention is high.

• *Tolerance tests* (Table A26.7), sometimes referred to as plasma appearance tests, are also conducted on the subject *in vivo*. In these tests, the concentration of the nutrient is measured both in fasting plasma and in plasma after an oral pharmacological dose of the nutrient (e.g. zinc and manganese). The response is enhanced in cases of nutrient depletion because the intestinal absorption of the nutrient is assumed to increase in a nutrient deficiency state. Use of pharmacological doses limit the usefulness of these tests because they may be handled differently by the gastrointestinal tract than physiological levels of the nutrient.

Examples of other functional *in vivo* tolerance tests include the relative-dose-response for vitamin A, and for chromium, changes in an oral glucose tolerance test after chromium supplementation. Both the relative dose response (RDR) and the modified relative dose response (MRDR) assays are used to estimate liver stores of vitamin A, and can be used to identify those individuals with marginal vitamin A deficiency. Details of these two tests are given in Table A26.7. Unlike the RDR, only one blood sample is required for MRDR test.

• In vitro *tests of* in vivo *functions in tissues/cells* isolated and maintained under physiological conditions; tests related to host defence and immunocompetence (e.g. measurement of total lymphocytes as index of protein-energy malnutrition) are the most widely used assays of this type. Total lymphocyte count is derived from the percentage of lymphocytes multiplied by the white blood cell count and divided by 100.

26.2.3 Functional physiological tests

This category of tests assesses the physiological performance of an individual *in vivo* and may includes tests of immune competence, taste acuity, night blindness, and muscle function. As well, growth and developmental responses such as lactation, sexual maturation, and cognition, can also be assessed. None of these tests are specific and hence must be used in conjunction with biochemical tests to identify the nutrient deficiency involved.

• *Immunocompetence* can be assessed by the delayed cutaneous hypersensitivity (DCH) response test. It involves injecting a battery of specific antigens intradermally in the forearm and noting the induced response. The recall skin test antigens commonly used are: purified protein derivative (PPD), mumps, trichophyton, *Candida albicans*, and dinitrochlorobenzene (DNCB). In healthy persons re-exposed to recall antigens intradermally, the T cells respond by proliferation and release of soluble mediators of inflammation. This produces an induration (hardening) and erythema (redness), the diameter of which is generally measured 24 or 48 hours after the antigen injection. In malnourished persons with protein-energy malnutrition and/or nutrient deficiencies such as vitamin A, zinc, iron, and pyridoxine, these skin reactions are often decreased, but are reversed after nutritional rehabilitation. Many other non-nutritional factors such as certain disease states, hormones, age, circulation problems and electrolyte imbalances, confound the interpretation of skin test reactivity.

• *Taste acuity* is impaired in mild zinc deficiency and hence has been used as a functional index of zinc status. Several methods for testing taste acuity have been used. Evaluation of taste acuity is generally based on the detection and/or recognition thresholds for each taste quality: salt, sweet, bitter, and sour. The detection threshold is defined as the lowest concentration at which a taste can just be detected; the recognition threshold is the lowest concentration at which the quality of the taste stimulus can be recognized. In some studies, recognition taste threshold of only one taste quality (salt) have been determined; perception to saltiness is said to be especially compromised by zinc deficiency.

• *Night blindness* arising from a deficit in dark adaptation is an early sign of vitamin A deficiency. It can be assessed *in vivo* using a rapid dark adaptation (RDA) test. The test requires a light-proof box, a light source, a dark, non-reflective work surface, a standard X-ray view box, and sets of red, blue, and white discs. For the test, subjects are light-adapted for a fixed time (1 minute), and then asked to separate out the white and blue discs as fast as possible. The time taken to achieve 100% accuracy of sorting is recorded (in seconds). The test is usually repeated three times to allow for learning and standardization. It is not appropriate for preschool children and is not sensitive enough to detect early signs of vitamin A deficiency.

• *Muscle function tests* assess changes in muscle contractility, relaxation rate, and endurance. Such changes are said to precede body composition changes that occur when protein stores are reduced and muscle catabolism take place during protein-energy malnutrition.

• *Growth* in terms of stature and/or weight can be used as an index of nutritional status in children as discussed in Section 26.1.2. When rate of change in stature and/or weight (i.e. growth velocity) is required, measurements must be taken over at least six months on the same child to provide the necessary precision. Changes in body composition indices (see Section 26.1.4) can also be assessed.

• *Cognitive function* is used increasingly in relation to iron and zinc deficiency. Measures employed include IQ-test performance in older children and the Bayley Scales of Infant Development for infants. These tests must be used in studies with a double-blind randomized supplementation design to confirm a relationship between cognitive function and a nutrient deficiency.

26.2.4 Evaluation of laboratory tests

The observed values for the laboratory tests discussed above can be compared with:

• *Reference distribution* This is usually generally defined by percentiles compiled from a reference sample of healthy persons participating in a national nutrition survey. The observed value of an individual is then compared with the percentile distribution of data from persons matched by those factors known to influence the measurement (e.g. age, sex, race, physiological status, etc.).

• *Reference limits* These can also be based on percentiles. For example, in the United States NHANES II data: 'normal' values or those above the reference limit, were defined as >10th percentile for haemoglobin, >5th percentile for mean cell volume, <90th percentile for erythrocyte protoporphyrin, and >10th percentile for transferrin saturation. No data are available, however, from national nutrition surveys for the distribution of reference values for most of the functional physiological tests because they are not feasible in large-scale nutrition surveys. Consequently, they are generally evaluated by monitoring their improvement serially, during a nutrition intervention program. Notable exceptions are growth and body composition indices.

• *Cutoff points* They are generally based on ranges associated with clinical signs, or impairment in a biochemical or physiological function reported in the literature; they may be age, race, and/or sex specific, depending on the laboratory index used. Sometimes, several cutoff points are used to define levels of 'risk' of deficiency such as 'high risk', 'medium risk', and 'low risk' or as 'deficient', 'low', 'acceptable', and 'high'.

26.3 CLINICAL ASSESSMENT

Clinical assessment consists of a routine medical history and a physical examination to detect physical signs (i.e. observations made by a qualified examiner) and symptoms (i.e. manifestations reported by the patient) associated with malnutrition. These assessment procedures are normally used in community nutrition surveys and in clinical medicine. They are most useful during the advanced stages of nutritional depletion, when overt disease is present.

26.3.1 Medical history

In clinical medicine, the medical history can be obtained by an interview with the patient and/or from the medical records. For community surveys, a questionnaire is generally administered in a household or site interview. The medical history usually includes a description of the patient, and relevant environmental, social, and family factors, as well as specific data on the medical history of the patient and his/her family. Details of food allergies and food intolerances are also obtained. An example of data obtained in a medical history is given in Table 26.3.

This information is used to establish whether a nutrient deficiency is likely to be primary, arising from inadequate dietary intake, or secondary in origin. In the latter, the diet is potentially adequate but conditioning factors such as drugs, dietary components, and/or disease states interfere with the ingestion, absorption, transport, utilization, or excretion of the nutrient(s). Respondent bias may occur during the conduct of the medical history. In general, voluntary information given by the patient tends to be less biased than answers to specific questions on past medical history. Consequently, it is preferable to use open-ended questions to elicit such information.

Table 26.3 Example of information obtained from a medical history

Nutrient intake	Anorexia
	Actual intake
	Gastrointestinal tract malfunction affecting intake, digestion, or absorption
Underlying pathology with nutritional effects	Chronic infections or inflammatory states
	Neoplasia
	Endocrine disorders
	Chronic illnesses: pulmonary disease, cirrhosis, or renal failure
End-organ effects	Oedema/ascites
	Weight changes
	Obesity
	Muscle mass relative to exercise status
Miscellaneous	Catabolic medications or therapies: steroids, immunosuppressive agents, radiation, or chemotherapy
	Genetic background: body habitus of parents, siblings, and family
	Other medications: diuretics, laxatives
	Food allergies: food intolerances

Reproduced by permission from Cerra FB. Assessment of nutritional and metabolic status. Chapter 3. In: *Pocket manual of surgical nutrition*, p. 25. St Louis: CV Mosby Co, 1984.

26.3.2 Physical examination

In the physical examination, physical signs and symptoms related to malnutrition are investigated; an abbreviated list is presented in Table 26.4. A detailed description and photographs of the physical signs recommended by the WHO Expert Committee on Medical Assessment of Nutritional Status can be found in the Assessment of Nutritional Status of the Community (Jelliffe, 1966).

Table 26.4 Physical signs and symptoms related to malnutrition

Normal appearance	Signs associated with malnutrition
Hair Shiny; firm; not easily plucked.	Lack of natural shine; hair dull and dry; thin and sparse; hair fine, silky, and straight; colour changes (flag sign); can be easily plucked.
Face Skin colour uniform with a smooth, pink, healthy appearance; not swollen.	Skin colour loss (depigmentation); skin dark over cheeks and under eyes (malar and supraorbital pigmentation); lumpiness or flakiness of skin of nose and mouth; swollen face; enlarged parotid glands; scaling of skin around nostrils (nasolabial seborrhoea).
Eyes Bright, clear, shiny; no sores at corners of eyelids; membranes are a healthy pink and are moist. No prominent blood vessels or mound of tissues or sclera.	Eye membranes are pale (pale conjunctivae); redness of membranes (conjunctival injection); Bitôt's spots; redness and fissuring of eyelid corners (angular palpebritis); dryness of eye membranes (conjunctival xerosis); cornea has dull appearance (corneal xerosis); cornea is soft (keratomalacia); scar on cornea; ring of fine blood vessels around cornea (circumcorneal injection).
Lips Smooth, not chapped or swollen.	Redness and swelling of mouth or lips (cheilosis); especially at corners of mouth (angular fissures and scars).
Tongue Deep red in appearance; not swollen or smooth.	Swelling; scarlet and raw tongue; magenta (purplish) colour of tongue; smooth tongue; swollen sores; hyperaemic and hypertrophic papillae; atrophic papillae.
Teeth No cavities; no pain; bright.	May be missing or erupting abnormally; grey or black spots (fluorosis); cavities (caries).
Gums Healthy; red; do not bleed; not swollen.	'Spongy' and bleed easily; recession of gums.
Face Face not swollen.	Thyroid enlargement (front of neck); parotid enlargement (cheeks become swollen).
Skin No signs of rashes, swellings, dark or light spots.	Dryness of skin (xerosis); sandpaper feel of skin (follicular hyperkeratosis); flakiness of skin; skin swollen and dark; red swollen pigmentation of exposed areas (pellagrous dermatosis); excessive lightness or darkness of skin (dyspigmentation); black and blue marks resulting from skin bleeding (petechiae); lack of fat under skin.
Nails Firm, pink.	Nails are spoon-shaped (koilonychia); brittle and ridged

Table 26.4 *(Continued)*

Normal appearance	Signs associated with malnutrition
Muscular and skeletal system Good muscle tone; some fat under skin; can walk and run without pain.	Muscles have 'wasted' appearance; baby's skull bones are thin and soft (craniotabes); round swelling of front and side of head (frontal and parietal bossing); swelling of ends of bones (peiphyseal enlargment); small bumps on both sides of chest wall (on ribs)—beading of ribs; baby's soft spot on head does not harden at proper time (persistently open anterior fontanelle); knock-kees or bow-legs; bleeding into muscle (musculoskeletal haemorrhages); persons cannot get up or walk properly.
Cardiovascular system Normal heart rate and rhythm; no murmurs or abnormal rhythms; normal blood pressure for age.	Heart rate above 100 (tachycardia); enlarged heart; abnormal rhythm; elevated blood pressure.
Gastrointestinal system No palpable organs or masses (in children, however, liver edge may be palpable).	Liver enlargement; enlargement of spleen (usually indicates other associated diseases).
Nervous system Psychological stability; normal reflexes.	Mental irritability and confusion; burning and tingling of hands and feet (paresthesia); loss of position and vibratory sense; weakness and tenderness of muscles (may result in inability to walk); decrease and loss of ankle and knee reflexes.

Source: From Christakis G (1973). Nutritional assessment in health programs. *American Journal of Public Health*, 63 (suppl.) 1–82. With permission of American Public Health Association.

The World Health Organization has classified the most common physical signs into three groups: (1) signs indicating a probable deficiency of one or more nutrients; (2) signs indicating probable long-term malnutrition in combination with other factors; and (3) signs not related to nutritional status. Generally in community surveys, only those signs in group (1) should be sought in the physical examination.

To assist in identifying specific nutrient deficiencies, the physical signs (and symptoms) are often grouped, combinations varying with age, race, country, environment, etc. Generally, the greater the number of signs present within a specific group, the larger the probability that the individual has a specific nutrient deficiency. The signs within a group can be classified into three categories, designated as high, moderate, and low risk. Individuals with either a specified combination of signs, or sometimes, a single sign in the high risk category, would be considered at high risk of developing or having a specific nutrient deficiency.

The physical examination as a technique for assessing nutritional status has certain limitations which must be recognized. In cases of mild and moderate deficiency, such as occur in industrialized countries, signs are frequently non-specific occurring with more than one nutrient deficiency and/or induced by non-nutritional factors. As well, they may be two-directional, occurring during both deficiency and recovery (e.g. enlarged liver in protein-energy malnutrition and during its treatment), and/or multiple, co-existing with other nutrient deficiencies. Examiner inconsistencies may also be a source of error, but can be minimized by training examiners and standardizing the criteria used to define the signs. In most cases, signs should be recorded as positive or negative and not in terms of severity.

FURTHER READING

1. Frisancho AR. *Anthropometric standards for the assessment of growth and nutritional status.* Ann Arbor: The University of Michigan Press, 1990.
2. Gibson RS. *Principles of nutritional assessment.* New York: Oxford University Press, 1990.
3. Gibson RS. *Nutritional assessment a laboratory manual.* New York: Oxford University Press, 1993.
4. Jelliffe DB. *The assessment of the nutritional status of the community.* World Health Organization Monograph No. 53. WHO, 1996.
5. Lohman TG, Roche AF, Martorell R (eds). *Anthropometric standardization manual.* Champagne, IL: Human Kinetics Books, 1988.
6. Pilch SM, Senti FR (eds). *Assessment of the iron nutritional status of the U.S. population survey based on data collected in the second National Health and Nutrition Examination Survey, 1976–1980.* Life Sciences Research Office, Federation of the American Societies for Experimental Biology. Maryland: Bethesda, 1984.
7. Shetty PS, James WPT. *Body mass index. A measure of chronic energy deficiency in adults.* Rome: FAO Food and Nutrition Paper 56, 1994.
8. WHO (World Health Organization). Use and interpretation of anthropometric indicators of nutritional status. *Bulletin of the World Health Organization* 1986; **64**: 929–41.

Appendix

Table A26.1   Minerals: static biochemical tests

Test	Comments
Calcium: serum (plasma should not be used). Flame atomic absorption spectrophotometry (AAS). Fluorometric titration with calcein as indicator and EGTA as titrant.	Insensitive test: levels strongly homeostatically control led—only fall after prolonged period of deprivation. Abnormal levels indicative of pathological rather than nutritional problems. Levels vary slightly with age and sex.
Serum ionized calcium Ion-specific electrodes.	Physiologically active form of Ca in blood—makes up 50% of Ca in plasma. Levels relate to disturbances in Ca metabolism. Low levels in hypoparathyroidism and vitamin D deficient rickets. Elevated levels in hyperparathyroidism or during chronic renal haemodialysis.
Phosphorus: serum. Colorimetric procedure—modification of molybdenum blue procedure of Fiske and Subbarow (1925).	Non-haemolysed samples must be used. Low levels in disorders of renal tubule reabsorption of phosphate (e.g. Fanconi syndrome). Levels vary with age.
Magnesium: serum (Plasma should not be used). Flame AAS.	Non-haemolysed samples must be used; slight diurnal variation. Insensitive test: only falls in severe deficiency. Hence used to confirm Mg deficiency in presence of clinical signs and symptoms. Levels vary with age and sex.
Leucocyte or mononuclear blood cell magnesium. Graphite furnace AAS.	In experimental animals, levels reflect cardiac and skeletal muscle. Mg content of leucocytes varies with cell age. Mg concentration in leucocytes higher than mononuclear blood cells.

Table A26.2 Trace minerals: static biochemical tests

Test	Comments
Chromium: serum/plasma. Graphite furnace atomic absorption spectrophotometry (AAS). Neutron activation analysis. Trace-element free vacutainers and siliconized needles must be used for blood collection.	Normal healthy adult levels range from 0.0019 to 0.0038 µmol/l—very close to detection limit of modern AAS. Validity as index of suboptimal chromium status is uncertain.
Urinary chromium in 24-hour sample. Graphite furnace AAS.	Urine major excretory route for absorbed Cr. Values accepted as accurate when <1 µg/day for normal healthy adults. Levels reflect changes induced by recent excessive dietary intakes rather than changes produced by chromium deficiency. Levels affected by exercise.
Copper: serum/plasma. Flame AAS.	Insensitive test: only fall in severe deficiency—used to confirm Cu deficiency in presence of clinical signs and symptoms. Elevated levels with use of oral contraceptive agents, pregnancy, infection or stress. Levels vary with age and sex.
Iodine: in 24-h urine sample or casual urine sample. Digest sample in chloric acid. Measure iodine content by its catalytic action in the reduction of ceric ammonium sulphate (yellow) to the cerous (colourless form) (stable—does not need refrigeration).	Reflects iodine intake on a population basis. Not suitable for an individual. Four cutoff points proposed for assessing the severity of iodine deficiency disorders: <0.16 Severe IDD; 0.17–0.40 Moderate IDD; 0.41–0.79 Mild IDD; ⩾0.8 µmol/l No deficiency
Selenium: serum/plasma. AAS with Zeeman background correction. Fluorometric method. Instrumental neutron activation. Trace-element-free vacutainers for blood collection.	Levels respond to short-term changes in Se intakes; also reflect Se status in populations with relatively constant Se intakes. Levels vary with age: independent of sex in children.
Whole blood selenium. As above.	Levels reflect chronic Se status.
Urinary selenium in 24-h sample. Fluorometric method.	Urine major excretory route for absorbed selenium. Levels reflect recent dietary intake unless Se intakes are very low. Some diurnal variation.
Hair selenium via instrumental neutron activation analysis.	Levels reflect chronic Se status provided Se-containing antidandruff shampoos have not been used. Adventitious Se in these shampoos is not removed by washing.

Table A26.2 (*Continued*)

Test	Comments
Toenail selenium via instrumental neutron activation analysis.	Levels may reflect Se status 6–9 months prior to collection. Validity requires confirmation.
Zinc: serum/plasma. Via AAS. Trace-element free vacutainers for blood collection.	Insensitive: homeostatically controlled only falls in severe deficiency. Non-specific—low in infection/stress and disease states with hypoalbuminaemia. Levels vary with age, sex, time of day, length of time prior to separation of serum, position of subject, fasting status of subject. Cutoff points for risk of Zn deficiency fasting: $<10.7\,\mu mol/l$; non-fasting $<9.95\,\mu mol/l$.
Hair zinc via AAS or instrumental neutron activation analysis.	Low in chronic zinc deficiency in children. Levels vary with age, sex, season. Tentative cutoff points for risk of Zn deficiency in children: summer $<1.07\,\mu mol/g$; winter $<1.68\,\mu mol/g$.

Table A26.3   Fat-soluble vitamins: static biochemical tests

Test	Comments
Vitamin A: serum retinol. Colorimetric method based on Carr–Price reaction.	Non-haemolyzed sample must be used. Fasting samples not necessary.
Fluorometry. High performance liquid chromatography (HPLC) reverse phase.	Insensitive test: only reflect liver stores when severely depleted or excessively high—otherwise homeostatically controlled. Levels vary with age, sex and race. Stress decreases levels.
Avoid exposure to bright light if stored for prolonged periods. Should be stored under nitrogen and frozen below $-40\,^{\circ}$C.	
Carotenoids: serum. HPLC	Reflect current intake of carotenoids. May be useful as a secondary index of vitamin A deficiency when dietary carotenoids provide only source of vitamin A.
Vitamin D: serum 25-hydroxy-vitamin D. HPLC + competitive protein binding assay.	Levels reflect total supply of vitamin D from endogenous and exogenous sources. Most abundant circulating metabolite of vitamin D. Levels reflect vitamin D content of liver. The major storage site of vitamin D. Levels vary with age, sex, exposure to solar ultraviolet light. Clinical signs of vitamin D deficiency occur with levels <3.0 nmol/l; toxicity >500 nmol/l.
Vitamin E: serum tocopherol. Gas–liquid chromatography (GLC). HPLC: reverse phase.	Levels highly correlated with serum cholesterol and total lipids. Thus, serum tocopherol/lipid ratios often used. Ratios <0.6 mg total tocopherol/g serum lipids indicative of deficiency. Levels vary with age, physiological state, analytical method.

Table A26.4 Water-soluble vitamins: static biochemical tests

Test	Comments
Thiamin: in 24-h urine sample. Urinary thiamin relative to creatinine excretion in casual urine samples.	Reflects recent dietary intake rather than body stores especially when intakes are excessive. At lower intakes only small changes in thiamin excretion occur. Levels vary with age.
Fluorometric thiochrome procedure or high performance liquid chromatography (HPLC).	Age-specific interpretive criteria are necessary
Riboflavin: in 24-h sample. Urinary riboflavin relative to creatinine excretion in casual urine samples.	Reflects recent dietary intake rather than body stores. Non-specific: varies with physical activity, sleep, environmental temperature, bed-rest, use of oral contraceptive agents.
Fluorometric method. Microbiological method using *Ochromonas danica*. HPLC. Competitive binding protein methods.	
Niacin: Urinary *N'*-methylnicotinamide. *N'*-methyl-2-pyridone-5-carboxylamide. Use fasting casual urine samples. Fluorometric assay. HPLC.	20–30% of nicotinic acid excreted as *N'*-methylnicotinamide; 40–60% as 2-pyridone. Ratios 2-pyridone/*N'*-methyl nicotinamide <1.0 indicative of niacin deficiency; 1.0–4.0 acceptable. Ratio independent of age. Not appropriate for pregnant or diabetic subjects.
Niacin index: ratio of erythrocyte nicotinamide adenine dinudeotide (NAD) to NADP. Method uses cycling mixture of thiazolyl blue and phenazine methosulphate and addition of ethanol and alchohol dehydrogenase.	Ratio erythrocyte NAD to NADP <1.0 may identify subjects at risk of niacin deficiency.
Pyridoxine: plasma pyridoxal 5-phosphate. Cation-exchange HPLC. Cation-exchange open column chromatography plus fluorometric assay.	Primary form of circulating vitamin B_6 in plasma: measure of active coenzyme form of vitamin B_6. Levels increase with decreasing B_6 intake but decrease with increasing protein intakes. Values >30 nmol/l indicative of adequate status in adults.
Urinary 4-pyridoxic acid in 24-h sample (2-methyl-3-hydroxy-4-carboxy-methylpyridine). Urinary 4-pyridoxic acid relative to creatinine excretion in casual urine samples.	40–60% of vitamin B_6 excreted as 4-pyridoxic acid. Levels reflect dietary intakes of B_6. Levels vary with age, sex, pregnancy. Tentative cutoff points mg/day: <0.5—marginal or inadequate. ⩾0.8 acceptable vitamin B_6 status.

Table A26.4 (*Continued*)

Test	Comments
HPLC with fluorometric detection. Multiple ion-exchange chromatography followed by fluorometric assay.	
Folate: serum/plasma. Microbiological technique using *Lactobacillus casei*. Radioimmunoassay. HPLC.	Non-haemolysed samples must be used. Main folate derivative in serum is methyltetrahydrofolate. Reflects recent dietary intake rather than body stores. Levels vary with age, smoking status, oral contraceptive agents. Cutoff points indicative of negative folate balance <6.8 nmol/l.
Red blood cell. Microbiological technique using *Lactobacillus casei*.	Polyglutamate forms of folate present. Reflect body folate stores. Levels vary with age, smoking status and in females with pregnancy, parity, and oral contraceptive use. Cutoff points indicative of depleted folate stores <368 nmol/l; folate deficiency <322 nmol/l; folate deficiency anaemia <227 nmol/l.
Vitamin B$_{12}$: serum. Microbiological technique using *Lactobacillus leichmanii, Euglena gracilis* or *Ochromonas malhamensis*. Radioimmunoassay.	20% vitamin B$_{12}$ in serum attached to transport protein-trans cobalamin (TC)II; remainder is glycoprotein B$_{12}$ binder—TCI and TCIII. Levels vary with age and sex. Very low levels (i.e. <74–59 pmol/l) indicative of vitamin B$_{12}$ deficiency; moderately low values (111–148 pmol/l) not specific for vitamin B$_{12}$ deficiency: may also occur in iron deficiency.
Ascorbic acid: serum. Spectrophotometric methods using: 2, 6-dichloroindophenol, α, α'-dipyridyl or 2, 4-dinitrophenylhydrazine. Fluorometric methods. HPLC.	Fasting blood sample essential. Can be used to reflect body ascorbic acid content in individuals with chronically low intakes. Levels affected by cold or heat stress, trauma, oral contraceptive agents, infection, smoking. Levels higher in women than in men. Cutoff values: low levels 11.4–17 µmol/l; deficient <11.4 µmol/l.
Leucocyte. HPLC after deproteinization with 6% metaphosphoric acid.	Reflect tissue stores. Preparation and assay difficult—must ensure complete separation of platelets from leukocytes. Cutoff points <11.4 nmol/10^8 cells associated with clinical signs of scurvy.
Urinary ascorbic acid: 24-h sample required. Spectrophotometric methods shown above.	Reflects recent dietary intake. Not very sensitive; low specificity.

Table A26.5 Enzymes: functional biochemical tests

Test	Comments
Thiamin: erythrocyte transketolase (ETK) activity. Transketolase is a thiamin pyrophosphate dependent (TPP) enzyme which catalyses two reactions in the pentose phosphate pathway. In thiamin deficiency, basal level of ETK activity is slow. After addition of TPP enzyme activity is enhanced = 'TPP' effect.	ETK activity varies with age of erythrocytes, certain disease states (e.g. cancer) and drugs. Interpretive criteria: activity coefficients (AC) 1.0–1.15 acceptable; 1.16–1.20 low; >1.20 deficient.
Riboflavin: erythrocyte glutathione reductase (EGR) activity. Glutathione reductase is a nicotinamide adenine dinucleotide phosphate (NADPH) and FAD-dependent enzyme which catalyses oxidative cleavage of the disulphide bond of oxidized glutathione to form reduced glutathione. In riboflavin deficiency, basal level of EGR is low and *in vitro* stimulation by FAD rises.	Single measures indicative of long-term riboflavin status. EGR AC independent of gender but may vary with age, presence of B_6 deficiency, Fe deficiency anaemia, uremia, concentration of FAD used in assay, and age of erythrocytes. Degree of elevation of EGR AC is not indicative of severity of deficiency. Tentative interpretive criteria: <1.2 acceptable; 1.2–1.4 low; >1.4 deficient.
Pyridoxine: alanine aminotransferase (AlaAT) activity in erythrocytes. Aspartate aminotransferase (AspAT) activity in erythrocytes. Both aminotransferase enzymes transfer the amino group from their respective amino acid to ketoglutarate forming L-glutamate and the keto acid corresponding to the original amino acid (i.e. for AlaAT = L-alanine; for ASPAT = L-aspartate).	Reflect long-term vitamin B_6 status: degree of elevation of AlaAT AC or AspAT AC is not indicative of severity of deficiency. AlaAT more sensitive to B_6 deficiency than AspAT and more stable, but should not be used for pregnant women or those using OCAs. More difficult to measure and less stable during storage *in vitro* than AspAT. Interpretive criteria: AlaAT AC ≤ 1.25 acceptable; >1.25 inadequate. For AspAT AC ≤ 1.5 acceptable; >1.5 inadequate.
Copper: erythrocyte superoxide dismutase. Cytosol superoxide dismutase (Cu, Zn-SOD) contains both Cu and Zn, found in cytosol and erythrocytes and other cells. Each molecule contains 2 g-atoms each of Cu and Zn. Enzyme acts as a scavenger of O^{2-}	More sensitive to Cu depletion than serum Cu or ceruloplasmin.
Selenium: erythrocyte glutathione peroxidase (GSHPx). Se-containing enzyme which helps to protect cell against lipid peroxidation damage.	GSHPx activity can only be used to assess Se status when dietary intakes are habitually low (e.g. New Zealand) because its activity plateaus at blood Se values >1.27 μmol/l. Activity varies with age, sex, race, physical activity, and exposure to antioxidants.

Table A26.6 Changes in blood components: functional biochemical test

Test	Comments
Vitamin A: retinol-binding protein (RBP) in serum. RBP is the carrier protein for retinol with a single binding site for one molecule of retinol. In vitamin A deficiency RBP secretion is blocked leading to its accumulation in the liver. Hence, liver RBP levels are high whereas serum levels are low.	Low specificity: also falls in protein and zinc deficiency, and cystic fibrosis. Normal levels are very low, difficult to measure, and not clearly defined.
Iron: haemoglobin. Iron is an essential component of haemoglobin—the oxygen carrying pigment of the red blood cells. Each haemoglobin molecule is a conjugate of protein (globin) and four molecules of haem. In iron deficiency anaemia the concentration of haemoglobin in the red blood cells is reduced.	Insensitive-only falls in severe iron deficiency when anaemia is present. Non-specific: also falls in chronic infections, protein-energy malnutrition (PEM), vitamin B_{12} or folate deficiency. Levels vary with age, sex, race, diurnal variation and smoking.
Ferritin in serum/plasma. Ferritin enters serum by secretions from reticuloendothelial system. Serum ferritin concentrations parallel total body storage iron.	Most sensitive index of iron deficiency: only index that can reflect a deficient, excess, and normal iron status. Specific: only falls in iron deficiency. Levels vary with age, sex; elevated in infection.
Free erythrocyte protoporphyrin. Protoporphyrin is a precursor of haem. When iron stores are exhausted, protoporphyrin IX accumulates in the developing erythrocytes because haem synthesis is impaired.	Protoporphyrin levels increase progressively in the second stage of iron deficiency. Infection and lead toxicity also elevate levels. Levels vary with age and sex.
Transferrin receptor in serum/plasma. Soluble transferrin receptor can be detected and quantified via ELISA.	Receptor synthesis is up regulated in iron deprived tissues. Concentrations are increased before free erythrocyte protoporphyrin (FEP) and mean cell volume (MCV). Levels remain normal in liver disease and inflammation.
Iodine: thyroid-stimulating hormone (TSH). Iodine is essential for the synthesis of thyroid hormones. Serum or whole blood TSH levels directly reflect availability and adequacy of thyroid hormone. TSH can be assayed via ELISA from both dried whole blood spots on filter paper and serum.	Best diagnostic test for determination of hypothyroidism. Elevated TSH in newborn or infant blood indicates that level of thyroid hormone is inadequate. Interpretive criteria 20–25 mU/l whole blood or 40–50 mU/l serum indicative of congenital hypothyroidism.
Thyroglobulin (Tg) in serum. Inadequate intakes of iodine induce proliferation of thyroid cells which results in hyperplasia and hypertrophy and thus enhanced turn over of thyroid cells. Hence, Tg is released into serum and levels become elevated. Assayed via ELISA.	Levels vary inversely with iodine intake. Interpretive criteria: 10.0–19.9 ng/ml mild, 20.0–39.9 ng/ml moderate, > 40.0 ng/ml severe deficiency (children and adults).

Table A26.7 Load and tolerance: functional biochemical tests

Test	Comments
Pyridoxine: tryptophan load test. Pyridoxal phosphate is a coenzyme for kynureninase in the tryptophan–niacin pathway. L-Isomer of tryptophan (2 g) used as a loading dose. It causes an increased excretion of metabolites of kynurenine pathway. Xanthurenic acid measured in urine at baseline and over 24-h period postload.	Not appropriate for pregnant subjects and those taking oral contraceptive agents (OCAs). Tentative cutoff points: >50 mg/24 h— marginal; <25 mg/24 h—acceptable.
Magnesium: load test. Basal urinary Mg measured in three 24-h urine samples. Mg administered over 8 h intra- muscularly (infants) or intravenously (adults). Mg excretion measured over 24 or 48 h period postload.	Cutoff points vary: Retention values >20–50% said to be indicative of suboptimal Mg status.
Zinc: oral zinc tolerance test. Plasma zinc measured at baseline and at hourly intervals for five hours post-dose of 25–50 mg Zn as zinc acetate. Test said to reflect zinc absorption which increases in zinc deficiency.	Use of pharmacological doses of Zn limits its usefulness. Elevated response after depletion and after repletion has been observed limiting validity of this test.
Vitamin A: relative dose response (RDR). In vitamin A deficiency, retinol–binding protein (RBP) accumulates in liver as apo RBP (i.e. RBP not bound to retinol). After dose of vitamin A, latter binds to apo RBP in liver and holo RBP (RBP bound to retinol) is released from liver causing rapid increase in serum retinol. Baseline blood sample taken and then oral vitamin A dose given. After 5 h second blood sample taken and RDR (%) calculated.	More sensitive index of marginal vitamin A status than using serum retinol. RDR > 14–20% indicative of marginal vitamin A status. Low RDR values with malabsorption, liver disease, and severe PEM.
Modified relative dose-response assay. Similar to RDR but uses an analogue of retinol, 3,4-didehydroretinol (DR). A single dose of DR is given orally. DR binds to accumulated apo RBP in the liver and is released into the serum as holo RBP. After 4–6 h the molar ratio of DR : retinol is determined in serum via HPLC.	Requires only one blood sample. Serum can be frozen and stored for later analysis. Need at least 200 μl serum/plasma. Free DR is unstable so extracts must be protected from light. Children with DR : retinol ratios ⩾ 0.060 said to have marginal vitamin A status.
Plasma retinol-binding protein response test. Plasma RBP measured at baseline and 5 h after oral dose of 600–1000 μg vitamin A. Plasma RBP concentration determined via radial immunodiffusion or by ELISA. Percentage increase in plasma RBP from baseline is calculated ΔRBP (%) = [RBP (maximum) − RBP (baseline)]/RBP baseline × 100.	High ΔRBP value compatible with functional vitamin A deficiency. Further validation required to assess its validity for marginal vitamin A deficiency and for older children and adults.

Part VI: Life stages

Pregnancy and Lactation

Elizabeth Johnston

27.1 Pregnancy

Pregnancy is a time of rapid growth and development for the fetus and increased nutrient needs for the mother. Proper nutrition prior to conception is essential in order to minimize the risk of birth defects in the fetus, while adequate nutrition during pregnancy has long been thought to play a key role in decreasing the number of low birth weight infants.

Biologists define three periods of development *in utero*. The first lasts from conception to the end of the second week and is usually described as the period of implantation; from the third week to the end of the eighth week is the period of organogenesis; from the ninth week to birth is a period of growth. While the conceptus is relatively insulated from environmental factors during the period of implantation, the period of organogenesis can be affected by either a deficiency or excessive intake of nutrients. For example, a relative deficiency of folic acid during the period of neural tube closure may result in improper closing of the neural tube resulting in the defect known as spina bifida. Adequate folic acid intake (400 µg/day) is therefore important prior to pregnancy as well as several weeks after conception. On the other hand, excessive intakes of vitamin A as retinol (over 3 mg/day) may lead to malformations in the infant (i.e. they are teratogenic); consequently high levels should be avoided during the time of organogenesis.

27.1.1 Weight gain

Adequate maternal weight gain, along with length of gestation and pre-pregnant weight have a significant and predictable effect on the birth weight of the infant. Low birth weight (<2500 g) is associated with increased infant mortality and increased risk for disabilities. Recommendations for maternal weight gain are frequently based on maternal pre-pregnant body mass index (BMI) with underweight women advised to gain more weight during pregnancy while overweight women are advised to gain less (Table 27.1).

Short women should gain at the lower end of the range and adolescents may need to aim for the upper end of the range. Even obese women must gain a minimum amount of weight (6 kg) in order to optimize the chances for a healthy birthweight. All pregnant women should be encouraged to eat at regular times throughout the day and avoid periods of fasting or dieting.

Weight gain in the first trimester is approximately 1–2 kg total but thereafter it averages 0.4 kg per week. The composition of the weight gain by the end of pregnancy is shown in Table 27.2. In the second trimester much of the weight gain is used for an increase

Table 27.1 Recommended weight gains for women with varying pre-pregnant body mass indexes (BMIs)

Recommended total gain	
BMI	Kilograms
< 20	12.5 minimum
20–25	11.5–14.0
> 25	6.0–11.5
Twins	16.0–20.0

Table 27.2 The distribution of maternal weight gain at 40 weeks gestation

Weight gain distribution (grams)	
Fetus	3300–3500
Placenta	650
Increase in blood volume	1300
Increase in uterus and breasts	1300
Amniotic fluid	800
Fat stores and additional fluid retention	4200–6000
Total	11 550–13 550

in the mother's plasma volume and the laying down of fat stores while in the third trimester the emphasis is on the increase in weight of the fetus. Women who gain excessively in the first half of pregnancy should be advised to slow their rate of gain but not eliminate it during the remainder of the pregnancy. Excessive maternal weight gain is detrimental; it has been associated with fetal macrosomia, late delivery dates and increased chances of labour problems and Caesarean section.

It has been assumed that the extra fat stored during pregnancy is valuable during lactation but a recent study indicated that there was no relationship between milk volume and maternal BMI. Even very thin mothers were able to produce large volumes of milk.

27.1.2 Energy

Throughout pregnancy an additional 250 MJ (60 000 kcal) are theoretically required to cover the increase in foetal and maternal tissue as well as the increase in basal metabolic rate. Physical activity may decline as pregnancy progresses so it is difficult to predict actual energy needs. Careful studies in Scotland, England, Netherlands and elsewhere have found that on average, women were not eating their expected energy requirement; they were only eating around 100 kcal/day extra. The theoretical increase per day during the second and third trimesters of pregnancy is two to three times this level of intake. This suggests that

Table 27.3 Recommended daily nutrient intakes during pregnancy

Nutrient	USA	Canada (a)	UK	Australia
Protein (g)	60	75	51	51
Vitamin A (µg)	800	800	700	750
Vitamin D (µg)	10	5	10	(c)
Vitamin E (mg)	10	8	(c)	7
Vitamin C (mg)	70	40	50	60
Thiamin (mg)	1.5	0.9	0.9	1.0
Riboflavin (mg)	1.6	1.3	1.4	1.5
Niacin (NE)	17	16	13	15
Folate (µg)	400	385	300	400
Vitamin B_{12} (µg)	2.2	1.2	1.5	3.0
Calcium (mg)	1200	1200	700	1100
Magnesium (mg)	320	245	270	300
Iron (mg)	30	13 (b)	14.8	22–36
Zinc (mg)	15	15	7	16
Iodine (µg)	175	185	140	150

(a) Values given for third trimester. (b) Based on assumption stores are adequate; if stores are inadequate, recommend 23 mg. (c) No recommendation set.

the increased intake of food may be insufficient to provide for the increased need for specific nutrients (e.g. calcium, folate and iron); hence foods in pregnancy should be nutrient-dense. Recommended intakes of selected nutrients are shown in Table 27.3.

27.1.3 Protein

Some additional protein is needed for growth of both maternal and fetal tissue. But the small extra amounts, estimated to average 10 g of reference protein per day by the United States and 6 g/per day across pregnancy by the United Kingdom and the FAO/WHO/UNU Committee, are covered adequately by a normal diet.

27.1.4 Minerals

Calcium, iron and zinc are the main minerals of interest during pregnancy. The infant is born with approximately 28 g of calcium which must come from the mother's reserves if sufficient calcium is not consumed during pregnancy. There are case reports in the literature which indicate that for a minority of women pregnancy may represent a drain on the body's store of calcium and subsequently increase susceptibility to osteoporosis. However, in the majority of cases if calcium needs are not met by an increased intake of dietary calcium and calcium is removed form maternal stores either during pregnancy or lactation, calcium balance and bone density are restored by 12 months postpartum.

Iron nutriture is a complex and emotional issue for many professionals dealing with the nutritional aspects of pregnancy. While some studies indicate that iron deficiency is associated with increased risk of prematurity and low birth weight infants, many investigators suggest that the fetus can take whatever it needs from the mother's iron stores in order to satisfy its own requirements. However, pregnancy is a drain on a woman's iron stores and most physicians recommend routine supplementation with iron. The United States and Australian recommended dietary intakes indicate that a supplement of iron is necessary for pregnant women. Recent research, however, suggests that iron absorption increases significantly as pregnancy progresses, from an absorption rate of 7% at 12 weeks gestation to 66% at 36 weeks gestation. If the mother enters pregnancy without iron deficiency, sufficient iron can usually be obtained from the diet alone provided the diet contains adequate amounts of meat and vitamin C to enhance the absorption of iron.

Zinc requirements are increased during pregnancy and women consuming iron supplements may be at particular risk since iron to zinc ratios exceeding 3:1 can impair zinc absorption. Zinc is required for DNA and RNA synthesis. Flesh foods such as meats and fish are good sources of readily available zinc; nuts and legumes are also good sources but zinc is less available. Strict vegans (who eat no foods of animal origin) may have difficulty obtaining adequate absorbable dietary zinc because of the high insoluble fibre and phytate content of their diets, components known to inhibit zinc absorption.

27.1.5 Vitamins

Vitamin needs increase during pregnancy and lactation in order to meet the needs of the growing fetus and the demand of supplying nutrients in the breast milk. Adequate folic acid is most important in the first weeks after conception at the time of neural tube closure and requirements remain high throughout pregnancy because of continued cell proliferation. Current recommendations for folate suggest a minimum intake of 400 µg prior to and during pregnancy. Food sources are leafy green vegetables, legumes and whole wheat grains. An increasing number of foods are being fortified with folic acid. Supplements are recommended in some countries.

Since vitamin B_{12} is found only in foods of animal origin it should be supplemented for women who eat all plant diets. The only vitamin which does not have an increase in the recommended nutrient intake during pregnancy is vitamin A. Vitamin A is important for its role in cell differentiation; however, there is concern that high dosages (>3000 µg retinol daily) are teratogenic, causing central nervous system and heart defects. Pregnant women are still encouraged to consume dark green or dark orange vegetables in order to obtain sufficient β-carotene but liver is no longer widely advocated as a desirable addition to a pregnant woman's diet because its vitamin A content is considered too high (10 000–10 500 µg retinol/100 g beef liver). Recommended intakes for vitamin A are in the vicinity of 800 µg retinol/day. Recent data suggest that adequate vitamin A status may reduce transmission of the human immunodeficiency virus from mother to infant.

27.2 COMMON COMPLAINTS

27.2.1 Morning sickness

Morning sickness is a common problem associated with pregnancy especially in the first trimester and for a minority of women it lasts throughout the pregnancy. Morning sickness may be related to heightened olfaction sensitivity. It is generally associated with a good clinical outcome. The best dietary advice seems to be to eat small frequent meals. Various dietary approaches have been suggested to reduce this unpleasant symptom of early pregnancy, but there is no conclusive evidence of their benefit. Most pregnant women prefer to avoid strong food odours.

27.2.2   Constipation

Constipation is a frequent annoyance in pregnancy resulting from the hormonal effects on muscle tone and possibly the ingestion of iron tablets. A diet rich in insoluble fibre, regular exercise and a high fluid intake help to lessen constipation.

27.2.3   Heartburn

Heartburn is common in pregnancy because of relaxation of muscle tone of the sphincter at the top of the stomach and pressure of the fetus on the stomach which permit reflux of stomach acid into the oesophagus. To avoid heartburn it is advisable to remain upright after a meal, to eat only small quantities at a time, avoid spicy foods and take fluids and foods at different times.

27.3   LIFESTYLE FACTORS

27.3.1   Exercise

Physical exercise during pregnancy appears to be beneficial in improving fitness, preventing gestational diabetes and reducing stress. However, it should be moderate and not increase core body temperature beyond 38 °C. Intense exercise such as marathon training may reduce infant birth weight.

27.3.2   Alcohol

Consumption of alcohol is contraindicated during pregnancy although it is unlikely that an occasional alcoholic beverage with a meal will do any harm. Because of perceived difficulties in obtaining accurate answers in retrospective or prospective epidemiological studies and the unethical nature of clinical trials, it is unlikely that a maximum acceptable level of alcohol will be determined. Consequently, the conservative view is to avoid all alcohol during pregnancy. Excess alcohol consumption causes fetal alcohol syndrome which is characterized by mental and physical retardation. Facial deformities include a short nose, low nasal bridge, short eyelid opening and a small head circumference.

27.3.3   Cigarette smoking

Smoking during pregnancy has a significant impact on the birth weight of the infant. The more tobacco smoked the greater the birth weight deficit. Women who smoke more than 20 cigarettes a day experience a decrease in birth weight of approximately 200–250 g.

Smoking is also thought to increase the risk of spontaneous abortion, premature birth and sudden infant deaths. Haemoglobin levels are usually higher in smokers as a result of increased carboxyhaemoglobin, giving the false impression that dietary iron status is adequate. In fact, smokers often have lower levels of several nutrients including vitamin C and folate.

27.3.4 Caffeine

Caffeine is known to cross the placenta and the fetus has a limited ability to metabolize it. While it has not been shown to be teratogenic in humans, dietary recommendations advise pregnant women to limit their intake to under 400 mg daily (4 cups of coffee or 10 colas). Aversion to coffee is common in pregnancy.

27.3.5 Drugs

Extreme caution is needed before any drug is taken during pregnancy and lactation. Medicines should be consumed only on the advice of a physician. This includes over the counter drugs, such as aspirin, which has been shown to affect fetal circulation and could lead to maternal iron deficiency through irritation of the gastric mucosa. Cannabis and cocaine intake during pregnancy have adverse effects on fetal growth and development.

27.4 LACTATION

Lactation should be considered the normal continuation of the reproductive cycle. In North America approximately 50–60% of newborn infants are initially breast-fed. Other industrialised countries such as Australia have up to 90% of new mothers initiating breast-feeding. In all nations, higher rates of breast-feeding are associated with increased maternal education and age.

27.4.1 Physiology of lactation

The majority of women who want to breast-feed their babies can do so. Lactation is still possible with inverted nipples, small breasts or multiple births. Milk is produced in direct response to the amount of infant suckling (Fig. 27.1). The suckling infant stimulates the mother's pituitary gland to release prolactin, a hormone needed to induce the cells in the breast to synthesize milk. These milk-producing cells then synthesize most of the protein, some of the fat and sugars and combine them with nutrients, including vitamins and minerals, from the mother's bloodstream. The pituitary releases a second hormone, oxytocin, which is responsible for releasing the milk from the cells into the ducts which carry the milk to the nipple of the breast. This 'let-down reflex' is affected by anxiety so mothers who are nervous or embarrassed by breast-feeding may have difficulty providing their infants with sufficient nourishment. Daily milk volumes vary from approximately 500 ml during the first week of lactation to an average of 750 ml once lactation is well established.

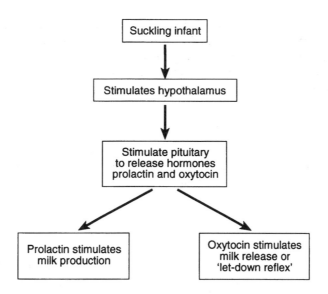

Fig. 27.1 Mechanism for milk production and 'let-down'.

27.4.2   Nutrient needs during lactation

Energy needs increase significantly during lactation to cover the amount of energy in the breast milk, approximately 2.6 MJ (630 kcal) in 750 ml of breast milk, as well as to allow for the energy to produce the milk. Most authorities suggest that some of the required needs of lactation should come from the mobilization of fat stores laid down during pregnancy. Hence, recommended dietary intakes are in the range of 2 MJ (400–500 kcal) with the additional required energy coming from mobilized fat stores. However, lactating women should not assume that their fat stores will decrease and they will lose weight automatically. Many studies indicate that breast-feeding is not associated with weight loss unless it continues for long periods of time (6–12 months). Postpartum weight retention may be more closely related to changes in eating behaviour and physical activity rather than the method of infant feeding.

Requirements for many of the other nutrients during lactation are mostly similar to requirements during pregnancy but there is a sustained need for calcium and a lower requirement for folate. Because breast milk is considered rich in vitamin A (670–700 µg/l) vitamin A recommendations are higher (Table 27.4), as are vitamin C and zinc. Mothers who are vegans are advised to take vitamin B_{12} supplements to ensure normal milk levels for the baby (1 µg/l). On the other hand, levels of vitamins K and D are low in breast milk. Infants are given vitamin K by a one time injection at birth, and in high latitude countries vitamin D by supplements beginning at two weeks. During lactation, the lack of normal menstrual flow results in reduced iron needs. Breast milk is low in iron (although high in bioavailability) so demands for this nutrient are lower during lactation compared with pregnancy.

Table 27.4   Recommended daily nutrient intakes during lactation

Nutrient	USA (a)	Canada (b)	UK	Australia
Protein (g)	65	71	56	61
Vitamin A (µg)	1300	1200	950	1200
Vitamin D (µg)	10	5	10	(c)
Vitamin E (mg)	12	9	(c)	9.5
Vitamin C (mg)	95	55	70	60
Thiamin (mg)	1.6	1.0	1.0	1.2
Riboflavin (mg)	1.8	1.4	1.6	1.7
Niacin (NE)	20	17	15	18
Folate (µg)	280	285	260	350
Vitamin B_{12} (µg)	2.6	1.2	2.0	2.5
Calcium (mg)	1200	1200	1250	1200
Magnesium (mg)	355	265	320	340
Iron (mg)	15	13	14.8	12–16
Zinc (mg)	19	15	13	18
Iodine (µg)	200	210	140	170

(a) First 6 months of lactation. (b) First 4 months of lactation. (c) No recommendation set.

FURTHER READING

1. Barrett J, Whittaker P, Williams J, Lind T. Absorption of non-haem iron from food during normal pregnancy. *BMJ* 1994; **309**: 79–83.
2. Dunne F, Walters B, Marshall T, Heath D. Pregnancy associated osteoporosis. *Clin Endocrin* 1993; **39**: 487–90.
3. Durnin JVGA. Energy requirements of pregnancy: an integration of the longitudinal data from the five country study. *Lancet* 1987; **2**: 1131–3.
4. Erick M. Battling morning (noon and night) sickness. New approaches for treating an age-old problem. *J Amer Dietet Assoc* 1994; **94**: 147–8.
5. Kalkwarf, H, Specker B. Bone mineral loss during lactation and recovery after weaning. *Obstet Gynecol* 1995; **86**: 26–32.
6. Prentice A, Goldberg G, Prentice A. Body mass index and lactation performance. *Eur J Clin Nutr* 1994; **48**: S78–S89.
7. Rees JM, Worthington-Roberts B. Position of the American Dietetic Association: nutrition care for pregnant adolescents. *J Am Dietet Assoc* 1994; **94**: 449–50.
8. Report of a Joint Food and Agriculture Organization/World Health Organization/United Nations University Expert Consultation. *Energy and protein requirements*. Geneva: WHO, 1985.
9. Semba R, Miotti P, Chiphangwi J, Saah A, Canner J, Callabetta G, et al. Maternal vitamin A deficiency and mother-to child transmission of HIV-1. *Lancet* 1994; **343**: 1593–7.

28
INFANT FEEDING
Donna Secker and Stanley Zlotkin

Interest in infant feeding centres around two principal objectives: the promotion of normal growth and brain development and the prevention of illness during the first years of life. Infants grow and develop rapidly in the first two years, making them particularly vulnerable to nutritional inadequacies. Breast-feeding followed by the introduction of a wide variety of solid foods provides the best opportunity for optimal growth and health during infancy. By two years of age, the infant should be consuming a variety of foods from the adult diet to ensure a nutritionally balanced intake.

It has been proposed that altering dietary patterns in infancy could reduce the risk of developing chronic illnesses such as premature atherosclerosis, hypertension, diabetes mellitus or obesity later in life. There is no scientific support for the effectiveness of this strategy primarily because it has never been shown that eating patterns or levels of serum cholesterol, blood pressure or body weight established in infancy persist into adulthood.

28.1 VALUE OF BREAST-FEEDING

Human milk is specifically composed to meet the nutritional requirements of the human infant and is considered the optimal nutrition source for healthy newborns, as well as many newborns with medical conditions. Breast-feeding provides immunological protection which is greatest during the early months, but increases with the duration of breast-feeding. Although more difficult to quantify, the psychological benefit of early and prolonged physical contact contributes to the development of a strong mother–infant bond. Other benefits include convenience, safety and cost. With the exception of vitamins D and K, breast milk produced by adequately nourished mothers provides all the nutrients needed by a normal healthy full-term infant for the first four to six months of life.

Recent studies have provided good evidence that even in developed countries breast-feeding protects against gastrointestinal and respiratory infections, reduces the risk of otitis media (inflammation of the middle ear), and reduces the incidence of food allergy in infants with a genetic predisposition. Breast-feeding does not appear to decrease the incidence of atopy (clinical forms of inherited hypersensitivity) in infants not at increased risk. There is also fair evidence that breast-feeding plays a role in preventing insulin-dependent diabetes mellitus (IDDM), particularly for those with genetic markers of increased risk. In addition, there is documentation that the mean values for cognitive development in populations of children who were breast-fed are slightly higher compared to bottle-fed infants from similar environments.

28.2   FORMULA-FEEDING

When an informed mother chooses not to breast-feed, the only acceptable alternative is a commercial infant formula. Manufacturers continue to modify their products in an effort to emulate human milk, and although they provide less than the optimal benefits of human milk they are nutritionally adequate for the first year of life. The standard formula choice is a cow's milk-based formula, containing skim milk powder, lactose and a variable blend of oils. Soy-based formulas made from soy protein, vegetable oils and glucose polymers ($\pm$ sucrose) are available for infants of vegetarian families, infants with galactosaemia or lactose intolerance, or those suspected to have an allergy to cow's milk protein. Lactose-free cow's milk-based formulas are also available for infants with lactose intolerance. 'Follow-on' or transition formulas are designed for the second six months of life and while nutritionally superior to cow's milk during this time, they provide no nutritional advantages over regular iron-fortified infant formulas. Homemade formulas from evaporated milk are nutritionally incomplete and are not recommended.

28.3   VITAMIN AND MINERAL SUPPLEMENTATION

With the exception of vitamins D and K, human milk from well-nourished mothers provides all the nutrients required for the first four to six months of life. Routine administration of intramuscular vitamin K at birth has eliminated vitamin K deficiency. Commercial infant formulas are fortified with vitamins and minerals. Therefore supplements are unnecessary.

28.3.1   Vitamin D

Human milk contains very little vitamin D. Therefore an additional source is recommended for exclusively breast-fed infants who may not be exposed to sunlight. Vitamin D needs will be met from occasional exposure to small amounts of sunlight, or prophylactic supplementation with 400 IU vitamin D/day. Infants at risk for vitamin D deficiency and the development of nutritional rickets are those who are dark-skinned, exclusively breast-fed, living at northern latitudes, or weaned to vegan diets. Naturally occurring dietary sources of vitamin D are rare (liver, oily fish), while only milk and margarine may be fortified with vitamin D in some countries. With increasing use of sunscreen and avoidance of sun exposure due to the risks of skin cancer, the potential for vitamin D deficiency may be higher.

28.3.2   Iron deficiency

Iron deficiency is most common among infants between the ages of 6–24 months. The major risk factors for iron deficiency anaemia in infants relate to socioeconomic status and include the early consumption of cow's milk, inadequate funds for appropriate foods, and poor knowledge of nutrition. Other high-risk groups include low birth weight and premature infants and older infants who drink large amounts of milk (1 litre/day) or juice and eat little solid food. The importance of preventing rather than treating anaemia

Box 28.1   Strategies for the prevention of iron deficiency anaemia

- Exclusive breast-feeding during the first 4–6 months
- Introduction of iron-fortified infant cereal, other iron-rich foods (e.g. strained meats) and enhancers of iron absorption (vitamin C, e.g. fruit) from 6 months
- Use of iron-fortified formula for infants weaned early from the breast or formula-fed from birth
- Delaying introduction of unmodified cow's milk until at least 9–12 months of age.

has been accentuated by findings that iron deficiency anaemia may be a risk factor for developmental delays in cognitive function and that this delay is irreversible with iron therapy and persists into early childhood (Box 28.1).

28.3.3   Fluoride

Fluoridation of the water supply has proven to be the most effective, cost-efficient means of preventing dental caries. In areas with low fluoride levels in the water source, fluoride supplements are recommended. The increased availability of fluoride (fluoridated water, foods or drinks made with fluoridated water, toothpaste, mouthwashes, vitamin and fluoride supplements) has resulted in an increasing incidence of very mild and mild forms of dental fluorosis in both fluoridated and non-fluoridated communities. This sign of excess fluoride intake has led to modifications in fluoride recommendations including later introduction and lower doses of fluoride supplements, and caution to parents of young children to use small amounts, and discourage swallowing of toothpaste. Dental fluorosis has not been shown to pose any health risks and while there may be mild cosmetic effects, the teeth remain resistant to caries.

28.4   COW'S MILK

The use of unmodified cow's milk before 9–12 months of age is not recommended. In comparison to human milk and iron fortified formula, cow's milk is higher in nutrients such as protein, calcium, phosphorus, sodium and potassium and significantly lower in iron, zinc, ascorbic acid, and linoleic acid (Table 28.1). Nutrients in solid foods emphasize these excesses and deficiencies, so that cow's milk-fed infants receive a higher renal solute load and are at greater risk of eating an unbalanced diet. In particular, the risk for iron depletion and iron deficiency anaemia is higher because the iron content of cow's milk is low and not readily bioavailable, and its absorption may be impaired by the high concentrations of calcium and phosphorus and low concentration of ascorbic acid in cow's milk. In addition, intestinal loss of (blood) iron in the stool is associated with cow's milk-feeding in the first 6–12 months of life. Reduced-fat milks should not be given before one year of age because of insufficient essential fatty acid content and the high renal solute load that the infant receives when he or she drinks larger volumes to satiate hunger.

Table 28.1 Nutrient content of human milk, formula and cow's milk per liter

Nutrient	Human milk Mature	Formula			Cow's milk 3.3% fat
		Cow's milk based[a]	Soy-based[a]	Follow-on[b]	
Energy (kcal)	750	670	670	670	640
Protein (g)	11	15	20	19	32
Fat (g)	45	36	37	30	36
Carbohydrate (g)	71	72	69	82	48
Sodium (mmol)	7	8	12	12	22
Potassium (mmol)	13	18	20	24	40
Chloride (mmol)	11	13	13	16	27
Vitamin D (µg)	<1	10	10	10	9[d]
Iron (mg)[c]	0.5	1.5/11	12.5	12	0.4

[a] Average value of 7 brands. [b] Average value of 3 brands. [c] Non-fortified/iron-fortified. [d] If fortified.

28.4.1 Association between cow's milk and incidence of diabetes

The aetiology of insulin-dependent diabetes mellitus (IDDM) appears to require both genetic predisposition to an autoimmune destructive process and exposure to environmental triggers. Several infant feeding practices have been investigated as possible environmental factors for genetically predisposed individuals, including early exposure to cow's milk protein (or early termination of breast-feeding) and solid food, and the ingestion of soy protein. The following cautionary recommendations have been issued:

(1) the endorsement of breast-feeding as the primary source of nutrition during the first year of life for all infants;

(2) for infants with a strong family history of IDDM, breast-feeding and avoidance of commercially available cow's milk and products containing intact cow's milk protein for the first year of life;

(3) for non-breast-fed infants, the use of commercial cow's milk-based infant formulas and the avoidance of soy-based formulas.

28.5   FRUIT JUICE

Infants may drink excessive amounts of fruit juice for a variety of reasons including their preferences, parental health beliefs, behavioural feeding difficulties, and financial limitations. If juice consumption decreases the infant's appetite for solid foods, energy and nutrient intakes (e.g. fat, protein, calcium, vitamin D, iron, zinc) can be inadequate, leading to poor weight gain, nutrient deficiencies and failure-to-thrive. Chronic diarrhoea can also occur in association with malabsorption of the juice's fructose and sorbitol and/or the low fat content of the infants' diets.

28.5.1   Nursing caries (decay)

The cause of extensive tooth decay in infants is multifactorial in nature and includes feeding practices such as putting an infant to bed with a bottle of carbohydrate-containing liquid (including milk or formula), the frequent use of pacifiers dipped in sugar, syrup or honey and bottle-feeding past 12 months of age. Acids produced by bacteria that ferment dietary carbohydrate attack the teeth (both erupted and non-erupted) particularly during sleep when saliva secretion is decreased. Infection or severe tooth decay may warrant tooth extraction. Early loss of primary teeth can lead to problems with speech articulation and chewing. Bedtime bottles are unnecessary but if used should contain only plain water.

28.6   INTRODUCTION OF SOLIDS

At some point in time exclusive breast-feeding no longer meets a growing infant's energy and nutrient needs and complementary foods must be added. These additional foods are not intended to replace or interfere with breast-feeding. The timing and type of complementary foods is variable, reflecting the numerous cultural foods and practices of society. Despite broad cultural diversity, most paediatric groups are fairly consistent in recommending that breast milk should be given exclusively for the first 4–6 months and that complementary food should be introduced after this time. Recommendations are based on issues related to nutritional need, physiological maturation, behavioural and developmental aspects of feeding, immunological safety and environmental influences. Most evidence suggests that introduction before two 2–3 months or later than 6 months has more risks than benefits.

Because infants require a good source of iron around 4–6 months of age, the most commonly used first food is iron-fortified infant cereal. Although the permeability of the infant's intestinal tract to foreign proteins has diminished by this age, it is considered practical to reduce the allergenic load as long as possible. Gluten, one of the more common allergens, is found in wheat, rye, oats and barley but not rice or maize. Therefore, for theoretical reasons, rice cereal is considered the most appropriate first cereal. Because each new food constitutes a potential allergic challenge, the introduction of one new food every two to three days is advised, using single rather than mixed foods initially. Infants at high risk for allergies are generally introduced to new foods more cautiously. Pureed or finely mashed vegetables and fruits are introduced next at 5–6 months; pureed meats, fish and poultry around 6–7 months of age. When an infant begins to make lateral motions of the jaw, chewing should be encouraged by increasing the texture of foods to included mashed table foods. An infant who is not encouraged to chew at this time may have trouble later accepting anything but fluids and purees. Between 9 and 12 months of age, finger foods should be introduced to encourage self-feeding. The size, shape and texture of the food should be considered because they influence the infant's ability to safely chew and swallow without choking (Table 28.2).

28.6.1   Food-related asphyxiation

The greatest risk of choking and aspiration on food occurs in children under the age of 4 months, with a significant peak in the 12–24 month age group. Small, round, smooth

Table 28.2 Introduction of solids

Age	Food	Reasons for introduction
4–6 months	• Iron-enriched infant cereal	Provides iron at a time when iron depletion may occur
6–9 months	• Pureed vegetables • Pure fruit and juices	Provides a sources of vitamins, minerals and energy Introduces new flavours. Starts good eating habits
	• Pureed meat, fish, poultry • Egg yolk • Yoghurt, cottage cheese • Pureed, cooked legumes	Provides additional protein vitamins and iron for rapid growth
	• Dried bread products	Encourages chewing when teeth erupt
9–12 months	• Mashed 'family' foods without sugar, fat, salt	Introduces textures
	• Finger foods such as peeled fruit pieces, cooked vegetable pieces, dry toast, mild cheese	Encourages chewing, coordination and independence
12 months	• Egg white	Earlier introduction might precipitate an allergy

foods such as smoked sausages, grapes, nuts, candies, raisins, seeds, peas, kernel corn and popcorn are most dangerous as they can slip prematurely into the pharynx and with a quick gasp for breath and drawn downward and become lodged in the airway. These foods are not recommended before 3–4 years of age unless they are cut into smaller pieces. Highly viscous foods, such as peanut butter, can plug the airway and should not be served by themselves. In addition to the shape and texture of foods, environmental factors such as distractions or inadequate supervision during eating increase the risk of food asphyxiation.

28.7 ASSESSING NUTRITIONAL ADEQUACY

In general, it is assumed that an infant's nutritional status is normal, and nutritional needs are being met, if he or she has a normal rate of growth, drinks adequate amounts of breast milk (or suitable formula or milk for age) and eats a variety of age-appropriate foods from each of the food groups. When nutritional status or growth is questionable the infant's intake should be evaluated in comparison to established national or FAO/WHO (Food and Agriculture Organization/World Health Organization) recommended nutrient intakes or allowances.

28.7.1 Energy and nutrient requirements

Due to their rapid rate of growth and higher metabolic rate, energy requirements for infants are higher than at any other time of life. Existing recommendations of 115 to

95 kcal/kg per day are based on intakes of healthy infants either breast-fed or formula-fed. Recent studies using the doubly labelled water technique have facilitated measurements of total energy expenditure of infants. Evidence from these studies suggest that current recommendations overestimate infants' energy requirements.

When an infant's energy requirements are met from a well-balanced diet the risk of other nutrient deficiencies is minimized. Intakes of individual nutrients which fall between 70–100% of recommended levels do not necessarily indicate a deficiency, as recommendations (with the exception of energy) are set at the mean requirement, plus two standard deviations to ensure that the needs of almost all infants are met.

28.7.2   Monitoring growth

Postnatal growth and central nervous system development are most rapid during the first year of life. The typical infant doubles his or her birth weight during the first four to five months and triples it in the first year. By two years of age a child has grown to half of their adult height. Plotting serial measurements of length-by-age and weight-by-length can be used to compare growth to normative values for healthy infants. Normal growth is indicated by weight-for-length and length-for-age tracking along similar percentiles or growth channels. When length-for-age and weight-for-length percentiles are disproportional or weight and/or height measurements cross more than two percentiles downwards, investigation of potential nutritional imbalances is indicated.

In interpreting an infant's growth, it is important to consider the data source for the growth chart used. The American National Center for Health Statistics Growth Charts (endorsed by WHO as the world-wide reference growth curves) are based on data collected primarily from formula-fed infants, or infants breast-fed for a short period of time. A recent cohort study has demonstrated that the growth rate of infants who have been breast-fed for more than three months is slower than that of formula-fed infants (or infants breast-fed for less than three months) from similar socioeconomic and ethnic backgrounds. Behavioural development, activity level and morbidity were not different between the groups of infants, suggesting the slower growth rate was of no nutritional significance. When this slower growth pattern of otherwise healthy and thriving breast-fed infants is misinterpreted as 'growth faltering' it can lead to unnecessary concern about the adequacy of breast-feeding, and interfere with the promotion of exclusive breast-feeding for the first four to six months of life. Until the best outcome measures are determined for assessing which growth rate is optimal, there is uncertainty about whether 'bigger is necessarily better'.

28.8   COMMON FEEDING PROBLEMS

28.8.1   Food allergies

Adverse food reactions are divided into two general categories: food intolerance and food allergy. A true allergic reaction to a food involves the body's immune system. In the paediatric population estimates of prevalence range from 1% to 8%, with the highest frequency in the first year of life. The risk of developing food allergies is largely related to genetic predisposition and the age at which the food is introduced, with the chance of sensitization greatest in the first year of life. Young infants are especially prone because their immature intestinal system is more permeable to absorption of food allergens and lacks local immunity defences. Most allergens are proteins of large molecular size. Therefore, food allergy commonly presents in infancy with the first introduction of milk, egg or peanuts. Along with soy, nuts and wheat these foods are responsible for about 95% of food allergies in infants and toddlers. It is rare for an infant to have allergies to more than two or three foods.

Management of food allergies involves strict avoidance of the allergenic food and requires careful reading of food labels to detect hidden sources. Sensitivity to many foods disappears within a few years, therefore retesting and rechallenging with the offending food should occur at regular intervals. Allergies to peanuts, nuts, fish and seafood are the most severe and tend to be life-long (Box 28.2).

28.8.2 Cow's milk protein allergy

Cow's milk protein is the most important food allergy trigger in infancy with estimations of prevalence ranging from 1–5%. The decision of which formula to use should consider the type and severity of the allergic reaction to cow's milk protein. Studies have revealed that 15–50% of milk sensitive infants also react to soy. However, in questionable or mild reactions to cow's milk protein, soy formulas may be tried as they are less expensive and more palatable than the alternatives. High-risk infants or highly allergic infants should be cautiously fed a formula containing cow's milk protein hydrolysates in which the proteins are extensively reduced in size. Rare reactions to these formulas have been reported in highly allergic infants who are then fed elemental formulas. Newer formulas with partially hydrolyzed protein are less expensive and more palatable than the hypoallergenic hydrolysate formulas. However, they contain a significant percentage ($\sim$20%) of peptides in the allergenic range. Although they may be useful for infants not known to be at risk they should not be used for infants who have already developed cow's milk protein allergy. Goat's milk has some similar antigens to cow's milk and is not recommended.

28.8.3 Lactose intolerance

The majority of adverse reactions to foods do not involve the immune system and are known as 'food intolerance'. The most common food intolerance in infants is lactose

Box 28.2 Strategies for reducing the incidence and severity of allergy in high-risk infants

- Prolonged breast-feeding
- Prolonged breast-feeding plus maternal avoidance of commonly allergenic foods during pregnancy and lactation
- Use of protein hydroysate formulas in non-breast-fed infants
- Delayed introduction of solids until at least 4 months, and preferably 6 months, especially for foods that are hyperallergenic

intolerance. Congenital lactase deficiency is extremely rare while primary hypolactasia is more common due to a normal developmental decrease in lactase activity. Lactose intolerance can develop in infants secondary to intestinal mucosal damage caused by gastroenteritis, malnutrition, cow's milk protein enteropathy, coeliac disease, giardiasis, bacterial overgrowth, inflammatory bowel disease, or drugs. Common symptoms include gas, cramps and explosive diarrhoea. Diagnosis is best obtained using the non-invasive breath-hydrogen test. Infants with lactose intolerance should be changed from a cow's milk formula to either a lactose-free cow's milk formula or a soy formula. Infants beyond 9–12 months of age can be given cow's milk treated with β-galactosidase (LactAid®) or a soy milk fortified with vitamin D. Infants with primary intolerance may be able to tolerate small amounts of lactose-containing foods. Following secondary intolerance, re-introduction of small amounts of lactose should be tried at regular intervals to return to a balanced diet as soon as possible.

28.8.4   Dietary management of acute diarrhoea

In developed countries, the typical infant with acute diarrhoea is well nourished, presents with mild to moderate dehydration and has a viral-induced diarrhoea with low electrolyte losses. In developing countries, children with acute diarrhoea are more likely to be malnourished and severely dehydrated with a bacterial-induced diarrhoea with high electrolyte losses. Oral rehydration therapy (ORT) which combines the use of oral electrolyte solutions (OES) with early refeeding has proven to be safe and efficacious for restoring and maintaining hydration and electrolyte balance in infants with mild and moderate dehydration, including those with vomiting. Oral electrolyte solutions containing specific concentrations of carbohydrate, sodium, potassium and chloride promote fluid and electrolyte absorption while fluids such as juices, soft drinks, tea, jello or broth do not. Human milk is well tolerated during diarrhoea and may reduce its severity and duration; therefore breast-feeding should continue throughout the diarrhoea with additional fluids given as OES. Early and rapid refeeding should occur as soon as rehydration is achieved and vomiting stops (ideally within 6–12 hours of beginning treatment) as infants treated with ORT and early refeeding have reduced stool output, shorter duration of diarrhoea, and improved weight gain. Routine change to lactose-free or diluted feedings is unnecessary in well-nourished infants with mild to moderate gastroenteritis. Factors that appear to increase the risk of developing lactose intolerance include younger age, malnutrition, bacterial diarrhoea, prolonged diarrhoea before treatment, and a greater degree of dehydration on assessment. Starchy foods are well tolerated as the initial foods for refeeding. Use of a low-residue diet (commonly called the BRAT diet: bananas, rice, applesauce or apple juice, and tea or toast) can theoretically worsen the clinical state as it supplies less than one-half of an infant's daily energy and protein needs.

28.8.5   Constipation

Breast-fed and non-breast-fed infants receiving an adequate diet are rarely constipated. When constipation occurs during infancy, it is usually due to inadequate intake of fluids or carbohydrate. Guidelines for the dietary management of constipation in infants less than six months old include ensuring an adequate fluid intake ($\geqslant 150$ ml/kg) and increasing carbohydrate intake by adding 10–20 g of sucrose or dextrose per litre of fluid feeding. In addition to the above, small amounts of prune juice and/or increasing the cereal, fruit and vegetable (fibre) content of the diet may be helpful for infants older than six months.

28.8.6 Fat intake

Dietary fat modifications recommended for adults are not applicable to infants. In contrast, a high fat diet ($\sim 50\%$ of energy from fat) helps to meet the infants requirements for energy and fatty acids. Restricting dietary fat may lead to inadequate energy intake and jeopardize growth and development. There is no consistent evidence that use of a fat-reduced, cholesterol-lowering diet in infancy decreases the risk of atherosclerosis in adulthood.

28.8.7 Vegetarianism

While the low saturated fat and high fibre content of vegetarian diets offers advantages to the health of adults, their bulky nature and low energy-density can restrict the amount of food energy that infants (with their limited stomach capacity and higher needs for accelerated growth) can consume. With careful planning, a properly selected vegetarian diet can meet all requirements of growing infants and children. However, the risk of nutritional deficiencies increases if the variety of foods making up the diet is very restrictive (e.g. macrobiotic, Rastafarian), and/or if supplementation and medical supervision is avoided.

Most vegetarians will continue breast-feeding well into the second year of life. Problems of nutritional inadequacy in the infant (e.g. vitamin B_{12}) are likely to occur if the mother's diet is very restricted, if prolonged breast-feeding is not supplemented around 4–6 months of age, or if infants are prematurely weaned on to an unsuitable breast milk substitute. Vegan infants who are weaned from the breast before 1 year of age should receive a commercial soy formula.

In infants consuming a macrobiotic diet, a clear relationship has been demonstrated between diet, nutrient intake and physical and biochemical evidence of deficiency for several nutrients including iron, vitamins B_{12}, D, and riboflavin. Slower growth rates (peaking between 6–18 months) and higher incidence of nutritional diseases such as rickets, kwashiorkor and anaemia have been reported. Macrobiotic diets consist of unpolished rice, pulses and vegetables with small additions of fermented foods, nuts, seeds and fruits; animal products are not consumed. Even less restricted vegetarian diets typically have a high content of phytates and other modifiers of mineral (e.g. iron, zinc, calcium) absorption which are associated with a higher prevalence of rickets and iron deficiency anaemia.

FURTHER READING

1. American Academy of Pediatrics. Infant feeding practices and their possible relationship to the etiology of diabetes mellitus. *Pediatrics* 1994; 94: 752–4.

2. Bock A, Atkins F. Patterns of food hypersensitivity during sixteen years of double-blind placebo controlled food challenges. *J Pediatr* 1990; **117**: 561–7.

3. Brown KJ, Peerson JM, *et al*. Use of nonhuman milks in the dietary management of young children with acute diarrhea: a meta-analysis of clinical trials. *Pediatrics* 1994; **93**: 17–27.

4. Davies PSW, Ewing G, Lucas A. Energy expenditure in early infancy. *Brit J Nutr* 1989; **62**: 621–9.

5. Dewey KG, Heinig MJ, Nommsen LA, Peerson JM, Lonnderdal B. Growth of breast-fed and formula-fed infants from 0 to 18 Months: The DARLING Study. *Pediatrics* 1992; **89**: 1035–41.

6. Feightner JW. Prevention of iron deficiency anemia in infants. In: *The Canadian guide to clinical preventative health care*. Canadian Task Force on The Periodic Health Examination. Ottawa: Health Canada, 1004: 244–55.

7. Hendricks KM, Badruddin SH. Weaning recommendations: the scientific basis. *Nutr Rev* 1992; **50**: 125–33.

8. Jacobs C, Dwyer JT. Vegetarian children: appropriate and inappropriate diets. *Am J Clin Nutr* 1988; **48**: 811–8.

9. US Department of Health Human and Services. Management of acute diarrhea. Oral rehydration, maintenance and nutritional therapy. *Morbidity and Mortality Weekly Report* (MMWR) 1992; **41**(RR-16): 1–20.

10. Rogan WJ, Gladen BC. Breast-feeding and cognitive development. *Early Human Develop* 1993; **31**: 181–93.

11. Stallings Harris C, Baker SP, Smith GA, Harris RM. Childhood asphyxiation by food. A national analysis and overview. *JAMA* 1984; **251**: 2231–5.

12. Wang EL. Breast feeding. In: *The Canadian guide to clinical preventative health care*. Canadian Task Force on the Periodic Health Examination. Ottawa: Health Canada, 1994: 232–43.

CHILDHOOD AND ADOLESCENCE

29.1 CHILDHOOD

Cynthia Tuttle

Childhood is usually regarded as the period between 2 and 10 years. The linear growth of pre-pubertal children occurs at a relatively constant rate of about 6 cm per year. The median heights and weights of girls and boys are very similar; they increase from approximately 87 cm and 12 kg at age 2 years, to approximately 137 cm and 32 kg at age 10 years. However, individual children may show considerable variation because some children grow faster than others. Even in childhood, boys tend to have slightly greater lean tissue mass (kg) and a lower proportion of body fat than girls.

Children are a potentially vulnerable group since they are entirely dependent upon parents or caregivers for all nutritional needs. Inadequate intakes of energy and essential nutrients may compromise growth and development to an extent which may have lasting consequences. In many developing countries such malnutrition is still widespread (see Chapter 17). However, in most relatively affluent societies where a wide variety of foods are available, growth and development usually occurs quite satisfactorily without detailed dietary advice. Obesity, rather than undernutrition, is the major nutrition-related disorder. An important consideration is that eating habits determined in childhood may be important determinants of chronic disease in later life.

29.1.1 Monitoring growth and development

A child's growth is assessed primarily by monitoring height and weight. A number of different growth charts are available. Those based on data from the United States National Center for Health Statistics (NCHS) are widely recommended for both children and adolescents (aged 2–18 years) because data collection procedures were well standardized and fully documented and the large and representative population attained their full growth potential (see Fig. 29.1). Longitudinal data from the Fels Research Institute were utilized to devise appropriate charts for infants from birth to 36 months. These charts are based on nude weights and recumbent lengths. There are several limitations including that the serial measurements were based on a relatively small number (720) of middle class white infants and the majority of these infants were predominantly formula-fed. As there are discrepancies between the growth velocities of breast-fed and formula-fed infants it has not yet been established with certainty whether these charts are appropriate

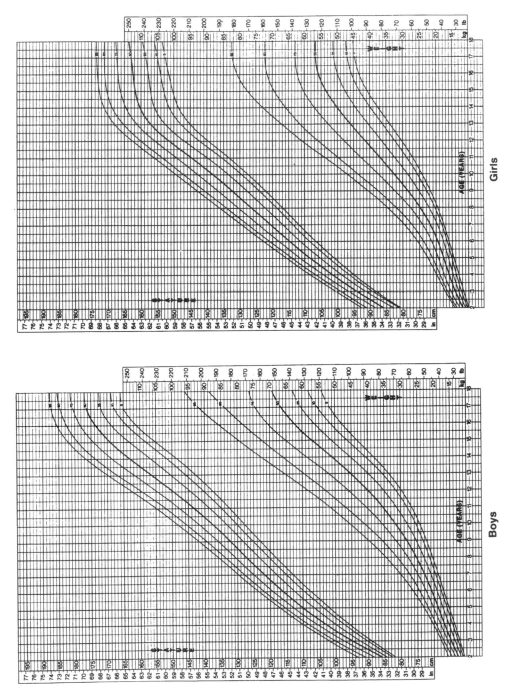

Fig. 29.1 Growth charts for boys and girls aged 2–18 years. *Source: Children are different: developmental physiology.* 2nd ed. Johston TR, Moore WM, Jeffries JE (eds). Columbus, Ohio: Ross Laboratories 1978; 20–1.

for monitoring the growth of breast-fed infants. Growth velocity charts based on longitudinal data, in which the same children are measured at regular intervals have also been constructed for older children and adolescents. These are useful adjuncts to the NCHS charts based on cross-sectional data which may provide unreliable assessments at the individual level because of the variable ages at which growth spurts occur (see Fig. 29.2).

29.1.2 Energy requirements and macronutrient intakes

Energy requirements for childhood are given in Table 29.1. Requirements differ accord-ing to body size and composition, growth rate and level of physical activity but in most societies, provided dietary guidelines are followed, the healthy child is usually the best judge of how much to eat. A controversial aspect of nutritional recommendations in this age group concerns the intake of fat, an important energy source in childhood. The increasing rate of obesity in young children (see Section 29.1.4) and the concern that habitual use of high fat foods in childhood may lead to a retention of this practice in later life and consequently an increased risk of coronary heart disease have led to the

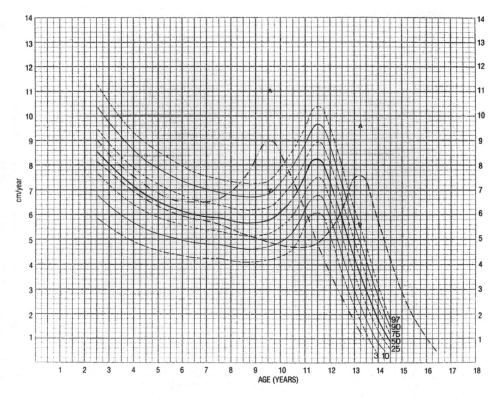

Fig. 29.2 Height velocity for girls.
Source: Tanner J, Davis PSW. *J Pediat* 1985; **107** (used with permission.)

Table 29.1 Estimated average energy requirements for chidren aged 3–10 years

Age (yrs)	Average weight (kg)		Intake/kg of body weight (kJ[kcal]/kg/day)		Estimated average requirements (MJ[kcal]/day)	
	Boys	Girls	Boys	Girls	Boys	Girls
3	15.3	14.9	405 [97]	384 [92]	6.23 [1490]	5.73 [1370]
4	17.0	16.8	395 [94]	365 [87]	6.73 [1520]	6.12 [1460]
5	19.3	18.9	370 [88]	345 [82]	7.19 [1720]	6.48 [1550]
6	21.7	21.3	350 [84]	320 [76]	7.57 [1810]	6.77 [1620]
7	24.2	23.8	325 [78]	295 [71]	7.92 [1890]	7.05 [1680]
8	26.8	26.6	305 [73]	275 [66]	8.24 [1970]	7.28 [1740]
9	29.7	29.7	290 [69]	255 [61]	8.55 [2040]	7.51 [1790]

Source: World Health Organization. *Energy and protein requirements*. Report of a joint FAO/WHO/UNU meeting. Technical report series 724. Geneva: WHO, 1985.

suggestion that intake of fat should be reduced in childhood. The counter-argument suggests that a low fat diet in childhood may provide insufficient energy for normal growth and development. The recommendation of several expert committees is that fat intake should be gradually reduced after the age of 2 years so that by the age of 5 years fat should provide around 30–35% total energy, approximately that recommended for adults. Reduced fat milks (2%) and milk products are not recommended until after the age of 2 years, and lower fat varieties only after the age of 5 years. The early acquisition of persisting dietary practices and the beginning of fatty streaks and plaques in the arteries of children provide cogent arguments for the introduction of diets low in saturated fatty acids as early as possible.

There is also debate as to whether children should have a high fibre intake. A high fibre diet may enhance satiety to an extent that total energy intake, and consequently growth, will be compromised. There have been reports of children failing to achieve their growth potential as a result of excessive intakes of fibre-rich carbohydrate but there is no convincing evidence to suggest that the problem is a widespread one. During childhood, carbohydrate should provide 40–50% total energy. A variety of fruits, vegetables, breads and cereals are advised since they provide a range of essential micronutrients and dietary fibre as well as carbohydrate. Sucrose and other extrinsic sugars are acceptable in moderate amounts but should, when possible, be consumed with meals (see Section 29.1.5). Added fibre (bran) and fibre-enriched breakfast cereals and breads are not recommended in childhood because in addition to the satiety-inducing properties the absorption of calcium, zinc and iron may be reduced.

Adequate protein intakes are readily achieved by children in relatively affluent countries following dietary guidelines.

29.1.3 Vitamin and mineral issues in childhood

Recommended intakes for some important nutrients for children are shown in Tables 29.2 and 29.3. While specific nutrient deficiencies in childhood are widespread

Table 29.2   Selected reference nutrient intakes for children

Age (yrs)	Vit. A (µg retinol/ day)	Folate (µg/day)	Vit. C (mg/day)	Vit. D (µg/day)	Calcium (mg/day)	Iron (mg/day)	Zinc (mg/day)
1–3	400	70	30	7	350	6.9	5.0
4–6	500	100	30	–	450	6.1	6.5
7–10	500	150	30	–	550	8.7	7.0

Source: Dietary Reference Values for Food Energy and Nutrients for the United Kingdom, 1991.

Table 29.3   Age-adjusted prevalence of overweight in children 6–11 years from national surveys in the United States

Dates	Boys		Girls	
	85th percentile	95th percentile	85th percentile	95th percentile
1963–5 (NHES)	15.2	5.2	15.2	5.2
1971–4 (NHANES I)	18.2	6.5	13.9	4.3
1976–80 (NHANES II)	19.9	7.9	15.8	7.0
1988–95 (NHANES III)	22.3	10.8	22.7	10.7

NHES, National Health Examination Survey; NHANES, National Health and Nutrition Examination Surveys. Adapted with permission from Troiano RP, Flegal KM, Kuczmarski RJ, Campbell SM, Johnston CL. Overweight prevalence and trends for children and adolescents. *Arch Pediatr Adolesc Med* 1995; **149**: 1085–91.

throughout the developing world, the majority of children in most relatively affluent countries can achieve all their nutrient needs by following dietary guidelines and eating an adequate number of servings from each food group (see Chapter 33). However, when food choice is restricted for any reason, and especially among those families who are at socioeconomic disadvantage, there may be a risk of developing a deficiency of one or more nutrients. For example, in New Zealand iron deficiency anaemia appears to be relatively common amongst Maori and Pacific Island children. The relative importance of infection and iron deficiency in causing this problem has not been established. Nevertheless, in public health nutrition programmes in such communities it is important to monitor iron intake and status and to ensure adequate intakes of haem iron and/or enhance bioavailability from breads and cereals (see Chapter 9).

Children who consume two to three servings each day of milk and milk products (e.g. yoghurt and cheese) should achieve sufficient calcium intakes. True milk allergy is rare and when it does occur, usually disappears by 3 years of age. These children may require fortified soy products. Children who refuse milk often eat milk products (e.g. yoghurt, custard, cheese). Canned fish with bones (sardines, salmon), whole grain cereals, beans, nuts, green vegetables and tofu are alternative sources of calcium, although calcium from plant sources may be less bioavailable than from dairy foods where the presence of lactose enhances calcium absorption.

29.1.4   Childhood obesity

Childhood obesity appears to be increasing in some countries (Table 29.4). Transient overweight in early childhood is probably not an important health issue but when obesity persists throughout childhood there may be important consequences. Obesity may contribute towards a distorted sense of self-worth and body image and tension at school and at home. Obesity continuing throughout childhood may continue into adolescence and adult life. Overall development may be adversely effected. Genetic factors, physical inactivity and excessive food intake are important causative factors. Encouraging a general increase in physical activity and a reduction in energy-dense convenience foods and confectionery products are the cornerstone of management. A social and physiological environment which encourages such behaviour patterns also provide the best means of avoiding obesity. Rigid weight-reducing diets are not suitable for children (see also Chapter 16).

29.1.5   Dental caries

Dental caries (or decay) usually begins in the enamel on the tooth surface, but may progressively destroy the hard tissues of the teeth. In many countries, about half of 5-year-olds experience some tooth decay. Dental caries are appreciably reduced by fluoridation of water supplies, topical applications of fluoride and regular brushing of teeth with a fluoride toothpaste (see Chapter 10.5). The prevalence is usually highest among families of low socioeconomic status. Frequency and manner of consumption of foods rich in sucrose and other non-milk extrinsic sugars appear to be important determinants of dental caries. Drinks containing sugars sipped over a long period of time and sweet foods nibbled gradually rather than consumed straightaway appear to be major contributors to the development of dental caries, especially when such foods are consumed in between meals and before bed. Therefore, children should be encouraged to have sweet foods at meal times. Water is the preferred drink at bedtime. Sugar-free medications are usually available and are especially important if used in the long-term and at night before bedtime. There is not convincing evidence that total amount of sugars consumed is related to dental caries. Starch appears to be associated with dental caries risk only when finely ground, heat treated and eaten frequently but the impact is less than that associated with sucrose and other non-milk extrinsic sugars.

29.1.6   Other nutrition-related health issues in childhood

The perception of food allergy amongst parents is sometimes a reason for withholding foods from children. A true food allergy is relatively uncommon and results from an immune response to a specific food protein which may cause asthma, diarrhoea, vomiting, abdominal pain, urticaria (hives), eczema or possibly irritability and hyperactivity. A food intolerance may cause similar symptoms without producing an immune response. Skin testing may be helpful in diagnosing allergies but a careful diet history, elimination and re-introduction of the suspected food are usually essential components of the investigation of a child believed to have a food allergy. Milk, wheat, eggs and maize are considered to be the most frequent causes of this relatively uncommon problem, but allergies to chocolate, oranges, soy products, legumes, fish, beef, pork, strawberries and peanuts have been reported. Peanut allergy differs from most of the others in that the reaction can be serious, sometimes even fatal.

A number of children nowadays are vegetarians or even vegans through their own choice or because their parents have chosen these dietary practices for them. Vegetarian children, who usually consume dairy products and eggs, though not meat, fish or food products derived from them, can fairly readily achieve adequate intakes of energy and essential nutrients. However, vegan children who also exclude eggs and dairy products may have considerable difficulty in achieving sufficient energy and sufficient amounts of vitamin B_{12}, iron, calcium and zinc. Their diets require careful planning and sometimes supplementation with additional quantities of these essential nutrients. There is some evidence that vegan children do not achieve their full growth potential even if they do not show clinical evidence of nutrient deficiencies.

Some foods, or substances in foods, have been associated with behavioural problems in children, especially with hyperactivity. Salicylates, nitrates and some other preservatives and food colourings have been implicated. Elimination and rechallenge diets may have a role in the investigation of such problems but a full clinical assessment is also essential to exclude other causes of hyperactivity and behavioural problems.

29.1.7 Eating patterns in childhood

The likelihood that dietary practices acquired and established in childhood will persist in later life is probably the most important justification for promoting dietary guidelines in childhood since most children in affluent societies are healthy most of the time and achieve adequate adult height. The traditional situation in which the mother provides all, or most, of a child's food at home has been eroded. Nowadays, both parents are often at work all day and there is considerable reliance on convenience foods at home, at school and after school, snacking throughout the day and fast food. Among many young parents the skill of attractively presenting appropriate foods has been lost and for children the lure of high fat, sugary, energy-dense and nutrient-poor foods and confectionery advertised on televi- sion by fast food chains and confectionery manufacturers has become overwhelming. Skipping breakfast has been identified as a growing problem among school-age children because it appears that they may not compensate for that loss of energy and nutrients at other meals. Many schools are also now selling foods, often of poor nutritional quality, for the express purpose of generating revenue. Establishing appropriate nutrition education in schools and for young parents represent a great challenge for practising nutritionists.

FURTHER READING

1. Department of Health. *The diets of British schoolchildren*. London: HMSO, 1989.
2. Gregory JR, Collins LD, Davies PS, *et al. National diet and nutrition survey: children aged* $1\frac{1}{2}$ *to* $4\frac{1}{2}$ *years*. Vol 1: Report of the diet and nutrition survey. London: HMSO, 1995.
3. National Health and Medical Research Council. *Dietary guidelines for children and adolescents*. Canberra: Australian Government Publishing Service, 1995.

29.2 ADOLESCENCE

Stewart Truswell

Biologically, adolescence is the time of life when growth is completed and individuals become sexually mature. The timing of the growth spurt and the onset of sexual function which occur at the start of adolescence, vary considerably between individuals. This can cause unhappiness and embarrassment in those who develop behind or in front of the main group of their peers. Adolescence may be taken as usually between 13 and 17 years in girls and between 15 and 21 years in boys. This means that in a co-educational school, at 13–14 years the girls are adolescents but not yet the boys, while in a place of work or college people of 19 years are adults if they are female and still adolescents if they are male (i.e. their growth is not yet completed).

Between the ages of 10 and 20 years lean body mass goes up from (average) 25–63 kg in boys and 22–42 kg in girls. Body fat goes from (average) 7–9 kg in boys and from 5–14 kg in girls. Total body calcium goes from about 300 g in both boys and girls to over 1000 g in boys and 750 g in girls.

There are of course social as well as biological aspects of adolescence:

- Young people assume the major control over what they choose to eat.
- They are intensely involved with the opinions and activities of their peers.
- They come under pressure to drink alcohol, to smoke (or not smoke), and to experiment with psychotropic drugs.
- They may be persuaded that the ideal body shape is very thin or they may aim for athletic achievement.
- They are not interested in food and nutrition except as part of a cult or fashion. They often feel the need to adopt different food habits from their parents.

29.2.1 Energy intakes

Many adolescents for a time eat more than at any other stage in their lives, more than the adult members of their families. This big energy intake has been recorded in many different countries by the methods described in Chapter 25. In girls, the growth spurt (peak height velocity) is usually around age 12 years and peak energy intakes have been recorded between 11 and 18 years. In boys, peak height velocity is usually around 14 years and highest energy intakes have been recorded between 13 and 18 years. Only a small proportion of the extra food is needed to provide the energy for growth, which is estimated to be 5.6 kcal (23.4 kJ)/gram of weight gain and corresponds to only about 1% of energy intake at 15 years. The extra energy is evidently used for the typical high level of physical activity of these young people who are at nearly adult size but more active than most adults. These energy intakes correspond quite well with recent measurements of energy expenditure using the doubly labelled water method (Chapter 5). However, there is a tendency for adolescent females and males to under-record their food intakes and presumably they either forget some snack foods or drinks or they would be embarrassed to write down such a large intake. Physical activity ratios (i.e. total energy expenditure/BMR) from the (so far limited) doubly labelled water studies are high at around 1.85 in adolescent males and 1.7 in adolescent females, higher than in adults. (In the typical housewife in Table 5.7 this ratio was 1.5 × BMR.)

Table 29.4 United Kingdom nutrient intakes for calcium and iron (1991) and mean energy intakes by IDECG (1996)

Age (yrs)	Energy (MJ)[a]		Calcium (mg)[b]		Iron (mg)[b]	
	Boys	Girls	Boys	Girls	Boys	Girls
7–10	8.2	7.3	550	550	8.7	8.7
11–14	10.2	8.4	1000	800	11.3	14.8
15–18	11.7	8.6	1000	800	11.3	14.8
Adults (19–50)	Around 13	Around 10	700	700	8.7	14.8

[a] Mean energy intakes for 17–18 years and energy expenditures of adults from Scrimshaw NS, Waterlow JC and Schürch B. Energy and protein requirements. *Eur J Clin Nutr* 1996; 50 (suppl. 1).
[b] Reference nutrient intakes for calcium and iron from Dietary Reference Values for Food Energy and Nutrients for the United Kingdom, 1991.

29.2.2 Inactivity and slimming

While the average adolescent is physically active, a minority have low energy intakes. Either they are trying to slim or they are not interested in sport or other exercise. In affluent communities up to half (and sometimes more) of adolescent females reply to questionnaires that they have dieted to lose weight and up to 20% of adolescent girls can be graded 'underweight', although mostly not seriously so. There is much less restrained eating and underweight in adolescent boys.

There are three important consequences of low energy intakes in adolescent girls:

1. They may not achieve their requirement for iron, which approximately doubles with the onset of menstruation especially if they avoid meat: 9% of 15-year-old girls in an Australian survey had subnormal plasma ferritin (see Chapter 9).

2. They may not achieve their requirement for calcium, which is increased at the time that bones should be elongating with linear growth (see Table 29.3). The result of this may be a relatively low peak bone mass which is thought to be a risk factor for osteoporosis in later life.

3. They may not achieve their full genetic potential in height, especially if they use cigarette smoking as a way of controlling food intake.

29.2.3 Severe eating disorders

Adolescent girls are the subgroup of the population in which anorexia nervosa and bulimia nervosa most commonly occur in affluent countries; their incidences average around 1%. These disorders are described in Chapter 21, in which Dr Fairburn observes that 'whilst dieting is common, few people develop an eating disorder'.

Overweight and obesity occur in a small percentage of adolescents, male and female. The policy for this excess adiposity in adolescents should stress the great value of regular, enjoyable exercise rather than restricting food before growth is completed. The exercise doesn't have to be competitive team sport but can be dancing, aerobics, walking, ice skating, cycling, etc. Overweight at this age too is a challenge for prevention of obesity later on. Prevention of obesity is much easier than cure. (Obesity and overweight are dealt with systematically in Chapter 16.)

29.2.4 Food and drink habits of adolescents

Several facets of eating behaviour are different or more pronounced in adolescents than at other ages and can cause concern or annoyance in the older members of their family:

* Missing meals, especially breakfast
* Eating snacks and confectionery
* Eating 'fast', take-away meals
* Eating unconventional meals—combinations of foods that other members of the family do not approve of
* Distinctive likes and dislikes for foods
* High consumption of soft drinks
* The start of alcohol consumption

Alcohol consumption is the most dangerous of the new food habits. The combination of inexperience with drinking alcohol and inexperience with car driving can be lethal! Although nutritionists may disapprove of soft drinks as not as nutritious as milk or as containing too much sugar, these objections are trivial against the risk of drink driving by adolescents.

It has been common for the older generation to complain about the bad food habits of adolescents yet these young people are in general more physically fit than their parents and are often growing taller. Their unconventional food habits are a response to the loosening of structure in their lifestyle, to experimentation; the need to assert themselves and response to peer pressure. They generally, with their parents' help, manage to combine enough of the essential nutrients in their own individual way.

Adolescence is a transitional stage. In a few years' time the young person will usually be living with a partner or spouse. They will have to work out a compromise set of food habits with him or her and settle down to re-establish the eating behaviour of a new family. It is at this stage that education about nutrition for health has more chance of an impact than during adolescence.

FURTHER READING

1. Crawley H. The energy, nutrient and food intakes of teenagers 16–17 in Britain. *Brit J Nutr* 1993; 70: 15–26.
2. Crawley H, Shergill-Bonner R. The nutrient and food intakes of 16–17 yr old female dieters. *J Hum Nutr Diet* 1995; 8: 25–34.
3. Department of Health. *The diets of British schoolchildren*. London: HMSO, 1989.
4. Moynihan DJ, *et al.* Dietary sources of iron in English adolescents. *J Hum Nutr* 1994; 7: 225–230.
5. National Health and Medical Research Council. *Dietary guidelines for children and adolescents*. Canberra: Australian Government Publishing Service, 1995.
6. Scrimshaw NS, Waterslow JC, Schürch B. Energy and protein requirements. Proceedings of an IDECG Workshop. *Eur J Clin Nutr* 1996; 50: (suppl. 1).
7. Truswell AS, Darnton-Hill I. Food habits of adolescents. *Nutr Revs* 1981; 39: 73–88.

30
SPORTS NUTRITION

Christine Thomson

Nutrition is the basis for supplying and regulating energy in all forms of physical activity and can play a significant role in optimizing performance. General nutritional goals are those for maintaining good health as well as specific needs of athletes for training and competition. There are no magic foods or supplements which on their own promote sports performance or substitute for a nutritionally balanced diet. However, in some circumstances diet may play a greater role, such as in endurance exercise, and for the female athlete, and where there is a need to control weight and body composition.

30.1 THE TRAINING DIET

Probably the most significant impact that sports nutrition has on performance is indirectly by allowing athletes to train to their optimal level and therefore to reach full potential through training. A poorly nourished athlete will not be able to continue with a strenuous programme, thus hindering endurance and performance.

The training diet must contain adequate energy and carbohydrate to sustain training, but also adequate intakes of all other nutrients; iron and calcium are most likely to be critical. For most athletes with large daily energy expenditures and food intakes, selection of a balanced varied diet should ensure nutrient intakes in excess of even the highest estimated needs. However, those who restrict daily energy intake to less than 8.4 MJ (2000 kcal) must eat more carefully to meet recommended levels of some micronutrients. The training diet should follow general nutrition guidelines, but greater emphasis may be placed on different nutrients for athletes participating in different sports events.

30.1.1 Energy

The major nutritional consideration for athletes is an increased requirement for energy to compensate for the increased expenditure through exercise. The extent of the increase will depend on body size, age, sex, type of sport and training volume, intensity and frequency. Inadequate energy intake can lead to chronic fatigue, weight loss, and impaired physical performance.

30.1.2 Carbohydrate

Dietary guidelines (see Chapter 33) recommend that all individuals eat plenty of high carbohydrate and fibre foods to maintain a healthy weight and to protect against cardiovascular disease. However, for athletes, carbohydrates have more immediate benefits for exercise performance through maximization of muscle glycogen stores. Carbohydrate is the major fuel for moderate to high intensity exercise. Research has shown a direct relationship between the level of muscle glycogen at the beginning of exercise and capacity for endurance, and that glycogen synthesis after exercise is directly related to the amount of dietary carbohydrate. A high carbohydrate training diet should therefore enhance endurance performance.

The benefits of maximizing glycogen stores immediately before endurance competition have received a lot of attention, and procedures will be outlined in Section 30.2.1. Of perhaps greater importance is the maintenance of glycogen stores of endurance athletes in daily training, as the ability to sustain prolonged intensive sessions on successive days will depend on how well the muscle glycogen levels are restored between sessions. Dietary carbohydrate intake of athletes in general training programmes should contribute 50–65% of total energy. However, endurance athletes undertaking several hours of training daily may need 500–600 g carbohydrate daily or 8–10 g/kg body weight. Some carbohydrate should be consumed as soon as possible after training sessions as this has been shown to enhance glycogen resynthesis.

30.1.3   Protein

Athletes engaged in strength and power events have traditionally consumed high protein intakes, believing that they are necessary for muscle synthesis. The conventional scientific view has been that protein needs of athletes do not differ significantly from those of non-exercising individuals, but research during the past two decades indicates that endurance and weight-lifting exercise significantly alters protein metabolism resulting in greater requirements.

During endurance exercise protein may contribute 5–10% of the energy expended, and somewhat more if muscle glycogen stores are depleted. Therefore, protein needs are higher than recommended dietary intakes. Similarly, strength athletes attempting to increase muscle mass have greater protein needs, particularly during the initial period of weight-training and muscle building. Current recommendations are for daily protein intakes of 1.2–1.4 g/kg body weight for endurance athletes, and 1.4–1.8 g/kg for strength and speed athletes.

In practical terms, athletes already consume 1.2–2.0 g/kg body weight per day because of their high energy intakes so the protein needs of all athletes are easily met by a mixed diet which supplies 12–15% of total energy as protein and adequate energy. Although a diet deficient in protein will lead to loss of muscle tissue, there is little evidence that excess protein will result in greater muscle synthesis. Nor is there evidence to support the use of amino acid supplements, or that they have the muscle-development potency of anabolic steroids. In spite of this, many strength athletes continue to ingest large quantities of high protein foods and expensive supplements. Potential hazards of this practice include the higher levels of fat present in many high protein foods, increased fluid loss in urine because of increased urea formation, and increased urinary calcium excretion caused by increased intake of sulphur-amino acids which may contribute to loss of bone mass in females.

30.1.4   Fat

Fat is an important energy source, but the ability of muscle to utilize fat as an exercise fuel is limited. Factors that influence the use of fat as muscle fuel include duration and intensity of exercise, glycogen stores, the degree of fitness and composition of the diet. During low intensity exercise (20–40% $\dot{V}O_2$ max) and the latter stages of endurance exercise, fat is an important substrate for energy production. Training results in physiological adaptations in the body that promote fat utilization, thus sparing the limited carbohydrate stores and delaying exhaustion. Research carried out during the last few years indicates that if an athlete has trained and adapted to a moderately high fat diet, performance may not be impaired.

30.1.5   Vitamins and minerals

Vitamins and minerals have numerous functions in the body, and many are involved in physiological processes which play an important role in exercise. B vitamins are essential for carbohydrate and fat metabolism, and folic acid and vitamin B_{12} are required for the formation of red blood cells. Of the more than 20 minerals needed by the body, two are of particular importance especially for female athletes: iron is essential in oxygen transport, while calcium is the major bone mineral.

Vitamins and minerals are found in a wide variety of foods and most athletes obtain adequate amounts from a balanced diet. Nevertheless, many athletes use vitamin and mineral supplements in the belief that they will enhance performance, yet extensive research has not shown beneficial effects in the absence of deficiency. However, some female athletes such as gymnasts, body builders, ballet dancers, and others on weight-reduction regimes who consume less than 4.2 MJ (1000 kcal) of energy daily, and those who avoid certain foods may be at risk of inadequate intake of some vitamins and minerals. Some athletes may have greater requirements of certain vitamins, such as vitamin E for high altitude mountain climbers, and vitamin C for the prevention of upper respiratory tract infections in endurance athletes.

30.1.6   Fluids and electrolytes

Water is one of the most important nutrients for physical performance, yet is often neglected in training. The amount of water lost through sweating depends on the severity of physical activity, as well as on the environmental temperature. Dehydration, which occurs with the loss of more than 1% of the body weight in water, hinders performance, interferes with co-ordination, motivation, and concentration, and reduces endurance. Blood volume is reduced when fluid loss reaches 2–3% body weight, which in turn places a significant strain on circulatory function, and impairs the capacity for both exercise and thermoregulation. Adequate hydration is achieved by balancing water loss with water intake, and can be maintained by ensuring full hydration prior to exercise especially in hot conditions, consuming small volumes (150 ml) every 15–20 minutes during exercise, and rehydrating after exercise. Thirst is not a good indicator of fluid requirements.

The efficacy of fluid replacement depends upon the rate of gastric emptying of the fluid, which is in turn affected by the composition and temperature of the fluid, the volume consumed, the work rate of the exercise and the ambient temperature. For events lasting under 1–2 hours, replacement with water is satisfactory, but events lasting longer require some carbohydrate replacement. High carbohydrate drinks take longer to empty from the stomach, delaying fluid absorption; however, they do supply energy at a faster rate. The composition of the rehydration fluid will therefore depend upon the relative importance of replacing water and/or carbohydrate. Sports drinks containing 5–10% carbohydrate as glucose or glucose polymer are at least as efficient in preventing dehydration as water and are more efficient in preventing fatigue due to carbohydrate depletion. Some athletes may tolerate and benefit from higher concentrations of carbohydrate.

Electrolyte replacement may be necessary only when prolonged sweating occurs on successive days, as dietary and kidney adjustments are sufficient to replace losses. A fall in blood levels of sodium (hyponatraemia) may occur occasionally in ultra-endurance athletes, probably due to intakes of large volumes of water causing dilution of sodium in body fluids and excessive losses in sweat. This can be prevented by using sports drinks which contain a small amount of sodium (10 mmol/l), which also enhances the absorption of water and glucose.

30.2 THE COMPETITION DIET

Dietary practices before and during competition can influence performance by helping to prevent energy depletion, dehydration and disturbances in electrolyte balance, while nutritional strategies immediately post-competition enhance recovery.

30.2.1 Pre-competition nutrition

For endurance competition lasting over 90 minutes (marathon, triathlon, 100 km cycle, tournaments), various glycogen supercompensation or carbohydrate loading regimes have been used to increase muscle glycogen stores substantially. These are based on work of scientists in the late 1960s who demonstrated that:

(1) optimizing muscle glycogen stores before endurance competition resulted in greater endurance capacity;

(2) high carbohydrate diets resulted in greater muscle glycogen resynthesis after exercise; and

(3) muscle depleted of glycogen by strenuous exercise could be 'supercompensated' with glycogen beyond original pre-exercise levels, if a high carbohydrate intake was maintained.

These findings led to the classical training and diet regime which included depletion of muscle glycogen stores, a low carbohydrate diet phase, and a high carbohydrate diet prior the event. This programme almost doubles muscle glycogen levels, but is rather rigorous and no longer recommended. Today, a modified procedure is recommended that eliminates the low carbohydrate and depletion phases and is equally effective in enhancing muscle glycogen. A normal diet is consumed during training until three days before endurance competition when the carbohydrate intake is increased to 70–80% of total energy intake, and training is gradually reduced. This method fits more easily into training programmes and has fewer side effects.

30.2.2   Pre-competition meal

The objective of the pre-competition meal is to maximize the body's energy reserves, to start competition well hydrated, and to avoid the sensation of hunger during an event while allowing for a relatively empty stomach to prevent discomfort. A suitable meal consists of 1.3–4.2 MJ (300–1000 kcal) of easily digested familiar and enjoyable carbohydrate foods and should be consumed two to three hours prior to competition. Foods with low glycaemic index are of value in providing a prolonged, sustained supply of carbohydrate. Plenty of fluids should be included up until the start of competition. Commercially available liquid meals are useful for athletes who experience gastrointestinal discomfort due to pre-competition nerves, or if time does not allow for a meal prior to the start of the event.

30.2.3   During competiton

The role of nutrition during competition is to avoid glycogen depletion, to minimize dehydration, and to maintain adequate electrolyte balance. The role of carbohydrate/electrolyte drinks in endurance events has already been discussed. These drinks are also beneficial for athletes participating in sports such as soccer, and in multiple event competitions and tournaments.

30.2.4   Recovery nutrition

Athletes who train for extended periods of time will substantially deplete their muscle glycogen stores. To restore fluid balance and to promote glycogen resynthesis, fluids and carbohydrate should be consumed within an hour of finishing competition and regularly thereafter. Carbohydrate intakes of 50–150 g (or 1–2 g/kg body weight) are recommended. High glycaemic index foods may facilitate glycogen replacement during the first 24 hours. Alcohol should be avoided until rehydration has been achieved.

30.3   WEIGHT MANAGEMENT

Nutrition plays a key role in weight management and in achieving a body composition within the optimal range for a particular sport. In sports such as distance running, cycling, cross-country skiing and triathlons, low body weight and body fat are considered important for biomechanical reasons. In others such as gymnastics, ballet, springboard diving and body building, body shape and composition are important for aesthetic reasons. In sports with specific weight categories such as wrestling, boxing, lightweight rowing, weight and power-lifting, judo and martial arts, athletes compete in weight divisions below their normal body mass, attempting to gain an advantage in strength over other competitors.

This desire to lose weight and reduce body fat, with pressure from coaches and parents to achieve extremely thin physiques, and lack of guidance in safe methods of weight loss leads many athletes to use undesirable and sometimes dangerous methods of losing weight in an unrealistically short time. These include dehydration through diuretics and saunas, use of laxatives, and very low-energy diets.

Weight loss should be no more than 0.5–1 kg/week. If the diet is too restrictive, the intake of food may not be sufficient to meet requirements of some nutrients, particularly iron and calcium, and may not provide sufficient energy to sustain training. Dehydration due to initial abrupt losses of water is a major hazard associated with the rapid weight loss practices of wrestlers, boxers, and rowers. Rapid weight loss may also affect body composition, causing unhelpful losses of lean body tissue rather than fat. Constant preoccupation with weight can lead to eating disorders such as anorexia nervosa and bulimia (discussed in Chapter 21), and a high incidence of these disorders is found in ballet dancers and rhythmic gymnasts. A further consequence of preoccupation with weight and body image, and with constant dieting is amenorrhoea, and its effect on bone mass (see Chapter 8.1.6).

Large body mass may be advantageous in events such as in heavyweight and sumo wrestling, weight-lifting, and long distance swimming in cold water, by contributing to stability, force development, protection, and thermal insulation. In weight- and power-lifting, the main objective is to gain lean body mass and muscle bulk. This can be achieved with an appropriate weight-training programme supported by a high-energy training diet with a high carbohydrate, adequate protein and moderate fat content. Protein supplementation is neither effective nor necessary to promote muscle mass.

30.4 SPECIAL CONCERNS FOR THE ATHLETE

30.4.1 Calcium and athletic amenorrhoea

Athletic amenorrhoea refers to the absence of regular menstruation in sportswomen and is emerging as a serious concern for the female athlete. There is an increasing incidence of amenorrhoea or oligomenorrhoea (irregular menstruation), particularly among endurance runners, rhythmical gymnasts and ballet dancers. These athletes usually have low body fat stores and low oestrogen production. They consume low-energy diets often lacking in dairy products resulting in inadequate dietary calcium. Low oestrogen levels cause loss of calcium from the bone, loss of bone mass and strength. These athletes have a high risk of stress fractures as their bones become weak and brittle, and an increased risk of osteoporosis in later life (see Chapter 8).

There are many contributing factors to this condition of which diet is only one. Poor nutrition in general, and more specifically, low-energy, fat and calcium intakes, vegetarian diets (especially avoidance of red meat), and excessive intakes of fibre have been associated with the condition. Other factors which contribute to the onset of amenorrhoea include high level of training, low body fat and body weight, premenstrual training, late menarche and emotional stress.

30.4.2   Iron and the athlete

Iron is a component of haemoglobin (Hb) in the blood and of myoglobin in muscles that transport oxygen, and of mitochondrial cytochrome oxidative enzymes which play an important role in aerobic exercise. Iron deficiency appears to occur more frequently among sports people, especially endurance athletes. This however should not be confused with 'sports anaemia': low Hb levels which result from the haemodilution effect of an expanded plasma volume, an adaptation to endurance exercise and not a true iron deficiency anaemia.

Individuals with iron deficiency anaemia generally lack energy, are easily tired, may feel light-headed, and may find themselves short of breath after relatively minor activities (see Chapter 9). Training may fail to achieve the improvement expected, or performance may be reduced. Possible causes of iron deficiency in athletes include:

- inadequate dietary iron caused by very restrictive weight-reducing diets or diets which eliminate red meat;
- diminished iron absorption in some athletes;
- destruction of red blood cells and degradation of haemoglobin as a result of mechanical haemolysis caused by weight-bearing exercise;
- increased iron losses due to menstruation in females, sweat losses, gastrointestinal bleeding, and haematuria.

Although treatment initially requires iron supplements, a good diet is sufficient to maintain iron status once it is back to normal. The consumption of oral iron supplements as a preventative measure is not recommended because of the potential danger of iron overload.

30.5   DIETARY SUPPLEMENTS AND NUTRITIONAL ERGOGENIC AIDS

In certain circumstances dietary manipulation may improve performance directly. Correction of a nutritional deficiency which has impaired performance, by additional intake of that nutrient, will naturally restore performance. On the other hand, in some situations nutrient supplementation in amounts above normal requirements may improve performance in the absence of deficiency, such as high carbohydrate dietary supplements and sports drinks for endurance events.

The word ergogenic means 'work enhancement' or 'work improvement'. For a long time, athletes have experimented with substances to try to enhance performance in order to obtain a competitive edge over their opponents. Nutritional ergogenic aids are characterized as those that contain nutrients greatly in excess of recommended intakes and greater than amounts normally provided by food, that claim to provide an ergogenic effect mainly through pharmacological rather than physiological processes, and that usually have some theoretical basis for their recommendation rather than documented scientific evidence. They are generally not supported by sports nutritionists.

A multitude of these supplements are available to athletes, ranging from megadoses of vitamins to compounds such as carnitine, ginseng, coenzyme Q_{10} and caffeine. Athletes are very susceptible to powerful marketing strategies aimed at convincing them of the

Table 30.1 Nutritional goals for physically active individuals

1. To enjoy food and pleasure of social eating opportunities.
2. To achieve and maintain the appropriate body weight and body fat level for their sport by balancing energy intake and exercise.
3. To achieve requirements of all nutrients, including any increase in requirements that might arise as a result of their exercise programme.
4. To prevent dehydration during exercise by drinking sufficient fluid before during and after exercise.
5. To provide adequate carbohydrate fuel for exercise activities and to promote recovery between sessions.
6. To incorporate nutritional practices that promote long-term health, and reduce the risk of chronic disease patterns of affluent western countries.

Source: Adapted from Burke L. Food selection and guidance for physically active people. *Asia Pacific J Clin Nutr* 1995; 4 (suppl. 1): 39–44.

benefits of such products, yet scientific evidence of an ergogenic effect is usually lacking. In the absence of deficiency, research shows that most of these substances are ineffective; any alleged improvement in performance can probably be attributed to psychological or placebo effects.

There are a few substances such as caffeine, carnitine, sodium bicarbonate, and more recently, creatine, which have shown positive effects on performance in some but not all studies. However, in general these substances are acting as drugs rather than nutrients and their use is not recommended. Optimum sports performance is better achieved through sensible dietary strategies rather than through the use of single nutrient supplements which may cause harmful side effects. There is a need for well-controlled research to answer questions relating to the effects of some of these dietary aids on performance and health.

Athletes can gain the most out of their genetic potential and training by consuming a balanced diet of natural foods that contain the required amounts of nutrients. For some athletes such as endurance athletes, female athletes and those needing to control weight and body composition, diet may play an even greater role. Table 30.1 outlines six goals common to all physically active individuals who wish to reach their potential, whether at an international or at a personal level.

FURTHER READING

1. Burke L, Deakin V. *Clinical sports nutrition*. Sydney: McGraw-Hill Book Company, 1994.
2. Coyle EF. Substrate utilization during exercise in active people. *Am J Clin Nutr* 1995; **61**: 968S–79S.
3. Lemon PWR. Do athletes need more dietary protein and amino acids? *Inter J Sports Nutr* 1995; 5: S39–S61.
4. Pearce J. *Eating to compete*. Auckland: Heinemann, Reid, 1990.

31

NUTRITION AND AGEING

Caroline Horwath

Nutrition interacts with the ageing process in numerous ways and the risk of nutrition-related health problems increases in later life. This chapter provides an overview of why nutrition is important in old age, what happens to our bodies as we age (including how digestive function changes with advancing years), and the nutritional needs and status of older adults. It also highlights some of the special issues arising in nutrition–disease relationships in old age.

31.1 WHY IS NUTRITION IMPORTANT IN OLD AGE?

There is a world-wide increase in the proportion of people in the older age groups. In developed countries, the proportion of the population aged 65 years and older ranges from around 12% to 14% in North America, Australia and New Zealand, to around 16% to 19% in Western Europe. By 2020, it is predicted that in some countries such as Japan, people over 65 years will make up nearly one in four of the population! (See Fig. 31.1.) Although the proportion of older adults is considerably smaller in the rest of the world, more than half of the world's population aged 60 years and over lives in developing countries, and by the year 2020, this figure will be approaching three-quarters (see Table 31.1). This dramatic increase in the proportion of older adults in the population results from a combination of lengthening life expectancy (in Western countries, life expectancy has almost doubled this century!) and declining birth rates. Gains in life expectancy are largely the result of better hygiene and nutrition, and advances in medical science (e.g. antibiotics). Rapidly growing older populations are of major concern since older people are disproportionately large consumers of costly health and welfare resources. In most developed countries, currently only about 5% of the over-65s are institutionalized (i.e. live permanently in residential homes, hospitals or nursing homes). However, population ageing means that the number of older people living in institutions is also rapidly increasing.

For a variety of physical, social and psychological reasons (Table 31.2), older adults are widely considered to be a group at particular risk of nutritional problems, either as a result of impaired food intake or reduced nutrient utilization.

Several of the health problems and bodily changes experienced by older adults which have long been attributed to the 'normal ageing process' are increasingly being recognized as linked to lifestyle or environmental factors. Good nutrition and other lifestyle factors, such as exercise, are vital to ensuring that more people can look forward to long and healthy lives, and that in later life people can continue to live as independently as possible within the community.

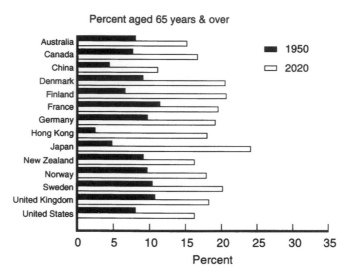

Fig. 31.1 The older population in selected countries, 1950, and the projections for 2020. *Source*: New Zealand now: 65 plus. Wellington: Statistics New Zealand, 1995.

Table 31.1 Ageing indicators for the world and major areas, 1950–2025

Region	Median age (yrs)				% aged 65+			
	1950	1975	2000	2025	1950	1975	2000	2025
World	23.4	21.9	25.9	31.1	5.1	5.7	6.8	9.7
Developed countries	28.2	30.4	36.4	40.8	7.6	10.7	13.7	19.0
Developing countries	21.2	19.3	23.7	29.6	3.8	3.8	5.0	8.0
Africa	18.6	17.5	17.7	22.2	3.2	3.1	3.1	4.1
Asia	21.9	20.1	25.7	32.5	4.0	4.1	5.8	9.6
Latin America	19.7	19.1	24.2	30.3	3.3	4.1	5.4	8.6
North America	30.0	28.6	36.6	41.1	8.1	10.3	12.8	19.9
Europe	30.5	32.4	37.6	42.9	8.7	12.3	14.9	20.1
USSR	24.7	29.1	33.0	36.4	6.1	9.5	11.7	14.8
Oceania	27.9	25.6	30.9	35.8	7.5	7.5	9.5	13.9

Source: El-Badry MA. World population change: a long range perspective. *Ambio* 1992; **21**: 18–23.

31.2 WHAT HAPPENS TO OUR BODIES AS WE AGE?

Changes in body composition, physical performance and organ system function occur in all of us as we grow older. However, there exists wide variation between people in the degree to which functions decline. The older people become, the more dissimilar they become from their contemporaries of the same chronological age. There can also be

Table 31.2 Potential contributors to nutritional problems in older people

Physical factors
- Reduced total energy needs
- Declining absorptive and metabolic capacities
- Chronic diseases
- Poor appetite
- Changes in taste or odour perception
- Poor dental health
- Reduced salivary flow
- Difficulty in swallowing
- Lack of exercise
- Physical disability (restricting the capacity to purchase, cook or eat a varied diet)
- Side effects of drugs (anorexia, nausea, altered taste, drug–nutrient interactions)
- Restrictive diets
- Alcoholism

Social and psychological factors
- Depression
- Loneliness
- Social isolation
- Bereavement
- Loss of interest in food or cooking
- Memory loss
- Food faddism

Socioeconomic factors
- Low income
- Inadequate cooking or storage facilities
- Limited nutrition knowledge
- Lack of transport
- Shopping difficulties
- Cooking practices that result in nutrient losses (e.g. soaking vegetables)
- Inadequate cooking skills (particularly in men)

considerable variability in the rate at which different changes occur within the same person. Some of this variability in functional decline may reflect heterogeneity in true rates of ageing; however, other factors which can accompany ageing seem to be of major importance. These include lifestyle factors such as poor nutrition, physical inactivity and smoking, and the development of disease. Each of these factors can contribute to deterioration in function (e.g. of cardiovascular, lung or endocrine functions), thereby accelerating one's apparent 'rate of ageing'. For example, decreased renal filtration rate and declining cardiovascular function have been observed in longitudinal studies such as the Baltimore Longitudinal Study of Ageing. However, after careful exclusion of people with kidney disease or heart disease, respectively, no consistent declines in function with age remained. Thus, the apparent declines in average functional indices of the study group members as they aged were due to inclusion of people with defined disease rather than to the ageing process *per se*. Similarly, neither can the declines in lean body mass (see Table 31.3) and increases in body fat (see Fig. 31.2) which tend to occur as people

(a)

(b)

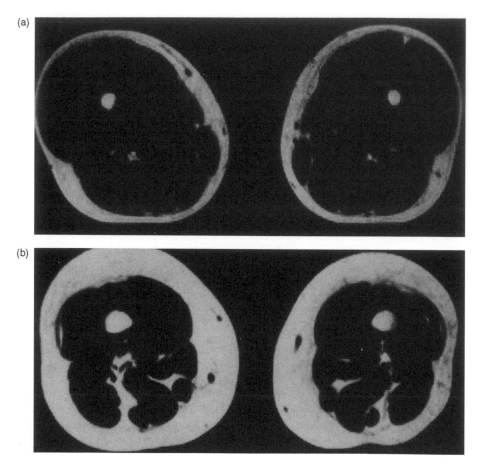

Fig. 31.2 Magnetic resonance images of the thigh showing differences in total muscle, intramuscular fat, subcutaneous fat, and bone between (a) a young woman athlete (age 20 years, BMI 22.6) and (b) an elderly sedentary woman (age 64 years, BMI 30.7). *Source*: Evans WJ, Meredith CN. Exercise and nutrition in the elderly. In: Munro HN and Danford DE (eds). *Nutrition, aging and the elderly*. New York: Plenum Press, 1989.

grow older be entirely attributed to the ageing process *per se*. A major contributor to these changes is the increasingly sedentary nature of people's lifestyles as they grow older in Western countries, illustrated in Fig. 31.3 by the decline in average energy intakes and expenditures of men with increasing age. Reduced physical activity leads to loss of muscle and the resultant declines in basal metabolic rate. Declining glucose tolerance and increasing blood pressure with advancing age are also linked with physical inactivity, increasing levels of obesity, and a more abdominal distribution of body fat. So although ageing appears to be an inevitable, natural process programmed into the genes, many of the changes that occur in our bodies as we grow older are at least partly the result of lifestyle or environmental factors. As such, they may be amenable to modification. In other words, we can adopt lifestyle habits such as regular exercise and healthy eating that will slow functional declines and compositional changes within the limits set by genetics.

Table 31.3 Total body protein (kg) in a cross-sectional study of men and women

	Young (20–29 yrs)	Middle-aged (40–49 yrs)	Elderly (70–79 yrs)
Men			
Muscle protein	4.54	3.80	2.50
Non-muscle protein	8.32	8.20	8.60
Total protein	12.86	12.00	11.10
Women			
Muscle protein	1.85	1.94	1.11
Non-muscle protein	7.23	6.53	6.10
Total protein	9.08	8.47	7.21

Source: Cohn SH, Vartsky D, Yasumura S, Sawitsky A, Zanzi I, Vaswani A, *et al.* Compartmental body composition based on total-body nitrogen, potassium and calcium. *Am J Physiol* 1980; **239**: E524–30.

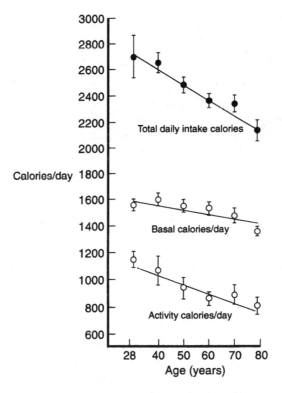

Fig. 31.3 Daily energy intake and expenditure in healthy men of different ages. (Values are means with standard deviations; cross-sectional data.) *Source*: McGandy RB, Barrows CH, Spanias A, Meredith A, Stone JL, Norris AH. Nutrient intakes and energy expenditure in men of different ages. *J Gerontol* 1966; **21**: 581–7.

Good nutrition may, by delaying or slowing disease processes, help people to reach their maximum life span potential...but can it extend it further? Read on...

31.3   SECRETS OF LONG LIFE?

For thousands of years, the search for eternal life and youth has captured people's imagination. In about 1750, George Cheyne, physician to Samuel Johnson, David Hume and Alexander Pope, wrote 'An essay of health and long life' in which he is emphatic that:

Nothing conduces more to Health and Long Life, than Abstinence and plain Food, with due Labour. Most chronical diseases proceed from Repletion... Without due Labour and Exercise, the Juices will thicken, the Joints will stiffen, the Nerves will relax, and on these disorders, Chronical Distempers and a crazy old Age must ensue. ...this [lessening the diet gradually with age] is a powerful means to make their old age Green and Indolent, and to preserve the remains of their Senses to the very last.

The similarities to recommendations derived from the latest research on ageing are remarkable! Currently Japan can claim the greatest life expectancy in the world. Genetics does not appear to be the explanation (mortality patterns change as Japanese migrate to Hawaii), but diet, in particular the low fat intake among even Westernized Japanese people, may play a role. Conversely, life span (the maximum number of years of life attainable) does not appear to vary among populations and has not changed over time. The extraordinary ages (150 years and older) claimed by inhabitants in several remote areas of Russian Georgia and southern Ecuador, and in the Hunza River region of the Himalayan mountains in Pakistan, have been found to be gross exaggerations.

Currently, the only nutritional manipulation shown to increase life span has been a drastic restriction of food intake in laboratory rats. Restriction of food intake in the early weeks of rats' lives, or even during adulthood, increased life span by as much as 60%. The restriction of energy intake required to produce such effects is around 25–40% of voluntary consumption. However, this corresponds to restriction of the food intake of a human infant, kept in an isolated environment away from infections for 20–25 years, to an amount that would permit the infant during that time to grow to about the size of a 1-year-old child. Clearly there is no direct application to humans.

To return to the question of whether nutritional changes can extend the human life span further—so far the answer is No. Attention is increasingly being focused, however, on the potential role of antioxidant nutrients in protecting against several chronic conditions that increase in prevalence with age, such as heart disease, cancer, arthritis and cataracts. Some individuals take vast quantities of antioxidant supplements in the hope that these may represent the secret of long life and eternal youthfulness. Antioxidant nutrients represent one aspect of the body's defence mechanisms against free radical damage. However, there is no evidence as yet that taking antioxidant supplements will slow the ageing process in humans.

31.4   DIGESTIVE FUNCTION IN OLD AGE

Changes in gastrointestinal function with age may alter nutritional needs. Impaired digestive or absorptive capacities for macronutrients were reported in hospitalized or institutionalized older people but these deficiences reflected the effects of medications or disease states rather than age itself. Most gastrointestinal functions remain relatively intact with increasing age, partly because of the large reserve capacity of the intestine, pancreas and liver.

Altered or reduced taste perception which occurs with ageing may influence enjoyment in eating. Although reduced salivary flow and dry mouth can be a problem for some older people, these are usually the result of the side effects of drugs or the presence of disease, rather than being an inevitable part of the ageing process. Decreased thirst sensation can also contribute to the problem of a dry mouth. Difficulty in swallowing occurs in some older adults if nervous function is disturbed.

Perhaps the most important change in gastrointestinal function with ageing is the reduction in gastric acid output in a subgroup of older people who have atrophic gastritis. Atrophy of the stomach mucosa becomes more common with ageing and appears to affect about one-third of those over 60 years. The result is lowered secretion of acid, intrinsic factor and pepsin, which if sufficiently severe, can reduce the bioavailability of vitamin B_{12}, calcium, iron and folate.

31.5   Do Nutritional Needs Change as We Age?

Several countries have published recommendations for nutrient intakes for adults over 50 years (e.g. the United States and Britain), and Australia has figures for men aged 64 years and older, and for postmenopausal women (i.e. 54 years and over). Until more specific information becomes available on the nutritional requirements of older adults, these broad age groupings will have to suffice for the entire heterogeneous older population. (See Chapter 33 for a more extensive discussion of requirements and recommended intakes.) How are the nutritional needs of older adults currently thought to differ from those of younger adults?

Older adults have reduced needs for energy and, as a result, presumably the B vitamins which are involved in energy metabolism, and postmenopausal women have lower needs for iron, as a result of cessation of menstrual blood losses. These differences are reflected in lower recommended nutrient intakes for older adults. The lower energy needs of older adults are the result of declines in metabolic rate (secondary to reduced lean muscle mass) and in activity levels. Neither of these changes are inevitable; indeed, it can be argued that morbidity and mortality could be lowered if lean body mass and physical activity were maintained at more youthful levels rather than diminished in older persons. The greater food intake needed to balance a higher energy expenditure is more likely to ensure adequate intakes of essential nutrients. If older adults consume low energy intakes, then it is important that the foods they eat be nutrient-dense, rather than low nutrient-density foods such as those high in sugars, fats or alcohol.

The body's requirements for iron are lowest in old age; however, other factors in the lives of many older people can increase the risk of iron deficiency. Such factors include chronic blood loss from ulcers or other disease conditions, poor iron absorption due to reduced stomach acid secretion, or medications like aspirin which can cause blood loss.

Calcium needs are also higher in oestrogen-deprived postmenopausal women and this is reflected in increased recommendations for calcium intakes. The importance of an

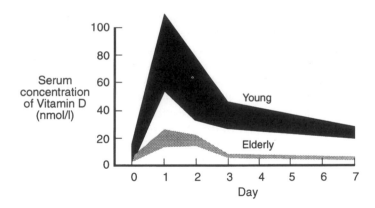

Fig. 31.4 Serum concentrations of vitamin D in healthy young and elderly adults in response to whole-body exposure to a dose of simulated sunlight on day 0. *Source*: Holick M. Vitamin D—new horizons for the 21st century. *Am J Clin Nutr* 1994; **69**: 619–30.

abundant calcium intake throughout life in protecting against osteoporosis, particularly for women, is discussed in Chapter 8.1.6.

There is also evidence accumulating that older adults may have greater needs for vitamin D, vitamin B_{12} and B_6, and lower needs for vitamin A than their younger compatriots. For example, factors that contribute to enhanced likelihood of impaired vitamin D nutriture in old age include the reduced capacity of older skin to synthesize previtamin D_3 (see Fig. 31.4), impaired hydroxylation of vitamin D_3 by the kidneys and reduced sun exposure. It has been estimated that in both the United States and Great Britain about 30–40% of older patients with hip fractures have inadequate levels of vitamin D. In older adults who are housebound or have extremely limited sunlight exposure (e.g. some of those in nursing homes), administration of a low dose vitamin D supplement (10 µg/day) is advisable. On the other hand, low serum vitamin A levels appear to be rare among older adults despite a high prevalence of dietary intakes below current recommended levels. So current recommendations for vitamin A may be unnecessarily high for older adults.

Overall, most older adults need to obtain the same intakes as younger adults for most vitamins and minerals, but usually in substantially lower overall food intakes. Thus a nutrient-dense diet is a high priority in old age.

31.6   A LOOK AT THE EATING HABITS OF OLDER ADULTS

A number of general conclusions can be drawn from studies of dietary intake conducted amongst older populations around the world. Contrary to the popular 'tea'n'toast' myth, it appears that most older adults outside institutions eat reasonably well. Energy intakes fall with advancing age (Fig. 31.3), but average protein intakes still generally remain well above recommended levels. The dietary patterns of older adults have generally been found to be similar to those of younger adults, with fat, saturated fat, and refined carbohydrate intakes above recommended levels, and complex carbohydrate and fibre intakes below recommended levels.

However, there are some subgroups within the older population v
likely to be consuming poor diets, and some nutrients for which there
of inadequate intakes. These nutrients are calcium, zinc, magnesium, vitam..
folate. The low calcium intakes of many older people, particularly women, ..
important implications for bone health. Poor zinc status is an important issue in view of
the apparent contribution of deficient zinc nutriture to delayed wound healing and
impaired immune response in older adults. Both the SENECA (Survey in Europe on
Nutrition and the Elderly, a Concerted Action) study and the Boston Nutritional Status
Survey have added considerably to our knowledge of the vitamin status of older adults.
In the SENECA study, 23% had biochemical levels suggesting subclinical vitamin B_6
deficiency. More than half of the people aged over 60 years in the Boston survey had
vitamin B_6 intakes below two-thirds of the recommended allowance. This is cause for
concern because of the documented effects of vitamin B_6 deficiency on immune function.
Low folate intakes are common and may be linked via elevated plasma homocysteine,
with vascular disease.

The two factors most consistently linked with poor dietary intake in old age are low
socioeconomic status and, among older men, living alone. Compared with men living with
a spouse, older men living alone tend to have a poorer fruit and vegetable intake, and more
frequently choose less nutrient-dense, easy-to-prepare foods which also tend to be higher
in fat and lower in fibre. Limited cooking skills and reduced motivation when cooking just
for one are probably important contributors. Institutionalized older people and those living
independently in the community but restricted in their mobility also tend to be at higher
risk of poor dietary habits. Lack of social contact, loneliness, being less active both socially
and physically, and recent bereavement are also associated with poor dietary intake. It is
probable that a rich and varied lifestyle and maintenance of positive interests lead to better
dietary quality through an improvement in life satisfaction, a better social support network,
and a lessening of the impact of some of the negative life events associated with growing
older. In fact, participation in fewer activities outside the home is linked with higher
mortality in old age. Other negative influences on dietary intake in old age are physical
disability, problems with chewing, shopping difficulties and depression. Loss of teeth and
poorly fitting dentures clearly reduce chewing efficiency.

Signs of poor nutrition in an older individual include recent weight loss, missing meals,
infrequent grocery shopping, depression, loss of appetite or declining food intake due to
digestive problems, taste changes and chewing or swallowing difficulties.

Low fluid and fibre intakes are common, and together with low activity levels,
contribute to the common problem of constipation, particularly in institutions. Factors
which place older people at risk of dehydradon are outlined in Chapter 7.1.5.

Daily intakes of fruits, vegetables, whole grains and dairy products as well as the
inclusion in the diet of lean meat, fish, poultry and legumes will ensure provision of
those nutrients found to be most 'at risk' in the diets of older people.

31.7   NUTRITION–DISEASE RELATIONSHIPS IN OLD AGE

One way nutrition affects longevity is via its role in disease prevention. The role of diet
in some chronic diseases is discussed elsewhere (see e.g. Chapters 18–20). Outlined here

are some special issues in older adults and differences in nutrition–disease relationships from those in younger adults.

It is often assumed that lifestyle changes to improve health are no longer worthwhile in old age, that the remaining years are not sufficient to reap the benefits of modifications which are often thought to lead to a reduction in enjoyment of food. Certainly, very restrictive diets may impair the adequacy of dietary intake. However, benefits can be gained from nutrition education and lifestyle change in old age. In several studies, a high proportion of older men and women were found to make dietary changes, often for health reasons, thus challenging the stereotyped view of older adults being 'set in their ways'.

The incidence and prevalence of coronary heart disease are highest in the older population, with established heart disease in up to 25% of older men. Smoking, hypertension and diabetes continue to be important risk factors for heart disease during old age, and the prevalence of diabetes and impaired glucose tolerance rises steeply with age. Intervention trials clearly demonstrate that the health advantages of stopping smoking and managing hypertension remain in old age. Dietary approaches to the management of hypertension (i.e. weight reduction in the overweight, sodium restriction, limitation of alcohol) are particularly relevant for older adults because they are more susceptible to severe adverse drug reactions and may be more responsive to sodium restriction. There also appear to be even stronger grounds for sodium restriction in older women on the basis of studies demonstrating a markedly increased obligatory urinary calcium loss and thus a higher dietary calcium requirement on high sodium intakes. Halving salt intakes (currently around 140 mmol sodium/day) can lower dietary calcium needs by about a third. Non-insulin-dependent diabetes in older adults should be managed by weight reduction and hypoglycaemic agents. Even moderate weight reduction has been shown to have benefits for diabetic control in older people. Limited data suggest that older adults are as responsive to drug and dietary treatment of high cholesterol levels as younger adults. It seems appropriate to consider biological rather than chronological age when deciding whether an individual should be given dietary advice to lower cholesterol levels. Someone who is generally healthy and appears likely to have a reasonable life expectancy should not be denied dietary advice. In fact, the absolute risk attributable to high cholesterol levels actually increases with age (i.e. the difference in absolute rates of disease between those with highest risk factor levels and those with lowest risk factor levels). However, more research is needed on the effects of cholesterol lowering in older adults, and cholesterol lowering in people over 80 years would not seem worthwhile.

In Western societies the common pattern of weight gain up to the age of around 50 to 60 years means that overweight and obesity are common problems in old age. However, rather than being an inevitable part of growing older, this pattern is linked with sedentary lifestyles. The health implications of being overweight in old age are controversial, however, it appears that overweight may be somewhat better tolerated by this group than by younger adults. This is reflected in wider acceptable BMI ranges for older adults in some countries (e.g. New Zealand), but not others (e.g. the United States). Being overweight still increases the risk of hypertension, diabetes and hypercholesterolaemia during old age, but to a lesser extent than in earlier life. Overweight and obesity can also aggravate arthritis and impair physical mobility. On the other hand, heavier women have a lower risk of hip fracture. This is partly due to 'padding' and better muscles, but may also be due to maintenance of higher oestrogen levels from the conversion of precursor steroids to oestrogen in adipose tissue.

A fairly recently noted link between nutrition and disease in older people is that between the antioxidant nutrients and risk of cataracts (a clouding of the lens of the eye resulting in diminished vision). Cataracts afflict nearly half of the American population aged 75–85 years, and are a major cause of blindness world-wide. The main contributors to cataract formation appear to be photooxidative damage and osmotic stress in the lens of the eye. It has been found that the highest risk of cataract is among individuals with low intakes of vitamin C, vitamin E and carotenoids. Osmotic stress due to high glucose levels is believed to be why people with diabetes are particularly prone to cataracts.

Constipation and diverticular disease are common problems, and awareness of the need to increase fibre intake is high, as reflected in widespread use of unprocessed bran supplements in older populations. However, it is preferable for fibre intakes to be increased through the consumption of a variety of cereals and vegetables rather than relying on extensive use of bran supplements. These may have adverse effects on the bioavailability of zinc and calcium, which may be marginally supplied in the diets of many older adults.

Severe nutrient deficiencies clearly impair both brain and immune function, and researchers are exploring the possibility that long-term moderate (subclinical) nutrient deficiencies also produce memory impairments or declining immunity in older adults. On the other hand, dementia can also have nutritional consequences. Dementia may lead to difficulty in shopping or cooking, or an older person with dementia may forget to eat or experience changes in taste, and may even not recognize food or eat non-food items.

For most older adults, probably the single most important health message is to achieve or maintain at least moderate levels of physical activity. There are numerous health benefits from exercise in old age: cardiovascular, musculoskeletal and psychological benefits, improvements in fat and carbohydrate metabolism, and promotion of good bowel function. There are similarities between the deterioration accompanying ageing and that occurring with physical inactivity. Randomized controlled trials demonstrate that high-intensity strength training exercises are an effective and feasible means of preserving bone density while improving muscle mass, strength and balance in old age.

31.8   Supplements for Older Adults

The use of supplements in the United States, Canada, Australia and New Zealand is widespread amongst older men (35–60%) and women (45–79%). Advertisers often target older people, claiming their products prevent disease or promote longevity. Unfortunately, the nutrient supplements most commonly used are rarely those in shortest supply in the diet, and furthermore supplement users generally tend to have better dietary intakes than non-users. Particular concerns are the risk of supplement interference with drug absorption in an age group that heavily consumes both prescription and over the counter drugs, and some evidence suggesting that vitamin A may be toxic at lower levels of intake in older than in younger adults.

There are, nevertheless, some indications for supplement use by older adults: nutritional doses of vitamin D by those who cannot get adequate sunlight exposure (i.e. hands, arms and face exposed to non-burning doses of sunlight for 15–30 minutes most days), calcium for osteoporosis prevention, or general multivitamin and mineral supplements (at recommended intake levels) for those with very low food intakes (i.e. less than 5 MJ/day). But a well-balanced diet will provide most healthy older people with the nutrients they need, and for those whose food intakes are very low, the more important priority is to identify and try to correct any underlying physical or psychosocial reasons for eating problems or poor nutritional state (see Table 31.2).

31.9 Drug–Nutrient Interactions

Older adults use more prescription and over the counter medications than any other age group, and are often taking several drugs at once. There are a number of ways by which drugs can affect nutrition, usually increasing nutrient need. Many drugs can reduce appetite, produce nausea, gastrointestinal disturbances, or alter the senses of taste or smell and hence affect food intake; long-term laxative use can impair intestinal function; and laxatives and diuretics can lead to severe loss of potassium. As many as 30% of older adults complain that drugs change their sense of taste.

31.10 Conclusions

Logically preventive measures to reduce diet-related disease should begin early in life; however, that is not to say that lifestyle modifications are worthless in old age. Improvements in diet and maintenance of exercise can benefit health regardless of age. Behavioural risk factors (e.g. not regularly eating breakfast, lack of regular physical activity, overweight, smoking) have been shown to remain predictors of 17-year mortality even at older ages (i.e. 70+). As the older population is more heterogeneous than any other age group, individual judgement is critical in deciding on the advisability of dietary and lifestyle changes. Physiological, psychological and sociological factors need to be considered. At one extreme are independent, vigorous, healthy people in their seventies, eighties and even nineties. At the other extreme are patients who are dependent and have multiple diseases and limited reserves. For the latter, advice to change diet or lifestyle may be inappropriate; a more important focus being attention to function and quality of life. However, it is often overlooked that although life expectancy at birth may only be to the mid to late-70s, at age 65 men and women in developed countries still have a life expectancy of some 15 and 19 years, respectively. Furthermore, at age 75 these life expectancies are around 9 and 11 years, respectively, and it is likely that improvements in nutrition would make these years healthier, more active and independent.

Further Reading

1. Evans WJ, Campbell WW. Sarcopenia and age-related changes in body compositon and functional capacity. *J Nutr* 1993; **123**: 465–8.

2. Hartz SC, Rosenberg IH, Russell RM, eds. *The Boston nutritional status survey*. London: Smith-Gordon & Co, 1992.
3. Horwath CC. Dietary intake studies in elderly people. *World Rev Nutr Dietet* 1989; **59**: 1–70.
4. Kaplan GA, Seeman TE, Cohen RD, Knudsen LP, Guralni KJ. Mortality among the elderly in the Alameda County Study: behavioural and demographic risk factors. *Am J Pub Health* 1987; **77**: 307–12.
5. Russell RM, Suter PM. Vitamin requirements of elderly people: an update. *Am J Clin Nutr* 1993; **58**: 4–14.
6. Welin L, Svardsudd K, Ander-Peciva S, Tibblin G, Tibblin B, Larsson B, *et al*. Prospective study of social influences on mortality: the study of men born in 1913 and 1923. *Lancet* 1985; i: 915–18.
7. Working group on the Nutrition of Elderly People of the Committee on Medical Aspects of Food Policy. *The nutrition of elderly people*. London: HMSO, 1993.
8. World Health Organization. Report of a WHO Study Group. *Epidemiology and prevention of cardiovascular diseases in elderly people*. WHO Technical Report Series 853. Geneva: WHO, 1995.

Part VII: Clinical and public health

32
FOOD HABITS
Helen Leach

Many of the topics which form the chapters of this book represent specializations in the subject of human nutrition. Structurally speaking, they can be slotted into compartments within the overall framework of this scientific discipline. The study of food habits, however, might best be viewed as the exploration of a relatively unbounded field lying outside the construction of nutrition, but impinging on it at many points.

32.1 STUDYING FOOD HABITS

A number of social scientists also locate their subject matter in this broad field of food habits: the American school of nutritional anthropology (e.g. Bryant, Fitzgerald, Jerome, Robson); a group of social anthropologists and sociologists interested in symbolism and structural order in food habits (e.g. Lévi-Strauss, Douglas, Nicod); anthropologists committed to more materialist explanations of food habits (e.g. Harris, Mintz); sociologists, economists and social historians concerned with explaining change in food habits (e.g. Mennell, Burnett, Charsley); and social psychologists who have an interest in the interface between cultural beliefs and individual behaviour, as they affect food preference (e.g. Rozin).

Historically the science of human nutrition developed in tandem with other medical sciences. At a clinical level, therefore, it has concentrated on the individual, and at a policy level, on the population, using epidemiological studies as a starting point. It has made by far the greatest progress with the biological aspects of human nutrition, and with the development of effective treatment of nutritional disorders in individuals. But in those aspects of human nutrition where individuals cease to behave as biological organisms or as members of biological populations, nutrition as an explanatory and applied science has had much less success. Of course humans have to eat to survive, the environment constantly sets limits on food production, and populations will continue to show change in genetic factors affecting metabolism, but where humans exhibit any choice at all in what they eat, what they select is more likely to be socially influenced than the result of a biological craving, environmental determinism, or idiosyncratic whim.

In discussing food habits, therefore, a definition must be used that stresses the socially influenced food-related behaviour of humans as members of groups. Murcott's usage of the phrase 'food habits' as 'a provisional, convenient and inclusive shorthand to cover the widest possible range of food choice, preferences, meal patterns and cuisines' will be followed here.

32.2 WHO CHOOSES?

There can be no denying that in the course of a human lifetime, the decision whether to ingest a particular food item lies ultimately with the individual (except in cases of forced or tube feeding). Infants are particularly adept at exercising the right to reject food. But the power to decide what food items are made available for the selection process, and in what form, frequently lies beyond the individual. For the baby, the mother usually decides what should be offered, starting with the decision of either breast milk or formula. But her choice on behalf of the baby is usually influenced by advice from female relatives, or health professionals. In the case of the former, this permits a family tradition of infant feeding to be passed on, compatible with the beliefs of the family's ethnic group and with their religious affiliation. A nurse's or doctor's advice will normally reflect the society's prevailing scientific paradigm concerning infant nutrition, for example, that solids should not be introduced until a certain age or that certain foods should be avoided.

The growing child has little control over the household menu, though at certain times (such as illness or the celebration of milestones in development), the person responsible for food acquisition and preparation will deliberately produce an item known to be the child's favourite. In some cultures, gender and position in the family may affect what is offered to each child in both quantity and variety. Similarly, the menu selected for the household may be strongly influenced by the preferences of a senior adult member. In societies where it is traditional for women to cook for their families, the desire to please their husbands may dictate the dishes they prepare for the whole household. Finally in old age, any former control over the menu may be lost through institutionalization or displacement from the kitchen by a younger household member. Thus, for many humans, selection of food is subject to significant constraints for much of their lifetime, despite the apparent freedom of the individual to eat as they choose.

32.3 SOCIAL AND CULTURAL INFLUENCES ON FOOD CHOICE

It is not surprising then that the cook, food purchaser, housewife or househusband, indeed any member of a group who makes food choices on behalf of that group, is sometimes referred to in research literature as the 'key kitchen person' (KKP), focal person, or gatekeeper, terms which recognize their pivotal role in the diet and food habits of their group. What social factors influence their choice of food to prepare? The broad answer is that they select according to the unwritten rules or norms of the culture to which they belong. Even when they respond to the food preferences of a particular member of their group, they are choosing items, composing them into dishes, and combining the dishes into menus within particular culinary traditions.

Culinary traditions operate at many levels from small kin-based group traditions to the nearly global culinary styles of Western cultures. In some isolated Third World situations, only one culinary tradition may be relevant, but for most First World groups, food providers and KKPs choose to work within the tradition which they see as most appropriate for a particular eating situation. For many important social occasions, the family culinary tradition of the organizers and chief participants will be followed. The significance of the occasion (e.g. wedding breakfast, Christmas dinner, religious festival) and the desire for a successful outcome usually constrain the menu within the traditional family or community pattern.

Even at this lowest organizational level, the family pattern of eating may be distinctive from that of its neighbours, though both may belong to the same ethnic and religious group and occupy the same socioeconomic position. Family food habits may be comparatively resistant to change in places where culinary knowledge and skills are learned primarily within the household and passed down between generations. Marriage residency practices, such as the wife joining her husband's extended family in a single household, may work to suppress change and reinforce the distinctiveness of the family tradition. Non-Western societies incorporate many different forms of household structure, depending on family lifecycle and kinship system. Each type will have a distinctive pattern of decision making relating to food.

Urbanized communities also feature a wide range of household arrangements, from two-parent two-generational families to groups of unrelated young adults. Food habits here are influenced by the background and social network of the group member who becomes the KKP for each main meal. If that person learned culinary skills in his or her own family setting, many of these will be transferred to the new household and applied according to the type of meal. However, in urbanized Western societies, such knowledge is frequently acquired outside the home (e.g. from the formal education system). For most of this century, cooking training in schools has been motivated by the goals of 'good nutrition' and has been responsible for reinterpreting Western culinary traditions within a scientific paradigm. There is ample evidence, however, that after schooling is complete, recipe repertoire is influenced by interaction with peers, within social networks, and by the media.

Magazines, newspapers, and television reflect an amalgam of culinary traditions depending on the contributing sources. A locally based food-writer for a monthly newspaper column may work within a regional food tradition, combining new variants with well-established and familiar dishes. A national or internationally distributed magazine may offer more cosmopolitan fare, strongly influenced by international food fashion trends. But there is little research on whether these fashions have a lasting impact on household food habits. For example, will the currently fashionable grain couscous become an important cereal in cosmopolitan cuisine, or will it be as short-lived as the fondue party?

The twentieth century trend to a cosmopolitan culinary repertoire has probably been influenced by the range of dishes cooked in the commercial kitchens of restaurants and fast-food outlets, and sampled as part of the phenomenon of 'eating out'. For the household member who is not actively involved in food preparation, eating out means more choice is possible from an extended menu. For the KKP, the responsibility for selecting food for others is removed, along with control over the dishes on the menu, and their composition. However, the characterization of restaurants and other food outlets into well-defined categories, such as vegetarian, wholefood, seafood, Italian, Thai, Cantonese, or other specified ethnic type, suggests that consumers still prefer to choose their food from an identifiable culinary tradition, even if it is not that of their own birth culture.

Thus, for the purpose of food and menu selection, many Western households operate within multiple layers of culinary traditions, not simultaneously, but moving between them from meal to meal, through the weekly cycle, and the annual calendar of festive occasions. Perhaps the unwritten rules for deciding which culinary tradition is appropriate, are part of evolving culinary traditions in their own right.

32.4 FOOD HABITS IN NUTRITION PRACTICE

From the viewpoint of the nutritionist offering clinical advice to an individual, it is clearly important to know how the patient relates to the KKP of the household where he or she normally resides. Without the informed support of the KKP, long-term dietary modification is unlikely to occur. And even with that support, pressure from other members of the household or a high status member, might frustrate any change.

It is also valuable for the nutritionist to have some knowledge of the culinary tradition from which most of the patient's meals are derived. Any modification of intake must be compatible with that tradition. We tend to categorize other traditions by their starch staple and typical flavouring substances. But culinary traditions are more than just the combinations of dishes/recipes that characterize and distinguish the eating patterns of particular human groups. They also include the rules for selecting and preparing food for consumption (such as butchering practices and preservation techniques), rules for composing the menu according to an acceptable structure of courses, and the rules or norms concerning eating behaviour (e.g. time, location, participants). As with all human social behaviour, these rules or norms are culturally transmitted. They are not immutable, but variation and innovation tend to take place more frequently within the structure than radical alteration of the overall framework. Culinary traditions also include the non-nutrient related meanings of food, including those that concern ethnic identity, values and religious beliefs.

Within certain traditions, there is strong social pressure to prepare and serve more food on occasions than might be considered nutritionally desirable. In such instances, the food is satisfying more than biological needs, and the participants are well aware that it is carrying a coded message concerning social relationships and value systems. For example, the Oglala Sioux of Pine Ridge Reservation in South Dakota require participants at communal high feasts to eat beyond satiety, and to bring containers for the removal of left-overs. Since their culture values generosity as the most important of four cardinal virtues, overindulgence is a statement about the generosity of the host, and an affirmation that this virtue is more highly regarded by the Oglala than by Euro-Americans.

Similarly on the Polynesian island, Tikopia, the anthropologist Raymond Firth observed that 'true hospitality consists in placing before a man more than he can possibly eat and then commanding him at intervals to continue when he shows signs of flagging'. In this Polynesian culture, which typically rates hospitality as an important virtue, the guest eats beyond satiety, regarding it as offensive to the host as well as shameful and embarrassing to confess to still being hungry. Food is used throughout Polynesia to confirm an agreement made between parties, and failure to partake could be interpreted as a sign that one party intends to break the contract.

Particular foods may encode metaphysical meanings which completely transcend any nutritional value. For the Christian taking communion, the wafer and the wine are clearly not food, but have been spiritually transformed. For modern Oglala Sioux Indians, ritual eating of dog involves equally complex ritual, reminding participants of the dog's role in

Sioux cosmology, and symbolizing all that is Indian in Oglala culture. The rejection of the dog as a food item by Euro-Americans adds to its symbolic importance for the Oglala, to the degree that the ceremonial stature of the dog feast has increased as Indian identity has been threatened. If dog consumption carried a health risk, a nutritionist who advised its avoidance would be threatening both group identity and religious belief.

Not all foods carry such complex spiritual meanings. However, under pressure, minority groups may encode particular items or dishes/recipes as markers of identity, when formerly they functioned simply as everyday food. Such is the case of 'soul food' in the United States. The pork and chicken products which provide the meat component of soul food, such as necks, backs, feet and giblets, were originally eaten because they were rejected by wealthier white consumers and were therefore cheaper. In one Southern case study it was found that middle socioeconomic class black households described them as 'black people's food', and ate them not for their cheapness but as a marker of ethnic identity. Lower socioeconomic class black and middle class white families classified them as 'poor people's food'. Lower class whites avoided them as 'nigger foods'. These food items have acquired a status ranking and racial connotation that is perceived differently according to the socioeconomic status and ethnicity of the various groups in the case study. It would be difficult for a nutritionist to change the usage or non-usage of these foods by any of the groups concerned because of their acquired load of non-nutritional meanings.

For many societies, food choice is constrained by religious proscription. Many of these food taboos are of such antiquity that they are written into the formal teachings of the religion (such as the Jewish and Hindu dietary laws which proscribe pork or beef). However, more recent dietary regimes based on particular philosophical or ethical principles have evolved food taboos of equal force for their adherents. As a secular movement, vegetarianism has been important for nearly two centuries, throughout this period drawing for justification on the accumulating data from the science of nutrition. Not surprisingly, nutritionists faced with evidence of health benefits from vegetarian diets for adults, have treated the movement with respect. However, the twentieth century has seen the development of far more restrictive dietary regimes allied to the 'health food' movement and the Western preoccupation with weight reduction. Food symbolism is highly developed in these regimes, with the polarization of 'natural' = healthy, versus synthetic = dangerous constantly reworked and elaborated by those who benefit commercially from sales of diet books and the approved foods. For the clinical nutritionist, disentangling the pseudoscientific justifications and powerful symbolism of these restrictive and potentially damaging diets is a major challenge. Furthermore, the social networks into which adherents of 'fad' or extreme diets are drawn for mutual support are likely to counteract what is perceived as criticism by the health professionals.

32.5 CHANGING FOOD HABITS IN THE MODERN WORLD

So far, this introduction to food habits has stressed the inbuilt tendency to conservatism within a culinary tradition, the individual's lack of control over food choice at various periods in his or her life, and the symbolic loading on certain foods which may exert powerful pressure against any change in usage or avoidance. Taken together these factors explain why nutritional advice aimed at individual or group level may be listened to politely (because of the status of the health professional), but not subsequently enacted.

At the same time, the success of multinational food companies provides ample evidence that throughout the world, even within highly conservative and symbol-rich culinary traditions, some substantial changes have occurred in diet during the twentieth century. These have included the introduction of many new food items, and even new menus borrowed from other traditions. Food manufacturers have invested heavily in research on food acceptance, and have realized that restrictive rules affecting food habits apply to meals rather than snacks. This observation, also made by Michael Nicod from his structuralist study of working class food habits in Britain, led to his definition of the meal as a structured food event, and the snack as an unstructured event. Although meals have courses which must be served in a prescribed order and contain certain food categories, for snacks, consumers are free to eat the items in any order or combination, at any time and with or without company. It is not surprising then that snack food manufacturers have had a global impact, because their promotional advertising does not have to confront long-established culinary norms. The lack of structure in snacking behaviour has allowed it to become a global arena where multinationals compete with new products, or old ones, newly packaged.

Nutritionists have had some success in promoting snacks with lower fat and sodium content, but realize that because snacking is usually supplementary feeding, their long-term objectives can only be met by dietary reform of meals, the area in which the multinationals have made much less headway. It has taken several decades to achieve public acceptance of pizza or burger-based main meals, when these items were originally conceived of more as snacks. Fast-food outlets have had to supply additional items such as potatoes, salads, and even desserts, to meet the public's norms of what constitute 'proper' meals.

The key to effecting change in meal composition is to provide substitutions for existing elements without threatening the overall structure. Studies of dietary change in indigenous societies following contact with Europeans have shown that the way in which the new foods are slotted into existing native classification systems is a useful guide to their acceptability. The most rapidly accepted foodstuffs are those that are judged similar to existing foods, in attributes such as taste, appearance, style of preparation, or growth habit. In many Pacific Island cultures, plants closely related to species already grown were the most rapidly incorporated, for example the West Indian root crop *Xanthosoma* sp., which was predictably classified as a form of taro (*Colocasia esculenta*). South American cassava (also known as manioc) and solanum potatoes were similarly acceptable because they could be grown like traditional yams, arrowroot, and sweet potatoes. With no cereal precedent in Polynesia, maize took much longer to be slotted into local culinary and horticultural traditions. In most Pacific cultures more than one starch staple was available, although they were seldom served at the same meal. This choice may have increased their readiness to accept the new staples introduced by Europeans. Monostaple cultures seem much more resistant to change. The depth of their attachment to their single staple may often be seen in the extension of the word used for the staple to mean food in general.

In some culture contact situations, foods that were initially disliked, but were essential to avoid starvation, eventually gained acceptance. This is reflected in the vernacular names which give evidence of the crucial classification process. Faced by the loss of the symbolically and nutritionally important buffalo, the Oglala Sioux initially rejected government beef rations from cattle held in corrals as smelling offensive and no substitute for buffalo meat. Under pressure, they compromised by turning loose the cattle, and then hunting, butchering and ritually feasting on them as though they were buffalo. Cattle acquired buffalo terminology and became Indian.

The message for nutritionists from such studies of culture contact is that the structural elements of culinary traditions are highly resistant to change. It is precisely these elements that in giving stability and continuity, define the tradition. Where dietary change has occurred, it has involved substitution of new foods for old within the indigenous food system, using the classification process as a guide to how the new food is to be used. Judging from historical studies, actual structural changes involving things like course order and essential elements, may take a century or longer. If thought nutritionally desirable, reform at such a fundamental level might be expected to add a new dimension to the notion of long-term planning! Ultimately, nutritionists must translate their findings into recommendations that will work within the culinary tradition, not against it.

FURTHER READING

1. Bryant CA, Courtney A, Markesbery BA, de Walt KM. *The cultural feast: an introduction to food and society.* St Paul, MN: West, 1985.
2. Charsley SR. *Wedding cakes and cultural history.* London: Routledge, 1992.
3. Douglas M (ed). *Food in the social order: studies of food and festivities in three American communities.* New York: Russell Sage Foundation, 1984.
4. Harris M. *Good to eat: riddles of food and culture.* London: Allen and Unwin, 1986.
5. Leach HM. Changing diets—a cultural perspective. *Proc Nutr Soc NZ* 1993; **18**: 1–8.
6. Messer E. Anthropological perspectives on diet. *Ann Rev Anthropol* 1984; **13**: 205–49.
7. Murcott A. Sociological and social anthropological approaches to food and eating. *World Rev Nutr Dietet* 1988; **55**: 1–40.
8. Robson JKK (ed.). *Food, ecology and culture: readings in the anthropology of dietary practices.* New York: Gordon and Breach, 1980.
9. Sharman A, Theophano J, Curtis K, Messer E (eds). *Diet and domestic life in society.* Philadelphia: Temple University, 1991.
10. Truswell AS, Wahlqvist ML (eds). *Food habits in Australia.* North Balwyn, Australia: René Gordon, 1988.

33

NUTRITIONAL RECOMMENDATIONS FOR THE GENERAL POPULATION

Stewart Truswell

Nutrition research often generates results which may be translated by the researchers themselves or the media into potentially confusing and conflicting messages. It is therefore critically important for governments, who develop food and nutrition policies, for those involved in health and nutrition education, and for consumers to have authoritative nutrition recommendations which represent consensus opinions of expert nutrition scientists. There are two major sets of recommendations: (1) recommended nutrient intakes; and (2) dietary goals and guidelines.

Recommended nutrient intakes (RNIs) or recommended dietary allowances (RDAs) are the first and older set. They are based on authoritative quantitative estimates of human requirements for essential nutrients. The earliest set that included micronutrients (only a few) was issued by the nutrition committees of the old League of Nations in 1937. The best known series of recommended intake numbers for essential nutrients, the United States Recommended Dietary Allowances, were first published in 1943 and have been revised nine times since. Many of the larger countries have their own national set of recommended nutrient intakes. In poor countries, food and nutrition policy must concentrate on striving to reach the RNI for as many people and as many nutrients as possible. But in affluent countries achievement of intakes near the RNIs can be taken for granted except in persons who are sick. More recently there has been the recognition that in most relatively affluent societies inappropriate intakes of macronutrients are involved in the aetiology of several important chronic degenerative diseases. Since the 1960s many countries have developed *dietary goals* which provide macronutrient targets aimed at achieving reductions of these diseases and *dietary guidelines* which help consumers to select from the many choices of foods in adequate diets to give better chances of long-term health. The variety of food products in affluent countries is bewildering. There is a Tower of Babel of nutritional breakthroughs, promises, adverts and threats. The whole food system needs signposts—guidelines to healthier food products and combinations that can be used in national food and nutrition policy, and in product development by food companies.

33.1   RECOMMENDED NUTRIENT INTAKES

The original US National Research Council's RDAs (1943) were a 'tentative goal toward which to aim in planning dietaries'. They were later described in the 1964 edition as designed to afford a margin of sufficiency above average physiological requirements to cover variations among practically all individuals in the general population. Essentially the same definition continues in the 1989 edition. RDAs are 'the levels of intake of essential nutrients that, on the basis of scientific knowledge, are judged by the Food and Nutrition Board to be adequate to meet the known nutrient needs of practically all healthy persons'.

Recommended nutrient intakes (RNIs) is being used here as the general term for recommended intakes of essential nutrients. Many different names are in use for these dietary standards (translated into English as needed): recommended dietary allowances (USA), recommended nutrient intakes (Canada), recommendations for the nutrient supply (Germany), recommended dietary intakes (Australia), dietetic daily recommendations (Guatemala), recommended nutritional contributions (France), and the newest term, dietary reference values for nutrients (UK).

All these names are used in different countries' reports for essentially the same numbers, which have two main functions:

1. They set the standard for an adequate intake of each essential nutrient for groups of the population. They advise people how much, on the average, they should aim to eat of these nutrients. They have a prescriptive or health promotional role.

2. They also serve as the reference unit for each essential nutrient. We need them because human (adult) requirements for individual nutrients range one billionfold (10^9), from about $1\,\mu g$, for vitamin B_{12}, through $1\,mg$ for thiamin and about $1\,g$ for calcium to about $1\,kg$ for water (Table 33.1).

Table 33.1   Approximate adult daily requirements for some essential nutrients

Adult daily requirements (rounded)	Essential nutrients
$1–10\,\mu g$	Vitamin B_{12}, vitamin D, vitamin K, chromium
$\sim 100\,\mu g$	Biotin, iodine, selenium
$200\,\mu g$	Folate, molybdenum
$1–2\,mg$	Vitamin A, thiamin, riboflavin, vitamin B_6, fluoride, copper
$5–10\,mg$	Pantothenate, manganese
$\sim 15\,mg$	Niacin, vitamin E, zinc, iron
$\sim 50\,mg$	Vitamin C
$300\,mg$	Magnesium
$\sim 1\,g$	Calcium, phosphorus
$1–5\,g$	Sodium, chloride, potassium, essential fatty acids
$\sim 50\,g$	Protein (8–10 essential amino acids)
$50–100\,g$	Available carbohydrates
$1\,kg$ (litre)	Water

Why does each country have a different set of these numbers? On close examination they are mostly similar and sometimes the same (Table 33.2). Some simply translate RNIs from another (major) country into another language. One reason for differences is that some RNIs are older and do not incorporate recent research. Another is that different age subgroups are used in the table and/or different reference weights or energy intakes are used to calculate those RNI which are originally expressed per kg body weight or per MJ. There remain a minority of nutrients only over which different groups of experts interpret the (incomplete) research data in different ways (e.g. calcium, iron, vitamin C).

Somewhere the idea originated that individual nutrient requirements are distributed in a statistical normal (Gaussian) curve—it is in the 1973 FAO/WHO Energy and Protein Requirements Report—and the RNI is then set at two standard deviations above the average of all individual requirements for each nutrient (i.e. at about the 95th percentile). But this idea did not appear in the USRDA reports until the 1989 (10th) edition, which states 'With the possible exception of the protein requirement, however, there is little evidence that requirements for nutrients are normally distributed. The distribution of the iron requirement for women, for example, is skewed. In this report (USRDA, 1989), therefore, each nutrient is treated individually...'

Most countries' reports have only one set of numbers of recommended intakes for different age and sex subgroups and for pregnancy and lactation. But another four related levels or numbers for each nutrient are needed to evaluate nutrient intakes in nutritional work. Some national reports of nutrient recommendations provide or discuss one or more of these.

Table 33.2 Recommended nutrient intakes (per day) in five national sets, and from WHO, comparing the numbers for men*

Nutrient	USA 1989 (age 25–50)	Canada 1990 (age 25–49)	Australia 1990 (age 16–64)	Germany 1991 (age 25–51)	UK 1991 (age 19–50)	WHO 1965–92 (age 15–50)
Protein (g)	58	61	55	59	45	55
Vitamin A (mg)	1.0	1.0	0.75	1.0	0.7	0.6
Vitamin D (µg)	10	3.5	–	5.0	–	2.5
Vitamin E (mg)	10	9	10	12	(7)	–
Thiamin (mg)	1.5	1.1	1.1	1.3	1.0	1.2
Riboflavin (mg)	1.7	1.4	1.7	1.7	1.3	1.8
Niacin (mg)	19	19	19	18	17	19
Vitamin B_6 (mg)	2.0	1.8	1.3–1.9	1.8	1.4	–
Folate (µg)	200	220	200	300	200	200
Vitamin B_{12} (µg)	2.0	2.0	2.0	3.0	1.5	1.0
Vitamin C (mg)	60	40	40	75	40	30
Calcium (mg)	800	800	800	900	700	400–500
Iron* (mg)	10	9	7	10	8.7	9.0
Zinc (mg)	15	12	12	15	9.5	9.4
Iodine (µg)	150	160	150	200	140	120–150
Selenium (µg)	70	25–50	85	20–100	75	40

* Values for women are the same or lower except for iron for which recommendations for (non-pregnant) women of reproductive age are higher than for men. WHO, World Health Organization.

33.1.1 A lower diagnostic level for assessing adequacy of nutrient intake

Since the RNI of a nutrient is adequate to meet the nutritional needs of practically all healthy people it is more than most people need. It cannot, therefore, be used directly to evaluate records of people's food intake, or if it is, there will be a misleading impression of inadequacy. Different approaches have been used to define a diagnostic level. Some have simply used two-thirds of the RNI.

Beaton in Canada has demonstrated a statistical probability method: the further the intake is below the RNI, the greater the probability it will be inadequate for any individual (with the parameters different for each nutrient). In 1991, the United Kingdom introduced the concept of the lower reference nutrient intake, which is defined as two standard deviations below the average of individual requirements. (This assumes, of course, that the frequency distribution of individual requirements is Gaussian for all nutrients—which we know is not always so.) Table 33.3 shows some sets of proposed lower diagnostic levels of nutrient requirements.

33.1.2 An upper level to control high dosage of supplements

Some people are enthusiastic about nutrient supplements or even believe that if a little of a vitamin does you good, more will be even better for you. Consumers and pharmacists

Table 33.3 Lower levels for evaluating risk of nutrient inadequacy for younger men

Nutrient	New Zealand 1981	Nordic 1989	Australia 1990	UK 1991
Protein (g)	35	49		
Vitamin A (μg)	600	600	600	300
Vitamin D (μg)	–	–	–	
Vitamin E (mg)	3.5		3–5	
Thiamin (mg)	0.4	0.8	0.8 (0.08/MJ)	0.6
Riboflavin (mg)	1.0	0.8	1.0 (0.1/MJ)	0.8
Niacin (mg)	5	12 (NE)	9–12	11
Vitamin B_6 (mg)	1.25	1.3	1.2	1.1
Folate (μg)	50 (as 'free')		200 ('as total')	100
Vitamin B_{12} (μg)	1.0		0.6–1.2	1.0
Vitamin C (mg)	10	10	10	10
Calcium (mg)	400	400	(550)	400
Magnesium (mg)	200			190
Iron (mg)	5	7	(5)	4.7
Iodine (μg)	100		75	70
Zinc (mg)	8		8	5.5
Sodium (mmol)			30	25
Potassium (mmol)			30	50
Selenium (μg)			30	50

The New Zealand figures are termed 'minimum safe intakes'; the Nordic figures are termed 'lower limits for intake of nutrients'; the Australian figures are termed 'lower diagnostic level intake'; the UK figures are termed 'lower reference nutrient intake'. NE = niacin equivalents.

need guidance about the level that becomes too much. It has long been known that vitamin A (retinol) and vitamin D can be toxic in some people at chronic intakes only about 10 times the RNI. There used to be a general rule that fat-soluble vitamins (like A and D) can be toxic but water-soluble vitamins not. The discovery that moderately high doses of (water-soluble) vitamin B_6 supplements causes peripheral neuropathy and that generally safe vitamins can be toxic in patients with kidney failure demolished this illogical idea. Table 33.4 shows two opinions on the start of undesirable or toxic intakes.

There is fair agreement on levels for vitamins A, D, B_6, iron, iodine and selenium and poor agreement on levels for thiamin, riboflavin, folate and vitamin C. The upper levels of niacin are used therapeutically for some hyperlipidaemias.

33.1.3 Estimated average requirement

This has to be the recommendation for energy (calorie) intake of a group. If the average energy requirement is provided for a group multiplied by the number in the group some will have more than they need and some less but these will balance out. But if the RNI concept used for other nutrients were used for energy, the energy provision would be that of those with the highest energy intakes and excessive for the majority. Estimated average requirements for protein and micronutrients are included in the United Kingdom 1991 dietary reference values.

33.1.4 Optimal intake range for some essential nutrients

There is accumulating evidence, largely based on epidemiological studies, that intakes of some nutrients well above the RNI may have beneficial effects. High intakes of vitamin C may reduce the risk of stomach cancer and generous intakes of vitamin E may be associated with lower rates of coronary heart disease and certain cancers. Intakes of folate above the RNI prevent the fetal malformations of neural tube defect if taken by the mother around the time of conception and for the month after. Larger than recommended

Table 33.4 Two opinions on thresholds of undesirable or toxic intake levels of nine major micronutrients expressed in mg/day (and multiple of RNI)

	Nordic 1989		Australian 1990	
Vitamin A (mg)	7.5	(7.5)	20 [10*]	(20[10*])
Vitamin D (mg)	0.5	(50)		
Vitamin E (mg)	350	(35)	200	(20)
Niacin (mg)	3000	(190)	merges into therapeutic use	
Vitamin B_6 (mg)	200	(100)	200 or less	(100)
Vitamin C (mg)	1000	(17)	500	(12)
Iron (mg)	100	(10)	100	(10)
Iodine (mg)	1.0	(6.6)	2.0	(13)
Selenium (mg)	0.2	(3)	0.5	(7)

* In pregnancy.

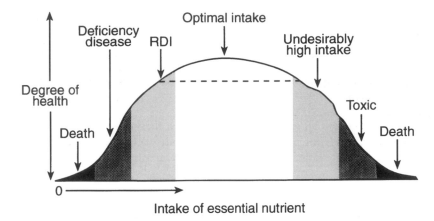

Fig. 33.1 The concept of optimal intake above the *recommended nutrient intake* (RNI). Ingestion of the RNI should guarantee no deficiency disease, but beyond the RNI there may still be additional health benefits (e.g. partial protection from a degenerative disease). The top of the dome beyond the RNI is then the optimal intake range. RDI in the figure = RNI.

amounts of folate may also reduce the risk of coronary heart disease by reducing homocysteine levels. It is not yet possible to accurately quantify the optimal intake of such nutrients, but against this background the term 'recommended' may not be the best word for some nutrients. The RNI for protein for younger men (Table 33.2) is 45–60 g/day but most men in developed countries eat around 100 g protein/day and with it obtain other important nutrients (iron, calcium, zinc, vitamin B_{12}, etc.). We do not want to recommend that men should halve their protein intake. The concept of an optimal range for some nutrients may therefore be useful (Fig. 33.1).

So we now have five different numbers for requirements of essential nutrients in use or seriously proposed. Most of them have more than one technical term even in the English language (Table 33.5). They need careful management by the international agencies and national committees. Concise, easily memorized and distinctive names for these five levels may not yet be agreed on but anyone who makes serious use of requirements numbers for essential nutrients should try and understand them.

33.2 DIETARY GOALS AND GUIDELINES (DGGs)

There do not appear to be authoritative definitions of the terms 'dietary goals' and 'dietary guidelines'. However, the former has been used in an attempt to direct national policy—what foods the nation should consume and provide. They are therefore addressed to bureaucrats and professionals. An example is 'Increase the consumption of complex carbohydrates and naturally occurring sugars from about 28% to about 48% of energy intake'. The term 'dietary guidelines', is usually used for advice to individuals, written in reader-friendly language for ordinary people, although they should be backed up by technical explanations which may include quantitative expression of the guideline.

Table 33.5 Different terms for requirements of essential nutrients (in ascending order of magnitude)

R1	Lower diagnostic level of essential nutrient.	EU: lowest threshold intake; UK: lower reference nutrient intake (LRNI).
R2	Average nutrient requirement of a subgroup of the population.	UK: estimated average requirement (EAR), this is the recommended intake for energy.
R3	Classic prescriptive recommended nutrient intake.	USA: RDA; UK: reference nutrient intake (RNI); **Canada**: recommended nutrient intake (RNI); **Australia**: recommended dietary intake, EU: population reference intake, etc.
R4	Suggested optimal range of intake of a nutrient.	Intake that gives 'high level wellness' or reduced risk of one (or more) degenerative disease(s).
R5	Undesirably high intake or start of toxic level of a nutrient.	Nutrient imbalance, lower intake than toxic. Toxicity at lower intakes for some physiological states (e.g. pregnancy) and people with some diseases (e.g. renal). Lower toxic levels for chronic than acute ingestion.

An example is 'Eat plenty of breads and cereals (preferably wholegrain), vegetables (including legumes) and fruits'. This guideline is expressed in food groups, which ordinary people are more familiar with than nutrients. Some of the major points contrasting dietary goals and guidelines with RNIs are shown in Box 33.1.

When dietary goals are expressed in quantitative terms it is important to be clear whether the cut-off numbers refer to populations or to individuals. A WHO (1990) report, *Diet, nutrition and the prevention of chronic diseases* proposed population nutrient goals. It suggests that the population goals for saturated fatty acids (SFAs) should be between 0% and 10%. This does not mean that every individual should eat less than 10% of dietary energy as SFAs. If a population's mean SFA intake is, say 9%, individuals could be eating between 5% and 14% energy as SFAs. Examples of dietary goals for fat and carbohydrate are given in Chapters 1 and 2.

Dietary guidelines have been published in over 20 countries, starting with the Nordic countries in 1968 (Table 33.6). In several of these countries there have been new editions or publications since the first appearance of dietary guidelines. In some countries (e.g. United States and United Kingdom) there are several sets of dietary guidelines, published by different expert groups. These are general dietary guidelines. There are also specialized guidelines that have been prepared by organizations concerned with heart diseases, cancer, and diabetes and vegetarian societies. Among these sets of dietary guidelines there is almost complete agreement on the six recommendations shown in Box 33.2, though the wording may differ slightly from one set to another.

A second group of guidelines is more controversial and less widely recommended. These give advice about polyunsaturated fats, dietary cholesterol and 'refined', 'extrinsic',

Box 33.1 Dietary goals and guidelines (DGGs)

- DGGs aim more to reduce the chances of developing chronic degenerative diseases than to provide enough of the essential nutrients (that is the purpose of RNIs).
- DGGs often start, not from zero intake (as do RNIs), but from the present (estimated) national average diet (and food habits).
- RNIs deal with essential nutrients; DGGs deal more with macronutrients and can also include other components in foods that are not nutrients in the classic sense (e.g. water, dietary cholesterol, dietary fibre, caffeine, fluoride).
- DGGs deal not with energy requirements but with optimal proportions of the energy-yielding macronutrients.
- DGGs are not usually expressed as micronutrients but as macronutrients, foods or food groups, or even as eating behaviour. They are not usually expressed as weight of substance per day. If expressed quantitatively this is mostly as percentage of total energy, that is, nutrient density (e.g. total fat should be 30% of total dietary energy).
- DGGs are targets for the population to aim for some time in the future (e.g. by the year 2000 or, as it gets nearer 2010). RNIs by contrast should be eaten now and (on the average) every day.
- RNIs give separate numbers for males and females and different age subgroups, but DGGs often appear to give the same advice to every man, woman and child.
- Although most RNIs are relatively well established scientifically and depend ultimately on short-term physiological experiments, DGGs are more provisional, based on indirect evidence about the complex role of food components in the cause of multifactorial diseases with long incubation periods. They rely more on epidemiological evidence than do RNIs.
- Although there is never more than one RNI report in a country, there can be several sets of DGGs in a large country at any one time.

Table 33.6 Countries with dietary guidelines by order of first appearance

1968	Nordic	1983	Denmark, UK
1976	Canada	1984	Eire, Japan
1977	USA, Quebec	1985	Netherlands, Germany
1979	Australia	1987	South Korea, Finland
1981	France, Sweden, Norway	1988	Hungary, Latin America, Italy
1982	New Zealand	1989	India, Singapore

'added' or 'concentrated' sugars (i.e. not sugars in fruits and milk). On sugar there is the widest range of opinions. Canada recommends 55% of energy from a variety of carbohydrate sources and does not single out sugar as particularly undesirable. Japan and South Korea do not mention sugar either. At the other end of the range the Nordic countries and Singapore advise restriction of refined sugar to less than 10% of energy. Thus, there are many different guidelines concerning sugar consumption including:

Box 33.2   Dietary guidelines for which there is almost complete agreement

> 1. Eat a nutritionally *adequate* diet composed of a *variety* of foods.
> 2. Eat less *fat*, particularly *saturated* fat.
> 3. Adjust energy balance for body *weight* control—less energy intake, more exercise.
> 4. *Eat more* wholegrain cereals, vegetables and fruits. In other words, eat more foods containing complex carbohydrates and fibre.
> 5. Reduce *salt* intake.
> 6. Drink *alcohol* in moderation, if you do drink.

- do not increase sugar consumption
- decrease sugar (not quantified)
- eat only a moderate amount of sugar and sugary foods
- cut down sugary snacks and sweets between meals

A third group of recommendations appears only in a small number of guideline sets:

- drink plenty of fluids each day,
- drink fluoridated water (or fluoride tablets),
- make sure you get enough calcium or milk,
- preserve (by good food preparation) the nutritive value of foods,
- eat three good meals a day,
- do not eat too much protein,
- eat foods containing iron,
- reduce intake of salt-cured and smoked foods,
- limit caffeine intake, and
- eat happily for a happy family life.

33.3   DIETARY GUIDELINES FOR CHILDREN

A WHO symposium on health issues for the twenty-first century, held in Kobe, Japan in 1993 considered that although countries could share their recommended nutrient intakes (RNIs), dietary guidelines will be most effective if the target groups are defined. New Zealand has different reports from the Department of Health, with dietary guidelines for infants and toddlers (1994), children (1992) and adolescents (1993). Australia has separate dietary guidelines for children of all ages from the National Health and Medical Research Council (1995). These reports allow for fuller consideration of the advantages and practice of breast-feeding and the nutritional problems of adolescents. There is also concern that relatively low fat diets are unsuitable for young children who start life with a 53% fat diet while they are exclusively breast-fed.

33.4   CAN RECOMMENDED NUTRIENT INTAKES AND
DIETARY GOALS BE COMBINED?

Recommended nutrient intakes and dietary goals or guidelines have usually been developed by different committees and published in separate reports both at the national and international level (i.e. WHO). A few countries have RNIs but no dietary goals or guidelines. There is, however, no reason why reference standards for essential nutrients (RNIs) and recommendations for other food components cannot be published in the same report. This has been done by the Nordic countries (1989), Canada (1990), United Kingdom (1991) and France (1992). But in these reports the two different types of standards and recommendations are presented in different sections of the report and in different ways. In the United Kingdom Report, three numbers (lower reference intake, cf. Table 33.3, estimated average requirement and reference nutrient intake, cf. Table 33.2) are given for 11 age groups by sex and for pregnancy and lactation for the essential nutrients, while for fat (as an example of a dietary guideline component) the recommendation is for the whole population and only a single quantitative recommendation is given (except for *cis*-polyunsaturated fatty acids).

33.5   DIETARY GOALS AND GUIDELINES IN DEVELOPING COUNTRIES

Dietary guidelines were introduced to deal with the nutritional problems of affluent countries. In low-income countries the major nutritional problem is that large sections of the population cannot afford or cannot grow enough food to meet all their family's requirement for essential nutrients. There are, however reasons why dietary goals and guidelines have a role in developing countries:

- Diet-related, non-communicable diseases in developing countries account for an increasing share of national mortality.
- Low-income countries cannot afford to add the burden of medical care of premature degenerative diseases to their already overstretched health budgets.
- Preparation and production of dietary guidelines is a low cost measure.
- The affluent middle class in a country such as India may be only 5% of the population but this means some 40 million people (more than many whole nations) who play a key part in the national economic development.

For India, Gopalan has proposed two sets of guidelines. For the 'relatively poor' majority, diets should be least expensive and conform to tradition and cultural practices as far as possible. Some legumes (pulses) should be eaten along with the high cereal diet, with some milk and leafy vegetables each day. For affluent Indians, he recommends restriction of energy, and of fat (especially ghee), sugar and salt, with emphasis on unrefined cereals and green leafy vegetables in the diet.

For Latin America, a set of general goals has been drafted *Guias de alimentacion bases para su desarrollo en America Latina* (1988). They have to be converted into focused guidelines for different segments of the population. Fat, for example, should be 20–25% of energy, so some groups need to be helped to eat more fat, whereas other sections of society need to bring their fat intake down.

33.6 INTEGRATING RNIs AND DGGs IN NUTRITION PROMOTION

Health professionals and, of course, those who shop and cook for the family have in practice to integrate what they read or hear about foods that provide essential nutrients and foods that fit the dietary guidelines. Teaching sets of food groups have been used since the 1940s to translate RNIs into foods, such as the four-food group plan: (1) cereal group; (2) vegetables + fruit, (3) meat, or alternatives, and (4) the milk group. There have been many attractive posters showing the four, or more, food groups. Can dietary guidelines be integrated in the same poster and nutrition education pamphlet? A partial answer to this challenge is the nutrition education pyramid, blocks or plate (Fig. 33.2).

33.7 REFERENCE NUMBERS FOR NUTRITION LABELLING AND FOOD STANDARDS

For nutrition labelling of foods it is nowadays standard practice for manufacturers to print statements like:

One standard serving (30 g) of this food provides 22% of the recommended dietary intake of vitamin X.

The wording and the reference recommended dietary intake are laid down by food law, which is set by statutory bodies such as the Food and Drug Administration (FDA) in the USA, Ministry of Agriculture, Fisheries and Food (MAFF) in the UK, the ANZ National Food Authority in Australia and New Zealand. The same reference set is used in controlling permitted additions of micronutrients in food fortification (e.g. 'Up to 50% of the RDI of vitamin X may be added per reference quantity, e.g. 30 g, of food Y').

A particular selection of the recommended nutrient intakes is chosen for food standards and then enshrined in law. In the United States, this reference is called the 'US recommended daily allowance (US RDA)'. The numbers are the highest values for any age/sex subgroup of (non-pregnant, non-lactating) people in the 1968 (7th edition) of the US Recommended Dietary Allowances report. Most figures are for young men, iron is the figure for young women and for thiamin, niacin, iodine and magnesium they are based on the recommendations for adolescent males (see Table 33.7).

In Australia, the food law 'RDIs' (Table 33.7) are based on the highest 1991 Australian recommended dietary intakes for (non-pregnant, non-lactating) younger adults. This means the figures for younger men for all nutrients except iron, for which the lower end of the recommended range for younger women is used. For preformed niacin, 10 mg is set, assuming that the remainder of the requirements will come from tryptophan in proteins; for vitamin D the 10 µg advised for housebound people is the value used.

Some of the United States numbers now appear too high (e.g. 400 µg for folate and 6 µg for vitamin B_{12}). The current (1989) recommended dietary allowances for these are now 200 µg and 2 µg, respectively. There will, of course, appear to be more iron or vitamin C in a food if compared against the Australian, rather than the US RDA (Table 33.7).

The Scientific Committee for Food of the European Union proposed in 1992 that reference values of micronutrients for nutrition labelling in the European Union should

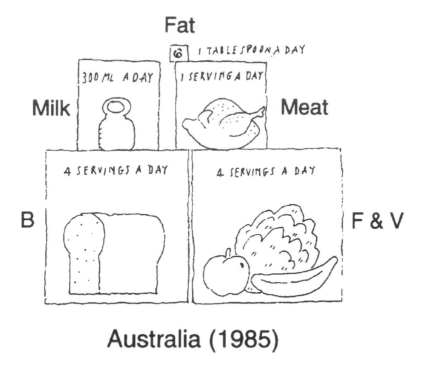

Australia (1985)

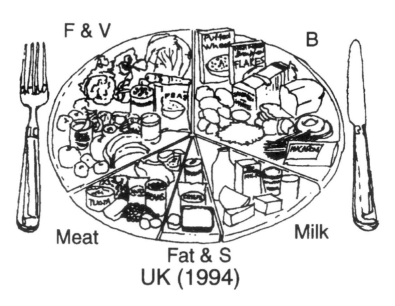

UK (1994)

Fig. 33.2 Visual expression of food guides that aim to integrate essential food groups and dietary guidelines. Area (or volume) represents amount you should eat: most of the cereal group and vegetables and fruits; moderately of meat and milk groups; sparingly of fat (and sugary food) groups. B, bread and cereal foods; F, fruit; Fat, fats; L, legumes; Meat, meat, fish or alternatives; Milk, milk, cheese, yoghurt, etc.; S, sugary foods, V, vegetables and salads.

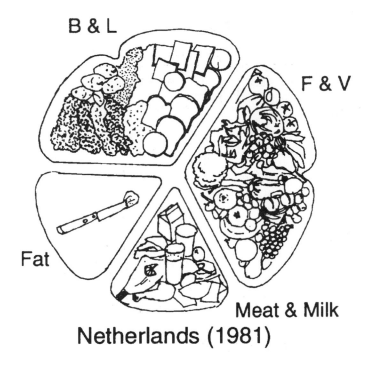

B & L

F & V

Fat

Meat & Milk

Netherlands (1981)

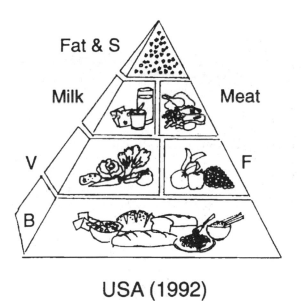

Fat & S

Milk

Meat

V

F

B

USA (1992)

Fig. 33.2 Visual expression of food guides that aim to integrate essential food groups and dietary guidelines. Area (or volume) represents amount you should eat: most of the cereal group and vegetables and fruits; moderately of meat and milk groups; sparingly of fat (and sugary food) groups. B, bread and cereal foods; F, fruit; Fat, fats; L, legumes; Meat, meat, fish or alternatives; Milk, milk, cheese, yoghurt, etc.; S, sugary foods, V, vegetables and salads.

Table 33.7 Reference standards for micronutrients for nutrition labelling and food standards

Nutrient	United States 'US RDI'	Australia ANZFA	EU Proposal
Vitamin A (μg)	1000	750	500
Thiamin (mg)	1.5	1.1	0.8
Riboflavin (mg)	1.7	1.7	1.3
Niacin (mg)	20	10	15 (NE)
Vitamin B_6 (mg)	2	1.6	1.3
Folate (μg)	400	200	140
Vitamin B_{12} (μg)	6	2	1
Vitamin C (mg)	60	40	30
Vitamin D (μg)	10	10	5
Vitamin E (mg)	30	10	–
Calcium (mg)	1000	800	550
Iron (mg)	18	12	7 (men) 14 (women)
Iodine (μg)	150	150	100
Magnesium (mg)	400	320	–
Phosphorus (mg)	1000	1000	–
Zinc (mg)	15	12	7.5

be the Average Requirements for adult men, except for iron. The committee reasons that this is a more realistic reference.

In practice, nutrient information on food labels is more likely to give values for components that are in dietary goals, rather than RNIs. If the national targets for total fat and saturated fat, fibre and sodium are 30% energy from fat, 10% energy from saturated fat, 30 g and 2.3 g, respectively and a rounded average energy intake of 10 MJ is assumed, the reference values are:

80 g for total fat, 27 g for saturated fat, 30 g for dietary fibre and 2.3 g for sodium.

Most members of the public are still a long way from being able to obtain useful information from labels of this kind and many attempts are being made to produce labels for packaged foods which will assist the shopper in making the most appropriate food choices.

References

1. Bengoa JM, Torun B, Behar M, Scrimshaw N. *Guias de alimentacion bases para su desarrollo en America Latina*. Guatemala City: INCAP, 1988.
2. Department of Health. *Dietary reference values for food energy and nutrients for the United Kingdom*. Report of the Panel on Dietary Reference Values of the Committee on Medical Aspects of Food Policy. London: HMSO, 1991.
3. Deutsche Gesellschaft für Eruährung. *Empfehlungen für die Nährstoffzufuhr*, 5 überarbeitung. Frankfurt/Main: Umschau Verlag, 1991.

4. Gopalan C. Dietary guidelines from the perspective of developing countries. In: Latham MC and van Veen MS (eds). *Dietary guidelines: Proceedings of an International Conference*. Ithaca, NY: Cornell International Monograph 21, 1989.

5. Health and Welfare Canada. *Nutrition recommendations*. The report of the Scientific Committee. Ottawa: Canadian Government Publishing Centre, 1990.

6. Hunt P, Gatenby S, Rayner M. The format for the National Food Guide: performance and preference studies. *Journal of Human Nutrition and Dietetics* 1995; 8: 335–51.

7. Nordisk Ministerrad. *Nordic nutrition recommendations*, 2nd ed. English version. Uppsala, Sweden: National Food Administration, 1989.

8. Report of a World Health Organization Study Group. *Diet, nutrition and the prevention of chronic diseases*. WHO Technical Report Series 797. Geneva: WHO, 1990.

9. Subcommittee on the Tenth Edition of the RDAs. Food and Nutrition Board. *Recommended dietary allowances*, 10th ed. Washington DC: National Academy Press, 1984.

10. Truswell AS, Dreosti IE, English RM, Rutishauser IHE, Palmer N (eds). *Recommended nutrient intakes*, Australian Papers. Mosman NSW: Australian Professional Publications, 1990.

FURTHER READING

1. Truswell AS. The philosophy behind Recommended Dietary Intakes: can they be harmonized? *European Journal of Clinical Nutrition* 1990; 44 (suppl. 2): 3–11.

2. Committee on Diet and Health, Food and Nutrition Board, National Research Council. *Diet and health: Implications for reducing chronic disease risk*. Washington, DC: National Academy Press, 1989, 749 pages.

3. Truswell AS. Evolution of dietary recommendations, goals and guidelines. *American Journal of Clinical Nutrition* 1987; 45: 1060–72.

34
Nutrition Programmes for Communities

Cynthia Tuttle and Vicky Scott

Nutrition issues continue to have a widespread impact on the health of individuals in communities throughout the world. The challenge becomes one of designing and implementing effective nutrition promotion programmes which will help to alleviate nutritional problems and thereby promote better overall health. This chapter will provide an introduction to nutrition programme design, implementation and evaluation at the community level.

34.1 Nutrition Programme Design

34.1.1 Defining the nutrition problem and conducting a needs assessment

The process of defining the nutrition problem depends upon observation and the collection of available data so the most urgent needs and concerns of a community can be identified. This involves gathering nutrition-related statistics including population demographics, geographical population distributions, economic and social characteristics, births, deaths and disease prevalence and incidence. This is combined with a subjective assessment of the existent social structures, resources and the perceived needs of communities. For example, agencies which provide food and nutrition services are identified, mass media messages examined, interviews conducted with local health professionals and community leaders and discussions may be held within the community group. With this information, planners should be able to identify effectively where potential opportunities or barriers exist and determine how prepared a community is for change.

34.1.2 Development of goals and objectives

Successful programmes are ones with clearly conceived goals and objectives. This means that national programmes and policies require regional and community input during conceptualization. Goals must be fixed, but the means by which they are achieved must be flexible so that adjustments can be made according to local conditions. Goals should be deemed to be measurable and achievable in the long term, but not necessarily realistic over a given time frame.

Objectives must answer the questions for *Whom, What, When* (within a reasonable time frame), and *To What Extent* (must be realistic). Health objectives usually require baseline data in order to be able to measure a difference in health indices. For example: 'To reduce the prevalence of anaemia, as measured by a haemoglobin less than 110 g/l, among children six months to four years of age attending health clinics by the year 2000.'

Behavioural objectives focus on the behaviour which is expected during or after the intervention effort. For example: 'By the end of the counselling session, all mothers will be able to name three foods which are high in iron.' Table 34.1 provides a list of key planning terms utilized in nutrition programme design.

34.1.3 Planning the programme

Goals and objectives are utilized as a guide for designing the intervention programme. Specific strategies, developed to meet the needs of the community, are then chosen to help bring about change. Some strategies simply provide information, others give people opportunities to practise healthy food behaviours, while there are some strategies which attempt to alter community environments. Consideration must include the budgetary

Table 34.1 Planning terms

Nutrition programme planning	A process of identifying and evaluating nutrition or health problems, setting goals and objectives and developing a plan of action to meet those established objectives.
Mission	Describes the general functions or services the organization performs.
Nutrition problem or need	A situation or condition which has a current or potential adverse effect on people's health and well-being.
Goal	Statements of outcomes which will have occurred when the need is met. It must be measurable.
Health objective	Statements of the results to be obtained as a means of achieving the goals. Focus on health indices and is stated in terms of a reduction of the problem to a specified degree in a specified period of time.
Behavioural objective	Sometimes called programme objectives, have as their outcomes a situation or condition which will affect achievement of the health objective. Focus is on behaviour change.
Milestones (process objectives)	Measures of activity or effort which can be used to monitor progress of objectives.
Programme evaluation	The process of determining the extent to which predetermined objectives and levels of operation are attained. It is a tool used to ensure that what is planned actually takes place and that the desired effect is achieved.

allotment for the programme, total numbers in the target population, equipment and materials required, facilities available, and the staffing needs for programme implementation. Other factors which could impact on the success of a nutrition intervention include awareness of the literacy level, knowledge and skills of the target population and barriers to programme access, such as the availability of transport, media resources, and the respondent burden.

34.1.4 Community participation

Experience has shown that when local people participate in all phases of programme development they are more likely to be involved and committed to maintaining changes. That is, programmes must be developed and managed locally so that they reflect local values. If programmes or policies are designed at a national level, local representatives need to be involved.

Assessing community needs by incorporating community input will help to prioritize problems appropriately. For example, although nutrition may be assumed to be a high priority in an area, if a high prevalence of diarrhoea exists in young children arising from unsanitary drinking water, the true priority may be to ensure a potable water system rather than nutrition education.

The use of peer counsellors or research assistants from the target population who have been specifically trained to implement the programme has been used successfully in many community nutrition intervention programmes. However, there will always be a certain amount of attrition among the trained staff, so well-planned programmes must include ongoing recruitment, training and an adequate reward scheme, monetary or otherwise.

34.2 COMMUNITY NUTRITION DEMONSTRATION PROJECTS

The Tamil Nadu Integrated Nutrition Project (TINP) in southern India provides a good example of a community-based intervention project. It highlights the success that can be achieved in combating malnutrition on a large scale through specific targeting of groups who are most in need. Because malnutrition is most prevalent during the weaning phase, the TINP project focused on children aged 6–36 months and was a large-scale nutrition project with a complex design including growth monitoring, supplementary feeding, nutrition education and health interventions.

The project was a time series design in that implementation was staggered amongst the 9000 villages taking part. This meant that some villages could serve as controls in the evaluation. Serious and severe malnutrition decreased by one half in the project villages. Participation rates were high; 90% of children were weighed monthly and 98% of the children who were eligible for the supplement, received it for a 90-day period. Only 7% of those who completed the feeding programme showed inadequate growth during the next six months.

An evaluation of one district after four years showed that immunization of children increased from 44% to 82%, registration for antenatal care rose from 54% to 70% and tetanus toxoid injections for pregnant women increased from 23% to 62%. The cost of the project was estimated to be less than half of that of a comparative programme, the National Integrated Child Development Scheme (ICDS).

The TINP project differed from other programmes because it targeted a small but extremely vulnerable age group and only provided supplements when needed. Adequate time was allowed for development, expansion and refinement of the project because it spanned six years rather than the typical three- or four-year period. Training of the workers was also more intensive, whereas the ratio of supervisors to workers (1 : 10) was much lower than other projects.

Community nutrition workers, with eight or more years of schooling, were recruited from the local villages and trained to weigh the children and monitor their growth on a monthly basis, provide short-term food supplements to those in need, deworm the children every four months, distribute vitamin A supplements biannually, and counsel mothers on nutrition as well as provide supplements for the diets of pregnant women in need.

At the same time, and in a co-operative way, health workers cared for women's health and the health of all other children. Specifically, they provided care prenatally and during childbirth, immunized pregnant women and children, distributed iron and folate supplements to pregnant women and monitored children's growth during the first six months of life. Women's working groups were also established in each village and longterm nutrition education strategies were employed to improve nutrition and health practices.

Many aspects of the TINP are relevant to other programmes. These include a narrower age focus, selective and short-term feeding, screening for early signs of malnutrition, the need to combine growth monitoring with nutrition education, supplementary feeding and health services, and the benefits of a project controlled by women who were well trained and supervised. Overall, this projects demonstrates that programmes which target resources can have a greater effect at a lower cost.

34.3   IMPLEMENTATION AND ADMINISTRATION

Another element for success is a stable, visible administrative structure with representation from different sectors of society, and support from the highest levels of local or national government. The purpose of such an administrative structure is to plan and co-ordinate nutrition activities which integrate with other sectors.

National nutrition goals are often not independent from other societal goals, and may not be important enough politically, for consideration by themselves. Most actions which influence nutrition come from sectors with other primary goals. Programme administrators, therefore, need to design strategies which will mobilize different agencies and government departments to function with a more integrated approach. They must make compromises in order to encourage individual sectors to include nutrition into their primary activities. Such compromises mean that actions rarely relate to nutrition directly but instead bring about improvement indirectly through actions such as improved water supplies and sanitation, new roads to improve food access and production of food crops for local consumption rather than monetary gain. Combating problems, such as malnutrition, therefore requires links with many agencies involved with rural development, primary health care, public administration, community organization, and political economy.

34.4 Evaluation

Successful programmes require a system to monitor whether they are meeting their objectives effectively and using resources and methods appropriately to achieve the stated goals. Evaluations are often used to determine future funding for a programme and whether modifications in design or implementation are required.

It is important to identify measures of success from the beginning so they can be tracked throughout a programme. Only essential indicators should be included in order to keep costs down and to avoid losing sight of programme goals and objectives through superfluous data. Measures of success need to relate to the type of programme being conducted and to the community involved.

Programmes may use one or more types of evaluation including formative, process, outcome and impact evaluations.

Formative evaluation (pretesting) assesses draft materials and strategies before implementation so that the most appropriate version can be selected and refined for the intended audience. Pretesting methods include:

1. *Readability testing*: estimating the reading level needed to understand written material.
2. *Focus group interviews*: carefully planned group discussions with 7–10 representatives of the target audience to provide insights on how materials or strategies are perceived.
3. *Surveys*: short questionnaires designed to reach many people.
4. *Personal interviews*: one-on-one, in-depth interviews.
5. *Theatre testing*: assessing audience reactions to audio or audiovisual materials.
6. *Gatekeeper review*: whereby other health professionals are asked to evaluate the effectiveness of materials or programmes.

Process evaluation monitors the internal workings of a programme. It examines the extent to which activities are being implemented and whether they are reaching the intended target group, as well as the quality of programme materials and components. Process evaluation can be achieved by keeping records of the type and number of activities conducted (including publicity) and the expenditures made. Observations and impressions, such as comments from programme instructors on the ease of delivering messages should also be documented. Participation and awareness are two indicators of target reach. Participation can be assessed either by keeping records of the numbers attending activities or requesting information; or it can be examined subjectively by observation. Brief questionnaires examining the value and relevance of information given, the level of difficulty and personal relevance, may also be used at the end of the activities to assess participant satisfaction and to identify any constraints and failures so that adjustments and/or improvements can be made, if necessary.

Outcome evaluation provides short-term results which usually relate to programme objectives, such as knowledge gains, attitude shifts, development of skills and intermediate changes in behaviour. These indicators are measured before a programme commences and are repeated at the end, in order to accurately determine the effectiveness of the programme. Policies which have been initiated during the programme and other institutional changes are also documented.

Impact evaluation focuses on long-term results and typically assesses programme goals, such as changes in health status which might include mortality and morbidity rates in a population, as well as more specific biological indicators such as biochemical and functional tests and a clinical assessment. All the indicators must be carefully selected to ensure they are responsive over the time frame of the programme and where appropriate, over the range of improvement expected. Although an important component of a comprehensive evaluation process, impact evaluations are rarely carried out because of the cost and time involved and due to the complexity of demonstrating that changes relate directly to the programme and not to other influences which occur with time.

34.4.1   An example of a community project in Finland

The North Karelia Project provides a good example of a research and demonstration project in an industrialized country.

Coronary heart disease (CHD) is a major cause of morbidity and mortality in many Western countries. Public health departments are therefore using demonstration programmes for CHD prevention as models for implementing their own programmes. These programmes are designed to minimize specific diseases using community input. The North Karelia Project is an important model because it is a pioneer community-based programme with over 20 years of follow-up. Furthermore, it has demonstrated that a reduction in risk factors for CHD can be achieved in communities.

The North Karelia Project began in 1972 in a province of eastern Finland. It developed as a consequence of a local petition calling for national aid to reduce the high CHD mortality rates. The project was subsequently launched with the aim of examining whether CHD risk factors could be reduced by a comprehensive community-based programme and whether this would be followed by a reduction in CHD morbidity and mortality. Strategies included an improvement in the detection and control of hypertension, a reduction in smoking, and promotion of diets lower in saturated fat and higher in vegetables and low fat products.

An office was established in the health department and local project advisory boards were set up with participation from various community agencies. A baseline survey identified the community's needs, and an inital awareness campaign commenced. Strategies and resources were also developed and local training activities were started.

Programme activites centred around improving services and changing behaviours and environments through the application of theoretical principles. Preventive services were improved by increasing the number of health centres and by establishing a hypertension register. Public health nurses were trained to identify high blood pressure and provide physician referral, follow-up monitoring, dietary and behavioural advice. Campaigns to educate people about their cardiovascular health were conducted through the media and via community groups and organizations such as worksites, schools, shops, commercial places and voluntary organizations.

Providing counter-arguments to strongly held beliefs was another persuasive strategy. The belief that high meat fat was necessary for hard-working individuals was disputed by pointing out that there were hard-working vegetarian lumberjacks and that the traditional diet for North Karelia had been low in fat compared to the present high fat diet. Attempts were also made to make low fat foods more available through collaboration with several food manufacturers, such as a local sausage factory and the county dairy.

Community-training programmes offered new skills and practices to the target population. A co-operative venture between the North Karelia Project and the local housewives' association, 'Martha', resulted in leaders demonstrating new cooking skills which were then practised by women in their village and presented to families as part of an evening social programme. Some organizational work occurred in the community through a 'lay leaders' weekend training programme where leaders were encouraged to be positive examples by practising healthy behaviours, by advocating for positive changes in the community and by disseminating information about the project.

The project was originally designed for 5 years, extended to 10, and finally broadened to include the prevention of other chronic diseases and health promotion activities and to focus on people other than the middle-aged. There have also been increased national activities in disease prevention, particularly for CHD in which the North Karelia Project has been actively involved. These include national antismoking legislation in the 1970s, nutrition policies and televised information on risk factor reduction.

The North Karelia Project undertook a comprehensive evaluation which included detection of CHD risk factors (serum cholesterol, blood pressure and smoking) in North Karelia and in a reference area. The results were based on well-standardized, comparable surveys of cross-sectional populations, aged 30–59 years. Risk factors fell markedly in the first five years in North Karelia, then decreased to a lesser extent in the next five years. Mortality due to CHD declined by 37% among men during the 1970s and 1980s, although the rate still remained one of the highest in the world. There was also a decline in risk factors in the neighbouring reference county during the first 10 years but the decreases were less than in North Karelia and were thought to be partly due to the flow-over effect of the project. A levelling off in the decline during the 10–15 year period brought about new nation-wide preventive activities which resulted in major declines in both serum total cholesterol and blood pressure at the 20-year follow-up. The reduction in serum cholesterol level corresponds with dietary change in saturated fat consumption, specifically with reduced milk fat consumption and increased intake of vegetable oils. Ischaemic heart disease mortality has declined by about 50% in Finland in the past 20 years.

The North Karelia Project has demonstrated a reduction in risk factors and broadened disease prevention strategies. Environmental changes now include menu-labelling in restaurants, labelling of healthy alternatives in supermarkets and policy initiatives such as the control of tobacco through vending machines. Self-help programmes for weight control, physical activity and smoking control are gaining interest because of their low cost and low intervention. There is also more involvement with community organizations such as workplaces and schools. Finally, the project accelerated national development in cardiovascular disease prevention strategies.

34.6 SUMMARY

Community-based nutrition promotion is about helping population groups overcome nutrition problems. This is achieved by involving local people actively in defining their common problems and needs, in setting goals and objectives, developing plans for change and in implementing and monitoring those changes.

FURTHER READING

1. Brems S. Target: Malnutrition results from Tamil Nadu. Mothers and children, *Bulletin on Infant Feeding and Maternal Nutrition* 1987; 6: 1–4.
2. Oshang A. *Planning and managing community nutrition work. Manual for personnel involved in community nutrition.* WHO Regional Office for Europe: Copenhagen, 1992.
3. *Pretesting in health communications.* U.S. Department of Health and Human Services, Public Health Service, National Institutes of Health, NIH Publication No. 84–1493, 1984.
4. Puska P, Nissinen A, Tuomilehto J, Salonen JT, Koskela K, McAlister A, *et al.* The community-based strategy to prevent coronary heart disease: conclusions from the ten years of the North Karelia Project. *Ann Rev Public Health* 1985; 6: 147–193.
5. Underwood BA. Some elements of successful nutrition intervention strategies. In: *Nutrition intervention stategies in national development.* New York: Academic Press Inc. 1983, pp 3–11.

35

DIETARY COUNSELLING

Sue Scarlet

Preceding chapters of this book have clearly illustrated the extent of scientific knowledge that now exists, identifying diet as a vital factor in maintenance of health and prevention of chronic disease. However, helping a client change his or her dietary habits goes beyond simply communicating knowledge as to what constitutes an appropriate diet for that person. It has been estimated that adherence to modified dietary regimens is approximately 30% with a range of 13–75%. This suggests that the process of dietary change is much more complex than is often appreciated.

35.1 THE NEED FOR DIETARY MODIFICATION

For the vast majority of clients who need to make dietary changes the changes recommended will be in line with national food and nutrition guidelines. Most of the discussion in this chapter focuses on this situation. Some medical conditions require dietary modifications which do not resemble national food and nutrition guidelines (e.g. a low potassium diet in end-stage renal failure or a high energy diet to replete a cancer patient). There are also situations where dietary modification is much more complex (e.g. in insulin-dependent diabetes or coeliac disease). In some situations failure to comply with diet results in immediate, harmful or life-threatening consequences, such as in a baby with phenylketonuria or a patient on dialysis who fails to comply with a fluid or potassium restriction. More frequently, when dietary modification is recommended in the management of conditions such as elevated cholesterol, hypertension, non-insulin-dependent diabetes, obesity, or a poor nutrient intake, the consequences of dietary non-compliance are less immediate. However, non-compliance may increase morbidity and shorten lifespan. Situations requiring dietary modification are outlined in Table 35.1. The reasons for dietary change and the consequences of not making such changes should be fully explained to the client. Until a client accepts the diagnosis and the need for change, dietary counselling will be ineffective.

If nutrition education is to go beyond merely handing over a pamphlet containing the relevant nutrition information, then time needs to be spent in which the nutrition educator establishes rapport with the client and begins to become familiar with the client's food behaviour. Factors to be considered when providing nutrition counselling are listed in Table 35.2.

Table 35.1   Examples of situations when dietary modification is required

Metabolic disorders, often diagnosed at birth or in a young child. Diet is the life-saving treatment.	e.g. phenylketonuria, galactosaemia, coeliac disease.
Diet combined with drugs or other medical intervention is a necessary part of an immediate life-saving treatment.	e.g. insulin-dependent diabetes, patients on dialysis.
Repletion of malnourished patients. Adequate nutrition repletion will increase chance of surviving surgery and/or improve quality of life.	e.g. in cancer or intestinal disease.
Diet alone or combined with drugs will control a diagnosed medical condition which would otherwise lead to serious morbidity and early mortality.	e.g. non-insulin-dependent-diabetes, hypertension, hyperlipidaemia.
Diets to control weight in obese people who may or may not have a disease associated with obesity.	e.g. hypertension.
Individuals who have no associated morbidity, but for whom changes in current eating habits would reduce morbidity later in life.	e.g. low calcium intakes in adolescent girls, inadequate diets in athletes, a high fat diet in an individual with a family history of coronary heart disease.
Nutritional deficiencies.	e.g. anaemia.
Elimination diets for diagnosis and control of food sensitivity.	
Diets as part of a test.	e.g. faecal fat.
Diets to deal with the side effects of drugs.	e.g. diets with increased potassium for patients on some diuretics.

Table 35.2   Factors to consider when providing nutrition counselling

- Diagnosis, biochemical results, height, weight, body mass index (BMI)
- Ethnic group
- Patient's acceptance of the diagnosis and the need for dietary change
- Previous dietary education for current or other problems
- Failed attempts at dietary modification
- Current eating habits
- Where food is purchased/obtained
- Food preparation skills
- Usual cooking methods
- Person responsible for cooking/purchasing food
- Other places food is eaten (e.g. work, socially)
- Social support for dietary changes
- Understanding and use of the English language

35.2   ESTABLISHING RAPPORT

Establishing a caring relationship is probably more influential in promoting learning and dietary behaviour change than any other aspect of the teaching/counselling process. The relationship a good educator establishes with the client has been described as one of 'unconditional positive regard'. This suggests a relationship without prejudice, including social prejudice, prejudice towards lifestyle factors identified and prejudice towards past failures at dietary modification. The relationship needs to be one in which the client and educator regard each other as equals. The educator must show empathy and demonstrate his or her desire to understand what the client is thinking and feeling.

At the start of the interview the educator introduces him or herself and explains why the interview is being carried out. It is also necessary to explain what is going to happen in the remainder of the interview, what they hope to achieve and time expectations. The client should be invited to discuss anything he or she feels is important before the interview proceeds.

35.3   The Diet History

Current eating habits are identified by finding out what is consumed in a typical day, investigating variations on a typical day and cross-checking food intake using a simple food frequency questionnaire. There are some exceptions to the rule; some clients' food intake will vary considerably from day to day and a typical day's intake will be difficult for them to describe, others are simply not aware of what they eat. In these cases food records will be more useful for identifying current food intake. Information on a typical day's intake is obtained by asking a series of neutral questions, for example:

'What time of the day would you normally first eat or drink?'

'What foods or drinks would you have at this time?'

'Are there any other foods you would have?'

'How much of each of these would you usually have?'

'When would you next eat or drink?'

Questions should be neutral and not leading. Leading questions indicate to the client that one answer is preferential to another. For example the question, 'Do you eat breakfast?', may indicate to the client that the educator believes eating breakfast is the norm and may influence the answer. During the interview the educator should avoid showing an emotional response to the information obtained. Both verbal and non-verbal responses must be avoided. For example, if the educator looks shocked or surprised by the amount consumed at an evening meal the client may be less open about discussing other dietary practices. Variations on a typical day's intake are most likely to occur at weekends, these should be investigated further. A simple food frequency questionnaire may be used to check the usual consumption of the following items: breads, cereals, fruits, vegetables, meats or alternatives, milk products, sugar, salt, fat, fibre, fluids, alcohol, takeaway foods, restaurant meals, high fat foods, sweet foods, snack foods, usual cooking methods and frequency of meals eaten away from home. Additional potentially useful aspects that may be identified in the interview include the person responsible for cooking the meals, previous attempts at dietary modification, health problems, current weight and height, weight history and familial weight patterns. The amount of detail established in the interview will vary depending on the objective of the interview. The interview must give the educator an insight into the environment in which eating occurs and help identify which dietary habits need to be changed. In some cases, the data gathered from the interview may be used to calculate usual energy or nutrient intake. In this situation information on amounts of food consumed will need to be more precise.

35.4 EDUCATION

Providing education and communicating knowledge may be part of the process of helping a client change eating patterns and food behaviours. Some people will already know what they should eat, for others knowledge of optimal dietary habits is lacking. At the very least, revision of appropriate dietary changes serves as a point to begin discussion on implementation of these changes. Education should be based at the level of comprehension of the client. For all clients education needs to be kept simple and relevant. People lead complex lives and are exposed to increasing amounts of information concerning all aspects of their lives. It is important not to overload the individual who may not share the educator's enthusiasm for nutrition information.

35.5 EDUCATION MATERIALS

Government health departments, organizations involved in heart disease, cancer and diabetes, nutrition foundations and the food and drug industry in most countries generate potentially useful education material. If using a pamphlet written by the food industry, the educator should carefully check that the information it contains is correct. Some educators with relevant expertise prefer to create their own educational material. The 'food pyramid' or the 'food plate' (see Chapter 33), printed as posters or pamphlets, are simple and very useful for general education on healthful eating. These are excellent tools as they focus on positive rather than negative aspects. It is the author's experience that many people referred for dietary counselling do not consume the minimum servings from one or more of the four food groups, and dietary counselling frequently begins by discussing the foods which should be increased. In addition to pamphlets and posters other useful education materials include food models, diagrams or photographs of plated meals, recipes or recipe books, food containers or labels, and in some areas, supermarket tours, run by dietitians, are available.

35.6 COUNSELLING

Before the educator discusses the undesirable eating habits that need changing, it is important to reinforce and show approval for those food habits that do not need changing:

'Since being informed about your diagnosis you have already made some very positive changes to your diet...'

'You have a good meal pattern and an excellent fruit intake'

'You did well to lose weight and maintain the weight loss for a year, before you had your recent relapse'

After providing some positive feedback it is then appropriate to discuss foods to avoid or foods or cooking methods that should be changed. The educator may begin with her or his judgement of what is most important. Finally, one or two goals for change should be selected for immediate implementation. For example, when comparing the usual dietary intake of a patient with hyperlipidaemia with the recommended intake, the educator may have identified the following possible changes:

(1) should include cereal and low fat milk for breakfast instead of a pie for morning tea,

(2) should increase fruit snacks and decrease cakes and sausage rolls,

(3) should change to a lower fat milk,

(4) should chose leaner meats and reduce the size of meat servings,

(5) should drink water or diet drinks instead of ordinary soft drink.

The educator and the client should decide on goals together. If the client is not committed to a goal or feels it is unachievable then this goal should not be a priority. In the above example educator and client may decide that goals (1) and (3) may be the simplest to achieve and result in the least disruption to family life. These can then be implemented first. Sometimes a compromise can be reached regarding a particular goal. For example, the goal may be to eat breakfast, but the client may feel that it is not acceptable to get up quarter of an hour early to do so. In this case a compromise may be reached when the client agrees to include a snack of yoghurt, fruit, muffins or a sandwich at the morning tea break.

35.7 BARRIERS TO CHANGE

Some discussion on barriers to the achievement of goals should be undertaken at this stage. 'What problems do you see in achieving this goal?' The goal of reducing meat servings at the dinner meal may mean the client has to regularly remind his partner to serve smaller amounts of meat. The goal of using a lower fat milk may mean buying two cartons of milk as other family members may not be prepared to make the change. The work place cafeteria may not provide fresh fruit and yoghurt, therefore the client will need to take this to work.

35.8 GOAL-SETTING

Goals should define food or lifestyle behaviours. The focus is on what the client actually has to do to achieve an improvement in health, such as weight loss or reduced lipid levels. Measurement of weight loss or biochemical results may not be particularly useful at this stage. For example, someone needing to lose weight may, at the time of first contact with the educator, be gaining weight. In such a person, initial small changes in food or exercise behaviour may slow or stop the increase. Measuring weight loss would not be a positive way to provide feedback; discussing achievement of behaviour change goals would be. Changes in blood lipid levels may be similarly slow to achieve. On the other hand, changes in blood pressure and blood glucose can occur quite quickly. In a client with non-insulin-dependent diabetes, blood glucose levels may drop with a decrease in food intake even before weight loss has occurred. These can be a useful way of providing positive feedback but the focus in the first instance must continue to be on the achievement of food and lifestyle behaviour change.

35.9 SELF-EFFICACY

Educators should guard against recommending a large number of changes at any one time and especially at the outset of counselling. Such an approach will often set the client up for failure. Setting small achievable goals has been recognized as important for enhancing a client's self-efficacy. Self-efficacy describes the level of confidence a client has in his or her ability to change behaviour. Successful performance of a behaviour increases a person's confidence in his or her ability to repeat the behaviour, whereas failure, especially repeated failure lowers confidence in his or her ability to make any sort of behaviour change.

35.10 SOCIAL SUPPORT

The inclusion of a family member or other support person at some of the education and counselling sessions should be encouraged. This is especially important if they are responsible for cooking or shopping or have influence over these activities.

35.11 RELAPSE COUNSELLING

Data show that lapses and relapses are an all too common part of any behaviour change. The educator needs to work with the client to anticipate and prevent dietary lapses. The client needs to be able to overcome minor slips of willpower before they become a total breakdown in self-control. Preparing the client to cope with relapse involves recognizing that relapse is a common problem. Next, the educator and client should identify situations which lead to relapse. Finally, discussion and practice with coping with these situations is needed. The educator may begin by explaining that the expectation of perfect dietary compliance is unrealistic. Abstinence from disallowed foods is frequently viewed by individuals from an all-or-nothing perspective. 'I ate one chocolate biscuit, I might as well eat the whole packet.' The educator and client should identify high-risk situations. Examples of these include social gatherings, emotional upheavals and feelings of boredom, stress and overwork. Prior to a dinner party or other social gathering, the educator may discuss with the client his or her intentions for coping. High-risk situations should not be avoided, merely seen as challenges in which to practise new behaviours. Lapses that occur should be discussed in the context of positive aspects of the eating behaviour which have continued. There should also be discussion as to how the situation may be handled differently should it arise in future. Education in stress management may also be part of the relapse prevention strategy.

35.12   MONITORING BEHAVIOUR CHANGE

Food records are a useful tool for the counselling process. Whether these are kept daily, several days each week or whether a one-off sample is kept depends on the nature of the nutritional problem being tackled and preference of the client. Food records help the client gain awareness of his or her own eating habits, as well as providing the educator with a basis for discussion at follow-up sessions. Additional recording tools that can be useful for specific clients include fat counters, fibre counters, and records on food intake and associated environmental factors.

35.13   FOLLOW-UP COUNSELLING

One session with a client is insufficient to promote long-term change in health behaviour. Follow-up counselling over a period of time allows the client to make behaviour changes in small steps and to cope with failure while support is available for relapse management. Dietary behaviour change is often easy for the first few weeks; after this time self-control declines and problems begin. The number of sessions needed will depend on characteristics of the client and the nature of the dietary problem. A minimum of three sessions is recommended, an initial session for assessment and education, a first follow-up visit to assess progress on goals, and a second follow-up visit to evaluate outcomes.

35.14   MOTIVATION TO CHANGE

Motivation can be understood as a person's present state or stage of readiness for change. The client may or may not be at a stage of readiness to change at the time of visiting the nutrition educator. The client may be less prepared to change if he or she has been coerced into seeing the educator by another person, such as the client's doctor. The educator needs to recognize that motivation to change is a dynamic state. There has been much recent research concerning the need to take into account the attitude of any individual towards the changes which are being suggested. There is little point in offering specific advice to someone who is not yet convinced of the need to make any changes in dietary intake. The various 'stages of change' are summarized in Table 35.3.

35.15   DISCHARGE

At the time of discharge from counselling there are three possible outcomes: First, an individual may have modified his or her eating habits successfully. Second, the person may have modified eating habits but is experiencing contined problems with relapse. Third, the individual may have been unable to make any dietary modification. In the first two instances a summary of goal achievement provides positive feedback prior to discharge. In all cases, the client should feel free to contact the educator if further information is required. There should always be an open invitation to return if problems arise or if the person feels that further counselling would be of benefit. A summary of the process of dietary counselling is shown in Table 35.4.

Table 35.3   'Stages of change' model

Stage	Characteristics
Precontemplation	No intention of changing behaviour in the foreseeable future. Unaware there is a problem and resistant to efforts to modify behaviour.
Contemplation	Awareness of a problem and seriously thinking about resolving it, but no commitment to take action in the near future.
Preparation	Stage of decision-making. Commitment to take action within the next 30 days and already making small behavioural changes.
Action	Subjects make notable overt efforts to change. In action stage if they have modified the target behaviour to an acceptable criterion.
Maintenance	Working to stabilize behaviour change and avoid relapse. In general, maintenance is sustaining action for at least 6 months.

Source: Greene GW, Rossi SR, Reed GR, *et al*. Stages of change for reducing dietary fat to 30% of energy or less. *J Am Dietet Assoc* 1994; **94**: 1105–10.

Table 35.4   A summary of the process of dietary counselling

1. Introduce interview
2. Identify medical problems and relevant history
3. Explain clearly the reasons for dietary modification and consequences of not carrying out dietary modification
4. Provide nutrition information using relevant education materials
5. Identify and discuss goals
6. Identify barriers to change*
7. Discuss relapse*
8. Monitor behaviour change
9. Provide adequate follow-up counselling
10. Show empathy
11. Enhance self-efficacy

*May occur in any order and may be discussed at follow-up sessions.

FURTHER READING

1. Holli BB, Calabrese RJ. *Communication and education skills, the dietitians guide*, 2nd ed. Malvern, PA: Lea and Febiger, 1991.
2. Greene GW, Rossi SR, Reed GR, *et al*. Stages of change for reducing dietary fat to 30% or less. *J Am Dietet Assoc* 1994; **94**: 1105–10.
3. Miller WR, Rollnick S. *Motivational interviewing: preparing people to change addictive behaviour*. London: Guilford Press, 1991.

Part VIII: Case studies

36
WAR IN FORMER YUGOSLAVIA: COPING WITH NUTRITIONAL ISSUES

Aileen Robertson and Philip James

The war in the Former Yugoslavia was the first time since the World War II that an emergency of such magnitude had occurred within Europe. In this chapter, therefore, an attempt will be made to show how fresh thinking in novel circumstances may bring a different perspective to the traditional approaches for the handling of emergencies in the Third World.

Bosnia-Herzegovina (BiH) was the republic in former Yugoslavia which became most dependent on international aid. Before the war, BiH had an estimated population of 4.3 million in 1992 which was approximately 45% Muslim, 35% Serb and 20% Croat. The majority of the 1.8 million Muslims lived in the regions of Sarajevo, Tuzla, Zenica and Bihac (Fig. 36.1). With the exception of the Bihac region, BiH was mainly industrial, with an economy heavily dependent on steel factories, hydroelectric plants and mining. As a result of the war these industries were completely destroyed and the production and distribution of food severely disrupted.

Political pressures forced the West to agree that something had to be done—but what? Political ineptitude and the failure to back up the recognition of Croatia with immediate military support amplified the fighting in Croatia and BiH and left the countries open to a brutal civil war. Suddenly large numbers of people were being slaughtered only a few hours' drive from Western Europe and in the West's holiday resorts. The media pressure to act was intense and organizations were urged to respond at any cost. Normally rational and caring people were projected into positions of extreme prominence where the drama of the crisis led to the emergence of individuals who responded by becoming dependent on the intensity and glamour of the media interest.

Famine, malnutrition and starvation are all emotive words which create sensational journalism. Thus, it soon became evident that the challenge for a nutritionist working in humanitarian assistance was how to avoid being corrupted by the barrage of emotional arguments and anecdotal stories which confronted us on a daily basis. The need for cool, calm and objective analyses, based on objective data and some understanding of nutritional needs, proved to be crucial in changing international perceptions of the role of nutritionists in crisis management. It is this process which will be demonstrated.

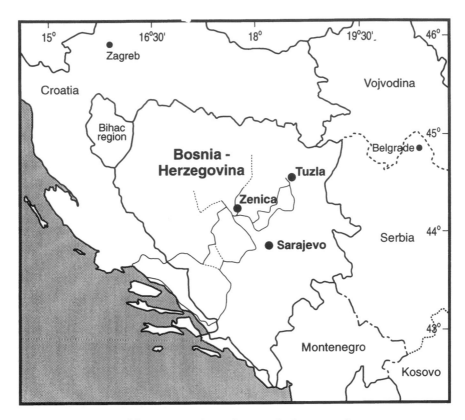

Fig. 36.1 A region of former Yugoslavia showing the location of Bosnia-Herzegovina.

36.1 EMERGENCY FOOD AID

The war in BiH started on 6 April 1992. The provision of food aid to the Bosnian people affected by the war began during the second part of 1992. The World Food Programme (WFP) had the prime responsibility for providing the food which was transported by truck, rail, air or sea by the United Nations High Commission for Refugees (UNHCR). The other UN organization involved was UNICEF, which has a special interest in children. The World Health Organization (WHO) is the UN organization traditionally responsible for advising all other agencies on issues related to the public health of the civilian population. The role of WHO is not normally crisis-response but rather the strategic issues of public health. However, the WHO office for the European Region in Copenhagen was asked for help because former Yugoslavia was part of the European Region of WHO.

The WHO Area Office for Europe therefore established an office in Zagreb, Croatia, to give public health advice during the emergency in former Yugoslavia. The first involvement of nutritionists in the war was in September 1992 after an emergency call from Sir Donald Acheson, the WHO Special Representative to former Yugoslavia. Sir Donald asked one of us (WPTJ) to provide immediate advice on the food needs of the besieged city of Sarajevo.

36.2   HOW MUCH ENERGY?

Our arrival in Zagreb confirmed that Sarajevo, a city of an estimated 380 000 people, was under siege by Bosnian Serb forces and that direct road transport to the capital had been cut off for almost six months. UN aeroplanes flying food aid into Sarajevo airport were being attacked regularly. Our calculations of UNHCR transport rates suggested that an average of 40 metric tonnes (MT) per day had been delivered to Sarajevo for the previous month of August 1992. The main questions were, therefore, (1) what were the true food needs of Sarajevo? and (2) if the figure of 40 MT was too low, how long would it take before the population became sick as a result of nutritional deficiencies?

Logistically, the UN believed that it was doing well to deliver 40 MT of food per day to Sarajevo. However, it immediately became clear that nobody knew the exact number of people in Sarajevo. Telephone calls, coming in hourly from the British Army patrols to the UNHCR in Zagreb, suggested that huge numbers of people were being displaced throughout Bosnia. They were walking over mountain tracks to avoid repeated ambush and gunfire in order to seek sanctuary in urban areas like Sarajevo. The number of people in Sarajevo was therefore likely to be larger than previously thought and likely to swell as the conflict continued to spread throughout Bosnia. As temperatures plummeted in autumn, with snow threatened within weeks, it was clear that the problems of providing emergency food aid would soon be exacerbated.

An immediate analysis of potential food needs for Sarajevo was required. Energy requirement calculations were based on a series of models of the likely population size, the age structure of the Sarajevan population, and the presumed physical activity of children and women who, we learned, were confined to the basements of apartment blocks under mortar and sniper fire; men were presumed to be very active in the front line of battle. The basis for estimating the energy needs of a population based on its age and sex structures, making allowances for physical activity, had just been developed. Thus, the daily tonnage needed in Sarajevo was estimated as 240 not 40 MT per day.

This calculation led to a complete re-evaluation of the transport of foods by the UN. It soon became clear that the UN operated a system of emergency food aid based on a crude estimate of energy needs and without any regard for the quality of the diet and whether the mineral or vitamin intakes were adequate. Within two to three days it was also apparent that the UN relief system was based on antiquated historical principles and UNHCR and aid workers were convinced that assumptions made from the experience of feeding free-living refugees in Africa, who sought additional food from the environment, could be applied to siege conditions in Yugoslavia. The knowledge of nutrition among the local decision-makers in WFP and UNHCR was rudimentary or non-existent. It was also evident that even their understanding of requisitioning needs was seriously flawed because we knew of the widespread prevalence of nutritional deficiency diseases in UN refugee camps throughout the Third World. Nevertheless, the UN organizations were very sensitive to any charges of professional incompetence and believed they knew what was required because they already successfully fed 20 million refugees daily throughout the world!

The very large change in estimated energy needs was politically charged; within four days Sir Donald Acheson, Baroness Chalker (the British Aid Minister who was visiting Zagreb at the time), and the UN negotiators in Geneva were involved. The specification of a different purchasing policy required a concomitant change in transport policy and an analysis of the situation for Lord Owen and Cyrus Vance who were negotiating in Geneva for the European Union and UN. They needed to know how much time could be allowed for negotiating a settlement while the blockade continued. Table 36.1 shows the estimates of the rate of weight loss of 380 000 people in Sarajevo, assuming a total siege, equitable family food distribution but preferential supplies to children and fighting men, and a 40 MT daily input of food by road.

Reference to the Leningrad siege of 1941–42 suggested that a weight loss of 20% was serious. It was estimated that children would die from November 1992 and women after Christmas. These estimates, after much debate about the advantage given to one or other of the warring factions, were released to the press. They led to dramatic changes in policy with an immediate release of millions of MREs (meals ready to eat) from army stores held by NATO in Frankfurt, a series of new NATO air exercises testing the usefulness of low and high altitude food drops, and the introduction of a high proportion of engineers

Table 36.1 Projected loss of weight and body mass index (BMI) in women in the Sarajevo siege

| | | Daily tonnage of food into Sarajevo | | | |
		40 MT		140 MT	
Estimated food supplied to young women (kcal/day)		375		1090	
Adjustment of activity from 1.64 × BMR to 1.35 × BMR		Yes		Yes	
Adjustment of BMR by week 1 with a fall of 15%		Yes		Yes	
		kg	BMI	kg	BMI
Weight and BMI at week	0	56.7	21.2	56.7	21.2
	4	49.0	18.3[a]	52.0	19.4
	8	43.3	16.2[b]	49.3	18.4[a]
Death imminent	12	38.2	14.2	46.8	17.5[a]
	16	33.4	12.5	44.6	16.6[b]
	20			42.5	15.9[c]
	24			40.5	15.1[c]

Note: These calculations assume two different inputs to a Sarajevo population of 380 000 with a normal population structure for Central Europe. On a 40 MT/day input, preferential feeding of children would be difficult and a 3-year-old child on a pro rata intake is predicted to lose nearly one-third of body weight within 1 month; their condition would then be very serious. On the 140 MT/day input to Sarajevo the children were estimated to receive 80% of their true needs and adolescent boys 75%.
   The predictions are based on adaptations in physical activity levels expressed as a ratio to the predicted BMR which in turn is assumed to fall in proportion to weight loss and in addition show a further adaptive fall of 15%.
BMR, basal metabolic rate; [a] 1st, [b] 2nd, [c] 3rd degrees of malnutrition as specified by James, Ferro-Luzzi and Waterlow (1988) for chronic states of energy deficiency; acute states have a worse prognosis.

into the British and French forces who sought to open up safe mountain routes through the deep snow and ice of winter. Hundreds of new trucks were then assigned to boost the input to Sarajevo to 240 MT daily while we at the World Health Organization began to worry about the escalating numbers of refugees fleeing through the mountains in sub-zero temperatures.

Professor Michael Golden (University of Aberdeen) followed WPTJ for a brief visit. Warmth, water, total food energy and specific nutrients were the sequential order of priorities as determined from calculations of estimated time to death if support was not available. It was clear that the operation would require continuous on-the-spot nutritional advice in Zagreb. A small group of nutritionists was therefore established in former Yugoslavia with a back-up team at the Rowett Research Institute in Aberdeen. Links were developed with non-governmental organizations (NGOs), the British and American Airforces and other groups involved in responding to the disaster. Professor Colin Mills headed the Health and Nutritional Status Advice (HANSA) Centre at the Rowett Research Institute and Professor Golden continued to provide a regular back-up service.

One of us (AR) transferred from the Rowett Institute to work with WHO in Zagreb during the last week of October 1992. The terms of reference we set were to establish a dynamic, responsive nutrition service able to provide rigorous professional advice to UN agencies, NGOs and local professionals involved with the public health issues in former Yugoslavia. A system of objective analyses of the nutritional state of the population and the quality of the diet being provided had to be established. AR was ably helped over the next two and a half years by other international nutritionists including Peter Halley (UK), Josephine Vespa (Canada) and Fiona Watson (UK).

36.3 Nutritional Surveillance: A Re-evaluation of Its Role in Wartime

The war was dominated by claims and counter-claims as sophisticated doctors manipulated the news with accounts of disaster, anaemia, deficiencies and illness on a daily basis in an attempt to divert aid to one or other region of Bosnia. Doctors also appeared at WHO in Zagreb pleading for anaesthetic kits, surgical packs, antibiotics and medicines which were flown in by the British in an attempt to keep the hospitals going throughout Bosnia. These supplies were smuggled across front lines over mountains, often on mule. Meanwhile, UNICEF had run out of all supplies of infant milk and were concentrating on bringing in immunization programmes to limit the anticipated epidemics and using a series of high profile media events to highlight the plight of children under sniper fire. Thousands of refugees were being made homeless daily and at a weekly conference the various agencies tried to cope with the spreading chaos, the incessant demands, the intensive political infighting, the elbowing for prestige and the long delays before supplies actually arrived. WHO was seen suddenly as a supplier of medicines and an epidemic early warning agency.

If the Sarajevan population was going to starve we needed some reference data immediately so that we could monitor weight loss. The mothers insisted that they would starve themselves first so the classic nutritionists' obsession with the welfare of only the under 5-year-olds was clearly flawed. By then criteria for adult 'chronic energy deficiency' had been established with Third World data. We determined to monitor adult BMIs as well as children's z-scores of weight-for-height, these two being seen as the simplest and most reliable indices of short-term deficits in food supply. These plans were greeted with scorn by the NGOs and UN bodies who saw this as academic dabbling in research in the throes of a crisis which called for action not surveys! Nevertheless, within days we were measuring children and mothers crowded into basements in Sarajevo. Everything had to be done from armoured personnel carriers with full military support and everybody wearing flack jackets, helmets, etc. as we carried scales and stadiometers from one block of flats to another whilst the battle continued in the foothills around the city and snipers fired on anybody who strayed into the area. The data were faxed to Zagreb, transferred to the Rowett in Aberdeen, recalculated, checked and displayed for submission to the next weekly inter-agency meeting. Suddenly we were established: the non-governmental agencies (NGOs) and UN agencies swapped stories and debated priorities in Sarajevo but immediately fell silent when a chart was displayed of z-scores or BMIs with standards and estimates from pre-war Croatia data of the likely weight loss in adults. The children were indeed being sustained in weight and height, despite appalling conditions with no heating, cooking fuel and light and in constant fear of their lives. Adults were, however, losing weight steadily but this merely reduced the overweight Yugoslavs to an ideal BMI range with a mean of 22–23!

Soon the UN, one warring party or another, or an NGO was demanding that we investigate a crisis in Tuzla, Zenica, Gorazde or Bihac so the issue now was how to cope with the demand for instant data. Slowly it was recognized by politicians and doctors that we could not be manipulated: we simply provided objective data with a careful and precise interpretation. We were constantly being told by the relief agencies that we did not understand the situation because their Third World experience had taught them the value of pragmatic solutions that worked. We, however, knew that data from the Third World were sparse and that little clear thinking had been applied to the prevalence of micronutrient deficiencies, to total energy needs, or to moving from crisis management to a programme for the long-term maintenance of displaced communities. The local medical services were also outraged by the arrogance of aid agencies applying Third World solutions to their sophisticated society. Our enquiry (see below) showed that over 90% of children had already been immunized once or more so the immediate obsession with immunizing children was misplaced: their immunization rates were far better than in the United States or United Kingdom! We, however, were concerned that the European Union, the United States or other countries were off-loading their excess food stocks as part of the aid programme without regard to nutritional issues. Thus, the European Union food parcel aimed to provide sufficient food for a family but was deficient in or devoid of numerous minerals and vitamins.

Four priorities therefore now emerged:

(1) rapid compositional estimates of foods in the pipeline for Yugoslavia with pragmatic solutions to make them nutritionally appropriate if, as expected, the war lasted months or more;

(2) establishing anthropometric measurement systems linked to the still functioning medical centres but based on proper population sampling;

(3) developing new approaches to assessing current household food stocks which were subject to widespread media manipulation and often the misleading selection of houses for the inspection of food status;

(4) a new approach to assessing the likelihood of mineral and vitamin deficiencies.

These issues, once dealt with, then led us to assess the long-term needs of former Yugoslavia.

36.4   THE QUALITY OF FOOD SUPPLY

The UN daily food ration was evaluated: it consisted of 450 g wheat flour, 30 ml oil, 60 g pulses, 40 g tinned meat/fish/cheese, 25 g sugar, 5 g salt and 3.5 g yeast. Complementary food items included fortified biscuits and dried skimmed milk. All food commodities were the cheapest available and so none of the items except the biscuits were micronutrient-fortified. Our calculations revealed the inadequacy of the diet currently on offer by the UN and indeed by the European Union.

We advocated specific changes to the basic food ration following the analysis of the nutrient composition of foods flown to Sarajevo over the previous month. These nutrients were expressed as a percentage of the dietary reference values per adult per day as set out in the then unpublished European Union's Population Reference Intakes (PRIs). The supplies of vitamins A, D, C, calcium, iron, folate and riboflavin were inadequate (Fig. 36.2). As an immediate practical response, solid fat replaced the cooking oil. There were two main reasons for this: there was a desperate shortage of fuel in the war-torn and snow covered Bosnia and solid fat could be spread on bread or biscuits and eaten

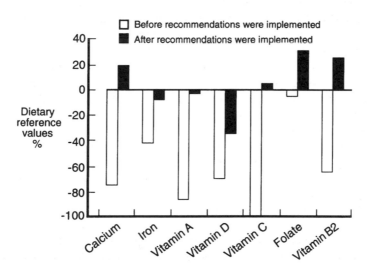

Fig. 36.2   Increase in nutrient levels of food ration following implementation of recommendations. The reference chosen was the then unpublished proposals from the Scientific Committee for Food, European Communities Commission, 1993.

even when there was no fuel for cooking; also, solid fat contributes the densest form of food energy and could also be fortified with vitamins A and D which were recognized to be in short supply.

We substituted the more energy-dense dried whole milk for the lower fat skimmed version. One 10-ton truck, struggling over an icy mountain pass with a load of dried skimmed milk, would supply only 330 000 kilocalories compared with a load of dried whole milk which provides 660 000 kilocalories. Thus, one truck carrying dried whole milk could feed 300 refugees compared with only 150 if skimmed milk were supplied.

The food basket provided by WFP was completely lacking in vitamin C so vitamin C deficiency was expected shortly. A fast and logistically viable method of safeguarding a population who had received no fresh fruit and vegetables for over six months was sought; however, a large stock of vitamin pills may have been available in Sarajevo. Dehydrated orange juice was therefore bought on our recommendation by UNHCR, UNICEF and various non-governmental organizations (NGOs).

The vitamin C present in the juice powder was also expected to enhance the absorption of the small amount of iron present in the WFP food basket. Iron deficiency anaemia was reported to be an increasing problem, although we had no strong evidence to support this. We did, however, consider that iron deficiency would be the first mineral deficiency to develop and therefore recommended that all wheat flour supplied to the former Yugoslavia should be fortified with iron. Flour was also to be fortified with calcium, thiamin and niacin.

Doctors also suggested that macrocytic anaemia was a problem so we proposed that yeast be used to supplement the basic WFP ration since yeast is a good source of folic acid and has the advantage of being a critical ingredient in bread-making. Bread is the stable food in BiH and so it was vital to allow the bakeries and the people to bake bread containing yeast.

A later re-analysis of the nutrient composition of the new food rations being sent to Sarajevo showed a marked improvement in the quantity of micronutrients being delivered (Fig. 36.2).

36.5 ANTHROPOMETRIC MEASURES

Traditionally, during 'emergencies' only children under 5 years of age are weighed and measured since they are considered the most vulnerable. Thus, the nutritional status of children under 5 years has acted as a proxy for the nutritional status of the whole population. We, however, decided that women of childbearing age, as the main carers, had to have their health monitored and maintained. We therefore embarked on a special cluster sampling scheme of women and their children based on a simple set of principles.

Cluster sampling was used as in many nutritional epidemiological studies, for example, to investigate immunization coverage and nutrition status in refugee camps. First, all the smallest geographical areas and local authorities in each region were identified and the area names listed alphabetically, together with their individual population numbers. The total number of areas were then randomly sampled to provide 30 clusters (the number of clusters in an area being proportional to its population size). Thirty clusters is the minimum number required to give a representative sample of the total population.

After selecting these 30 localities, permission was sought from the president of the local committee to carry out the survey. We randomly selected a household within the cluster area and then chose the adjacent house where necessary until the requisite number of children were obtained for each age group (i.e. 15 children aged 6 months to 5 years for anthropometric assessment together with their mothers; seven children aged 13–15 months for analysis of immunization coverage and four babies within each cluster aged less than 16 weeks to monitor infant feeding practices).

Figures 36.3 and 36.4 show a collation of data on children under 5 years of age and their mothers measured during the winter of 1992 and the summer of 1993 in many parts of Bosnia. The data confirmed the naivete of current thinking: the BMIs of the mothers, their differences and shifts, gave a far better perspective of food supplies than monitoring the children. However, the children's data were reassuring as well as politically essential to stop local politicians using alarmist anecdotal stories about starving children.

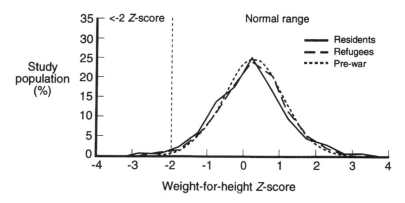

Fig. 36.3 Distribution of weight-for-height z-scores in 2503 Bosnian children aged 0.5–5 years.

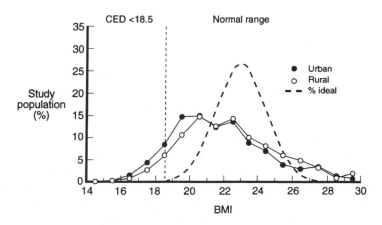

Fig. 36.4 Distribution of body mass index (BMI) in 2220 Bosnian mothers. CED = a BMI less than 18.5, is classified as energy-deficient.

565

A much higher percentage (12%) of resident mothers in Sarajevo and Zenica were classified as energy-deficient with a BMI below 18.5. The pre-war data suggested substantial weight losses and a large number of adult females, particularly those living in urban areas, had BMIs just above the critical cutoff point of 18.5 for undernutrition. Nevertheless, these findings refuted most of the alarmist accounts of mass starvation.

36.6 IN SEARCH OF THE MOST VULNERABLE

Having established that the rural community was relatively self-sufficient in food, we concentrated in the following months on the urban populations who tried to cope with flour and other raw ingredients on open fires when they were accustomed to electric cookers, microwaves and washing machines.

Nutritional status and household food security (see below) were longitudinally monitored in three besieged cities of BiH (Sarajevo, Zenica and Tuzla) from December 1993 to May 1994. The objectives were to provide early warning of deterioration and identify particularly vulnerable groups. A total of 398 households were included in the sample which covered 1469 household members. Additional samples of residents living in old people's homes (37 in Sarajevo and 233 in Tuzla) were added because we were concerned that the elderly might sacrifice themselves when food was scarce.

The percentage of the elderly with BMIs below 18.5 was much higher than expected and peaked at 15% in January 1994. (For an explanation of the significance of BMI < 18.5, see Table 36.1.) Elderly people living in the old people's homes also had a lower mean BMI and higher levels of undernutrition when compared with the elderly living with families or even alone but within the community. Weight change among adults and the elderly during the 1993 winter is shown in Fig. 36.5. With our aid concentrated on urban communities we now found weight loss was most severe among rural residents

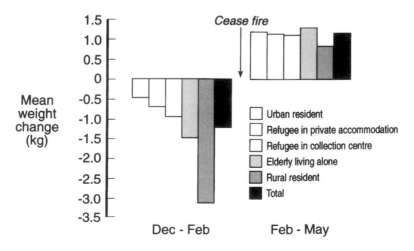

Fig. 36.5   Weight change in adults and the elderly by household group, December 1993–May 1994.

(3 kg)—but they still had the highest mean BMI (24) in February. Prior to one of the ceasefires (February 1994), trends in some of the nutritional indicators suggested that the situation was deteriorating. Although the mean BMI was still within normal limits, the percentage of men with a low BMI appeared to be increasing and a greater prevalence of low BMIs (i.e. <18.5), persisted in urban rather than rural groups with some households being particularly affected. After the ceasefire, a steady weight gain was noted in all groups.

36.7 Assessing Food Security

A number of approaches were devised to assess household food security. First, food stocks were measured by asking the woman of the household how much she had of each individual food item in the home that day. The total quantity of food stocks was divided by the number in the household to give a value in kilograms of food stocks per person. This indicator proved to show the same trend as the weight changes (Fig. 36.6). Zenica and Tuzla benefited much more from the ceasefire because both the humanitarian food convoys and commercial traffic could once again start to flow into central Bosnia whereas Sarajevo continued under siege. Another method was to assess the cost of a food basket estimated to meet 100% of a household energy needs for a month at black market prices (Fig. 36.7). Note the greater sensitivity to change of the black market food price compared with the food stock levels in the home shown in Fig. 36.6.

Both food security indicators (i.e. food stocks and the cost of food) proved to be more dynamic measures of changing circumstance than anthropometry, important though the latter is. Food aid, when scarce, should be targeted at those most in need on the basis of anthropometry but this approach was alien to ex-socialist Yugoslavia where the concept of equity meant that no matter how much or how little resources the state possessed

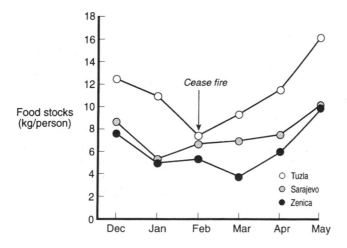

Fig. 36.6 Trends in quantity of household food stocks, December 1993–May 1994.

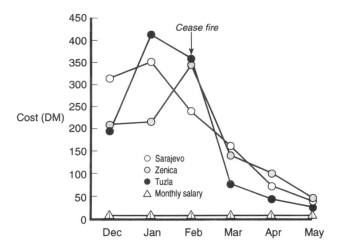

Fig. 36.7 Trends in monthly cost of food basket per person, purchased on the black market, December 1993–May 1994. The monthly food basket (per person) consisted of 3375 g flour, 0.225 l oil, 188 g sugar, 450 g beans and 300 g tinned meat.

everyone was entitled to an equal share. It was therefore very difficult to convince the local authorities to develop social systems to identify and then target food aid to the most vulnerable.

36.8 ASSESSING NUTRITIONAL DEFICIENCIES: PROTEIN AND MICRONUTRIENT ISSUES

One of the problems in an over-medicalized society like former Yugoslavia is that health is often seen only in terms of disease. Unwittingly, the doctors had created a dependency on drugs; neither doctors nor the population considered how to prevent disease. Before the war, doctors prescribed vitamin and mineral supplements routinely so the medical profession were convinced that widespread micronutrient deficiency must now develop in the population even if normal food were provided. Protein was also regarded as vital and needed in twice the amounts considered ample in the West. Most of these misconceptions stemmed from the fact that the recommended dietary reference values for protein and micronutrients are far too high in Central and Eastern Europe: the daily protein allowance for adults is 100 g and, as vegetable protein is considered to be inferior, only meat protein is thought to prevent the onset of protein deficiency.

Many agencies, especially those employing non-technical, non-trained relief staff, immediately responded to this plea for help from local doctors and supplied huge quantities of multivitamin tablets. Thus, seasoned relief workers from the Third World, when transferred to former Yugoslavia, relied on local 'expert' opinion and readily responded to the alarm of doctors siding with the Croatian, Serb or Bosnian view of the crisis. The truth was difficult to establish and all decisions on food needs were based on the 'judgements' of a galaxy of experts from NGO and UN agencies, none of whom had any grounding in the need for objective measures or a modern perspective of nutrition. Physicians in Sarajevo were convinced that micronutrient deficiencies and anaemia were especially prevalent. The likelihood of this was difficult to deny since, as far as we knew at the time, the only sources of micronutrients might have been the paltry amounts delivered in food to Sarajevo. The political sensitivity of the issues demanded formal assessment with biochemical analyses of nutritional status even though the immediate requirement was to establish the prevalence of anaemia. Therefore, a series of surveys was conducted, with Professor Colin Mills arranging with the British Air Force for the transport of frozen plasma samples from different parts of Sarajevo to Aberdeen where analyses were conducted by both Dr Iain Broom at the Royal Infirmary and by the Rowett.

Over 200 subjects were sampled from 30 clusters distributed in proportion to the population resident in each district of Sarajevo. The choice of the households was first by 'blind' scoring of the required number of clusters for each district on to a map. Then random numbers were used to choose the house, floor and family in each block of apartments closest to the chosen point. Streets under sniper fire were substituted with the street at right angles so no bias would be introduced in the assessment of households who had been under siege for 10 months.

As expected, in view of the very poor vegetable supply, plasma carotenoids were almost absent but vitamin A concentrations had not yet fallen below normal. The confined circumstances of the population, away from sunlight after 10 months of siege probably explained the prevalence of low plasma 25(-OH) vitamin D with 65% of the elderly showing levels below the acceptable minimum level of 25 mmol/litre. Thus, the use of these specific measures revealed the marginal haematological and biochemical status of this population.

The men's mean haemoglobin fell within the 10th to 20th centiles of United States and United Kingdom surveys but all age groups had a pronounced macrocytosis which probably related to the observed low plasma folate concentrations. Serum ferritin levels were reduced by 30–50% with 46% of women having a low serum ferritin (<20 mg/l); the ferritin status of children was also low.

It was easy to dismiss the usefulness of this survey once the data were available because the evidence did not show widespread frank deficiencies. Yet it played an important part in putting into perspective the true nutritional state of the population. It has to be recognized that such a survey would have been politically and perhaps logistically impossible in a Third World country. Nevertheless, new micromethods are becoming available and if simple tests for vitamin or mineral deficiency could be developed, analogous to the prick test for measuring haemoglobin, then this could revolutionize biochemical measures in the Third World and probably reveal a far more precarious nutritional state than is currently recognized.

In many Third World countries the only assessment of nutritional deficiencies is by monitoring clinical signs but this has been abandoned because of the considerable observer variability, the lack of specificity in many clinical signs and the need for substantial deficiency before the clinical features are manifest.

36.9 PUBLIC HEALTH ISSUES IN FORMER YUGOSLAVIA: INFANT FEEDING PRACTICES

Levels of exclusive breast-feeding were very low in former Yugoslavia before the war, and during 1993–4 our surveys confirmed that only 2–11% of mothers were exclusively breast-feeding. In the United Nations Protected Areas (UNPAs) in Croatia almost half (45%) of mothers gave their babies no breast milk at all because they felt that they produced insufficient milk of poor quality. Over one-third of the mothers gave their babies sugared tea and water between feeds and in all areas almost everyone followed a rigid feeding regimen.

Doctors believed that mothers were unable to breast-feed because (1) the stress of war stopped their milk production, (2) the mothers were too undernourished to produce milk and (3) milk quality would be poor because of the poor diet; mothers were frequently being diagnosed as anaemic. Even under normal conditions these ideas are dangerous but under war conditions lethal. Indeed, the poor rates of breast-feeding probably explain the high infant mortality. Even before the war, infant mortality in former Yugoslavia was among the highest in Europe, almost 25 deaths per 1000 live births compared with between 5–10 per 1000 in Western Europe. In Sarajevo, infant mortality probably increased during 1994 to around 27 deaths per 1000 live births and during a conflict the dependence on infant formula is clearly life-threatening. The supply of powdered milk in Sarajevo was hopelessly erratic and clean water, boiling facilities and disinfectants were rarely available.

All the evidence shows that mothers can breast-feed successfully under war conditions, that even undernourished mothers can produce a copious volume of milk with an adequate energy content and that its quality is likely to exceed artificial supplies. Yet, free supplies of infant formula were given as a magnanimous humanitarian gesture with governments, donors and NGOs all encouraging its distribution. This has detrimental short- and long-term effects on the morbidity and mortality of infants but helped infant formula companies establish a new market.

Given that the health risks to non-breast-fed babies, in terms of infection, are very high, mass education of health professionals and mothers was therefore urgently needed. During 1994 we therefore worked with the Ministry of Health and UNICEF to improve the levels of breast-feeding. Local groups for the promotion of breast-feeding were established, after training seminars for health professionals.

To evaluate the success of these training programmes, the surveys were repeated but this time they were carried out by local health professionals themselves and only supervised by WHO. The percentage of mothers exclusively breast-feeding increased dramatically from 1% in 1993 to 25% in 1994. Moreover, in 1994 only 13% were not breast-feeding at all compared with nearly half (42%) during 1993 (Fig. 36.8). Mothers, however, still believed that their babies required drinks of sweetened tea and water between feeds. So, whereas only about one-fifth of mothers were feeding their babies tea and/or water in 1993, there was a massive increase to 63% by 1994. This seems to be a response to local folklore. UNICEF and WHO distributed 30 000 leaflets to mothers through the Ministry of Health to encourage them to stop this unnecessary and potentially risky habit.

The claim that large numbers of children were undernourished led to great concern that, if not properly immunized, large numbers of children would succumb to infection.

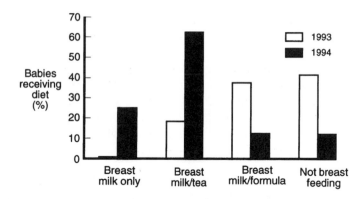

Fig. 36.8   Breast-feeding practice of mothers, comparison of 1993 with 1994.

Although national statistics showed that coverage with all vaccines was over 95%, this figure related only to the number of children who were specified by the doctors as eligible to receive vaccination and there was a large list of exclusions (e.g. for influenza, fever or infection). Data were therefore required urgently to establish the coverage rate so the estimate of immunization coverage was added to the anthropometric surveys.

The antituberculosis vaccine (BCG) coverage was almost universal (over 94%) and over two-thirds of the population sampled in Bosnia had received their first vaccination of DPT (diphtheria, pertussis and tetanus) and polio (OPV). However fewer than half had received all three doses and the level of measles coverage was very worrying considering that mortality rates increase dramatically when undernutrition is combined with measles epidemics.

On the basis of our results, NGOs applied for funds from USAID (US Agency for International Development) and were successful in obtaining major grants to undertake a massive 'catch-up' immunization campaign throughout central Bosnia in 1994. UNICEF and WHO also conducted training courses on the Expanded Programme for Immunization (EPI) for the local regional and district managers.

We then evaluated (Fig. 36.9) the impact of the NGO immunization campaigns and the UNICEF/WHO training programmes. During the 14 months from July 1993 to September 1994 there was a marked improvement in coverage (e.g. of the third DPT injection from 45% to 69%). Although the measles coverage rate doubled, the levels were still too low to prevent an epidemic of measles. Since measles mortality is linked to vitamin A deficiency, we also insisted that foods fortified with vitamin A should be included in the emergency ration. On the basis of this work, the Ministry of Health planned to create a permanent public health education system with mass media campaigns to improve vaccination rates.

36.10   DEVELOPING NUTRITION EXPERTISE IN MODERN PUBLIC HEALTH

Former Yugoslavia had an extremely well-developed health infrastructure with many highly qualified doctors but fewer and less well-trained nurses. There were almost no

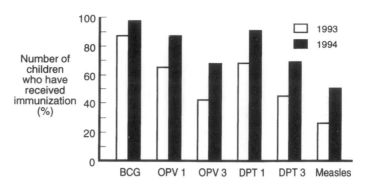

Fig. 36.9   Immunization coverage in a region of Bosnia, comparison of 1993 with 1994. Vaccinations: BCG, tuberculosis; OPV, polio; DTP, diphtheria, pertussis, ketanus. Data kindly provided by International Medical Corps, Zenica.

nutritionists; the medical concept of health was related to clinical diagnosis and treatment rather than to public health approaches and prevention. Everything, including normal physiological processes, tended to be medicalized. For example pregnancy, childbirth and breast-feeding were seen as the domain of the hospital clinician. The concept of healthy eating was poorly understood and doctors limited themselves to prescribing special therapeutic diets for clinical conditions such as diabetes, renal disease and liver problems. These doctors therefore demanded expensive drugs to treat the prevalent diet-related diseases such as heart disease, hypertension and non-insulin-dependent diabetes (NIDDM).

Although barely recognized by the public health professionals in Eastern Europe, these countries have the highest mortality and morbidity rates from diet-related chronic diseases in the world. Yet most professionals are concerned with the prevalence of infectious diseases (rates of which have dropped dramatically over the past 50 years) and with deficiency disorders associated with protein and micronutrient deficiency.

During the war, it was understandably impossible to engage health professionals in considering the ill-effects of diet in cardiovascular or chronic disease when the population may starve. We therefore developed a strategy which involved studying the impact of the war on patients suffering from NIDDM. We compiled a register of NIDDM patients with pre-war anthropometric and biochemical results and selected 55 patients in a systematic and random way. Each patient was then weighed and measured; blood pressure, levels of haemoglobin A1c(HbA1c), fasting blood glucose and serum lipids were also measured.

Before the war, two-thirds (60%) of the patients had been obese (BMI > 30) with a mean BMI of 31 ± 4.5. By January 1995, the mean BMI had fallen significantly ($p < 0.01$) to 27 ± 3.9 and only 17% were obese. The mean pre-war blood pressure was 154/92 (systolic/diastolic) and this reduced to 138/84 in January 1995. The proportion with values above 140/90 also fell from 51% to 30% in January 1995. High HbA1c levels (above 8%) also fell from 85% to 68%. These results therefore suggested that the glycaemic control of NIDDMs did improve during the war with weight loss and this probably also contributed to the fall in blood pressure.

In an effort to give a new public health perspective on nutrition we also held a course in Sarajevo in November 1994. This was the first of its kind in former Yugoslavia and provided training for 12 public health professionals in data collection, analysis and interpretation and how to apply these skills to gather public health information on the general population.

Course participants worked with the CDC/WHO computer software, EPI-INFO, for which an introductory booklet was produced in Bosnian. They examined their own daily food consumption, expressed it as nutrients, and then compared the calculations with WHO international nutrient goals. These nutrient goals form the cornerstone for the prevention and rational treatment of many chronic diseases. The participants came to see that chronic diseases were the largest single cause of the high morbidity and mortality rates in the former Yugoslavia and that these were preventable.

The public health professionals learned to design a questionnaire to collect information from households living in Sarajevo, Zenica and Tuzla. They then collected the infomation on income, savings, health status and access to water and heating, as well as household nutrition and food stocks. In six days they visited 150 elderly households, 150 resident/ refugee households and 63 households living in collective centres and, in order to measure the impact of the wintry conditions of 1994–5, the exercise was repeated at the end of February 1995. We hoped thereby to transfer our skills and the lessons that we had learned over the previous two years. This course was the culmination of our nutrition work in Bosnia.

36.11 CONCLUSION

A disaster with major nutritional implications in a relatively sophisticated country with an extensive medical service and within an easy drive from Germany presented completely unexpected challenges. The UN agencies involved applied their standard Third World approach only to find the basis of their whole operation challenged by politicians, relief agencies, the local population, the indigenous doctors and ourselves. We learned the vital role of rapid objective survey methods, of monitoring adult and elderly BMIs as well as children's weights, of challenging the very basis of current international feeding schemes and of devising novel approaches to food availability by monitoring black market food prices. Nutrition is taken for granted by the international aid community and indeed is often scorned since the issues seem simple and their solution requires money and practical societal help. Yet, the power to change thinking by the ruthless application of scientific analysis of nutrient requirements and nutritional status is now at last causing the whole basis of refugee feeding to be re-evaluated. The ignorance and neglect of nutrition by aid agencies, is now highlighted by the clear demonstration in former Yugoslavia that nutrition can matter, that objective nutritional data do change major policies, and that it is time to reconsider the low status of nutritionists in the UN. The benefits of linking nutritional field workers with academic centres through sophisticated communication systems should be recognized and can serve to bring political clout and a rational approach during the chaos of decision-making in the early phase of disaster relief. The link with modern public health thinking in nutrition has also been neglected too long and there is a clear need to change medical thinking on diet-related diseases in Central and Eastern Europe.

FURTHER READING

1. Acheson D. Health, humanitarian relief and survival in former Yugoslavia. *BMJ* 1993; **307**: 44–8.
2. Dean AD, Dean JA, Burton JH, Dicker RC. *EPI-INFO software version 5*. Atlanta: Centers for Disease Control, 1990.
3. European Communities Commission. *Reports of the Scientific Committee for Food* (31st series): *nutrient and energy intakes for the European Community*. London: HMSO, 1993.
4. James WPT, Schofield EC. *Human energy requirements: A manual for planners and nutritionists*. Oxford University Press, 1990.
5. James WPT, Ferro-Luzzi A, Waterlow JC. Definition of chronic energy deficiency in adults. Report of Working Party of IDECG. *Eur J Clin Nutr* 1988; **42**: 969–81.
6. UNHCR, MSF, WFP. *Quick nutrition survey among populations in emergency situations*. Geneva: UNHCR, 1991.
7. Watson F, Helsing E (eds). CITY UNDER SIEGE: Impact of two years of war on nutrition in Sarajevo—*Eur J Clin Nutr* 1995; (suppl.) **49**, Suppl 2.
8. World Health Organization. *Diet, nutrition and the prevention of chronic diseases*. Report of a WHO Study Group. Technical Report Series 797. Geneva: WHO, 1990.

37

THE ELIMINATION OF IODINE DEFICIENCY DISORDERS

Basil Hetzel

Iodine deficiency is now recognized as the most common preventable cause of mental defect in the world today. Estimates by the World Health Organization (WHO) indicate a massive population at risk—1.6 billion—with at least 20 million suffering from mental defect that is totally preventable by correction of iodine deficiency before pregnancy. The availability of effective technology for mass coverage with iodized salt or iodized oil has made elimination of this condition feasible. However, the establishment of effective public health programmes in developing countries has been delayed until the last decade. This case study examines the way in which a major change has occurred with the establishment of new momentum in public health programmes throughout the world.

In the early 1980s there was very little public health action to control iodine deficiency. It was clear that there was a big communication problem and that a new concept, beyond that of goitre and cretinism, was needed which would better reflect the increase in knowledge that had occurred over the preceding 25 years, particularly in relation to brain development. The term 'iodine deficiency disorders' (IDD) was proposed to denote all the effects of iodine deficiency on growth and development of a population which could be totally prevented by correction of iodine deficiency.

The announcement by WHO in 1980 of the global eradication of smallpox, also encouraged the acceptance of the goal of eradication (later changed to elimination) of IDD in view of the ready availability and effective mass distribution systems for iodized salt and iodized oil. Elimination is more appropriate for IDD because the conditions arise from a soil deficiency of iodine which will always be present and therefore addition of iodine to the diet will always be necessary.

Serious attention was given to the problem as worthy of priority in international nutrition by a Symposium at the Fourth Asian Congress of Nutrition, held in Bangkok in 1983. This led to an invitation in 1984 from the Sub-Committee on Nutrition (SCN) of the UN, through the Australian government, for the preparation of a state-of-the-art review of IDD and the possibility of successful prevention and control on a global basis. The report noted the great delay in the application of existing knowledge on IDD and its prevention, to the detriment of the many millions in developing countries who were suffering irreversible effects on brain development. To help bridge this gap, an expert consultative group of scientists and other public health professionals was proposed to assist in the development of IDD control programmes at national level.

37.1   THE INTERNATIONAL COUNCIL FOR CONTROL OF
IODINE DEFICIENCY DISORDERS (ICCIDD)

The decision to establish such a group, the International Council for Control of Iodine Deficiency Disorders (ICCIDD), was made in Delhi in March 1985, when the proposal was put to a group of ten consultants and advisers who were attending a WHO/UNICEF inter-country workshop on the control of IDD in South East Asia.

The ICCIDD now consists of a multidisciplinary global expert network of 400 scientists, public health administrators, technologists, communicators, economists and other experts, who are committed to assist national governments and international agencies in the development of national programmes for the elimination of IDD as a public health problem. More than half are from developing countries.

From the outset, the ICCIDD has worked closely with WHO and UNICEF. At the inauguration, notable messages of support were received from both the Director General of WHO and the Executive Director of UNICEF. The ICCIDD has been recognized as the expert group by the UN system. Since 1987 it has reported annually to the Sub-Committee on Nutrition (SCN) of the UN Administrative Co-ordinating Committee and now has official relations with the WHO as a non-government organization (NGO).

In 1987 a special IDD Working Group (IWG) was established by the UNSCN with the following functions:

1. Monitoring the prevalence and severity of IDD in countries throughout the world.

2. Facilitating the launching of programmes for the control of IDD.

3. Helping mobilize international resources to support such programmes.

4. Monitoring the progress of national IDD control programmes.

Since then, this group has met each year at the time of the SCN and full reports have been made to it by the ICCIDD. The IWG has become a major channel of communication on IDD and national control programmes. The meetings are attended by representatives both from multilateral agencies including WHO, UNICEF, World Bank, World Food Programme, World Food Council, and the Food and Agriculture Organization (FAO) and bilateral agencies (i.e. countries providing support for nutrition programmes: Australia, Belgium, Canada, Sweden, Netherlands, Denmark, Italy, Switzerland).

The ICCIDD itself has a governing board of 39 members with more than half from developing countries and the international agencies. The board meets annually, usually in conjunction with a regional meeting, or special workshop. The first meeting took place in Kathmandu, Nepal, in March 1986, when a review of all aspects of public health programmes was carried out. An executive was elected including chairman, vice chairman, executive director and secretary. The executive director position has been full-time, the others part-time. The global secretariat is in Adelaide, Australia, with a small office staff (two part-time secretaries and a part-time accountant).

From the outset, funding support has been provided by Australia through the Australian International Development Assistance Bureau (AIDAB, now AusAID) and by UNICEF and WHO, followed later by Canada through the Canadian International Development Agency (CIDA), the World Bank, the Swedish International Development Agency (SIDA) and the Dutch Co-operation Programme.

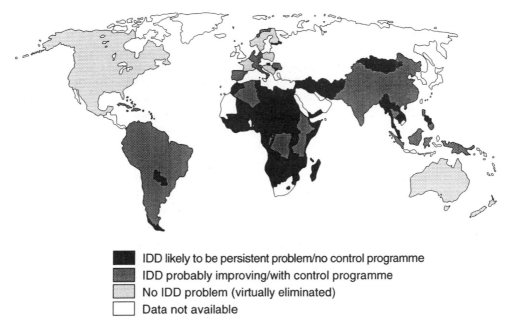

IDD likely to be persistent problem/no control programme
IDD probably improving/with control programme
No IDD problem (virtually eliminated)
Data not available

Fig. 37.1 Map of active progress of national IDD elimination programmes throughout the world. Countries are grouped into four categories. *Source*: Reprinted with permission from Report to 43rd World Health Assembly, Geneva: WHO, 1990.

The ICCIDD has regional co-ordinators for the Americas, Europe, South East Asia, Africa and East Asia including China. The regional co-ordinators take appropriate initiatives including consultancies in individual countries to expedite the development of national programmes. Since 1986, the ICCIDD has held with WHO and UNICEF a series of regional meetings designed to foster the development of national control programmes. These have occurred in Africa (twice), Asia (twice), Europe (twice), Latin America and the Middle East.

An overview of the status of national programmes throughout the world is shown in Fig. 37.1.

37.2 POLITICAL IMPACT AT COUNTRY LEVEL

In 1990, ministers of health of more than 160 governments, meeting in the World Health Assembly, adopted the goal of elimination of IDD as a public health problem by the year 2000. A further major step in securing a higher priority for expenditure on children's health and education was the World Summit for Children held at the UN headquarters on 30 September 1990. This was attended by 71 heads of state together with senior representatives of 88 other governments who signed a declaration and approved a new programme for the improved health and education of children throughout the world. The list of goals included the virtual elimination of IDD by the year 2000. This was an unprecendented commitment by heads of state to give priority to the needs of children.

The World Summit for Children in 1990 was followed by a further commitment by 60 heads of state who nominated delegations to the Policy Conference on Micronutrient Malnutrition held in Montreal, Canada (October 1991). The international Conference on Nutrition (Rome, December 1992) was attended by government delegations from 160 countries. The conference reaffirmed the goal of elimination of IDD by the year 2000.

This new level of political commitment at the national level has made the achievement of the goal of elimination of IDD much more likely than before. Examples are provided by Indonesia, the Philippines and China. In Indonesia, President Suharto announced a trebling of the expenditure on IDD control in January 1992. In the Philippines, President Fidel V Ramos, speaking at a national advocacy meeting on 'ending hidden hunger' in June 1993, noted recent progress in ensuring that no baby is born physically or mentally handicapped because of iodine deficiency and called on his government to fully support IDD elimination. In China, a national advocacy meeting on the elimination of IDD was held in the Great Hall of the People with the sponsorship of Premier Li Peng (September 1993). It is clear that the Chinese government has recognized the major hazard of the effects of iodine deficiency on early brain development in relation to its one-child family policy.

At a regional level, this commitment to the elimination of IDD has also been made by the South Asian Association for Regional Co-operation which includes Bangladesh, Bhutan, India, the Maldives, Nepal, Pakistan and Sri Lanka. It has also been made by the Organization for African Unity (OAU) in Cairo (1993) and the Organization of American States in Latin America (Bogota 1992).

The ICCIDD, together with WHO and UNICEF, is providing advice and help to national governments with the necessary expertise required for effective national IDD control programmes. As described previously, regional IDD working groups are now functioning throughout the world, attended by national government representatives for a regular review of their programmes.

From the perspective of a national government, the elimination of IDD can be seen to offer the following positive outcomes for the promotion of national health and development:

- increased child survival
- increased child learning
- improved women's health
- greater economic productivity
- greater livestock production
- better quality of life

The great increase in momentum of national programmes in the last five years is due to recognition by national governments of these great benefits.

Examples of progress include Bolivia where, in 1985, the mean goitre rate was 69.4%. Following an intensive programme of salt iodization with the formation of salt co-operatives, the goitre rate had fallen to 4.5% in 1994 with normal urine iodine excretion (see Section 10.3). In Bhutan in 1983 a national survey revealed a national mean goitre prevalence of 64.5% with cretinism to be seen in all districts. Following an extensive programme with iodized salt and iodized oil, the total goitre rate in 1992 varied from 18.4% to 45.9% with normal urine iodine excretion. Similar improvements have been observed in the Cameroon in Africa following an effective iodized salt programme, as indicated by a normal range of urine iodine excretion.

37.3 A Global Partnership

Despite the immense magnitude of the threat to human potential posed by iodine deficiency, great progress has been made through a global partnership which has now come into being between people, governments, agencies and the expert multidisciplinary network of the ICCIDD. Most recently, the salt industry has joined the partnership through a link established with the ICCIDD, while in 1993, the World Service Club, Kiwanis International, adopted through UNICEF the virtual elimination of IDD as their World Service Project for the next five years.

This case study has described the development of a global partnership through the creation of a non-government organization (NGO), the International Council for Control of Iodine Deficiency Disorders, based in Australia with the support of the Australian International Development Assistance Bureau (AusAID) and other international agencies. It demonstrates the application of nutritional science to health and development in developing countries. For this, the ICCIDD as a NGO has been essential, particularly as advocate with the major international agencies and with national governments.

It provides a model for other similar translations from nutritional science to international public health.

Further Reading

1. Hetzel BS. Iodine deficiency disorders (IDD) and their eradication. *Lancet* 1983; 2: 1126–9.
2. Hetzel BS. *The prevention and control of iodine deficiency disorders.* Report to the United Nations Administrative Co-ordinating Committee: Sub-Committee on Nutrition, Rome, 1988.
3. Hetzel BS. *The story of iodine deficiency: an international challenge in nutrition.* Oxford University Press, 1989.
4. Hetzel BS, Potter BJ, Dulberg, EM. The iodine deficiency disorders: nature, pathogenesis and epidemiology. *World Rev Nutr Dietet* 1990; 62: 59–119.
5. WHO/UNICEF/ICCIDD. *Global prevalence of iodine deficiency disorders.* Micronutrient deficiency information systems (MDIS) working paper no. 1. Geneva: WHO, 1993.

38

Nutritional Consequences of Poverty in Developed Countries

Winsome Parnell and Sarah Bethell

'It upsets me that I'm not feeding the kids the food I want to, and they want to eat'

Traditionally, the many nutritional consequences of poverty have been identified and discussed in the context of developing countries. Recently, however, developed countries, particularly those with changes in their economic environments, have begun to identify an increasing prevalence of poverty-related health issues. Nutritionists recognize the overriding effects of the economic, social and educational factors, which together can influence nutritional status. Research in this area has therefore had to encompass new definitions and methodologies to assess the magnitude of the problem and the multi-faceted causes in order to develop strategies to alleviate them. Specific definitions of poverty and deprivation are always made in relative terms (between the 'haves' and 'have-nots') and therefore only apply to the society or group under discussion. Poverty is defined in terms of money and equivalent income; deprivation refers to the lack of certain material items regarded as essential in that society. Different degrees of deprivation can occur over a range of income levels with low monetary income (below a defined 'poverty' level) not necessarily being associated with severe deprivation.

Social and material circumstances are known to affect health outcomes. However, it is difficult to ascertain whether food and nutrient intakes have actually been impaired by socioeconomic disadvantage and can therefore be viewed as a cause of poorer health. Research focus has mostly been to link socioeconomic factors with health outcome, or to a limited extent, to link food and nutrient intake with poverty.

The major areas of nutritional concern, specifically found to be related to poverty in developed countries include:

- energy intake: both undernutrition and overnutrition
- insufficient intake of some micronutrients (e.g. iron)
- more babies with low birth weight and fewer babies breast-fed

38.1 METHODOLOGY

The selection of appropriate methodologies to study the nutritional consequences of poverty is not easy. First, a definition of poverty needs to be developed which is appropriate to the specific population group under consideration. Many researchers have used purely economic definitions (e.g. a percentage of mean equivalent disposable household income). Others recognize that deprivation criteria should be part of the definition of poverty (e.g. lack of adequate housing, transport or clothing). The length of time a group or individual experiences deprivation will be a determining factor in the effects of poverty.

Second, in developed countries with adequate food supplies, the concept of hunger has been difficult to define. It is not an isolated outcome, but one consequence of the larger problem of poverty. Hunger can be cyclical, short term or long term; it is not just physiological need. From the debate has come the new term 'food insecurity'. Food insecurity may be said to exist when the availability of nutritionally adequate and safe foods or the ability to acquire adequate supplies of culturally acceptable foods in socially acceptable ways is limited or uncertain.

Methodologies need to be developed to assess the nutritional consequences of poverty in whole populations or in selected at-risk subgroups within a population. National food and nutrition surveys, such as the United States National Health and Nutrition Survey NHANES III, now endeavour to include specific measures of food insecurity at household and individual level, using short questionnaires in association with detailed dietary recalls. Studies targeted at at-risk subgroups require special consideration of their particular circumstances when developing the methodology. Participation may be affected by poor access to transport and telephones, language and literacy problems, along with a variety of other social stresses. Sensitivity to these issues, including those of confidentiality and privacy, must be taken into account.

A landmark study in this area was carried out in London in the early 1990s by Dowler and Calvert. Their report *Nutrition and diet in lone-parent families in London* describes the socioeconomic circumstances, food intake patterns and nutrient intakes of 200 lone-parent families, with the aim of identifying the most important factors which differentiate diets at higher or lower risk for long-term ill-health. Data collected included three-day weighed intake records for each lone parent and at least one child, a food-frequency questionnaire, and a taped, semi-structured interview. The main conclusion from this work was 'that poor material circumstances combined with severe constraints on disposable income are the main factors characterizing nutritional deprivation in lone parents, and sometimes their children'. The diets of parents (predominantly mothers) were affected more than chidren's diets, and patterns of food shopping and food management skills had little effect on nutritional outcome. 'These mothers are not bad managers who do not know how to look after their children. They face impossible odds in making ends meet, and the aim of policy should be to help them, not to blame them'.

A further example of a study recently conducted in this area involved a convenience sample of 40 European families in two locations in New Zealand. A questionnaire was developed and piloted to assess the many aspects of food security. Nutritional status was measured by means of weights and heights; nutrient intakes were measured by multiple 24-hour dietary recalls. This study also found the women in these families were the most nutritionally disadvantaged. Studies such as this provide a step forward in the development of useful methodologies in this area.

38.2 Undernutrition and Obesity

Studies of the growth rates and weight-for-height relationships of children in the 5 to 12-year-old age range, of varying socioeconomic circumstances, generally conclude that disadvantaged children have lower heights-for-age and are more likely to have lower weight-for-height. This suggests that undernutrition (insufficient energy intake) over a period of time does have a negative effect on children's growth in developed countries.

However, it is clear that obesity also occurs in socioeconomically disadvantaged children, although to a lesser extent than among those of wealthier backgrounds. Further research is necessary and must include measures of dietary intake, along with measures of growth patterns and income, in order to determine the role of nutrition in growth in developed countries.

Few studies on adults in developed countries have linked poor socioeconomic status with undernutrition. Undoubtedly, some extremely deprived men and women (e.g. the homeless) exhibit clinical signs of undernutrition. Prevalence studies do not appear to have been conducted among these groups. In contrast, extensive work has documented the inverse relationship between socioeconomic status and obesity amongst women; but this relationship has not been shown in men. While poverty has long been held to be a cause of obesity among women, recently the inverse has been suggested: that obesity will result in lower socioeconomic status, mediated through unequal work and partnership opportunities.

Although the relationship between obesity and lower socioeconomic status clearly exists, there is little evidence from food and nutrient data that excess energy intake is the main influencing factor.

Criticisms of the existing studies on the energy intakes of obese women focus on the fact that they are more likely than non-obese women to under-report food intake, and to eat less than their habitual intake during study periods. Until the problem of accurately determining energy intake among obese women is solved, no conclusions can be made about the primary cause of obesity in socioeconomically disadvantaged women. It may also be possible that the notion of 'habitual intake' is less applicable to socioeconomically disadvantaged women than wealthier women because their economic resource base is not stable and they experience times of feast and famine. Whether obese women of low socioeconomic status are less physically active than obese women of wealthier backgrounds is not known. Economic deprivation is, however, known to affect motivation and self-esteem, and it limits opportunities for many forms of recreational exercise (Fig. 38.1).

38.3 Heart Disease and Diabetes

Research has shown that the prevalence of coronary heart disease (CHD) and accompanying changes in risk and mortality rates appear to be influenced greatly by socioeconomic factors. Although CHD is more common in more affluent countries, it appears to have a higher incidence in less affluent subgroups of these countries. Overall, declining mortality rates have been largely at the higher end of the socioeconomic spectrum, and in some regions have risen amongst lower socioeconomic groups of men

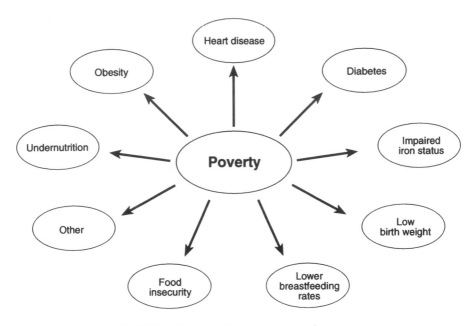

Fig. 38.1 Nutritional consequences of poverty.

and women. These differences have in part been attributed to different rates of high blood pressure and obesity. Blood pressure, within average community levels, is influenced by sodium intake. Lower socioeconomic conditions in childhood have also been linked to increased CHD risk in adulthood, both in women and men. This association has not been fully explained, but several studies provide some evidence to link nutritional status in childhood to subsequent CHD.

There is no obvious link between socioeconomic status and either quality or quantity of fat in the diets of men or women. However, there is clear evidence across all socioeconomic groups, that fat intake, particularly intake of saturated fat, is a significant dietary factor associated with the incidence of CHD (see Chapter 18.1.3). Many studies within developed countries document distinctive differences in eating habits and food choices between high and low socioeconomic groups, but this seldom has a profound effect on the contribution to energy intake from macronutrients including fat. Indeed, some authors conclude that there is a general uniformity of nutrient-density consumption patterns across different socioeconomic groups.

While obesity is one identified risk factor for CHD, it is also a major predictor in the onset of non-insulin-dependent diabetes mellitus (NIDDM), with both the duration and magnitude of obesity increasing the risk of development of NIDDM. Since obesity is associated with lower socioeconomic status, it would be expected that NIDDM will occur more frequently in groups of lower socioeconomic status. The incidence of NIDDM and impaired glucose tolerance were found to be inversely related to annual gross household income but not to a broader socioeconomic status (the Elley–Irving Index) in a multi-racial workforce study in New Zealand. The prevalence of insulin-dependent diabetes mellitus (IDDM) in children has been noted to be associated with material deprivation, but it has not been possible to link this with any particular nutrient. Recent research suggests that early exposure to cow's milk or diminished breast-feeding may be an important determinant of subsequent IDDM.

38.4   IRON DEFICIENCY

The aetiology of iron deficiency can be viewed as a negative balance between iron intake and iron loss. During the periods of rapid growth, iron balance is difficult to maintain (i.e. during infancy, early childhood, adolescence and pregnancy).

In infancy, lower iron status is associated with lower socioeconomic status, although iron deficiency occurs in all strata of society. Low iron status among adolescent girls of all socioeconomic groups is largely attributable to their increased dietary requirement of iron to balance the needs of growth and menstruation. Studies have not shown any difference in iron intakes amongst adolescent girls in low socioeconomic groups when compared to those from more affluent backgrounds. Women of childbearing potential in the United States have lower intakes of some nutrients, including iron, if they are of lower socioeconomic status. This can contribute to low iron status during pregnancy. Iron deficiency anaemia has been shown to be associated with poverty and to be linked with an increased risk of pre-term delivery and low birth weight.

38.5   LOW BIRTH WEIGHT

Low socioeconomic status is predictive of low birth weight (LBW) in most developed countries. A number of factors have been found to increase the incidence of LBW: cigarette smoking, low maternal weight gain during pregnancy, low prepregnancy weight, iron deficiency anaemia, alcohol intake, and possibly caffeine. Some of these factors are more prevalent in lower socioeconomic groups, and others are not. For example, cigarette smoking, which has a direct effect on the flow of nutrients across the placenta, is higher among low socioeconomic groups. Smokers have also been shown to eat less than non-smokers. Alcohol intake, however, has in some studies been higher among the wealthy.

Women for whom birth outcome is most at risk from a nutritional cause both enter pregnancy with a low body mass index (BMI) and do not gain sufficient weight during their pregnancy. Poor socioeconomic circumstances could contribute to this scenario, but no studies show that it is confined to such groups. Future studies may be able to discern if poverty has a significant influence on LBW because maternal nutrition has been impaired, rather than because, for example, smoking rates are higher, or other lifestyle factors, such as prenatal health care, are less than optimal.

38.6   BREAST-FEEDING

Social class is an important marker of breast-feeding success, which is more common in mothers of high socioeconomic status. Solo mothers, who are over-represented in the lower socioeconomic groups, are less likely to initiate or continue breast-feeding. The reasons for this are complex, but it is generally acknowledged that women need adequate support and encouragement to successfully breast-feed, and this help may be most limited amongst solo mothers.

38.7 BEHAVIOUR

The issue of whether inadequate nutrient intake and particularly hunger affect behaviour has been most studied among schoolchildren. After World War II, policy-makers in the United Kingdom and United States felt that food programmes for lunches and/or breakfasts in schools, would have a significant impact on school performance, including alertness, intelligence, educational attainment and general behaviour patterns. These programmes were made available regardless of socioeconomic circumstances, although those in higher socioeconomic groups were expected to pay. Fifty years on, when many such programmes have been reduced or dropped, hunger is again considered a problem among schoolchildren, and the reasons given are inadequate family income and lifestyle factors, such as time for food preparation and food habits. Thus, socioeconomic status is still believed to impact negatively on children's behaviour patterns. While many believe that nutrition is a significant issue, it is very difficult to disentangle the effects of the many disadvantaging factors of low socioeconomic status and how they impact on children's behaviour. Nutrition may well be one of these but few studies adequately address the issue in totality. For example, a study of 'perceived hunger' in schools in New Zealand found that the prevalence was higher in inner city areas and where ethnic diversity was greatest. No measures of behaviour at school were made, or of nutritional status. Reviews of school feeding programmes in the United States conclude that they have positive nutritional impact, but have not adequately evaluated such programmes in terms of their effect on academic performance. The fact that so many outcomes of poverty, in both the home and school environment, have the potential to influence behaviour of children, means that adverse food patterns and nutrition will always be a part of the spectrum to a varying degree. Generalizations regarding the circumstances of groups of children are probably inappropriate and only individual assessment of a child's circumstances will reveal whether nutrition needs to be improved.

38.8 FOOD INSECURITY

From the previous sections it can be concluded that it is difficult, in developed countries, to quantify the effect of poverty on nutritional status, both for methodological reasons and possibly because nutritional status is seldom profoundly affected. In addition, poor nutritional status is not confined to low socioeconomic groups.

Food security, however, is clearly difficult to achieve when economic status drops suddenly or when it is inadequate and remains so for long periods of time. To be food secure, individuals need more than adequate disposable income. They may need to overcome obstacles such as lack of transport, inadequate cooking or storage facilities and access to food which is culturally acceptable (see Fig. 38.2).

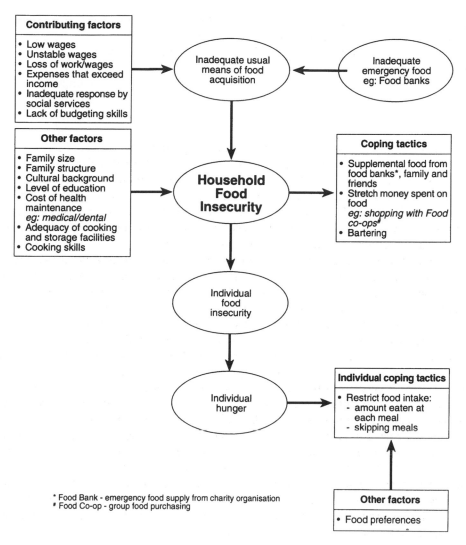

Fig. 38.2 Household food insecurity. *Source*: Adapted from Williams C, Dowler EA. *A working paper for the Nutrition Task Force Low Income Project Team*. London: Department of Health, 1994.

'I don't buy 5 kg of potatoes as I can't carry it.'

'I hope my husband will agree to give us the car.'

What is measurable is the growth of the many and varied programmes to alleviate shortage of food for groups of economically disadvantaged people. Food banks or pantries set up by charitable organizations are reported to have recently increased in number and size of operation in most developed countries. Their aim is to provide free food to the needy in an emergency or on a short-term basis. In some countries, government purchasing assistance such as 'food stamps' serve as a permanent or semi-permanent source of food income.

'It's hard to ask people for help. I don't want to be a burden.'

There is little dispute that the root cause of food insecurity has underlying socio-economic and political causes. These must be addressed by economists and politicians. What can nutritionists do? Many have attempted an educational approach, on the premise that budgeting and food preparation skills should be improved. In some instances this is helpful. But many communities of people in constrained circumstances vocalize their need to find solutions and coping strategies using their own skills and resources, along-side appropriate professional input.

Public health policy in many developed countries states that the effects of socio-economic disadvantage on nutritional well-being is a public health priority. Australia's Food and Nutrition Policy document opens thus: 'The Government's food and nutrition policy is to facilitate and support action through the entire food and nutrition system, in order to achieve better nutrition for Australians, especially for those most disadvantaged.' New Zealand's National Plan of Action for Nutrition lists 'Improving household food security' as a first priority, noting the need to establish baseline information on the current situation with respect to accessibility, acceptability and affordability of food.

It is now apparent that developed countries cannot assume that all segments of their population are food-secure. They need to document the prevalence of food insecurity and to monitor the prevalence of nutritional outcomes of food insecurity, including rates of obesity, iron status of women and infants, birth weights and breast-feeding rates. Every effort can then be made to develop and co-ordinate economic policies, educational strategies and social action to alleviate the nutritional consequences of poverty.

FURTHER READING

1. Bailey VF, Sherriff J. Reasons for the early cessation of breast-feeding in women from lower socio-economic groups in Perth, Western Australia. *Aust J Nutr Diet* 1992; **49**: 40–3.
2. Bartley M. Unemployment and ill health: understanding the relationship. *J Epid Comm Health* 1994; **48**: 333–7.
3. Dowler E, Calvert C. *Nutrition and diet in lone-parent families in London.* London: Family Policy Studies Centre, 1995.
4. Miller JE, Korenman S. Poverty and children's nutritional status in the United States. *Am J Epidemiol* 1994; **140**: 233–43.
5. Sobal J, Stunkard AJ. Socioeconomic status and obesity: A review of the literature. *Psychol Bull* 1989; **105**: 260–75.

39

CULTURAL SENSITIVITY IN NUTRITION EDUCATION: THE TONGAN EXPERIENCE

Barbara Guthrie, Soana Muimui-heata, Losa Moata'ane and Viliami Toafa

An important concept underlying research relating to culture and nutrition is an acceptance that ideas about health are social constructs that have meaning only within the context of a particular social group. It is therefore necessary to recognize that what it means to be healthy is culturally defined and that Western health services and scientifically based nutritional advice are cultural practices that people from other cultures do not inherently know or understand. Culture also influences decisions on what is illness and what is appropriate treatment.

39.1 INDIGENOUS HEALTH SYSTEMS

For many indigenous peoples two systems of medicine exist side by side: traditional medicine and Western medicine. Often, the belief system and culture of traditional medicine is familiar while the belief system and culture of Western medicine is strange and unfamiliar.

The science of nutrition arises from within the belief network or social construct of Western medicine where human beings are seen as having a molecular structure and where the meaning of illness can be sought at the molecular level (e.g. the role of bacteria, nutrient deficiencies or hormonal imbalance). In contrast, traditional views are very much tied up with spiritual beliefs and the most familiar method of assistance can be from a traditional healer.

Tongan traditional healers are called 'kau faito'o'. Their healing skills have been passed down through the generations within their own families. Faito'o never charge for their services, no appointments are necessary, they are available 24 hours a day, they work from their own homes and usually the whole family will attend when a family member visits a faito'o. Their motivation for undertaking this work is the privilege of being able to help and serve their community.

39.2 TONGAN PACIFIC ISLAND HEARTBEAT

This section presents a brief summary of the results of an evaluation using focus groups of two nutrition education materials: a pamphlet and a poster prepared for Tongan people. They illustrate what happens in nutrition education when resources are used which were developed with other purposes in mind. The pamphlet was originally produced by the Pacific Islands Heartbeat programme for a one-off Pacific Islands food festival. The origin of the logo on the front cover was a Pacific Islands art competition for school children. Resource development must allow for grass roots participation in defining the aims of the resources. Only then will concepts that have meaning and value to the target group be readily identifiable by them.

The front cover of the pamphlet is shown (Fig. 39.1); the background was cream in colour with the writing in a reddish brown. First impressions of the Tongan Pacific Island Heartbeat pamphlet were not favourable. The reasons given for the unfavourable responses included: the lack of colour and the lack of aesthetic appeal. One participant said, 'I would not pick it up or even look twice at it if it were in the supermarket...however because we are discussing it I will read it'. The graphics on the cover page were a mystery. Many thought it was an ethnic design but not Tongan. Most did not know it was a heart; the English title 'Heartbeat' did not automatically convey that meaning. Some who did recognize it as a heart thought that it looked diseased.

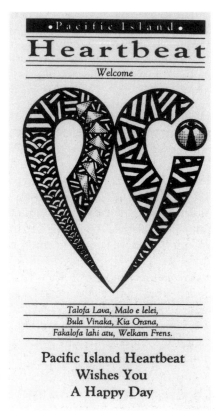

Fig. 39.1 Cover of Pacific Island Heartbeat pamphlet. Used with permission, National Heart Foundation of New Zealand.

Tongan cultural values were not taken into consideration for the photographs in the Pacific Island Heartbeat pamphlet. One photo was headed 'Food: We use it for special events' and showed a man and two women carrying food (Fig. 39.2). It was very clear to the participants that the adults in the photo were not Tongan and that their mode of dress was not appropriate for serving food, for, as one participant said, 'half naked women and men should never display food, especially at a special event'.

Special events, such as feasts, are the times when community traditions are at their strongest so that any errors in visual presentations will be readily noticed. It was further noted that the picture couldn't possibly be representing a special event because, as many participants said, 'Where is the pig?' (a pig is always served at a Tongan special event). In addition, there were bananas in the photo and they are foods that are not usually served at special events. Thus, the picture had also ignored the traditional Tongan cultural values of different foods. Pork is a traditional food accorded a high value and is an essential part of any feast. Yams also have a very high cultural status, as does giant taro.

On the next page was a very colourful drawing of a food shell based on the idea of the food pyramid (Fig. 39.3). The food shell was developed by the Pacific Islands Women's Project following food pyramid guidelines. This was received very favourably by the groups. They particularly appreciated that Pacific Island foods were clearly visible in the shell and that traditional foods were recognized as healthy foods. But some concepts were confusing: participants asked if fish is so good for you why is it in the 'eat moderate' group and not the 'eat most' group and why is white bread in the 'eat most' group?

The page on illustrations of cooking methods was misleading to the participants because in the translation from English to Tongan a new nuance was introduced which meant that some participants believed they were being asked to choose which of the

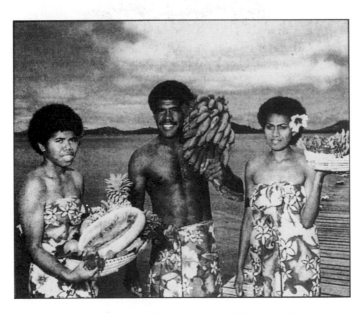

Fig. 39.2 Illustration from Pacific Island Heartbeat pamphlet entitled: 'Food we use for special events'. Used with permission. National Heart Foundation of New Zealand.

591

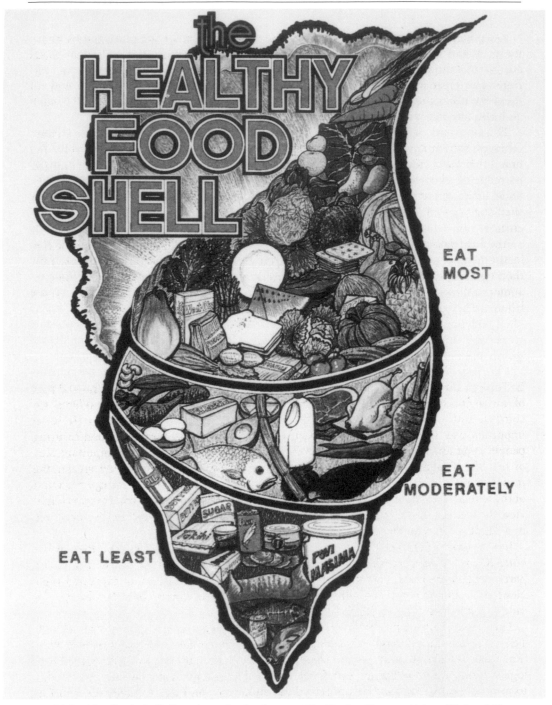

Fig. 39.3 The food shell (based on the food pyramid). Used with permission. National Heart Foundation of New Zealand.

cooking methods was actually the best method. These participants unanimously chose the umu (the traditional ground oven) over and above any of the other cooking methods and, in making this choice, were unaware of the underlying nutrition message on this page (i.e. to use low fat cooking methods). Some participants wanted to know why all the methods of food preparation referred to the *cooking* of foods when *raw* fish is such an important and valued part of the Tongan diet.

The last page of the Pacific Island Heartbeat pamphlet contained a list of Palangi (Western) concepts of things to do when shopping. There were several instructions: the first was headed: 'Take care' and this section contained six points, three of which related to reducing the use of coconut cream. All the groups expressed their difficulty in understanding why there was a coconut piece in the 'eat most' section of the healthy food shell and yet under 'Take care' they were being asked to cut back on the use of coconut cream.

Another shopping behaviour was 'Read the labels on food'. If the intention of this instruction was that shoppers should look for the nutrient content, (e.g. reduced fat), then the instructions were not sufficiently clear, as only one participant understood it. Some participants did not have any understanding of the instruction and asked, 'What label?'

39.3 FOOD AND CULTURE IN TONGA

In Tonga, as in many cultures, food is at the centre of social life. It plays an integral part of all major occasions and is a form of social interaction. Food is a vehicle for communicating customs and social status, kinship and social relationships. It is an important way to show love and respect, to share, to express hospitality and to bring people together. The provision of food in abundance and feasting is an important part of the life of many Pacific Islanders. The more food that is provided, the greater the respect being shown. To not eat food that is offered is regarded as rude and a rejection of the love and respect offered. It is, therefore, perhaps not surprising that Tongans might view the concept of a balanced diet, a notion that is at the heart of Western dietary advice in a slightly different way than Westerners.

In the poster (Fig. 39.4) the man is saying perhaps 'I am a little big' and then at the bottom our nearest translation is 'eat balanced meals or eat a balanced meal'. The participants were asked, What is a balanced meal? Several participants expressed their views of balance, such as, 'eat till you feel you can't take any more food', 'eat everything on the plates', 'eat till you drop'.

These ideas, although not in accordance with Western science, are in accord with Tongan beliefs that it is desirable, indeed respectful, to eat all food that is offered. So if 'Kai Palanisi ma'u pe' is giving the idea that there is a desirable way of eating, then it is logical from within the Tongan belief network for the participants to have interpreted this to mean a meal where food was provided in abundance and that everyone was very full after the meal. In addition, the concept would include ideas of the giving and receiving of love and respect.

The response groups were also asked their ideas on why the man was so big. All groups focused on the differing perceptions between Tongans and Palangi (Europeans) in terms

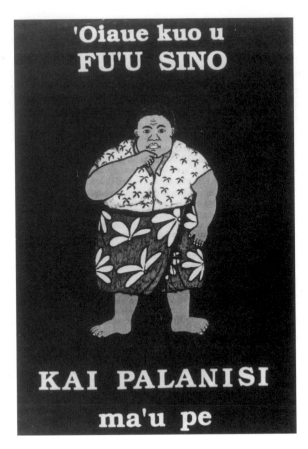

Fig. 39.4 Big Man poster. Used with permission.
Source: Occupation, Vol 2, No 2, October 1994.

of what is a healthy weight and size. 'A healthy weight is big, but not too big.' 'Healthy weight for the Palangi is too thin and overweight is considered to be too big but a Tongan healthy weight is probably in between this.'

The natural Tongan pattern of eating was given as a possible contributing factor to high body weight. This included: ideas of eating whatever is available, eating whenever you want to, eating now while you can, and the more that is available the more you eat. Other possibilities included family history 'Some families are all big so no matter how much they eat they all have a tendency to be too big', and the nature of life. 'God is the one who created us so He's the one who determines our body build. So He's the one who makes us big or small'.

39.4 CULTURALLY APPROPRIATE NUTRITION EDUCATION

In the scientific world, food guides are viewed as simple and reliable nutrition education tools that have been translated from the world of nutritional science into the world of the everyday person. Considerable debate and research have occurred over the best manner of presentation for food guides and the focus is usually on foods as opposed to nutrients. The successful preparation of nutrition education materials, however, requires more than the accurate translation of scientific principles into the language of the lay person. What has often been overlooked is that participants will only understand food guides if they have an understanding of the belief network that underlies the food guides.

Health, as it is understood in Western medicine, and the role of nutrients in food have little meaning in most traditional cultures. The world of science needs to acknowledge non-scientific belief systems if it is successfully to assist people of varying cultures. The starting point for the preparation of food guides must be the belief network of the intended user community and not the belief network of scientists.

FURTHER READING

1. Guthrie B, Muimui-heata S, et al. Kai fakamou'ui lelei: Tongan food choices, beliefs and education. *Occupation* 1994; **2**: 24–41.
2. Kinloch P. *Talking health but doing sickness: studies in Samoan health.* Wellington: Victoria University Press, 1985.
3. Muimui-Heata S, Guthrie BE. An evaluation of the Pacific Island Heartbeat pamphlet for Tongan people in New Zealand. *J NZ Dietet Assoc* 1993; **47**: 64–6.
4. Vainikolo F, Vivili P, Guthrie BE. Food consumption patterns and beliefs of Tongans living in Dunedin. *J NZ Dietet Assoc* 1993; **47**: 6–9.
5. Moata'ane LM, Muimui-Heata S, Guthrie BE. Tongan perceptions of diet and diabetes. *J NZ Dietet Assoc* 1996; **50**: 52–6.

Part IX: Nutritional immunology and nutrition support

40
NUTRITION AND IMMUNE DEFENCE

Bill Woodward

Nutritional immunology has its origins in the study of nutritional deficiency. A vicious cycle is the most common relationship between malnutrition and infection, and depression of immune functions is integral to this cyclic interaction (Fig. 40.1). Among children suffering protein-energy malnutrition (PEM) ranging from mild through severe, the interaction between nutritional deficit and infection is multiplicative and accounts for more than 50% of all deaths. A similar interaction is apparent between infectious complications and secondary malnutrition among critically ill hospitalized patients.

Nutritional deficits typically depress diverse immunological defences simultaneously. This observation is fundamental to an understanding of clinically meaningful depression in the functions of a multitiered and tightly integrated physiological system such as the immune system. Thus, no isolated immunological change can be considered paramount in the susceptibility of the malnourished to infection. Malnutrition-associated infections are caused most commonly by organisms that are normally harmless commensals. Such opportunistic infections (e.g. pneumonia caused by *Streptococcus pneumoniae* or *Pneumocystis carinii* and diarrhoea caused by various coliforms) develop whenever the balance is upset sufficiently between resistance and exposure to our normal human microflora. In addition, the risk of mortality following infection with pathogenic organisms (e.g. the measles virus) can be increased dramatically by nutritional deficit. Malnutrition-associated immunodepression is documented most extensively in relation to wasting PEM (i.e. marasmus, kwashiorkor and marasmic kwashiorkor) in the weanling stage of life.

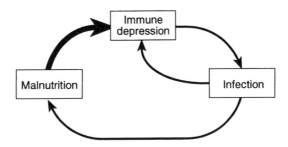

Fig. 40.1 The malnutrition–infection cycle depicted to include immunodepression as an essential component. The broad arrow represents the portion of the cycle on which the bulk of research effort has been expended. Many infections that are aggravated by malnutrition also induce immunodepression (e.g. measles) so a bidirectional connection links infection and immunodepression.

40.1 Outline of the Immune System

The immune system isolates and/or eliminates anything that can be identified as non-self. This includes microorganisms, tumour cells, non-living particulate matter and molecules such as bacterial toxins. An outline of the main barriers of the immune system is shown in Fig. 40.2, which shows the two main types of immune defence designated 'innate' and 'adaptive'.

Innate defence barriers are each effective against many different infectious organisms, and require no infectious (or other) challenge in order to become established at an effective level. Innate barriers comprise an essential first line of defence that limits entry, proliferation and colonization by microorganisms during the period of days required to generate the more potent adaptive responses. The latter, also termed 'acquired' immunity, exhibits specificity such that, for example, a response to the measles virus is ineffective against any other organism. In addition, adaptive immunity usually includes a component of memory that may persist for years and that permits a more rapid and powerful response to second and subsequent challenges with the same non-self agent. Vaccinations are designed to stimulate adaptive immunity to specific microorganisms.

The physical barriers include the epithelia (e.g. of the skin and of the respiratory, gastrointestinal and genitourinary tracts) and the endothelia of the vascular and nervous systems. These barriers not only impose an impediment to the penetration of microorganisms into the deeper tissues, but also possess the means to prevent adherence and colonization by microorganisms. Mucus, for example, limits microbial adherence to an underlying epithelial cell layer both through a physical washing action and through a biochemical strategy of competition for binding sites.

Phagocytosis is a process whereby cells ingest particles ranging in size from bacterial dimensions (0.5–1.0 μm) up to several micrometres in length. The major phagocytes include the neutrophil and the mononuclear phagocyte. Neutrophils are the most numerous circulating white blood cells in humans and the first motile defensive cell to congregate at a site of infection. The longer-lived mononuclear phagocyte follows as a second wave of phagocytic defence, manifesting as the blood monocyte that differentiates

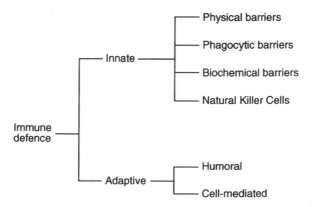

Fig. 40.2 An outline of the immune system illustrating the main barriers that impede the entry and facilitate the elimination of non-self biochemicals and particulate matter.

to become the macrophage in the extravascular tissues. Ingested particles are confined within an intracytoplasmic sac into which the phagocyte injects high levels of a variety of cytotoxic molecules. These include reactive metabolites of oxygen (e.g. hydrogen peroxide) that the phagocyte synthesizes only during and subsequent to phagocytosis, as well as a variety of preformed proteins that function, in part, by disrupting microbial electrolyte balance.

Diverse soluble proteins contribute to innate defence. For example, the complement system includes approximately 20 blood proteins that interact in a cascade of activation reactions yielding key mediators of inflammation. Although unpleasant, inflammation is a critical defence function designed to confine an infection for concerted immunological attack. Complement activation generates a peptide that attracts neutrophils to seek foci of infection by a process called 'chemotaxis'. Complement peptides also initiate reaction cascades, through vascular endothelial cells and mast cells, to release additional chemotaxins as well as vasodilators and mediators of increased vascular permeability. Activation of complement also yields a protein that enhances phagocytic rate by coating ingestible particles and promoting their adherence to plasma membrane receptor molecules displayed by phagocytes. These proteins are termed 'opsonins', and a variety of opsonins unrelated to complement (e.g. fibronectin) are normal constituents of blood plasma. Finally, complement stimulates a protein complex that can kill important disease-causing organisms, notably enteric Gram-negative bacteria.

The inflammatory response is promoted further through the release of soluble proteins, including interleukin (IL)-1, tumour necrosis factor-α and IL-6. These molecules are classified within the large and heterogeneous family of soluble immunoregulatory proteins collectively termed 'cytokines'. The inflammatory cytokines are endocrine hormones produced mainly by mononuclear phagocytes. These mediators augment the numbers and effectiveness of neutrophils, and stimulate the liver to secrete proteins into the plasma, designated 'acute phase', that provide immunological, antioxidant and anticoagulant protection (e.g. the third component of complement, caeruloplasmin and fibrinogen, respectively) as well as protection against the proteolytic enzymes released at sites of infection. In addition, IL-6, IL-1 and tumour necrosis factor-α mediate the fever response. Although unpleasant, an appropriately modest level and duration of fever is advantageous. Fever promotes neutrophil chemotaxis and, together with IL-1, promotes neutrophil microbicide and T cell lymphocyte responses. Another inflammatory cytokine, interferon-γ, is a paracrine hormone of lymphocytes that stimulates the phagocytic and microbicidal activity of mononuclear phagocytes. Thus, the inflammatory cytokines provide an important link between innate and adaptive defences.

Three distinct lineages of lymphocyte are recognized. The natural killer cell is a component of innate defence against viruses, tumour cells and, perhaps, some bacteria and fungi. The specificity and memory of adaptive immunity, however, reside in the lineages of lymphocytes designated B cells and T cells. B cells mature within the bone marrow, whereas T cells originate in the marrow but mature within the thymus.

When B cells are presented with non-self molecules (termed 'antigen' in the context of adaptive defence) which they can recognize, they proliferate and differentiate to give rise to antibody-producing plasma cells. There are five classes of antibody designated immunoglobulin (Ig) G, A, M, D and E, and their synthesis and release is the humoral response. Within mucosal epithelia, the humoral response is dominated by IgA. This immunoglobulin functions within the mucous layer by binding to microorganisms and antigen molecules as a blocking antibody that prevents adherence of the foreign agents to epithelial cells. IgG and IgM are produced mainly by plasma cells in the spleen and deep lymph nodes. Like IgA, these antibody classes can exert a blocking action, preventing attachment of viruses or toxin molecules to target cell receptors. In addition, IgM and some types of IgG can augment innate defences as opsonins and as activators of the complement cascade.

Most T cells belong to one or the other of two distinct subsets. These are distinguished on the basis of the mutually exclusive cell surface proteins CD4 and CD8. The CD8$^+$ lineage gives rise to cytotoxic T cells that kill virus-infected host cells or tumour cells. This is termed cell-mediated immunity (CMI) because the invading entity is an intact, living cell. In a second type of CMI response, the CD4$^+$ T cell releases cytokines, notably interferon-γ, that promote the ability of macrophages to kill particularly resistant organisms (e.g. tuberculosis bacteria), which have a propensity to penetrate host cells. Thus, CMI complements humoral immunity by providing protection against infectious agents that are beyond the reach of the antibody molecule, a defensive element that is confined to the extracellular space.

Most CMI and antibody responses are regulated by cytokines of CD4$^+$ T cells that stimulate proliferation and differentiation of B cells, T cells and mononuclear phagocytes. Although most CD4$^+$ T cells, therefore, are designated helper (Th) cells, some arc sct apart as 'inducers', thought to elicit differentiation of a subpopulation of CD8$^+$ T cells that suppresses adaptive responses. The balance among cytokines released by CD4$^+$ T cells appears to determine which type of adaptive response is generated in any particular case. For example, IL-12 and interferon-γ generally promote CMI but down-regulate antibody responses, whereas IL-4 exerts the opposite influence. Other cell types (e.g. CD8$^+$ T cells, macrophages and dendritic cells), also release many of the same cytokines. Although undoubtedly costly from a metabolic standpoint, such complexity permits a high degree of control over the nature and magnitude of adaptive immune responses.

A key feature of immunocompetence is the need for only a small initiating stimulus. For example, the spleen, lymph nodes and mucosal lymphoid aggregates (e.g. the tonsils) can concentrate minute quantities of antigen for presentation to lymphocytes that continuously recirculate through these sites. This promotes rapid expansion of those lymphocyte clones that are specifically required at a particular time, while permitting the economy of maintaining only small numbers of lymphocytes against irrelevant antigens. The same principle applies to innate defences (e.g. in the reaction cascade that activates complement). Thus, protective immunity can be generated without exposure to an overwhelming antigenic (infectious) load.

40.2   IMMUNODEPRESSION IN WASTING PROTEIN-ENERGY MALNUTRITION

Many physical barriers to infection appear compromised in protein-energy malnutrition (PEM). For example, failure to secrete acid in the stomach may contribute to overgrowth of Gram-negative bacteria in the small intestine. PEM also causes quantitative and chemical changes in mucous glycoproteins and this, in turn, may increase the risk that microorganisms will adhere to, and even colonize, mucosal epithelial cells, thus initiating infection.

Clearance of foreign particles from the blood is depressed in PEM, and this has been interpreted to reflect poor phagocytosis by hepatic and splenic macrophages. Blood clearance, however, provides only an indirect measure of phagocytic activity because factors such as blood perfusion, phagocyte numbers and capacity for opsonizing particles also control clearance rate. In fact, phagocytosis is largely unaffected in PEM on the part of both the neutrophil and the monocyte/macrophage.

Blood neutrophil numbers are also usually normal in PEM. Malnourished subjects, however, cannot sustain the elevated numbers of blood neutrophils seen in the well-nourished in response to infection, and often exhibit the opposite response, a particularly ominous sign in immunocompromised patients. In addition, the ability of the neutrophil to kill microorganisms is depressed in PEM, and this correlates with a depressed ability to generate toxic metabolites from molecular oxygen. In contrast to the neutrophil, mononuclear phagocyte numbers are low in PEM.

The classic clinical signs of infection, inflammation and fever, are attenuated in PEM. In the absence of infection, the blood concentrations of complement proteins often are only modestly depressed. In response to infection, however, malnourished patients cannot generate the necessary elevated levels of key complement proteins (e.g. the third component, C3). Instead, such patients often exhibit depression in complement protein concentrations. As well, production of inflammatory cytokines such as IL-1, tumour necrosis factor-α and IL-6, is depressed in PEM so that the protective benefits of fever and the hepatic acute phase plasma proteins are not available. As a result of these abnormalities there is reduced capacity both to attract phagocytes and lymphocytes (from their atrophied cellular pools) and to promote phagocytosis and destruction of microorganisms.

Despite the importance of the innate defences, resistance to infection requires the specificity and power of lymphocyte-mediated adaptive responses, either cell- or antibody-mediated. Lymphoid tissue throughout the body is profoundly reduced in PEM. The decrease in T cell numbers has attracted particular attention as an explanation for the key observation that, unlike the antibody response, cell-mediated immunity (CMI) is consistently depressed in PEM. Like CMI, however, most antibody responses require T cell help. Moreover, although B cell numbers in the blood are largely preserved in human PEM, B cells in the rest of the body are much depleted. The particular sensitivity of CMI to wasting PEM, therefore, presently defies explanation, although it is a very well-established phenomenon. CMI is depressed even in mild wasting PEM whereas it is usually unaffected by stunting malnutrition. A clear understanding of CMI in PEM is important because this type of response defends against organisms (e.g. tuberculosis bacteria) that penetrate host cells to become inaccessible to other immunological defence actions.

Levels of immunoglobulins (all classes) in the blood are normal or even elevated in PEM. Much of the antibody in the blood plasma, however, is a polyreactive type not characteristic of the mature, high-specificity antibody response. Consequently, blood immunoglobulin concentrations should not be interpreted (as is commonly done) to indicate humoral immunocompetence. At the same time, maintenance of this 'natural antibody' in PEM represents preservation of an early defence barrier which, for example, is the preferred opsonin for promoting phagocytosis of organisms such as staphylococci.

Mucosal diseases, such as pneumonia and diarrhoea, are much the most common infections among the malnourished, but there is little information pertaining to mucosal immune defence, including adaptive humoral immunity. It is clear, however, that levels of IgA antibody in mucous secretions are low in PEM. The main effect probably is not on the production of this class of antibody by the intestine and other mucosae. Rather, the transport of IgA across the mucosal epithelium to its site of action within the mucin layer is profoundly depressed in PEM.

Much of the information about lymphocytes and their responses in PEM derives from the study of blood, the most accessible tissue in the human being. The blood, however, contains only 2% of the lymphocytes in the body. Consequently, blood lymphocyte data are easily overinterpreted when extrapolating to compartments such as the spleen and lymph nodes in which adaptive immune responses take place. For example, a low ratio of cellular numbers within the $CD4^+$ T cell subset relative to $CD8^+$ T cells (CD4/CD8 ratio) commonly occurs in the blood in PEM. This has been widely interpreted as insufficiency of $CD4^+$ T cell help relative to $CD8^+$ suppressor and cytotoxic T cell capacity. The low blood CD4/CD8 ratio, however, is irrelevant to other lymphoid compartments and to thymus-dependent immunodepression, at least in experimental PEM.

Lymphoid involution is undoubtedly important to the depressed adaptive immunity of PEM, but is only one contributing factor. Imbalances among critical T cell subsets in PEM remain distinctly possible, and may relate to evidence of a reduced capacity for producing T cell cytokines including the critical endogenous T cell mitogen, IL-2.

40.3   IMMUNE DEFENCES IN PREVALENT MICRONUTRIENT DEFICIENCY CONDITIONS

Animal studies have contributed substantially to establishing the immunological consequences of micronutrient deficiencies. Such studies permit investigation of isolated deficiency conditions and provide an opportunity for control over the confounding factor of associated weight loss. Vitamin A, iron and zinc deficiencies are of special interest because of their prevalence among human beings.

Deficiency of vitamin A, the 'anti-infective vitamin', compromises innate and adaptive immunological barriers including mucosal epithelia, blood clearance, cell-mediated immunity and antibody responses. Even subclinical vitamin A deficiency increases the risk of infection, although lymphoid involution does not occur. Analysis of subclinical vitamin A deficiency in mice has shown overproduction of the cytokine, interferon-γ, by $CD4^+$ T cells. This is potentially a key to the poor antibody response in this deficiency condition.

Iron deficiency is reminiscent of PEM in its immunological effects, although thymus-dependent immunity is probably less severely affected. It is sometimes suggested that iron deficiency may protect against infection and that repletion increases susceptibility. Except in the case of malaria, however, this idea is not consistent with clinical experience, particularly if iron repletion is achieved by the oral route. Iron overload, however, can increase susceptibility to infection. This is partly attributable to saturation of plasma transferrin (with consequent inability to withhold iron from microorganisms) and, also, is partly because of immunodepression from cellular iron loading. Injection of iron, therefore, is not advised where immunocompetence and blood transferrin levels are both low (e.g. in neonates and in kwashiorkor).

The immunological impact of *zinc deficiency* is remarkably similar to that of PEM. Consequently, immunodepression in PEM is frequently attributed to zinc deficiency. In further support of this notion, it is often pointed out that zinc supplementation can improve the rate of immunological recovery during rehabilitation of children from PEM. During convalescence, however, there is a high zinc requirement for catch-up growth. No clear support exists for the idea that immunodepression in PEM is attributable to micronutrient deficiency.

40.4 LIPIDS

Some influences of lipids (e.g. on chemotaxis and microbicidal activity of neutrophils) appear to be mediated primarily through eicosanoids, whereas others (e.g. influences on the cytolytic activity of lymphocytes and macrophages) must be attributed to mechanisms such as modulation of membrane fluidity and signal transduction or alteration in the burden of lipid peroxides. Polyunsaturated fatty acids (PUFA) of ω6 and ω3 families complement one another in their influence on some immune functions (e.g. lymphocyte-mediated cytolytic activity) but appear antagonistic in relation to others (e.g. lymphocyte proliferation). The impact of lipids on adaptive immunity also appears to vary with state of health. Despite the obvious immunomodulatory power of lipids, therefore, few generalizations with predictive value have emerged.

Deficiency of ω6 essential fatty acids (EFA deficiency) generally induces depression in the inflammatory response and in the activity of phagocytes. Antibody responses, also, are generally depressed, but cell-mediated immunity has exhibited a spectrum of responses ranging from depression through enhancement in the artificial setting of experimental EFA deficiency. Divergent responses to diet on the part of cell- and antibody-mediated immunity, however, are a continuing theme in nutritional immunology, and this is also apparent in various experimental animals fed diets containing high levels of fat (e.g. exceeding 25% of calories) rich in ω6-PUFA. Generally, such experimental conditions depress CMI but are without effect on antibody responses. These observations may help to explain the association between consumption of a high proportion of calories as fat and susceptibility to metastatic tumours.

40.5 INTRAUTERINE GROWTH RETARDATION (IUGR)

Any insult causing placental insufficiency imposes the risk of giving birth to an infant that is small-for-gestational-age (e.g. less than 2500 g at term) and susceptible to opportunistic infections. The immunological features of this condition closely resemble those observed in post-weaning PEM although some features suggest a more severe immunodepression (e.g. a low blood lymphocyte count and low blood plasma immunoglobulin concentrations). In particular, studies both of animals and of human subjects emphasize the refractory nature of IUGR-associated immunoincompetence. Despite catch-up growth such immunodepression can persist into adulthood, although this may depend on additional eliciting factors, notably exposure to infectious agents.

IUGR appears to be a potent independent risk factor for adult degenerative conditions such as cardiovascular disease. Persistent immunodepression following IUGR, therefore, is best regarded as part of this larger syndrome thought to result from intractable endocrine derangements. Wasting PEM, if imposed sufficiently early in infancy, also can produce a depression in CMI that may persist for many years.

40.6 NUTRITIONAL DEFICIENCY CONDITIONS CAN STIMULATE IMMUNITY

Weaning and adolescent rodents subjected to stunting (not wasting) malnutrition by means of a low-protein diet, or through restricted intake of a complete diet (approximately 40% reduction in caloric intake below ad libitum), can exhibit increases in CMI, and parallel increases in resistance to selected pathogens, relative to animals given free access to a complete diet. Short-term fasting in obese humans and in rodents (i.e. periods of several days) also can stimulate immunity. In the rodent system, a parallel increase in resistance to pathogens has been demonstrated, and the main effect involves the macrophage independently of adaptive immunity. It is important not to misinterpret these experimental results to mean that the very-low-calorie diet (less than 800 kcal/day) will confer immunological benefit in the treatment of obesity. Weight reduction programmes are protracted in duration relative to a short-term fast, and their main impact immunologically is to place at risk diverse innate defences and CMI.

40.7 THERAPEUTIC APPLICATIONS OF SPECIFIC NUTRIENTS

Long-chain ω3-PUFA are of interest as antiinflammatory agents. Ingestion of several grams of fish oil daily for periods of several weeks or months has produced clinical improvements in patients suffering a variety of inflammatory conditions including psoriasis, ulcerative colitis and rheumatoid arthritis. Animal-based studies concur with generally more clear-cut results. Eicosapentaenoic acid ($20:5$ ω3) is usually implicated as the main antiinflammatory agent, acting at least in part through conversion to prostaglandin E_3 and leukotriene B_5. These compounds are less powerful inflammatory mediators than the corresponding eicosanoids from arachidonic acid (i.e. prostaglandin E_2 and leukotriene B_4). The latter eicosanoid, for example, increases vascular permeability and is a potent chemotaxin for neutrophils. ω3-PUFA are also thought to act by a non-eicosanoid-mediated mechanism to depress the synthesis of tumour necrosis factor-α, IL-1 and IL-6 by mononuclear phagocytes and lymphocytes.

Nutritional immunomodulation is also of interest in relation to chronic infectious conditions that characteristically induce multiple nutrient deficiencies. For example, daily vitamin A supplements can retard the development of AIDS in HIV-positive human beings. Low blood retinol levels are common among HIV-infected persons and effective levels of supplementation have been in the range of three to seven times the United States recommended dietary allowance (RDA).

Short-term immunostimulation through nutritional supplements can be achieved in critically ill patients (e.g. victims of burns or other physical injuries) who experience immunosuppression mediated by endogenous inflammatory cytokines. Pharmacological supplements of some nutrients (e.g. nucleotides, arginine and long-chain ω3-PUFA supplied as fish oil) appear effective in management. Pyrimidine nucleotides are considered to exert a direct, substrate-level influence in supporting proliferation of lymphocytes because these cells have a limited biochemical capacity to salvage these molecules for re-use. In contrast, arginine may act indirectly (perhaps through the polyamines, or somatotropin, or a complex neural network) to enhance T cell proliferative capacity. Enteral nutrition appears superior to parenteral delivery in promoting immunocompetence and reduced infectious complications among high-risk postoperative subjects.

40.8   RESPONSE OF INFECTIOUS AGENTS TO NUTRIENT DEFICIENCIES OF THE HOST

Microorganisms can play a pro-active role in the vicious cycle involving nutritional deficit and infection. For example, iron deprivation of the host enhances toxin production by the pathogen, *Corynebacterium diphtheriae*. Further, deficiency of at least some antioxidant nutrients can promote mutation to pathogenicity on the part of a normally avirulent organism. This occurs in a murine model combining selenium deficiency and infection with the widespread Coxsackie B enterovirus, and adds a new dimension to the field of nutritional immunology.

40.9   HEALTH PROMOTION

There is much interest in the immunomodulatory power of nutrients for the purpose of disease prevention among free-living, healthy human beings. For example, breast-feeding reduces the risk of infections among infants in both industrialized and non-industrialized settings. This is attributable, in part, to the diverse innate and adaptive immunological defence components in breast milk. Some of these defensive elements confer passive immunity, whereas it is suspected that others promote development of mucosal immunity in the suckling infant.

At the other extreme of the lifespan, supplementation with isolated micronutrients (e.g. vitamins C, E, or B_6), or with multivitamin/mineral preparations, can stimulate adaptive and innate immune defences, reduce the frequency of infection-related illness and increase responses to vaccination in the elderly. Supplements supplying only small multiples of the United States RDA have elicited responses so that the mechanism is probably a correction of subclinical nutrient deficiencies. In effect, the question has arisen as to the extent to which ageing-associated immunodeficiency is secondary to nutritional deficits. Alternatively, currently recommended intakes for numerous micronutrients may prove insufficient for maximizing immunocompetence in the elderly.

40.10   CONCLUDING PERSPECTIVE

Important applications are either in place or on the horizon. Measures of immunocompetence are helpful in identifying patients requiring nutritional support and in assessing the response to such support. Tests of proven value for these clinical purposes include the blood lymphocyte count and delayed hypersensitivity skin tests to antigens such as those of the tuberculosis bacterium. Moreover, assessment of immunocompetence may prove useful in establishing upper and lower safe limits of intake for nutrients and energy in health and disease. In this context, it is often suggested that a level of intake, beyond which immunodepression will occur, exists for all nutrients. For example, from the standpoint of immunocompetence, 50 mg daily is proposed as the upper safe limit for zinc intake by free-living adult human beings. The concept of optimum nutrient intake is intutitively attractive and also has modest support from studies of vitamin A, iron, selenium, iodine, vitamin E, ω-6 PUFA and total fat intake.

Immune functions are an integral component of the physiology of humans and animals. Thus, diet-induced immunological change is a component of an integrated, whole-body effort to adapt to the metabolic challenge imposed by altered intake of nutrients and/or energy. It follows, for example, that susceptibility to infection is the price for the adaptive benefits of diet-related immunodepression (e.g. support of the liver with biochemicals from involuting lymphoid organs). Appreciation of the basic physiology connecting diet and immunocompetence is foundational to a rational application of knowledge from the field of nutritional immunology.

FURTHER READING

1. Blok WL, Katan MB, Van Der Meer JWM. Modulation of inflammation and cytokine production by dietary (n-3) fatty acids. *J Nutr* 1996; **126**: 1515–33.
2. Bower RH, Cerra FB, Bershadsky B, Licari JJ, Hoyt DB, Jensen GL, *et al.* Early enteral administration of a formula (Impact^R) supplemented with arginine, nucleotides, and fish oil in intensive care unit patients: Results of a multicenter, prospective, randomized, clinical trial. *Critical Care Medicine* 1995; **23**: 436–49.
3. Hunt NH, Chaudri G. Nutrition and infectious disease. *Redox Report* 1995; **1**: 231–33.
4. Lee W-H, Woodward BD. The CD4/CD8 ratio in the blood does not reflect the response of this index in secondary lymphoid organs of weanling mice in models of protein-energy malnutrition known to depress thymus-dependent immunity. *J Nutr* 1996; **126**: 849–59.
5. Munoz C, Schlesinger MS. Interaction between cytokines, nutrition and infection. *Nutr Res* 1995; **15**: 1815–44.
6. Peck MD. Interactions of lipids with immune function. II: Experimental and clinical studies of lipids and immunity. *J Nutr Biochem* 1994; **5**: 514–21.
7. Spear-Hartley A. Sherman AR. Food restriction and the immune system. *J Nutr Immun* 1994; **3**(2): 27–50.
8. Stallone DD. The influence of obesity and its treatment on the immune system. *Nutr Reviews* 1994; **52**: 37–50.
9. Woodward B. Zinc, a pharmacologically potent essential nutrient: focus on immunity. *Canadian Med Assoc J* 1991; **145**: 1469.

41

ENTERAL AND PARENTERAL NUTRITIONAL SUPPORT

Madeleine Ball

41.1 THE NEED FOR NUTRITIONAL SUPPORT

In the mid 1930s, a Cleveland surgeon by the name of Hiram Studley looked carefully at a number of factors which he felt might contribute to the high death rate after stomach removal for ulcers. He found that the amount of weight a patient lost correlated with the death rate. We now know that excessive weight loss and malnutrition have a range of adverse effects which may cause death or prolong the recovery from illness or surgery. These include reduced muscle strength, reduced respiratory function, delayed wound healing and increased susceptibility to infection. Maintenance of good nutritional status is thus very important in sick people. However, people who are unwell may not be able to eat normally. Studies suggest that a significant proportion of patients are undernourished before entering hospital and many have signs of malnutrition when they leave. This is particularly true for patients with gastrointestinal disease and cancer, but undernutrition is also common in the sick elderly.

Malnutrition may result from reduced food intake and also from concurrent increased energy expenditure. The reasons for reduced intake may include confusion, lack of appetite, vomiting, or pain. Chemotherapy for malignant tumours can result in severe malnutrition due to side effects of the therapy. Food intake may also be contraindicated for patients who have a severe inflammatory bowel disease, as the bowel may need rest, or following surgery when the gut does not work properly or time is needed for recovery. Yet at this very time when they are not eating normally the patient's energy requirements are often actually increased above normal because of the hormonal responses to stress, a raised temperature and/or infection.

41.2 METHODS OF PROVISION OF NUTRITIONAL SUPPORT

Nutritional support can be provided in two main ways: (1) enterally, when the gut can be used, and (2) parenterally, if the gut cannot be used.

41.2.1 Enteral feeding

Enteral support includes providing feeds by mouth (liquidized if necessary) with frequent sip feeding or the use of special drinks which are fortified with products such as Caloreen (a glucose polymer) or milk powder to increase the energy content.

In another form of enteral nutritional support, nutrients are supplied into the gastrointestinal tract via a flexible tube passed down the nose or mouth into the stomach, duodenum or jejunum (nasogastric feeding).

Tubes can also be inserted directly into the stomach or small intestine from the outside through the skin and abdominal wall (Fig. 41.1).

Some indications for use of enteral tube feeds include:

- burns to the face
- unable to swallow
- unconscious
- severe nausea
- obstruction in the oesophagus

Originally, mashed food was given via such tubes, but now there are a wide range of commercial formulas available which can be given down fine, flexible, more comfortable tubes. The formulae are usually supplied to the hospital in sterile containers. The solution is transferred to a plastic container and administered down the tube usually as a continuous infusion and frequently using a regulator or pump. The formulas contain proteins, carbohydrates including glucose, fats, vitamins and minerals and can deliver 4–8 kJ (1–2 kcal) per ml.

A range of different preparations is available. The protein is generally casein, the fats may be medium- or long-chain triglycerides, and the carbohydrates include glucose and

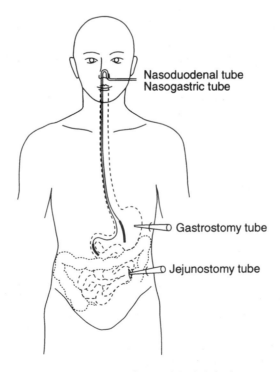

Fig. 41.1 Routes of enteral (tube) feeding.

glucose polymers (chain of glucose molecules). They require less digestion than the constituents of a normal diet.

Proprietary enteral feeds include the whole protein preparations mentioned above and also elemental diets. Elemental diets contain 'food' in its basic chemical form so that it requires very little digestion and they originate from diets developed for use in the American aerospace programme (hence 'space diets'); they are not palatable enough for oral use without modification. They are also concentrated (hypertonic) and tend to cause diarrhoea so that if given at all they should be sufficiently diluted and preceded by a 'starter' regime. The use of elemental diets with amino acids, rather than whole protein enteric feeds, is declining. Elemental feeds are considered only when hydrolysis within the gut is severely reduced, as in pancreatic failure, or where the absorptive capacity of the small intestine is very defective, as in the short bowel syndrome where there is a reduced amount of small bowel to absorb nutrients. Absorption may still not be complete, however, as some amino acids are better absorbed as dipeptides.

Enteral nutrition is generally safe and a valuable means of providing nutritional support, but it is important that the solutions are kept sterile and that the feeds are not given too rapidly. Monitoring of the blood will also be needed to check that the correct amount of salts and minerals are being provided and that there are no adverse effects.

41.2.2 Parenteral feeding

Tube feeding may be contraindicated in someone who has obstruction of the gastro-intestinal tract, fistulae between parts of the bowel, or immediately before and after surgery on the bowel. Patients with these problems are potential candidates for parenteral feeding, where nutrients are infused directly into a vein. This form of nutrition may sometimes be life-saving. Some indications for parenteral nutrition include:

- severe Crohn's disease (an inflammatory bowel disease)
- small bowel fistulae (communications between loops of the bowel)
- major surgery on the intestine, to allow bowel rest and healing
- severe pancreatitis
- severe malabsorption
- intractable vomiting.

When parenteral nutrition is the sole means of nutritional support this is termed 'total parenteral nutrition' (TPN).

41.3 DEVELOPMENT OF PARENTERAL FEEDING

World War II stimulated research into the metabolic changes induced by trauma and infection and the importance of nutrition in critically ill patients. Widespread interest in, and appreciation of, parenteral nutrition developed following the reports of Dudrick and colleagues who used a catheter into a large central vein to feed growing dogs, and malnourished infants and adults, and demonstrated that it resulted in good growth, positive nitrogen balance and improved health. Other important researchers involved in developing this form of feeding were Wretland and Cuthbertson.

The uses of parenteral nutrition now vary from short periods of nutritional support after surgery to more prolonged use, either as a supplement to other forms of nutrition, or on its own, total parenteral nutrition (TPN). An example of a need for prolonged parenteral nutrition is after a large portion of the small bowel has been destroyed or removed at surgery. In this situation, long-term parenteral nutrition may be needed, and this can now be provided in the patient's home.

The provision of nutrients directly into a vein (intravenously) instead of into the gut requires that these nutrients be in a form that can be utilized without the need for digestion. The solutions used nowadays generally consist of pure L-amino acids, glucose and a triglyceride emulsion, plus minerals, vitamins, and trace elements (if nutrition is for a prolonged period). The solutions must be sterile and are generally mixed into a large collapsible plastic bag. This prevents microbial contamination, and also prevents air being sucked into the vein when the bag (or bottle) is empty. The contents pass from the bag down a tube via a pump into a catheter which has been inserted into a large

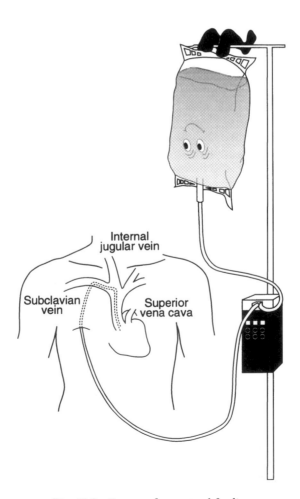

Fig. 41.2   Routes of parenteral feeding.

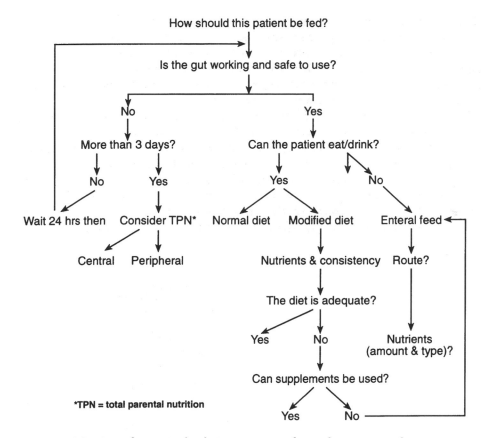

Fig. 41.3 Some factors in the decision process of providing nutritional support.

vein, usually the subclavian vein (which is under the clavicle) or the jugular vein (which is in the neck), as shown in Fig. 41.2.

A flow diagram which considers some of the factors in the decision process of providing nutritional support is given as Fig. 41.3.

41.4 NUTRIENT REQUIREMENTS OF ENTERALLY AND PARENTERALLY FED PATIENTS

Nutrient requirements differ according to the degree of nutritional depletion, the resting energy expenditure and the activity of the patient. In nutritionally depleted patients, who often have considerable and recent weight loss, the main aim is to restore lean body mass with or without fat. In patients with very high resting energy expenditure (hypermetabolism) and considerable nitrogen loss (hypercatabolism), for instance, after a severe road traffic accident, maintaining a balance may be difficult. The aim in these circumstances is initially just to reduce the losses. Figure 41.4 outlines some of the factors to be considered in determining energy and nutrient requirements.

Nutrient Requirements

Depend on - Age, sex, size, condition, infection

Energy requirements (compared to usual requirements as 100%)

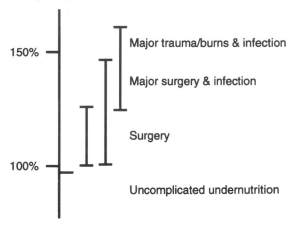

Major trauma patient may require 120-300 g protein and > 12.6 MJ.

Total energy expenditure = resting metabolic energy expenditure + diet induced thermogenesis + activity energy expenditure + stress.

Fig. 41.4 Indicators of nutrient and energy requirements for patients receiving nutritional support.

There is a requirement for macronutrients (carbohydrates, fats and proteins) to provide for energy and tissue-building, and for micronutrients (vitamins, minerals and trace elements) to provide structural components and enzyme cofactors. These come from body stores and ongoing nutrient intakes. The actual nutrient requirements will depend on the degree of previous depletion of body stores, possibly by a drawn-out disease process, and the ongoing effects of any disease state on the activity and basal metabolism of the person.

The nitrogen requirement for a moderately catabolic patient may be estimated at 15 g or more daily, and the regimen for enteral (or parenteral) feeding can be devised on this basis. Nitrogen will normally be given as protein for enteral feeds, with the exception of elemental diets which contain mixtures of amino acids. Some amino acids are better absorbed in peptide form so that giving pure amino acids may offer no nutritional advantage.

Tissue maintenance, repletion and nitrogen balance may be defective if any of the 40 or so essential nutrients is lacking. All must be supplied regularly, where possible on a daily basis. The correct amount of an essential nutrient may not be known, even for a normal subject, but if the minimum requirement is known then at least this amount should be given, unless there are specific contraindications.

Of the micronutrients, particular attention should be paid to the vitamins, trace elements, and essential fatty acids. The published recommendations for daily intake of vitamins, minerals and trace elements are often approximate (see Chapter 33 and chapters on individual nutrient classes). The variation in recommended intake reflects ignorance of the absolute daily requirements. In general, larger doses are required by the enteral than parenteral route, because only a fraction of the enteral amounts are absorbed. Among the trace elements, zinc, copper, chromium, and manganese are all essential, and zinc deficiency often occurs in patients with gastrointestinal disease. Lack of trace elements is of particular importance in patients on prolonged parenteral nutrition, although it should also be remembered that trace elements given in excess can be toxic. When zinc or copper are being given intravenously their circulating concentrations should be regularly measured. Since zinc and chromium are excreted via the kidneys, and copper and manganese through a biliary tract, it is important to take into account diseases of these organs that can reduce excretion of these trace elements.

41.5   Constituents of Parenteral Nutrition Regimens

41.5.1   Protein

Nitrogen is given in the form of amino acids, either as protein hydrolysates or more frequently as mixtures of synthetic L-amino acids. Hydrolysates of protein such as casein (Aminosol) provide a significant amount of their total nitrogen in the form of small peptides; synthetic amino acid solutions are preferable but are more expensive.

41.5.2   Energy sources

The ideal intravenous energy source should be rapidly utilized and have no abnormal side effects. A number of sources have been tried, but a mixture of glucose and triglycerides is probably the best for most patients. Since glucose provides about 17 kJ/g (4 kcal/g), it is necessary to administer a hypertonic solution to achieve an adequate intake of energy. Patients will tolerate 300–400 g of glucose a day but at this intake blood glucose must be monitored regularly and some patients will have to be given small injections of insulin. It is now considered that the overfeeding of lots of extra calories to improve nutritional status may not be effective and may be dangerous. Fat is most often given as an emulsion of 10% or 20% soybean oil (containing 2–5% glycerol and egg yolk phosphatides as an emulsifier). Lack of the essential fatty acids, linoleic and arachidonic acid which must be supplied because they are not made by the body, has been reported in patients who are fed parentally without regular fat infusion. Arachidonic acid is essential for the function of membranes and is a precursor of the prostaglandins which are chemicals that have many functions in the body. Patients who do not receive intravenous lipids can be given some fatty acids by rubbing an emulsion on to the skin.

Table 41.1 gives an example of energy and nutrient requirements for a 70 kg man fed by total parenteral nutrition (TPN).

41.5.3   Water and electrolytes

The amount of fluid required varies considerably with losses, especially those from the intestine which may be difficult to estimate. Although 2–3 litres a day is normal, up to

615

Table 41.1   An example of possible intravenous nutrient requirements of a 70 kg man fed by total parenteral nutrition (TPN)

Nitrogen (protein)*	12–17 g nitrogen ($\equiv$75–106 g protein)
Energy	165–210 kJ/kg body weight, i.e. 12.6 MJ
	(40–50 kcal/kg body weight, i.e. 3000 kcal)
Energy–nitrogen ratio	About 200 : 1
Energy source	Glucose and fat emulsion in roughly equal proportion
Sodium	70–100 mmol
Potassium	60–80 mmol
Magnesium	10–15 mmol
Calcium	7–10 mmol
Phosphorus	10–20 mmol
Other requirements	Water-soluble vitamins
	Vitamins A, D, K
	Essential trace elements; zinc, copper, manganese, etc.

*Nitrogen makes up about 16% of food proteins and it is often easier to measure protein as nitrogen and then multiply by 6.25 (see Chapter 4).

6 litres may be needed when losses are excessive. In severe acute disease such as trauma, major infection or intestinal obstruction, major maldistribution of fluid also occurs. In these circumstances, maintenance of an appropriate plasma volume takes precedent over other considerations in order to maintain circulation essential to healing and recovery.

41.5.4   Other constituents

These include minerals such as calcium and phosphate, the essential trace elements such as zinc and copper, and vitamins. The requirements for phosphate are often under-estimated, and low plasma phosphate may impair white cell function, contribute to muscle weakness, and produce osteomalacia. The trace elements which have been proven to be essential for humans include zinc, copper, manganese, iodine, chromium, iron, selenium and cobalt. During long-term parenteral nutrition, especially in patients with gastrointestinal disease, deficiency of these elements can occur, as they are not adequately replaced by chance contaminants in the intravenous solutions. Trace element solutions are available to correct these deficiencies, and if given in the correct form and amounts they are without side effects.

41.6   AREAS OF RECENT INTEREST

Interest has recently focused on the inclusion of glutamine in nutritional support regimes, the use of medium chain triglycerides and structured lipid emulsions, and the optimal content of ω3-fatty acids. Glutamine is considered beneficial for maintaining the health and function of the tissues of the gut, which may reduce infection occurring due to passage of bacteria through the gut wall. New lipid emulsions containing medium-chain triglycerides (triglycerides with fatty acids containing 6–10 carbon atoms) are of interest as they may be more easily metabolized, particularly in severely ill patients. ω3-Fatty acids are now considered necessary as they may be important in prostaglandin metabolism, but there is still debate as to the optimum amount that should be supplied (see Chapter 3.4).

FURTHER READING

1. Allison SP. The uses and limitations of nutritional support. *Clin Nutr* 1992; **11**: 319–30.
2. Broom J. Sepsis and trauma. In: Garrow JS, James WPT (eds). *Human nutrition and dietetics*. 9th ed. Edinburgh: Churchill Livingstone, 1993: 456–64.
3. Cerra FB. How nutrition intervention changes what getting sick means. *J Ent Parent Nutr* 1990; **14**: S164–9.
4. Pichard C, Jeejeebhoy KN. Nutritional management of clinical undernutrition. In: Garrow JS, James WPT (eds). *Human nutrition and dietetics*. 9th ed. Edinburgh: Churchill Livingstone, 1993: 421–4.
5. Splett P. Effectiveness and cost-effectiveness of nutrition care: a critical analysis with recommendations. *J Am Dietet Assoc* 1991; **91** (suppl.).
6. Thomas B (ed.). Enteral feeding. In: *Manual of Dietetic Practice*. 2nd ed. Oxford: Blackwell Scientific Publications, 1994: 65–79.
7. Truswell AS, Dreosti IE, English RM, Rutishauser IHE, Palmer N (eds). *Recommended nutrient intakes*. Australian Papers. Mosman, NSW: Australian Professional Publications, 1990.